YOU'VE JUST PURCHASED
MORE THAN
A TEXTBOOK

TO ACCESS YOUR RESOURCES, VISIT:

http://evolve.elsevier.com/Wold/geriatric

Evolve Student Learning Resources for Wold: *Basic Geriatric Nursing, 5th edition,*
offers the following features:

- Animations depicting anatomy, physiology, and procedures

- Answer Guidelines for Nursing Care Plan Critical Thinking Questions

- Answers and Rationales for Review Questions for the NCLEX® Examination

- Audio Glossary with pronunciations in English and Spanish

- Calculators for determining body mass index (BMI), body surface area, fluid deficit, Glasgow coma score, IV dosages, and conversion of units

- Concept Map Creator

- Fluids and Electrolytes Tutorial

- Resources for Older Adults

- Videos Clips of patient assessment

REGISTER TODAY!

To my mother, Esther Hoffmann,
and my father-in-law, Rev. W.R. Wold,
who always encouraged me and demonstrated
the resilience of older adults. May they rest in peace.
To my daughter Rebecca,
who helps keep me young at heart;
and to my husband Norm,
with whom I wish to continue to grow old.

Basic Geriatric Nursing

Gloria Hoffmann Wold, MS, BSN, RN
Nursing Instructor
Milwaukee Area Technical College
Milwaukee, Wisconsin

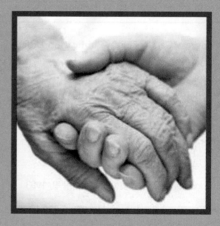

5th Edition

ELSEVIER
MOSBY

3251 Riverport Lane
St. Louis, Missouri 63043

BASIC GERIATRIC NURSING ISBN: 978-0-323-07399-8

Notice

Knowledge and best practice in this field are constantly changing. As new research and experience broaden our understanding, changes in research methods, professional practices, or medical treatment may become necessary.

Practitioners and researchers must always rely on their own experience and knowledge in evaluating and using any information, methods, compounds, or experiments described herein. In using such information or methods they should be mindful of their own safety and the safety of others, including parties for whom they have a professional responsibility.

With respect to any drug or pharmaceutical products identified, readers are advised to check the most current information provided (i) on procedures featured or (ii) by the manufacturer of each product to be administered, to verify the recommended dose or formula, the method and duration of administration, and contraindications. It is the responsibility of practitioners, relying on their own experience and knowledge of their patients, to make diagnoses, to determine dosages and the best treatment for each individual patient, and to take all appropriate safety precautions.

To the fullest extent of the law, neither the Publisher nor the authors, contributors, or editors, assume any liability for any injury and/or damage to persons or property as a matter of products liability, negligence or otherwise, or from any use or operation of any methods, products, instructions, or ideas contained in the material herein.

Library of Congress Cataloging-in-Publication Data

Wold, Gloria.
  Basic geriatric nursing / Gloria Hoffmann Wold. – 5th ed.
    p. ; cm.
  Includes bibliographical references and index.
  ISBN 978-0-323-07399-8 (pbk. : alk. paper) 1. Geriatric nursing. I. Title.
  [DNLM: 1. Geriatric Nursing–methods. 2. Aged. 3. Aging. 4. Nursing Care. WY 152]
  RC954.W58 2012
  618.97'0231–dc22

                                                                    2011010833

Previous editions copyrighted 2008, 2004, 1999, 1993

International Standard Book Number 978-0-323-07399-8

NCLEX®, NCLEX-RN®, and NCLEX-PN® are federally registered trademarks and service marks of the National Council of State Boards of Nursing, Inc.

Executive Editor: Teri Hines Burnham
Developmental Editor: Tiffany Trautwein
Associate Developmental Editor: Jennifer Shropshire
Publishing Services Managers: Hemamalini Rajendrababu and Deborah L. Vogel
Project Managers: Divya Krish and John W. Gabbert
Design Direction: Jessica Williams

Printed in China

Last digit is the print number: 9 8 7 6 5 4 3 2 1

Ancillary Contributors

Karen L. Amsden, RN, BSN, MSHA
Professor, LPN Coordinator
Jefferson College
Hillsboro, Missouri
Test Bank

Anna Allen Hamilton, RN, BSN, MS
Formerly, Instructor
McLennan Community College
Waco, Texas
Test Bank

Charla Hollin, RN
Nursing Program Director
Rich Mountain Community College
Mesa, Arizona
Audience Response System questions
TEACH PowerPoint slides

Laura Bevlock Kanavy, RN, BSN, MSN
Instructor, Practical Nursing Program
Career Technology Center of Lackawanna County
Scranton, Pennsylvania
*Rationales for Review Questions for the NCLEX®
   Examination*

Jennifer A. Ponto, BSN, RN
Instructor, Vocational Nursing
South Plains College, Lubbock, Texas
TEACH Lesson Plans

Reviewers

Margaret Barnes, MSN, RN
Assistant Professor
Indiana Wesleyan School of Nursing
RNBSN Post-Licensure Program
Florence, KY

Kathy Bredberg, MSN, RN
Vocational Nursing Program Director
Grayson County College
Van Alstyne, Texas

Belinda Douglas, MSN, PMHNP-BC, GNP-BC
Four Rivers Regional Nursing Director
Tennessee Technology Center - Ripley
Ripley, Tennessee

Phyllis Graves, RN, BSN
PN Educator
Waynesville Career Center
Waynesville, Missouri

Donna M. Kuenstler, MSN, RN
Director
Sul Ross State University
Vocational Nursing Program
Alpine, Texas

Christina A. Lamb, MSN, RN
Director of Practical Nursing Education
Bolivar Technical College
Bolivar, Missouri

Jennifer Lucsko, BSN, RN
Pediatric Specialty Clinic
Clinical Team Leader
Pediatric Endocrinology
Roanoke, Virginia

Carolyn W. Lyon, MSN, RN
Assistant Professor
Director of Practical Nursing Program
Jefferson College of Health Sciences
Roanoke, Virginia

Melaine Moore, PhD, MSN, RN
Associate Professor
Virginia Western Community College
Roanoke, Virginia

Teresa G. Newby, MSN, RN
Assistant Professor
Crown College
Saint Bonifacius, Minnesota

Jennifer Ponto, BSN, RN
Instructor
Vocational Nursing Program
South Plains College
Levelland, Texas

Beth Jackson-Rumbaoa, RN, BSN
Coordinator/Instructor PN Program
Boonslick Technical Education Center
Boonville, Missouri

Carmen Toca, RN, C
Assistant Coordinator/Instructor Skills Lab
Practical Nursing Program
Union County College
Plainfield, New Jersey

Laura Travis, MSN, RN
Health Careers Coordinator
Tennessee Technology Center at Dickson
Dickson, Tennessee

Elise Webb, MSN, RN
Allied Health Program Coordinator
Wilson Community College
Wilson, North Carolina

LPN/LVN Advisory Board

To the Instructor

Aging is neither good nor bad—it is a fact of life. It begins the day we are born and ends the day we die. We all have a different view of what getting older means. Children and adolescents rarely consider what it means to get old; old age is too far away and they are too busy living each day to worry about it. Young adults are too caught up in the daily struggle for survival and success to pay much attention to old age. Middle age brings a new awareness of the passing of time, particularly when one's parents slip into old age and then die. The reality of aging can no longer be denied when one becomes part of the oldest living generation of a family.

Today's world contains a larger percentage of middle-aged and older adults than ever before. This changing demographic presents an immense challenge to health care providers and society as a whole. Because nurses are at the frontline of health care delivery, they must be well prepared to recognize and respond appropriately to the needs of our aging population. The goal of this text is to give the beginning nurse a balanced perspective on the realities of aging and to broaden the new nurse's viewpoint regarding aging people so that their needs can be met in a compassionate, caring, and appropriate manner.

ABOUT THE TEXT

The fifth edition of *Basic Geriatric Nursing* presents the theories and concepts of aging, the physiologic and psychosocial changes and problems associated with the process, and the appropriate nursing interventions. The *LPN Threads* design has been revised and provides even more consistency among Elsevier's LPN/LVN textbooks. Many key features have been retained, including extensive coverage of cultural issues, clinical situations, delegation, home health care, health promotion, patient teaching, and complementary and alternative therapies. Numerous Critical Thinking exercises provide practice in synthesizing information and applying it to nursing care of the older adult.

LPN THREADS

The fifth edition of *Basic Geriatric Nursing* shares some features and design elements with other Elsevier LPN/LVN textbooks. The purpose of these *LPN Threads* is to make it easier for students and instructors to use the variety of books required by the relatively brief and demanding LPN/LVN curriculum. The following features are included in the *LPN Threads*.

- A **reading level evaluation** is performed on every manuscript chapter during the book's development to increase the consistency among chapters and ensure the text is easy to understand.
- The **full-color design**, **cover**, **photos**, and **illustrations** are visually appealing and pedagogically useful.
- **Objectives** (numbered) begin each chapter and provide a framework for content and are especially important in providing the structure for the TEACH Lesson Plans for the textbook.
- **Key Terms** with phonetic pronunciations and page number references are listed at the beginning of each chapter. They appear in color in the chapter and are defined briefly, with full definitions in the **Glossary.** The goal is to help the student with limited proficiency in English to develop a greater command of the pronunciation of scientific and nonscientific English terminology.
- **Key Points** at the end of each chapter correlate to the objectives and serve as a useful chapter review.
- In addition to consistent content, design, and support resources, these textbooks benefit from the advice and input of the Elsevier **LPN/LVN Advisory Board** (see p. vii).

ORGANIZATION

Unit One presents an overview of aging, examining the trends and issues affecting the older adult. These include demographic factors and economic, social, cultural, and family influences. The unit explores various theories and myths associated with aging and reviews the physiologic changes that occur with aging.

Unit Two includes a wide range of information on modifying basic nursing skills for the aging population. There is a strong focus on (1) health promotion and health maintenance for older adults; (2) age-appropriate verbal and nonverbal communication; (3) relevant nutritional and fluid needs, alterations in pharmacodynamics, and concerns related to medication administration for older adults; (4) health assessment of older adults; and (5) meeting safety needs of the older adults.

Unit Three addresses the psychosocial needs of the older adult through the nursing process.

Psychosocial care precedes physiologic care, reflecting the order in which the content is most often taught. Areas of content include (1) cognition problems, (2) self-perception and self-concept, (3) changing roles and relationships, (4) coping and stress management, (5) values and beliefs, and (6) sexuality.

Unit Four addresses the physical needs of the older adult through the nursing process. Areas of content include (1) safety, (2) hygiene and skin care, (3) elimination, (4) activity and exercise, and (5) sleep and rest. Units Three and Four both offer assessment, nursing diagnoses, and nursing interventions across care settings.

SPECIAL FEATURES

- **Nursing process** sections that provide a strong framework for discussing care of older adults in the context of specific disorders
- **Nursing interventions** grouped by health care setting (e.g., acute care, extended care, home care)
- **Special boxes** for critical thinking, clinical situations, health promotion, safety, patient teaching, complementary and alternative therapies, delegation, and more (see p. x)
- Increased **cultural content** on the impact of aging in various cultures
- Focus on **changing demographics** including Baby Boomers and the impact of their aging on health care
- Additional information on **home health** for both patients and caregivers
- **New Review Questions for the NCLEX® Examination** at the end of every chapter
- Updated **Laboratory Values** for Older Adults (Appendix A)
- The **Geriatric Depression Scale (GDS)** (Appendix B)
- A revised **dietary information** for older adults (Appendix C)
- Revised list of **resources on aging,** including relevant websites (Appendix D)
- **Bibliography** grouped by chapter and listed at the end of the book for easy access
- Free, built-in **Study Guide** with Answer Key (for instructors only) on Evolve

TEACHING AND LEARNING PACKAGE

FOR INSTRUCTORS

The comprehensive and free *Evolve Resources with TEACH Instructor Resource* include the following:
- **Test Bank** with approximately 525 multiple-choice and alternate-format questions with topic, step of the nursing process, objective, cognitive level, NCLEX® category of client needs, correct answer, rationale, and textbook page reference
- **TEACH Instructor Resource** with Lesson Plans, Lecture Outlines, and PowerPoint slides—with Audience Response System questions embedded—that correlate each text and ancillary component
- **Image Collection** that contains all the illustrations and photographs in the textbook
- **Answer Key** for the in-text Study Guide
- Tips for **Teaching English as a Second Language (ESL) Students**

FOR STUDENTS

The *Evolve Student Resources* include the following assets:
- **Animations** depicting anatomy, physiology, and procedures
- **Answer Guidelines** for Nursing Care Plan Critical Thinking Questions
- **Answers and Rationales** for Review Questions for the NCLEX® Examination
- **Audio Glossary** with pronunciations in English and Spanish
- **Calculators** for determining body mass index (BMI), body surface area, fluid deficit, Glasgow coma score, IV dosages, and conversion of units
- **Concept Map Creator**
- **Fluids and Electrolytes Tutorial**
- **Resources for Older Adults**
- **Video clips** of patient assessment

ACKNOWLEDGEMENTS

I would like to thank Teri Hines Burnham, Jennifer Shropshire, Tiffany Trautwein, Johnny Gabbert, and Jessica Williams—as well as the other staff at Elsevier—for their professional expertise, tenacity, insights, patience, and steady encouragement throughout the development of this edition.

To the Student

READING AND REVIEW TOOLS

- **Objectives** introduce the chapter topics.
- **Key Terms** are listed with page number references; and difficult medical, nursing, or scientific terms are accompanied by simple phonetic pronunciations.
- Each chapter ends with a *Get Ready for the NCLEX® Examination!* **section** that includes (1) **Key Points** that reiterate the chapter objectives and serve as a useful review of concepts; (2) a list of **Additional Resources** including the Study Guide and Evolve Resources; and (3) an extensive set of **Review Questions for the NCLEX® Examination** with answers located on the inside back cover and Answers and Rationales on Evolve.
- A complete **Bibliography and Reader References** in the back of the text cite evidence-based information and provide resources for enhancing knowledge.
- A **Glossary** of key terms provides definitions of all the terms that appear at the beginning of chapters.
- An in-text **Study Guide** includes *Critical Thinking and Application* sections and *Selected Activities by Chapter* with multiple choice, fill-in, and matching questions.

SPECIAL FEATURES

The following special features are designed to foster effective learning and comprehension and reflect the LPN Threads design:

 Clinical Situation boxes relate the text to patient situations and care scenarios.

Complementary and Alternative Therapies boxes address nontraditional and adjunct therapies.

Coordinated Care boxes address leadership and management issues for the LPN/LVN and include topics such as restraints and end-of-life care.

Critical Thinking boxes pose questions designed to stimulate thought and to help students develop and improve their critical thinking skills.

Cultural Considerations boxes provide advice on culturally diverse patient care of older adults.

Health Promotion boxes recommend quality-of-life tips for older adults.

Home Health Consideration boxes give essential information for home care for the older adult.

Medication tables provide quick access to information about medications commonly used in geriatric nursing care.

Nursing Care Plans with Critical Thinking Questions provide students with real-world examples of nursing care plans and encourage them to think critically about the given scenarios.

Patient Teaching boxes instruct and inform both older patients and their caregivers about health promotion, disease prevention, and age-specific interventions.

Contents

Trends and Issues

Objectives

1. Describe the subjective and objective ways that aging is defined.
2. Identify personal and societal attitudes toward aging.
3. Define *ageism*.
4. Discuss the myths that exist with regard to aging.
5. Identify recent demographic trends and their impact on society.
6. Describe the effects of recent legislation on the economic status of older adults.
7. Identify the political interest groups that work as advocates for older adults.
8. Identify the major economic concerns of older adults.
9. Describe the housing options that are available to older adults.
10. Discuss the health care implications of an increase in the population of older adults.
11. Describe the changes in family dynamics that occur as family members become older.
12. Examine the role of nurses in dealing with an aging family.
13. Identify the different forms of elder abuse.
14. Recognize the most common signs of abuse.
15. Describe approaches that are effective in preventing elder abuse.

Key Terms

abuse (p. 22)
chronologic age (krŏ-nŏ-LŎJ-Ĭk) (p. 2)
cohort (KŌ-hŏrt) (p. 8)
demographics (dĕm-ŏ-GRĂF-Ĭks) (p. 6)

geriatric (jĕr-ē-ĂT-rĬk) (p. 2)
neglect (nĬ-glĕkt) (p. 22)
respite (RĚS-pĬt) (p. 26)

INTRODUCTION TO GERIATRIC NURSING

HISTORICAL PERSPECTIVE ON THE STUDY OF AGING

Until the middle of the nineteenth century, only two stages of human growth and development were identified: childhood and adulthood. In many ways, children were treated like small adults. No special attention was given to them or to their needs. Families had to produce many children to ensure that a few would survive and reach adulthood. In turn, children were expected to contribute to the family's survival. Little or no concern was given to those characteristics and behaviors that set one child apart from another.

As time passed, society began to view children differently. People learned that there were significant differences between children of different ages and that children's needs changed as they developed. Childhood is now divided into substages (e.g., infant, toddler, preschool, school age, and adolescence). Each stage is associated with unique challenges related to the individual child's stage of growth and development. Because the substages are related to obvious

physical changes or to significant life events, this classification method is now accepted as logical and necessary.

Until recently, society also viewed adults of all ages interchangeably. Once you became an adult, you remained an adult. Perhaps society perceived dimly that older adults were different from younger adults, but it was not greatly concerned with these differences because few people lived to old age. In addition, the physical and developmental changes during adulthood are more subtle than those during childhood; therefore, these changes received little attention.

Until the 1960s, sociologists, psychologists, and health care providers focused their attention on meeting the needs of the typical or average adult: people between 20 and 65 years of age. This group was the largest and most economically productive segment of the population; they were raising families, working, and contributing to the growth of the economy. Only a small percentage of the population lived beyond 65 years of age. Disability, illness, and early death were accepted as natural and unavoidable.

In the late 1960s, research began to indicate that adults of all ages are not the same. At the same time, the focus of health care shifted from illness to wellness. Disability and disease were no longer considered unavoidable parts of aging. Increased medical knowledge, improved preventive health practices, and technologic advances helped more people live longer, healthier lives.

Older adults now constitute a significant group in society, and interest in the study of aging is increasing. The study of aging is expected to be a major area of attention for years to come.

WHAT'S IN A NAME: GERIATRICS, GERONTOLOGY, AND GERONTICS

The term geriatric comes from the Greek words "geras," meaning old age, and "iatro," meaning relating to medical treatment. Thus, geriatrics is the medical specialty that deals with the physiology of aging and with the diagnosis and treatment of diseases affecting the aged. Geriatrics, by definition, focuses on abnormal conditions and the medical treatment of these conditions.

The term gerontology comes from the Greek words "gero," meaning related to old age, and "ology," meaning the study of. Thus, gerontology is the study of all aspects of the aging process, including the clinical, psychologic, economic, and sociologic problems of older adults and the consequences of these problems for older adults and society. Gerontology affects nursing, health care, and all areas of our society—including housing, education, business, and politics.

The term gerontics, or gerontic nursing, was coined by Gunter and Estes in 1979 to define the nursing care and the service provided to older adults. The aim of gerontic nursing is "to safeguard and increase health to the extent possible and to provide comfort and care to the extent necessary." This textbook focuses on gerontic nursing. It addresses ways to promote high-level functioning and methods of providing care and comfort for older adults.

The objectives of this book are as follows:

- Examine some of the trends and issues that affect the older person's ability to remain healthy.
- Explore the theories and myths of aging.
- Study the normal changes that occur with aging.
- Review the pathologic conditions that are commonly observed in older adults.
- Emphasize the importance of effective communication in working with older adults.
- Explore the general methods used to assess the health status of older adults.
- Describe the specific methods of assessing functional needs.
- Identify the most common nursing diagnoses associated with older adults, and discuss the nursing interventions related to these diagnoses.

- Explore the impact of medication and medication administration on older adults.

The dictionary defines old as "having lived or existed for a long time." The meaning of old is highly subjective; to a great degree, it depends on how old we ourselves are. Few people like to consider themselves old. Old age seems to come later as we become older. A recent study reveals that people younger than 30 years view those older than 63 as "getting older." People 65 years of age and older do not think people are "getting older" until they are 75.

Aging is a complex process that can be described chronologically, physiologically, and functionally. Chronologic age, the number of years a person has lived, is most often used when we speak of aging because it is the easiest to identify and measure. Unfortunately, chronologic age is probably the least meaningful measurement of aging. Many people who have lived a long time remain functionally and physiologically young. These individuals remain physically fit, stay mentally active, and are productive members of society. Others are chronologically young but physically or functionally old.

When we use chronologic age as our measure, authorities use various systems to categorize the aging population (see Table 1-1). To many people, 65 is a magic number in terms of aging. The wide acceptance of age 65 as a landmark of aging is interesting. Since the 1930s, the age of 65 has come to be accepted as the age of retirement, when it is expected that a person willingly or unwillingly stops paid employment. However, before the 1930s, most people worked until they decided to stop working, until they became too ill to work, or until they died. When the New Deal politicians established the Social Security program, they set 65 as the age at which benefits could be collected, but the average life expectancy of the time was 63. The Social Security program was designed as a fairly low-cost way to win votes because most people would not live long enough to collect the benefits. If 65 was considered old then, it certainly is not now. If the same standards were applied today, the retirement age would be 77. However, for various reasons, society

Table 1-1 Categorizing the Aging Population	
AGE (YEARS)	**CATEGORY**
55 to 64	Older
65 to 74	Elderly
75 to 84	Aged
85 and older	Extremely aged
	or
60 to 74	Young-old
75 to 84	Middle-old
85 and older	Old-old

clings to 65 as the "retirement age" and resists political proposals designed to move the start of Social Security benefits to a later age. Despite the resistance, the age to qualify for full Social Security benefits is changing. Individuals born before 1937 still qualify for full benefits at age 65, but there are incremental increases in age for all persons born after that time. Individuals born in 1960 or later must wait until age 67 to qualify for full benefits. Reduced benefits are calculated for individuals who claim Social Security benefits after age 62 but before the full retirement age.

ATTITUDES TOWARD AGING

Before we look at the attitudes of others, it is important to examine our own attitudes, values, and knowledge about aging. The three Critical Thinking boxes that follow are designed to help you assess how you feel about aging.

? Critical Thinking

Your Views and Attitudes About Aging

- How many "old people" do you know personally?
- Do you think they are old, or do they think they are old?
- How do you personally define old?
- Why is getting old an issue today?
- Should Social Security laws be changed to reflect today's longer life expectancy?

Please complete the following statements. Write as many applicable comments as you can. *There are no right or wrong answers.*

A person can be considered old when _____.

When I think about getting old, I _____.

Growing old means _____.

When I get old I will lose my _____.

Seeing an old person makes me feel _____.

Old people always _____.

Old people never _____.

The best thing about getting old is _____.

The worst thing about getting old is _____.

Looking back at my responses, I feel that aging is _____.

? Critical Thinking

Your Values About Aging

Quickly name three older adults who have had an impact on your life. List five characteristics that you associate with each person. *There are no right or wrong answers.*

Person 1	*Person 2*	*Person 3*
Name _____	Name _____	Name _____
Relationship _____	Relationship _____	Relationship _____

CHARACTERISTICS:

1._____	1._____	1._____
2._____	2._____	2._____
3._____	3._____	3._____
4._____	4._____	4._____
5._____	5._____	5._____

Look at the characteristics you described, and think about the feelings you experienced as you considered these individuals. Do your feelings correspond to your attitudes about aging? Were these three people's characteristics similar or different? What do these characteristics say about your values?

Your Current Knowledge About Aging

Respond to the following questions to the best of your knowledge.

You are old at age _____.

There are _____ older adults in the United States.

Most older people live in _____.

Economically, older people are _____.

With regard to health, older people are _____.

Mentally, older people are _____.

Our attitudes are the product of our knowledge and values. Our life experiences and our current age strongly influence our views about aging and old people. Most of us have a rather narrow perspective, and our attitudes may reflect this. We tend to project our personal experiences onto the rest of the world. Because many of us have a somewhat limited exposure to aging, we are likely to believe quite a bit of inaccurate information. When dealing with older adults, our limited understanding and vision can lead to serious errors and mistaken conclusions. If we view old age as a time of physical decay, mental confusion, and social boredom, we are likely to have negative feelings toward aging. Conversely, if we see old age as a time for sustained physical vigor, renewed mental challenges, and social usefulness, our perspective on aging will be quite different.

It is important to separate fact from myth when examining our attitudes about aging. The single most important factor that influences how poorly or how well a person will age is attitude. This statement is true not only for others but also for ourselves.

Throughout time, youth and beauty have been desired (or at least viewed as desirable), and old age and physical infirmity have been loathed and feared. Greek statues portray youths of physical perfection. Artists' works throughout history have shown heroes and heroines as young and beautiful, and evildoers as old and ugly. Little has changed to this day. Few cultures cherish their older members and view them as the keepers of wisdom. Even in Asia, where tradition demands respect for older adults, societal changes are destroying this venerable mindset.

Cultural Considerations

The Role of the Family

Cultural heritage may work as a barrier to getting help for an older parent. Many cultures emphasize the importance of intergenerational obligation and dictate that it is the role of the family to provide for both the financial and personal assistance needs of older adults. This can lead to high stress and excessive demands, particularly on lower-income families.

Nurses need to recognize the impact that culture has on expectations and values and how these cultural values affect the willingness to accept outside assistance. Nurses need to be able to identify the workings of complex family dynamics and determine how decision making takes place within a unique cultural context.

[?] Critical Thinking

Caregiver Choices

- What expectations does your cultural heritage dictate regarding obligations to frail older family members?
- Who in your family culture makes decisions regarding the care of older family members?
- Should Medicare or insurance plans pay low-income family members to stay at home and provide care for infirm older adults?
- To what extent should family members sacrifice their personal lives to keep frail or infirm older adults out of institutional care?
- Can filial obligations be met in a society that provides little support or relief to caregivers?

For the most part, mainstream American society does not value its elders. The United States tends to be a youth-oriented society in which people are judged by age, appearance, and wealth. Young, attractive, and wealthy people are viewed positively; old, imperfect, and poor people are not. It is difficult for young people to imagine that they will ever be old. Despite some cultural changes, becoming old retains many negative connotations. Many people continue to do everything they can to fool the clock. Wrinkles, gray hair, and other physical changes related to aging are actively confronted with makeup, hair dye, and cosmetic surgery. Until recently, advertising seldom portrayed people older than 50 years except to sell eyeglasses, hearing aids, hair dye, laxatives, and other rather unappealing products. The message seemed to be, "Young is good, old is bad; therefore, everyone should fight getting old." It is significant that trends in advertising appear to be changing. As the number of healthier, dynamic senior citizens with significant spending power has increased, advertising campaigns have become increasingly likely to portray older adults as the consumers of their products, including exercise equipment, health beverages, and cruises. Despite these societal improvements, many people do not know enough about the realities of aging, and, because of ignorance, they are afraid to get old. Interestingly, some studies of the media have found that people who watch more television are likely to have more negative perceptions about aging.

GERONTOPHOBIA

The fear of aging and the refusal to accept older adults into the mainstream of society is known as **gerontophobia**. Senior citizens and younger persons can fall prey to such irrational fears (Box 1-1). Gerontophobia sometimes results in very strange behavior. Teenagers buy antiwrinkle creams. Thirty-year-old women consider facelifts. Forty-year-old women have hair transplants. Long-term marriages dissolve so that one spouse can pursue someone younger. Too often these behaviors may arise from the fear of growing older.

Ageism

The extreme forms of gerontophobia are ageism and age discrimination. **Ageism** is the disliking of aging and older people based on the belief that aging makes people unattractive, unintelligent, and unproductive. It is an emotional prejudice or discrimination against people based solely on age. Ageism allows the young to separate themselves physically and emotionally from the old and to view older adults as somehow having less human value. Like sexism or racism, ageism is a negative

belief pattern that can result in irrational thoughts and destructive behaviors such as intergenerational conflict and name-calling. Like other forms of prejudice, ageism occurs because of myths and stereotypes about a group of people who are different from ourselves.

The combination of societal stereotyping and a lack of positive personal experiences with the elderly affects a cross section of society. Many studies have shown that health care providers share the views of the general public and are not immune to ageism. Few of the "best and brightest" nurses and physicians seek careers in **geriatrics** despite the increasing need for these services. They erroneously believe that they are not fully using their skills by working with the aging population. Working in intensive care, the emergency department, or other high technology areas is viewed as exciting and challenging. Working with the elderly is viewed as routine, boring, and depressing. As long as negative attitudes such as these are held by health care providers, this challenging and potentially rewarding area of service will continue to be underrated, and the elderly will suffer for it.

Ageism can have a negative effect on the way health care providers relate to older patients, which, in turn, can result in poor health care outcomes in these individuals. Research by the National Institute on Aging reports that (1) older patients receive less information than do younger patients with regard to resources, health management, and illness management; (2) less information is provided to older adults on lifestyle changes such as weight reduction and smoking cessation; (3) limited rehabilitation is available for older adults with chronic disease, despite studies demonstrating that individuals older than 85 years do benefit from rehabilitation programs; and (4) only 47% of physicians feel that older adults should receive the same evaluation and treatment for acute illness as their younger counterparts.

Because an increasing portion of the population consists of older adults, health care providers need to do some soul searching with regard to their own attitudes. Furthermore, they must confront signs of ageism whenever and wherever they appear. Activities such as increased positive interactions with older adults and improved professional training designed to address misconceptions regarding aging are two ways of fighting ageism. The Nursing Competence in Aging (NCA) initiative, which was started in 2002, focuses on enhancing competence in geriatrics by expanding nurses' knowledge, skills, and attitudes. Research coming from this initiative can help nurses regardless of their area of practice. Becca Levy, a Yale University professor, found that young people who hold positive feelings toward the elderly live 7.5 years longer than those with negative perceptions of aging. On a purely self-serving basis, health care providers should work to stamp out ageism.

Age discrimination reaches beyond emotions and leads to actions. Age discrimination results in different

---

Box 1-1   Aging: Myth Versus Fact

MYTH
- Most older people are pretty much alike.
- They are generally alone and lonely.
- They are sick, frail, and dependent on others.
- They are often cognitively impaired.
- They are depressed.
- They become more difficult and rigid with advancing years.
- They barely cope with the inevitable declines associated with aging.

FACT
- They are a very diverse age group.
- Most older adults maintain close contact with family.
- Most older people live independently.
- For most older adults, if there is decline in some intellectual abilities, it is not severe enough to cause problems in daily living.
- Community-dwelling older adults have lower rates of diagnosable depression than younger adults.
- Personality remains relatively consistent throughout the life span.
- Most older people successfully adjust to the challenges of aging.

treatment of older people simply because of their age. Refusing to hire older persons, barring them from approval for home loans, and limiting the types or amount of health care they receive are all examples of discrimination that occur despite laws prohibiting them. Some older individuals respond to age discrimination with a passive acceptance, whereas others are banding together to speak up for their rights.

The reality of getting old is that no one knows what it will be like until it happens. But that is the nature of life—growing older is just the continuation of a process that started at birth. Older adults are fundamentally no different from the people they were when they were younger. Physical, financial, social, and political conditions may change, but the person remains essentially the same. Old age has been described as the "more-so" stage of life because some personality characteristics may appear to amplify. Old people are not a homogeneous group. They differ as widely as any other age group. They are unique individuals with unique values, beliefs, experiences, and life stories. Because of their extended years, their stories are longer and often far more interesting than those of younger persons.

Aging can be a freeing experience. Aging seems to decrease the need to maintain pretenses, and the older adult may finally be comfortable enough to reveal the real person that has existed beneath the facade. If a person has been essentially kind and caring throughout life, he or she will generally reveal more of these positive personal characteristics as time marches on. Likewise, if a person was miserly or unkind, he or she will often reveal more of these negative personality characteristics as he or she grows older. The more successful a person has been at meeting the developmental tasks of life, the more likely he or she will successfully face aging. Perhaps the best advice to all who are preparing for old age is contained in the Serenity Prayer:

O God, give us the serenity to accept what cannot be changed; courage to change what should be changed; and wisdom to distinguish one from the other.
                                                        Reinhold Niebuhr

DEMOGRAPHICS

Demographics is the statistical study of human populations. Demographers are concerned with a population's size, distribution, and vital statistics. Vital statistics include birth, death, age at death, marriage(s), race, and many other variables. The collection of demographic information is an ongoing process. The most inclusive demographic research in the United States is compiled every 10 years by the Bureau of the Census. The most recent census was completed in the year 2010. It will take some time for the full analysis of these data to be compiled.

Demographic research is important to many groups. Demographic information is used by the government as a basis for granting aid to cities and states, by cities to project their budget needs for schools, by hospitals to determine the number of beds needed, by public health agencies to determine the immunization needs of a community, and by marketers to sell products. The politicians of the 1930s used demographics to formulate plans for the Social Security program. Demographic studies provide information about the present that allows projections into the future.

One important piece of demographic information is life expectancy. Life expectancy is the number of years an average person can expect to live. Projected from the time of birth, life expectancy is based on the ages of all people who die in a given year. If a large number of infants die at birth or during childhood, the life expectancy of that year's group tends to be low. The life expectancy throughout history has been low because of environmental hazards, wars, accidents, food and water scarcity, inadequate sanitation, and contagious diseases.

- During biblical times, the average life expectancy was approximately 20 years. Some people did live significantly longer, but 40 years was considered a good, long life.
- By 1776, when the Declaration of Independence was signed, the life expectancy had risen to 35 years. It was not uncommon for people to live into their sixties.
- By the 1860s, at the time of the American Civil War, the life expectancy had increased to 40 years. The 1860 census revealed that 2.7% of the American population was older than 65 years.
- By the beginning of the twentieth century, the overall life expectancy had increased to 47 years, and 4% of the American population was 65 years of age or older. In a span of more than 2000 years, life expectancy had increased by only 27 years.
- During the twentieth century, the life expectancy of Americans has increased by approximately 29 years. A child born in the United States in the year 2004 has an average life expectancy of nearly 77.4 years.
- Projections indicate that a child born in 2010 will have a life expectancy of 78.4 years.

Since the beginning of the twentieth century, advances in technology and health care have dramatically changed the world, especially in industrialized nations where food production exceeds the needs of the population. Diseases such as cholera and typhoid have been eliminated or significantly reduced by improved sanitation and hygiene practices. Dreaded communicable diseases that at one time were often fatal (e.g., smallpox, measles, whooping cough, and diphtheria) are now preventable through immunization. Even pneumonia and influenza are no longer the fatal diseases they once were. Today, vaccines can be given to those who are at higher risk, and treatment can be given to those who become infected. It is hoped that changes in the geopolitical climate of the world will lessen the number of deaths resulting from war.

A longer life is a worldwide phenomenon. Almost 8% of the world's population is age 65 or older. Developed countries, including Japan, Australia, Canada, and Sweden, lead the world in longevity statistics. Germany, the United Kingdom, Switzerland, Norway, and France, including Jordan and South Korea, exceed the United States. The standing of the United States has declined over the last few decades, and the United States now ranks 49th among countries with large percentages of senior citizens. Some possible explanations for the disparity between the United States and other countries include higher levels of accidental and violent deaths, obesity, relatively high infant mortality, and the high cost of health care. Much of the world's net gain in older persons has occurred in the still-developing countries in Africa, South America, and Asia (Figure 1-1).

SCOPE OF THE AGING POPULATION

According to the U.S. Department of State, for the first time in recorded history, the number of people over age 65 is projected to exceed the number of children under age 5. In 2008, an estimated 39 million people,

or 1 out of 8 people, age 65 or older, lived in the United States. By 2050, this is expected to increase to 72 million people age 65 or older. This is 1 out of 5, or about 20% of the total population of the United States. Individuals older than 85 years now make up 4% of the entire U.S. population and represent the fastest-growing segment of the older population. We are becoming an increasingly older society (Figure 1-2).

GENDER AND ETHNIC DISPARITY

The Administration on Aging projects that minority populations will represent 26.4% of the older population by 2030, an increase from 16% in 2000. It is projected that by 2030, the white non-Hispanic population will increase by 77%. During the same time period, the percentage of minority persons of the same age cohort is expected to grow by 223% (Hispanics, 342%; African Americans, 164%; American Indians, Eskimos, and Aleuts, 207%; and Pacific Islanders, 302%).

The life expectancy is variable within the U.S. population. The populations of men and women are not equal, and in the older-than-65 age group, this disproportion is very noticeable. There are 22.4 million older women to 16.5 million older men. Women currently outlive men by approximately 7 years. Women

Life expectancy world map

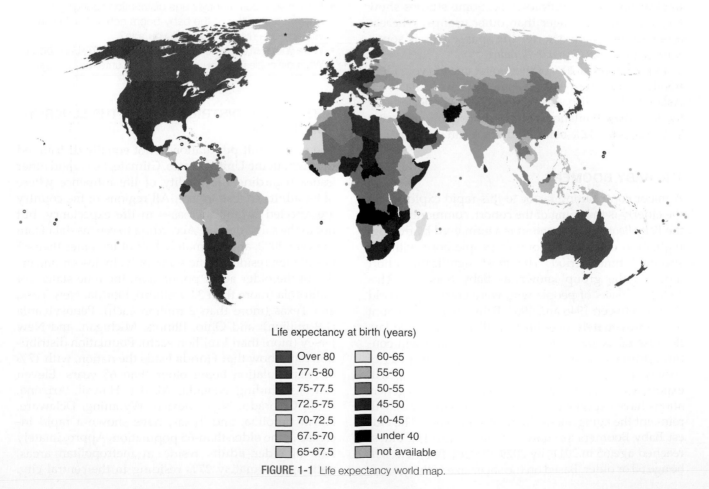

Life expectancy at birth (years)

Over 80	60-65
77.5-80	55-60
75-77.5	50-55
72.5-75	45-50
70-72.5	40-45
67.5-70	under 40
65-67.5	not available

FIGURE 1-1 Life expectancy world map.

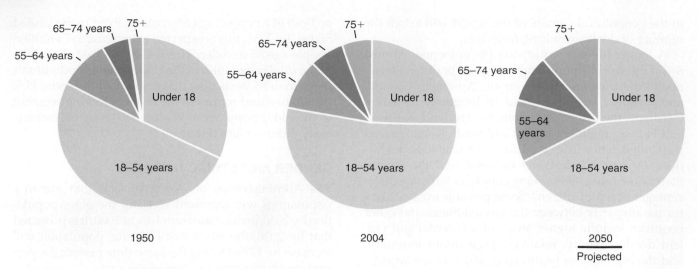

FIGURE 1-2 Percentage of population in five age groups: United States, 1950, 2004, and 2050.

tend to live longer than men, and whites tend to live longer than blacks, although disparities seem to be declining.

White women have the longest life expectancy, about 81 years. Black women have a life expectancy of about 76.9 years; white men, 76 years; and black men, 70 years. Because of the lack of precision in defining a Hispanic status (surname, country of origin, etc.), statistics for a Hispanic life expectancy are unclear and often contradictory. Some studies show Hispanics living longer than other groups, whereas other studies show shorter life spans. This is sometimes called the *Hispanic Paradox.*

In 2008, almost 20% of those over age 65 were identified as minorities. Approximately 9% were black, 3% Asian, and 7% Hispanic of any race. It is projected that by 2050 the population will be almost 40% minority: 20% Hispanic, 12% black, and 9% Asian.

THE BABY BOOMERS

A major contributing factor to this rapid explosion in the elderly is the aging of the cohort, commonly called the *Baby Boomers.* Age **cohort** is a term used by demographers to describe a group of people born within a specified time period. The most significant cohort today is the group known as Baby Boomers. This cohort consists of people who were born after World War II between 1946 and 1964. Baby Boomers account for approximately one-third of all Americans today. Because of its size, this group has had, and will continue to have, a significant influence in all areas of society. It remains to be seen whether this group will experience aging in the same way that previous generations have experienced changes or whether they will reinvent the aging and retirement experience. The oldest Baby Boomers are now in their sixties. The oldest reached age 65 in 2011. By 2029 all Baby Boomers will be age 65 or older. Based on the sheer size of this group,

the older population in 2030 will be twice the number it was in 2000. The implications of this for all areas of society, particularly health care, are unprecedented.

> **? Critical Thinking**
> **Demographics and You**
> - What impact will the changing demographics have on you personally?
> - How is your community's age distribution changing?
> - Are you a member of the baby-boom cohort? Is this an advantage or a disadvantage as you age?
> - Were you born after the baby boom? Before the baby boom? What difficulties do you expect to encounter as you age?

GEOGRAPHIC DISTRIBUTION OF THE ELDERLY POPULATION

The older adult population is not equally distributed throughout the United States. Climate, taxes, and other issues regarding the quality of life influence where older adults choose to live. All regions of the country are affected by the increases in life expectancy, but not to the same degree. According to census data from the year 2000, approximately half of the older-than-65 population reside in nine states only. In descending order of the older adult population, the nine states are California (more than 3.8 million); Florida, New York, and Texas (more than 2 million each); Pennsylvania (1.9 million); and Ohio, Illinois, Michigan, and New Jersey (more than 1 million each). Population distribution data show that Florida leads the nation, with 17% of its population being older than 65 years. Eleven states, including Nevada, Alaska, Hawaii, Arizona, Utah, Colorado, New Mexico, Wyoming, Delaware, North Carolina, and Texas, have shown a rapid increase in the older-than-65 population. Approximately 78% of older adults reside in metropolitan areas, with approximately 27% residing in the central city.

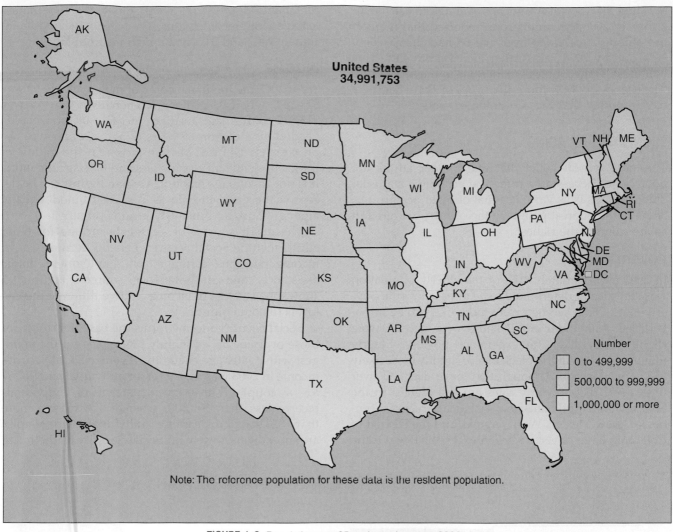

FIGURE 1-3 Population age 65 and over by state, 2000.

Only 23% of older adults reside in nonmetropolitan areas (Figure 1-3).

Statistical evaluation of minority populations reveals that groups tend to concentrate in a limited number of states. Half of elderly blacks live in New York, Florida, California, Texas, Georgia, North Carolina, Illinois, and Virginia; 70% of the Hispanic elderly live in California, Texas, Florida, and New York; and 60% of elderly persons of Asian, Hawaiian, or Pacific Island descent favor California, Hawaii, and New York. The majority of elderly people of Native American or Native Alaskan descent live in California, Oklahoma, Arizona, New Mexico, Texas, and North Carolina.

MARITAL STATUS

In 2008 three-fourths (75%) of men over age 65 were married compared to 57% of older women. The percentage of married individuals drops significantly as age progresses, but the percentage of the oldest old men who are married remains high at 55%. At age 65, 42% of women were widows compared with only 14% of men. By age 85, 76% of women were widows compared

to only 38% of men. The percentage of older adults who are separated or divorced has increased significantly to 11%. An increase in the number of divorced elders is predicted as a result of a higher incidence of divorce in the population approaching age 65.

The number of single, never-married seniors remains somewhat consistent at about 4% of the older-than-65 population.

EDUCATIONAL STATUS

The educational level of the older adult population in the United States has changed dramatically over the past three decades. In 1970, only 28% of senior citizens had graduated from high school. By 2008, 78% were high school graduates or more, and 21% had a bachelor's degree or higher. Twenty-seven percent of older men hold bachelor's degrees as contrasted with 16% of older women.

In addition to being better educated, today's older adult population is more technologically sophisticated. A Pew research study conducted in 2004 revealed that 23% of Americans over age 65 use the Internet. In 2006 the same group reported that Internet use among Americans over age 65 had increased to 34%, and by 2008 had further increased to 43%. This will most likely continue to increase in the near future because, as of 2009, more than 77% of Baby Boomers have reported that they are Internet users.

ECONOMICS OF AGING

The stereotypical belief that many older adults are poor is not necessarily true. The economic status of older persons is as varied as that of other age groups. Some of the poorest people in the country are old, but so are some of the richest.

POVERTY

In 2007 approximately 10% of the elderly population was statistically determined to be at or below the poverty level. Older women were more likely to be impoverished than older men. Those over age 75 were slightly more likely to experience poverty. Elderly minorities, particularly blacks, were slightly more likely to live in poverty. Although they have declined over time, as of 2008, poverty rates are still highest in the South. Mississippi, Louisiana, Alabama, Arkansas, Tennessee, New Mexico, West Virginia, and the District of Columbia have poverty rates in excess of 17%. Of the remaining elderly, 26% were statistically determined to have a low-income status, 33% were in the middle-income range, and 31% had a high-income status.

INCOME

As of 2007 the median income of men over age 65 was $24,142, whereas that for women over age 65 was $13,877 only. The median income of households headed by a person 65 years of age or older was approximately $43,159. Median income is the middle of the group with half earning less and half earning more. It is not an average amount. Median figures can be deceptive because income is not distributed equally among whites and minority groups (Figure 1-4).

The major sources of aggregate income for older adults include Social Security benefits earnings, asset income, pensions, earnings from employment, public assistance, and miscellaneous sources. Figure 1-5 shows the sources of income for five different income levels (income quintiles).

Social Security income forms the base of income for those over age 65, or slightly higher age for the youngest with a later age eligibility. Average Social Security income in 2008 was $1,079 for an individual and $1,761 for a couple. Thirty-seven percent of individuals receive less than $10,000, whereas 7% receive more than $20,000. Low-earning individuals and couples are more likely to rely on Social Security as the major

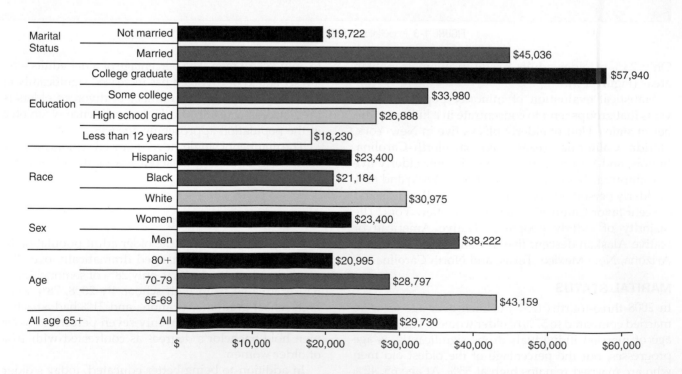

Median Household Income by Demographic Traits of Householder, 20087

Marital Status	Not married	$19,722
	Married	$45,036
Education	College graduate	$57,940
	Some college	$33,980
	High school grad	$26,888
	Less than 12 years	$18,230
Race	Hispanic	$23,400
	Black	$21,184
	White	$30,975
Sex	Women	$23,400
	Men	$38,222
Age	80+	$20,995
	70-79	$28,797
	65-69	$43,159
All age 65+	All	$29,730

Source: Both figures from CRS analysis of the March 2008 *Current Population Survey.*

FIGURE 1-4 Median individual income by demographic traits, 2007.

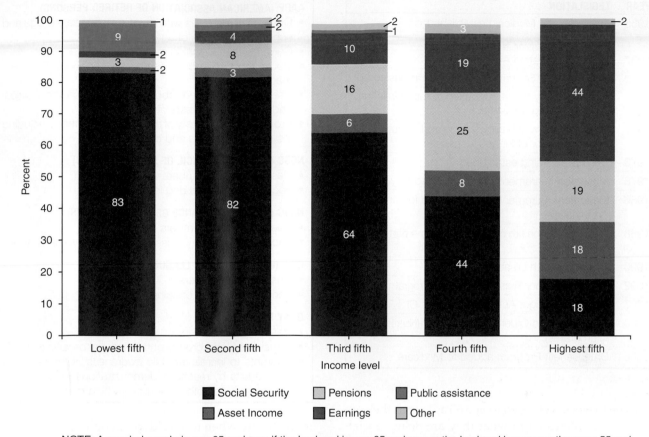

Sources of income for married couples and nonmarried people who are age 65 and over, by income quintile, percent distribution, 2008

FIGURE 1-5 Sources of income.

NOTE: A married couple is age 65 and over if the husband is age 65 and over or the husband is younger than age 55 and the wife is age 65 and over. The definition of "other" includes, but is not limited to, public assistance, unemployment compensation, worker's compensation, alimony, child support, and personal contributions. Quintile limits are $12,082, $19,877, $31,303, and $55,889 for all units; $23,637, $35,794, $53,180, and $86,988 for married couples; and $9,929, $14,265, $20,187, and $32,937 for nonmarried persons.
Reference population: These data refer to the civilian noninstitutionalized population.
SOURCE: U.S. Census Bureau, Current Population Survey, Annual Social and Economic Supplement, 2009

source of income. High earners are less reliant on Social Security.

An area of concern is that Social Security funding could become inadequate as the number of retirees drawing benefits increases, while the pool of workers paying into the system decreases. Plans to ensure the long-term survival of the Social Security program have been proposed by many both within and outside of the government.

Asset income, income derived from investments such as stocks, bonds, and other retirement accounts, has dropped drastically since 2008. The economic downturn has been compared in severity to the Great Depression of the 1930s. Many retirees and those near retirement lost a large percentage of the monies they had saved and invested for retirement. Many of those who invested personally and those who had their money in employer-directed programs were severely affected. These financial losses have forced many individuals nearing retirement to reconsider whether they can afford it.

In 2007 slightly more than one-third of people age 65 and older received pensions from public or private sources. People who worked for a governmental agency were much more likely to receive a pension than those who worked for a private industry or business. Not only are former government employees more likely to receive a pension, but also government pensions tend to be far more generous than those in the private sector. The median government pension in 2007 was $16,629, whereas the median private sector pension was $7,200 only.

Early retirement was popular from until about 1985. Since then the trend has shown more people working for pay after age 65. For those over 65 who work, the median wages in 2007 were $20,000. This is significantly less than what the person earned earlier in life and reflects a decrease in hours worked and in wages.

Earnings make up a substantial portion of income for many people over age 65. Those who are in higher income brackets, generally professionals, may

Table 1-2 Legislation That Has Helped Older Adults

YEAR	LEGISLATION
1965	Medicare and Medicaid established
	Administration on Aging established
1967	Age Discrimination Act passed
1972	Supplemental Security Income Program instituted
	Social Security benefits indexed to reflect inflation, cost-of-living adjustment
1972	Nutrition Act, which allows for providing nutrition programs for older adults, passed
1973	Council on Aging established
1978	Mandatory retirement age changed to 70 years
1986	Mandatory retirement age eliminated for most employees
1988	Catastrophic health insurance became part of Medicare
1990	Americans with Disabilities Act
1992	Vulnerable Elder Rights Protection Program
1997	Balanced Budget Act (Medicare Part C)
2000	Amendment to Older Americans Act (Nutrition programs)
2006	Drug Benefit Program added to Medicare

Box 1-2 Politically Active Senior Citizen Groups

AARP (AMERICAN ASSOCIATION OF RETIRED PERSONS)
- Consists of members who are at least 50 years of age and spouses regardless of age
- Currently has 30 million members
- Could have 76 million members when Baby Boomers reach age 50
- Uses volunteers and lobbyists to advance the political and economic interests of older adults
- Provides a wide variety of membership benefits, including insurance programs and discounts

NCSC (NATIONAL COUNCIL OF SENIOR CITIZENS)
- Has 4.5 million members
- Focuses on political and legislative issues

NASC (NATIONAL ALLIANCE OF SENIOR CITIZENS)
- Has two million members
- Focuses on a variety of issues of concern to older adults

OWL (OLDER WOMEN'S LEAGUE)
- Has 20,000 members
- Focuses on needs of aging women

GRAY PANTHERS
- Has 75,000 members
- Consists of local groups and a national organization
- Attempts to increase public awareness of the needs of older adults by means of demonstrations, door-to-door canvassing, and other attention-getting methods

continue to work well beyond age 65 as long as they are healthy and interested in what they are doing. Socialization, time away from a retired spouse, intellectual challenge, and a sense of self-worth are verbalized as reasons for working, particularly by those in the baby boom generation. Some Baby Boomers need to continue to work to maintain a standard of living they desire. Some need to work because they neglected to save enough for retirement or need to make up for losses in their investments. Those in lower income brackets may need to continue to work, or to seek work, to pay for necessities of life or a few luxuries.

Legislation and political activism among older people have helped improve the economic outlook for older adults (Table 1-2). Through activist organizations, older adults have united to consolidate their political power and to use the power of the vote to initiate programs that benefit them (Box 1-2). Over the past 25 years, these groups have done much to improve the economic welfare of older adults. The Federal Housing Authority and other lending agencies have proposed the use of reverse mortgages, which are plans that allow older adults to remain in their homes and receive monthly payments based on their equity in the property. Monthly income realized from these plans could range from as little as $100 to as much as several thousand dollars, depending on the value of the property and the age of the residents. This money could be a much-needed income supplement for older adults. Plans such as these are likely to become more common in the future when more elderly people recognize their economic benefits.

Older people may choose not to seek help, despite the availability of assistance programs designed to aid them. Many older adults are suspicious of "getting something for nothing" or are reluctant to disclose the details of their financial status, which is necessary to qualify for most assistance programs. Many older people feel that asking for help is humiliating. Some may fear they will lose what little they have if they seek assistance. Other older people have no difficulty seeking or, in some cases, demanding financial assistance or concessions. The term *greedy geezers* was coined to describe those older individuals who expect the government to provide more money and services or for businesses to provide discounts based on senior status. Factors that can affect the financial well-being of older adults are described in Box 1-3.

Sensitivity is needed when dealing with the financial issues of older adults. The Critical Thinking box on page 13 should help you assess your attitudes, and therefore your sensitivity, toward these kinds of situations. Many older adults who find it easy to talk about their intimate physical and medical problems are reluctant to discuss finances. Nurses may suspect financial need if an older person lacks adequate shelter, clothing, heat, food, or medical attention. When an economic problem causes real or potential dangers, nurses must be prepared to respond appropriately.

Box 1-3	Factors That Influence the Economic Conditions of Older Adults

- Many older adults bought their homes when housing costs and inflation were low. If they paid off their mortgages before retirement, their housing costs are limited to taxes, maintenance, and utility bills.
- The number of older adults who receive pensions is greater now than it will be in the future. The current changes in business conditions are resulting in the offering of smaller pensions to fewer employees.
- Older adults qualify for several tax breaks that are unavailable to younger people.
  - Most older adults pay no Social Security taxes, whereas younger working adults pay increasingly higher rates.
  - Social Security and government pensions are largely exempt from taxation.
  - Taxpayers older than 65 years of age can take extra tax deductions.
  - A one-time capital gains tax exclusion applies when the house is sold.
- Most older adults qualify for government income programs.
  - The income from Social Security exceeds the program contributions of most recipients.
  - Medicare covers 70% of medical costs.
  - Programs such as Social Security, SSI, Medicare, housing programs, and energy assistance provide an annual average of $9,000 per every older adult.

? Critical Thinking

Your Sensitivity to the Financial Problems of Older Adults

Respond to the following statements:
- Older adults control all of the money in the country.
- Most older adults are poor.
- Older adults have it easy; the younger working people have it rough.
- Older adults have too much political power, and they get too many benefits and entitlements.
- Older adults worked for what they are getting, and they deserve everything they receive from the government.
- A society that does not care for its older people is cruel and uncivilized.
- The property of older adults should be used to pay for their physical needs and medical care.

Because regulations covering assistance programs change often, it is difficult for older patients and the nurses trying to help them to keep current and up to date. Nurses may be called on to help older adults deal with the paperwork required when applying for assistance, to provide emotional support as they work through the frustration of bureaucratic processes, or to arrange transportation to the appropriate agencies. Nurses usually are not expected to be experts in this area, but they should know how to locate appropriate resources. Nurses working in community health should be aware of community agencies that provide assistance to older adults so that appropriate referrals can be made. Nurses working in hospitals and nursing homes can initiate referrals to social workers or other professionals who are knowledgeable about assistance programs. Most states and counties throughout the United States have services for the elderly or departments on aging. These are typically listed in the government section of a telephone directory. Many publish directories of resources available in their specific community.

WEALTH

Although many older people receive less cash on a yearly basis from Social Security and pensions than some younger individuals earn, a substantial number have accumulated assets and savings from their working years. Frugal lifestyles and self-reports by older adults of being "poor" must be viewed cautiously. Some individuals are truly impoverished, whereas others have significant estates to leave to their children or to charities.

Approximately 80% of households headed by a person older than 65 years of age own their homes. Of these homes, 68% are owned outright. In 2007 the median value of homes owned by older persons was $168,654 (with a median purchase price of $45,191). A home is usually an older person's largest asset. Many older people choose not to sell their houses because they fear they will have nowhere to live. Many prefer to remain "house rich and cash poor," making do on a limited income, rather than selling their homes. Economic reversals in recent years have led to a high foreclosure rate resulting in a glut of houses for sale. This makes a profitable sale of property by the elderly more difficult to achieve. Additional considerations regarding homeownership and housing options are discussed in more detail later in the chapter.

Economic well-being is usually measured in terms of income, which is the amount of money a household receives on a weekly, monthly, or yearly basis. However, this measurement is not always a reliable indicator of financial security in older adults. People older than 65 years of age generally have more discretionary income (i.e., money left after paying for necessities such as housing, food, and medical care) available than do younger people. Younger individuals, particularly those with growing families, may have a higher income, but they also have higher nondiscretionary demands.

HOUSING ARRANGEMENTS

When asked where older adults live, most people say that they live in senior citizen housing or nursing homes. They are wrong. More than two-thirds of older adults (68%) live independently in a family setting.

Twenty-seven percent live in modified but not institutional settings, including senior citizen housing, group homes, and apartments, or with family members. Approximately 5% of all older adults are institutionalized, and this percentage increases with advancing age. Only 1% of 65- to 74-year-old individuals are institutionalized. This rate increases to 4.7% with individuals 75 to 84 years of age and reaches 18.2% with people older than age 85.

Older individuals often try to keep their homes, despite the physical or economic difficulties in doing so. A house is more than just a physical shelter; it represents independence and security. The home holds many memories. Being in a familiar neighborhood close to friends and church is important. A sense of community is important to many aging people, who dislike the thought of leaving security for the unknown. The physical exertion and emotional trauma involved in moving can be intimidating, even overwhelming, to older adults. Moving to a different, often smaller, residence is a difficult decision, particularly when it involves giving up precious possessions because of the lack of space.

For some older people, keeping the family home is not a sensible option for many reasons. Many of the houses owned by older adults are in central cities with high crime rates. Expenses, including increasingly high property taxes and ongoing maintenance costs, often present excessive strain on older persons with limited financial resources. Home maintenance, including even simple tasks such as housecleaning, becomes increasingly difficult with advancing age or illness. Ownership may require more effort in terms of money and time than some older people possess; yet many struggle to remain independent and keep their houses.

Some older individuals remain in their own houses and refuse to give them up long after it is safe for them to be alone. They may be able to cope as long as family, friends, and neighbors are willing to help. However, if there is a change in their support system, dangerous, life-threatening situations may arise. Some older people try to live in their houses, despite broken plumbing, inadequate heat, and insufficient access to food. Families, health care professionals, and social service agencies may have to step in to protect the welfare of these aging individuals.

Some older people recognize the problems associated with living alone and decide to seek housing arrangements that are more in keeping with their needs and abilities. They may choose to move into an apartment, condominium, senior citizen complex, or some other type of housing. As the older adult population grows, a variety of new types of housing and living arrangements is evolving (Figure 1-6). The following Critical Thinking box should help you determine your attitudes toward housing for older adults.

? Critical Thinking

Your Attitudes Toward Housing for Older Adults

- Is it safe for older adults to remain indefinitely in their own houses?
- When should an older person sell his or her house?
- Once a house is sold, what are the best types of living accommodations for older adults?
- What kinds of alternative housing for older adults are available in your community?
- Should older adults live in housing that is separated from people in other age groups? Why? Why not?

Independent or **assisted-living centers** are becoming common. These centers combine privacy with easily available services. Most consist of private apartments that are either purchased or rented. For additional charges, the residents can be served meals in restaurant-style dining rooms and receive laundry and housekeeping services. Different levels of medical, nursing, and personal care services are available. Health care services may include assistance with hygiene, routine medication administration, and even preventive health clinics. Many centers have communal activity rooms, art-and-craft hobby centers, swimming pools, lounges, beauty salons, mini-grocery stores, greenhouses, and other amenities. Transportation to church, shopping, and other appointments is provided by some of these facilities. Most independent and assisted-living facilities are privately operated, and costs are significant. Some states offer subsidies to older individuals with limited resources because these living arrangements are often more cost-effective than other housing alternatives.

A study reported in the *Journal of the American Geriatrics Society* described an interesting alternative to assisted living—"Cruise Care." The article asserted that, with slight modifications for help with the activities of daily living, a senior citizen might be better off living on a cruise ship than in an assisted-living facility. The ship provides a higher employee-to-resident ratio, more activities, more and better choices of food, better scenery, and more companionship for a comparable price. Although not appropriate for individuals suffering from dementia, it might be an option (at least temporarily) for some adventurous seniors.

Life-lease or **life-contract facilities** are another housing option. For a large initial investment and substantial monthly rental and service fees, older persons or couples are guaranteed a residence for life. Independent residents occupy apartment units, but extended-care units are either attached to this apartment complex or located nearby for residents who require skilled nursing services. If one spouse needs skilled care, the other may continue to live in the apartment and can easily visit the hospitalized loved one. When the occupants die, control

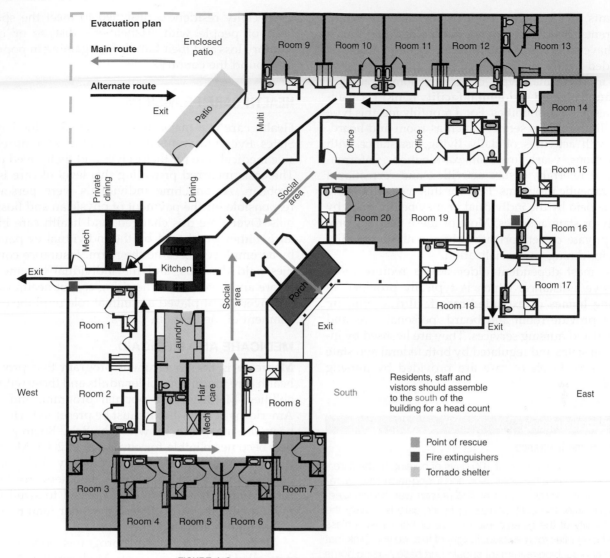

Evacuation plan

Main route

Alternate route

Enclosed patio

Exit

Patio

Private dining

Dining

Multi

Mech

Kitchen

Social area

Office

Office

Room 9   Room 10   Room 11   Room 12   Room 13

Room 14

Room 15

Room 20   Room 19

Room 16

Room 17

Exit

Porch

Room 18

Exit

Social area

Laundry

Hair care

Mech

Room 1

Room 2

Room 8

West

South

East

Residents, staff and vistors should assemble to the south of the building for a head count

■ Point of rescue
■ Fire extinguishers
■ Tornado shelter

Room 3

Room 4   Room 5   Room 6

Room 7

FIGURE 1-6 A living plan for CBRF with evacuation plan.

of the apartment reverts to the owners of the facility. The costs for this type of housing are high and may be out of the range of the average older adult. However, despite the costs, many find this option satisfactory because it meets their needs for independence, socialization, and services. Many find security in knowing that skilled care is easily available if needed.

Less-well-to-do people are more limited in their housing options. Some older adults qualify for **government-subsidized housing** if they meet certain financial standards and limits. Government-subsidized housing units may be simple apartments without any special services, or they may have limited services, such as access to nursing clinics and special transportation arrangements. Most communities are finding that the demand for these facilities exceeds the availability. Waiting lists and 1- to 2-year delays are common. Interpretation of government regulations is causing some concern with regard to senior citizen housing. Residences originally intended for older adults may be required to accept a

variety of medically disabled people, regardless of age. Some of these younger residents suffer from psychiatric or drug-related problems, and the presence of these individuals may leave older adult residents feeling threatened and fearful for their own safety and well-being.

Some older adults who are not related to each other are forming **group-housing plans**. In this type of arrangement, two or more unrelated people share a household in which they have private bedrooms but share the common recreational and leisure areas, as well as the tasks involved in home maintenance. Some communities offer services to help match people who are interested in this option. Roommates are selected so that the strengths of one individual compensate for the weaknesses of the other. In some cases, a large house may shelter 10 or more residents. Not all of these arrangements are limited to older adults. In some situations, younger adults who need reasonable housing may be included. By providing services for older adult residents, the younger residents are able to reduce their rental costs. Both younger and older individuals who have chosen this option report benefits from the extended-family atmosphere.

A more formal type of group home called a **community-based residential facility** (CBRF) is available in some communities. For a monthly fee, this type of facility provides services such as room and board, help with activities of daily living, assistance with medications, yearly medical examinations, information and referrals, leisure activities, and recreational or therapeutic programs. Fees for this type of housing may be paid by the individual or may be provided by county or state agencies. Most of these facilities provide private or semiprivate rooms with community areas for dining and socialization.

The most dependent older adults require more extensive assistance, which is typically provided in **nursing homes** or **extended-care facilities**. Nursing homes provide room and board, personal care, and medical and nursing services. They are licensed by individual states and regulated by both federal and state laws. Three levels of care are provided by nursing homes.

[?] Critical Thinking

Nursing Home Insurance

Medicare will pay for most of 100 days of nursing home care if admission follows a hospitalization and if long-term care placement is for the same reason as the person was hospitalized. After that time, the cost of nursing home care is usually the responsibility of the older person or his or her family, unless he or she qualifies for Medicaid. In light of this, do you think that people approaching retirement should purchase nursing home insurance? Why or why not?

Basic care facilities provide the level of care and supervision necessary to maintain the residents' safety and well-being. They provide assistance with activities of daily living, including hygiene, ambulation, nutrition, elimination, and other basic needs. This level of care is typically provided by nursing assistants and licensed vocational or practical nurses. *Skilled care facilities* provide skilled nursing care on a regular basis. Interventions, such as the administration of medication and skilled treatments or procedures that require the expertise of registered and practical nurses, are provided in this type of facility. Skilled care facilities also provide services performed by specially trained professionals such as speech, physical, occupational, and respiratory therapists. *Subacute care facilities* provide comprehensive inpatient care designed for individuals who have an acute illness, injury, or exacerbation of a disease process. Subacute care falls between the traditional care provided in an acute care facility and that provided in a skilled nursing home.

Specialty residences designed to meet the special need of people with Alzheimer's disease or other memory loss and their families are gaining in popularity around the country.

HEALTH CARE PROVISIONS

Health care is a major area of concern in the United States. Everyone wants the best and most comprehensive medical care for themselves and their loved ones. The costs incurred providing this level of care is the problem. At one time individuals were personally responsible for the payment of physician and hospital bills. Over time this changed, and health care insurance, either purchased by the individual or paid for by an employer, became the norm. Insurance companies paid the bills, and the individual became less aware and involved in the rising cost of health care.

Government played a minimal role until the establishment of Medicare in 1965's.

MEDICARE AND MEDICAID

Medicare is the government program that provides health care funding for older adults and those with disabilities. Medicare is a popular program, and most Americans believe that it must be preserved. This will be increasingly difficult when the Baby-Boom generation becomes eligible for coverage. In 2005, Medicare provided coverage for approximately 42.5 million citizens. By 2031, when all Baby Boomers are eligible for coverage, this number is expected to swell to 77 million citizens. Most Americans older than 65 years of age qualify for Medicare.

Medicare has four distinct programs, none of which pays all of the health care costs. Medicare **Part A** covers inpatient hospital care; extended care in a skilled nursing facility following hospitalization; some home health services such as visiting nurses and occupational, speech, or physical therapists; and hospice services, but only after the patient pays an initial deductible and any co-pay expenses. During the 1980s, Medicare instituted the **diagnosis-related group** (DRG) system in an attempt to contain hospital costs. Under this system, a hospital is paid a set amount based on the patient's admitting diagnosis. If the patient is discharged in fewer days than predicted, the hospital may keep the excess money. If the patient needs to stay longer than projected, the hospital must absorb the additional costs. Although DRGs have resulted in some cost reduction, they have also resulted in the quicker discharge of sicker people than in the past. Many older people are released from the hospital before they have actually recovered from their illnesses, placing an increased health care burden on families and home health agencies.

Medicare **Part B** is optional, but most people choose to obtain this coverage. This plan covers 80% of the "customary and usual" rates charged by physicians after deductibles are met. In addition to physicians' fees, services covered by Medicare Part B include medically necessary ambulance transport; physical, speech, and occupational therapy; home health services when medically necessary; medical supplies and equipment; and outpatient surgery or blood transfusions. The patient is responsible for the remaining 20% of the costs plus the difference between the actual fee and the government's "customary and usual" rate. The actual costs of medical care often exceed the amount that the government pays. Many elderly pay for private supplemental health care insurance to cover these expenses rather than pay these costs out of pocket.

In 1997 optional Medicare **Part C** coverage was made available to individuals who are eligible for Part A and enrolled in Part B. Medicare Part C includes "Advantage" or "Choice" plans, which allow beneficiaries to receive Medicare benefits through private insurance companies that are able to demonstrate cost savings. These plans involve enrollment in a private plan offered by a health maintenance organization (HMO), preferred provider organization (PPO), provider sponsored organization (PSO), private fee for service (PFFS) organization, or medical savings account (MSA). These plans are designed to cover total costs so that supplemental insurance coverage is not necessary. They do, however, limit the pool of available health care providers, and premiums vary depending on the plan selected.

Medicare **Part D**, prescription drug coverage, went into effect during 2006. It is a voluntary plan available to anyone enrolled in Part A or B of Medicare. Under Part D, prescription drugs are distributed through local pharmacies and administered by a wide variety of private insurance plans. In many plans, there is a significant gap between the cost of the drugs and the benefits provided. Individuals will need to be cautious when selecting coverage to ensure that they select a plan that is most cost-effective for their specific situation and needs. Elderly people who have high medication costs may experience the "donut hole." In 2010 an elderly person was expected to meet a deductible of $310, then pay a 25% co-insurance of up to $2,830. Once costs exceed that amount, the elder enters the "donut hole" and must pay the full cost of medication until out-of-pocket expenses reached $4,550. Costs drop to a set fee for generic ($2.50) and brand name ($6.30), only after this large amount is reached in a single year.

Supplemental Medicaid (Title 19) assistance may be available for those older adults who meet certain financial need requirements. Many of those who have assets do not qualify; they are left with a Medicare gap (or "medigap") that they must pay themselves. Many older people buy private medical insurance—often at unreasonable prices—to pay medical bills that are not covered by Medicare.

RISING COSTS AND LEGISLATIVE ACTIVITY

The costs of health care have increased dramatically in recent years. More money is spent on health care in the United States than in any other country in the world, yet health care is not provided for all U.S. citizens. Many other nations do a better job than the United States of meeting their citizens' health care needs.

During 2009 the Centers for Medicare & Medicaid Services (CMS) reported that approximately $2.5 trillion was spent on health care in the United States. This exceeds the amount spent on any other activity, including defense. This amount is expected to grow to $4.3 trillion by 2018. A significant proportion (close to one-third) is spent on the 13% of the population that is older than 65 years of age. These costs are staggering considering how quickly the number of older adults is increasing. To contain health care costs, there has been an upsurge in initiatives such as managed care and insurance reform. If we expect to continue to provide adequate health care in the future, we can expect to see more changes in the way health care is financed and delivered. This is a major, and often divisive, political issue.

The cost of Medicare alone has grown dramatically from $3 billion in 1967, the first year of funding, to $52 billion in 1983; $297 billion in 2004; $425 billion in 2009; and $528 billion in 2010. The Congressional Budget Office (CBO) projects it will reach $735 billion in 2015 and $1,038 billion (more than $1 trillion) in 2020 (Figure 1-7).

In December 2009, under highly charged political controversy, the United States Congress passed The **Patient Protection and Affordable Care Act** (**PPACA**). It was signed into law by President Barack Obama in 2010. The law includes numerous health-related provisions to take effect over several years. This 2,000-plus-pages legislative initiative includes major changes in health insurance, health care funding, student loans, and a wide range of spending considerations. The costs of these provisions are supposed to be offset by a variety of taxes, fees, and cost-saving measures.

There is a great deal of controversy because many specifics of the legislation and their ramifications are still unknown. Those in favor of the legislation cite expanded coverage, more competition among insurance companies, coverage of people with preexisting medical conditions and closure of the "donut hole" affecting senior citizens. Those opposed to the legislation cite cuts in Medicare funding, cuts to the Medicare Advantage program along with increases in the Medicare tax. They fear increased costs of health care, more taxes, decreased incentives to primary care physicians, and possible rationing of care as seen in single-payer plans such as those provided in Canada.

Legal challenges regarding the constitutionality of this bill were raised by several states. The legality of the bill may eventually require a ruling by the Supreme

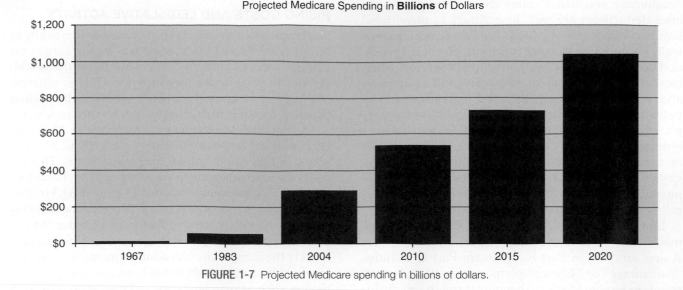

FIGURE 1-7 Projected Medicare spending in billions of dollars.

Court. This could be a drawn out process, and it remains to be seen what will happen in the interim. Health care providers should pay attention because this legislation is likely to have an impact on how health care is provided and funded.

COSTS AND END-OF-LIFE CARE

Not all older people use the available health care resources equally. Most health care services are consumed by the very ill or terminally ill minority, many of whom happen to be elderly. Studies by the Health Care Financing Administration indicate that 2% of the older-than-65 population receiving Medicare accounts for 34% of the costs. Overall, 72% of the total resources are used by only 10% of the aging population. More than 25% of the Medicare budget is used for terminally ill patients; 50% of all physicians' services, and 49% of all hospital days involve older Americans. Serious questions are being raised about the appropriateness of using intensive, expensive interventions to extend the lives of terminally ill older people.

Financial concerns are forcing health care providers and society to face ethical dilemmas regarding the allocation of limited health care resources. This is a highly emotional issue with no easy answers. Many people are alive today because of advances in medical technology. Some of those who benefit are young, whereas others are old. Some go on to lead lives of high quality; others never lead normal lives again. By virtue of their training, physicians are inclined to try to cure everyone. Most doctors do not feel comfortable allowing a patient to die, regardless of the person's age. Most doctors will use all available technology to save a life. Talking about death is not easy for anyone, including physicians. It is easier to avoid end-of-life issues than to take time for this difficult discussion. Many physicians are unwilling to take time away from other activities to have this discussion, particularly because they

can do only minimal billing for the time spent counseling the patient. In spite of these concerns, more physicians need to take time to have honest discussions with patients while they are competent to understand and make informed decisions.

Reputable authorities, ethicists, and politicians have widely differing points of view on this issue. Some believe that health care restrictions on older adults are the ultimate in age discrimination. Others argue that the benefits gained, which can usually be measured in months, do not outweigh the costs. Private citizens examining this dilemma are equally confused. Even those who believe that health care costs are excessive frequently want everything possible done to save their lives or those of their loved ones. This dilemma is moral, ethical, and legal, with no simple right answer. Part of the debate regarding health care reform involves differing viewpoints regarding end-of-life care. Perhaps this issue will encourage an honest national discussion among spouses, families, spiritual advisors, physicians, and other health care providers.

The Critical Thinking box is designed to increase your awareness and insight into these problems.

? Critical Thinking

Your Understanding of the Health Care Dilemma

- Should an 80-year-old person have a coronary bypass surgery at a cost of approximately $100,000?
- Should dialysis be provided to individuals older than 65? Older than 75? Older than 85?
- Should people older than 65 be candidates for organ transplants?
- Should a respirator be used on a terminally ill patient?
- Are feeding tubes a part of basic physical care, or are they extraordinary means?
- Should the individual, the family, or the physician decide the type and amount of medical intervention necessary?
- What should be the role of the government in health care?

ADVANCE DIRECTIVES

All adults who are 18 years of age or older and of sound mind have the right to make decisions regarding the amount and type of health care they desire. Because older adults are more likely to experience significant health problems, the question of what and how much medical care to administer must be addressed. Such important decisions are best made during a stress-free time when the individual is alert and experiencing no acute health problems. A person's wishes can best be communicated using advance directives, which are legally recognized, written documents that specify the types of care and treatment the individual desires when that individual cannot speak for himself or herself. Areas typically addressed in advance directives include (1) do not attempt to resuscitate (DNAR) orders, (2) directives related to mechanical ventilation, and (3) directives related to artificial nutrition and hydration.

Two formal types of advance directive are recognized in most states: (1) the durable power of attorney for health care and (2) the living will. Information about both of these is typically provided when a person enters the hospital. Each patient is expected to make a decision about the type and extent of care to be administered if his or her condition becomes terminal.

These written documents are designed to help guide the family and medical professionals in planning care. The family is often relieved to have this information when making difficult decisions during a stressful time. In general, advance directives are recognized and respected, but various agencies, individual physicians, or health care providers may have beliefs or policies that prohibit them from honoring certain advance directives. Individuals should discuss their wishes with their health care providers when these documents are written. Open communication reduces the chance of questions, conflict, or legal repercussions later. If irreconcilable differences exist between an individual and the care provider, changes in either the document or the care provider must be considered.

Durable power of attorney for health care transfers the authority to make health care decisions to another person, called the *health care agent*. The agent may act only in situations in which the person is unable to make decisions for himself or herself. Because the health care agent must be trusted to follow through with the older person's wishes, the agent specified in the document is usually a family member or friend. These wishes are specified in writing and usually witnessed by unrelated individuals to reduce the possibility of undue influence. Standardized legal forms are available to initiate a power of attorney for health care.

A living will informs the physician that the individual wishes to die naturally if he or she develops an illness or receives an injury that cannot be cured. Living wills prohibit the use of life-prolonging measures and equipment when the individual is near death or in a persistent vegetative state. Living wills go into effect only when two physicians agree in writing that the necessary criteria are met.

Usually, either of these documents is adequate to communicate one's wishes; both are not needed. Those who choose to initiate both documents should ensure that there is no conflict between the directions provided in each document. Either document can be revoked at any time. Directions to accomplish this are usually provided on the specific forms. An advance directive should be stored in a safe place where it can be located easily if the need arises. A safe deposit box is not recommended for this purpose. Ideally, family members and the family lawyer should know the content of the document and its location. An advance directive should be provided to the physician so that it becomes part of the patient's permanent medical record. These documents are often required and kept available for emergency situations when an individual resides in an institutional setting such as an independent or assisted-living apartment, community-based residential facility, or a nursing home.

Laws and specifics differ from state to state. Nurses should be aware of the legal standing of such documents in the particular state where they practice and should understand any legal ramifications engendered by these documents.

? Critical Thinking

Advance Directives

- How would you as a nurse approach a patient regarding initiation of an advance directive?
- Can a person who is diagnosed with Alzheimer's disease initiate a living will or durable power of attorney?
- What is the legal standing of these documents in your state?
- How do hospitals and extended care facilities identify a patient's advance directive?

IMPACT OF AGING MEMBERS IN THE FAMILY

The family is undergoing significant change in our society. Many factors, including increasing divorce rates, single parenting, and a mobile population, are creating a less stable, less predictable family structure. Blended families, extended families, and separated families all present challenges. In addition to these societal changes, the demographic changes discussed previously are having, and will continue to have, repercussions that we can only begin to appreciate (Box 1-4).

Families today face historically unprecedented situations. Because of the life span extension, it is not uncommon for four or five generations of a family to be

Box 1-4   Demographic Changes Affecting the Family

- Extended life spans are leading to more older family members.
- There are more people who are living with chronic conditions and who need some degree of care or assistance.
- The number of people in the younger generations is decreasing in proportion to the number of older members.
- There is an increasing number of widows who may be unprepared to provide for their own needs and who therefore need assistance.
- The role of women is changing. As women increasingly must work outside the home, many are attempting to meet the demands of their parents, home, children, and workplace.

Table 1-3   The Family

AGE (YEARS)	GENERATION
80+	Parents
60+	Children
40+	Grandchildren
20+	Great-grandchildren
Less than 20	Great-great-grandchildren

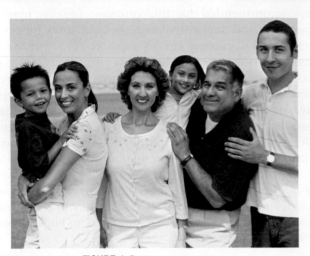

FIGURE 1-8 Three generations.

alive at one time (Figure 1-8). Until recently, this was an unheard-of occurrence. Using 20 years as a typical generation, a family might resemble one such as that described in Table 1-3. If the generation time is less than 20 years, even more generations might be alive at the same time.

PERSONAL REFLECTION

Some years ago, as death was approaching for a 91-year-old gentleman, his family gathered at the hospital. His wife of 69 years asked that "the children" come into the room. This sounded rather strange because "the children" were all in their 60s, the grandchildren were all mature adults, and the great-grandchildren were fast approaching adulthood. It sounded even stranger to me, because this older man was my grandfather, and my father was "the baby" of the family.

Gloria Wold

It is estimated that 80% of older adults who need care will receive assistance from their families. The problems encountered in such situations can differ widely, depending on the respective ages of the family members. In some families, the "children" who are attempting to provide care for the oldest members are likely to be older than 65 themselves. They may have health problems of their own that make care giving difficult or impractical.

Middle-aged family members often become the caregivers. The generation in their forties and early fifties is often called the "sandwich" generation because its members are caught in the middle—trying to work, to raise their own dependent children, and often, to provide assistance to one or two generations of aging family members. In some cases, they are also trying to help raise grandchildren by giving financial or physical assistance or both.

Although the financial, psychological, and physical demands of assisting aging relatives affect all family members, women are likely to be the most affected. It is estimated that 72% of the caregivers in the United States are female. Regardless of whether this is fair, women are the primary caregivers in the family (Box 1-5). Typically, sons contribute financially, but the brunt of the emotional and physical care burden falls to the daughters. It is estimated that as the population ages, women will spend more time caring for their parents than they did caring for their children.

Families try to help aging family members in a variety of ways. If the aging family member is able to live alone, families may demonstrate concern by visiting frequently and assisting with transportation to shopping and doctor appointments. Some prepare meals, do the heavy housecleaning, and make major home repairs. Running between two households and trying to maintain both can be mentally and physically exhausting to younger family members, but many are willing to help their loved ones in any way they can.

Box 1-5   Caregivers in the United States

- Average caregiver age is 46.
- 30% of caregivers who provide 40 hours of care each week are 65 years or older.
- 73% of caregivers are female.
- Average woman spends 18 years helping an aging parent.
- More than half of caregivers work full-time.
- Average age of care recipient is 77 years.
  - 40% are older than 75.
  - 24% are older than 85.

A family crisis may occur when the aging person is no longer able to live alone. Important decisions must be made. Most families who try to do the right thing find that there is no perfect solution. The two most common options are bringing the aging parent into the home of one of the children or placing the parent in a long-term care facility. There are problems and concerns with both of these options. It is essential that the family making this difficult decision consider many factors. The amount of care needed by the parent; the availability of a willing and able family member; the amount of available space in the child's home; the added financial burden of an additional household member; the wishes of the parent, the child, and the child's family; and the interpersonal dynamics within the family must be considered before a decision is made.

Children often take older parents into their homes when the older parents can no longer maintain their own houses or apartments. Although this arrangement works well in some families, in others it is problematic for everyone involved. The familiar roles and responsibilities often reverse when children step in and attempt to take care of their parents. This places the aging person into the role of the child, which he or she usually resents strongly. "Don't tell your mother what to do!" or "I'm still your father!" is often heard in aging parent-child interactions.

Loss of independence is probably the most significant issue that aging parents and their children must face. The aging family members have spent 40, 50, 60, or even 70 years making their own decisions as adults. As independent adults, they could make their own choices about where to live, what to do, and when to do it. They chose what to eat, obtained their food, and prepared it without interference. They went to bed when and where they chose. They went to places they wanted to go without asking anyone's permission. They had control of their lives. Independence is what being an adult is about. Most independent adults do not want to ask anyone for help.

As physical changes or diseases affect older adults, some or all of their independent function may be lost. Aging persons find it difficult to accept that they can no longer do the things they once did. It is also distressing for the family to watch their loved ones change. While the aging person tries to cope with these changes, the family tries to determine how to respond to these changes. If "the right thing to do" is not known, all family members begin to have mixed feelings and confusion. Feelings of grief, anger, frustration, and loss are common in all affected individuals.

When an aging family member moves in with a child's family, the dynamics within the home are unavoidably changed. The ability of the family to adapt and cope with an additional member of the household varies greatly from situation to situation. If all parties are agreeable to the move, and if the older adult can be given enough privacy to maintain independence, the blending of the older person into the child's home may be successful. Some families feel that a resident grandparent is rewarding and enriching. However, if the presence of the older person intrudes excessively on the family unit, the situation may be unpleasant for both the family and the older person.

If the older family member requires a substantial amount of physical care, the demands on family members can be intense. Regardless, many children feel duty-bound to care for their aging parents. This sense of obligation may be based on cultural, religious, or personal beliefs. If the children determine that they are unable to care for their parent and instead opt for nursing home placement, children often feel that they have failed in their responsibilities. This can lead to intense feelings of guilt, even if nursing home placement is the most realistic and reasonable option.

THE NURSE AND FAMILY INTERACTIONS

When we as nurses care for older adults, particularly in hospital or nursing home settings, we see the person only as he or she is now. We tend to forget that these people have not always been old. They lived, loved, worked, argued, and wept as each of us does. Often, the older adults we care for are very ill or infirm, and, as nurses, we tend to focus on their physical needs, cares, and treatments. In our preoccupation with our duties, we can easily lose our perspective of the older patient as both a person and a member of a family.

In hospitals and nursing homes, family members come and go. Some families show a great deal of interest and concern for their aging members, visiting regularly and interacting with the patient and the staff. This allows us to increase our understanding and appreciation of our patients as people. Other older individuals may never have family members visit them. They seem to be alone in the world, even though the charts list children and their telephone numbers for emergencies. Even in home settings, family attention and interaction vary greatly. In some households, a great deal of interest is given to each family member, whereas in others little or none is shown. Why do we see such a wide variation of family attention?

The answer often lies in family dynamics and processes that began long ago when the older adult was a young spouse and parent. Some families are very stable and cohesive. They are together often and share close, loving bonds. They have developed healthy methods for interacting, responding, and meeting each other's needs. Because of the strong bonds that have developed over many years, these families remain interested in and supportive of aging members.

Other families never develop the closeness that is ideal in a family. The family unit may have been disrupted by divorce, mental illness, or other serious problems. There may have been problems with **abuse**, alcoholism, or drugs. In fact, many families today are troubled by these problems, which may have been caused by the behavior of younger family members or by the behavior of the older person. Long-term problems that have developed over time do not go away when a person gets old. When the family unit is weak, supportive behavior from family members is unlikely.

Most families we interact with fall somewhere between these extremes. Few families are perfect, and few are terrible. Families are made up of human beings who respond to stress in many different ways. Coping with the stresses related to aging is difficult for both the aging individual and for his or her family. The behavior we see at any given time is the best that the person is capable of at that time. That does not mean that it is the best that he or she will be capable of at some other time. We as nurses need to examine the stresses affecting the family so that we can best respond to the needs of all family members. The Critical Thinking box should help you determine your stress factors.

? Critical Thinking

You and Your Family

Complete the following:
When my parents are unable to care for themselves, I will

_____.

If both my parents and grandparents were alive and in need of assistance, I would

_____.

If both my children and my parents needed help from me, I would

_____.

If my parents were in a nursing home, I would want the nurses to

_____.

When I grow old, I want my family to

_____.

SELF-NEGLECT

Abuse and **neglect** are usually something done to someone, but, unfortunately, self-neglect is a common problem in the older adult population. Self-neglect is more likely to be seen when an older person has few or no close family or friends, but it can occur despite their presence. Because our society has laws to protect the rights of adults, it may be difficult for concerned parties to intervene until a situation has reached critical or even life-threatening proportions.

Self-neglect is defined as the failure to provide for the self because of a lack of ability or lack of awareness. Indicators of self-neglect include the following:

1. The inability to maintain activities of daily living such as personal care, shopping, meal preparation, or other household tasks

2. The inability to obtain adequate food and fluid as indicated by malnutrition or dehydration
3. Poor hygiene practices as indicated by body odor, sores, rashes, or inadequate or soiled clothing
4. Changes in mental function such as confusion, inappropriate responses, disorientation, or incoherence
5. The inability to manage personal finances as indicated by the failure to pay bills or by hoarding, squandering, or giving away money inappropriately
6. Failure to keep important business or medical appointments
7. Life-threatening or suicidal acts such as wandering, isolation, or substance abuse

Self-neglect in the community is most likely to be recognized by neighbors and reported to the police, public health nurses, or social workers. It may also be suspected by emergency department nurses who see these individuals after they are found injured on the street, after a fire, or in some other state of distress.

Self-neglect is often connected with some form of mental illness or dementia. Once the problem is recognized, legal action through the courts may be needed to place the person in the custody of a family member or adult protective services.

ABUSE OR NEGLECT BY THE FAMILY

It is estimated that 10% of older adults will need some form of long-term care in the home. Attempts to meet these demands may be accompanied by high levels of stress for the caregivers. Increased demands on limited resources, physical exhaustion, or mental fatigue can result in deviant behaviors on the part of the caregiver. Inappropriate behavioral responses include abuse and neglect of the older family members. A Senate subcommittee that studied the problem of elder abuse estimated that as many as one million older Americans are being abused in some way by their families.

Intentional abuse occurs when any person deliberately plans to mistreat or harm another person. Abusive behavior cannot be justified at any time or in any way. Intentional abuse is most likely to occur in families with preexisting behavioral or social problems. High-risk families include those that have a history of family conflict and those with family members who have a history of violence or substance abuse, those with mental impairment of either the dependent person or caregiver (or both), and those with severe financial problems or unemployment.

Not all forms of abuse are intentional, but even unintentional abuse is devastating to older adults. Unintentional abuse or neglect is most likely to occur when the caregiver lacks the necessary knowledge, stamina, or resources needed to care for an older loved one. Often, the caregiver is an older spouse or an aging child who physically cannot meet the high-level care demands. Situations that trigger abuse are more likely when the older person requiring care is confused or needs continual care.

Continuous demands on caregivers can virtually make them prisoners within their own homes. Stress builds, leaving the caregiver feeling trapped, frustrated, or angry. Unable to cope with the stress of these continual demands, caregivers may strike out at older adults, lock them in a room, restrain them in a chair, or leave them unattended. When stress is high and the coping ability is low, caregivers may not be able to identify any better options. They may not intend to hurt the older person or may rationalize that they are doing it to only "keep Dad from hurting himself," but the end result is still abuse.

Abuse can be physical, financial, psychological, or emotional. Neglect and abandonment also constitute forms of abuse.

Physical Abuse

There are many types of physical abuse. Physical abuse is any action that causes physical pain or injury. Abuse may involve a physical attack upon a frail elderly person who is unable to defend himself or herself from younger, stronger family members. Older people may be locked in bedrooms, closets, or basements. Older women may be sexually abused or raped by caregivers or family members. Some older people are starved by family members or given food that is unsuitable or unfit for human consumption. Failure to provide adequate food or fluids also constitutes physical abuse. The inappropriate use of drugs, force-feeding, and the use of physical restraints or punishment of any kind are examples of physical abuse. Warning signs of physical abuse include bruising, lacerations, broken teeth, broken glasses, sprains, fractures, burn marks, wounds in various stages of healing, unexplained injuries, torn or bloody underwear, signs of vaginal trauma, delay in seeking medical treatment or history of "doctor shopping," and refusal by the caregiver to let visitors see the elderly person.

Neglect

Physical abuse involves one or more actions that cause harm. Neglect is a passive form of abuse in which caregivers fail to provide for the needs of the older person under their care. Neglect, whether intentional on unintentional, accounts for almost half of the verified cases of elder abuse. Neglect includes situations in which caregivers fail to meet the hygiene or safety needs of the older adult. Examples include situations in which a bedridden person is left wet and soiled with body wastes for days at a time without care or in which an older person suffers from exposure because he or she lacks adequate clothing for protection from the elements. Failure to provide necessary medical care may constitute neglect because, with no means of going to the doctor or pharmacy, the older person may suffer or even die.

However, it is not considered neglect if the mentally competent older person refuses treatment. Neglect may be deliberate on the part of the caregiver, or it may result from lack of knowledge, inadequate financial resources, or an insufficient support system. Neglect is not uncommon in situations where one elderly spouse cares for the other. In spite of the best intentions, the caregiving spouse may be unable to provide adequately for the needs of the more dependent partner.

Emotional Abuse

Even when physical abuse is absent and adequate physical care is provided, emotional abuse may be present. Emotional abuse is more subtle and difficult to recognize than physical abuse or neglect. It often includes behaviors such as isolating, ignoring, or depersonalizing older adults. Emotional abusers may forbid visitors and isolate the older person from more responsible and sympathetic friends or family members. They may prohibit the use of the telephone or interfere with communication by mail.

Emotional abusers can use verbal or nonverbal means to inflict their damage. Verbal abuse includes shouting or voicing threats of punishment or confinement. Emotional abusers often threaten older adults with all manners of horrors if they tell anyone about their plight. Displeasure, disgust, frustration, or anger can be communicated nonverbally through sighing, head shaking, door slamming, or other negative body language. Repeatedly ignoring what the older person has to say and avoiding social interaction with the individual are subtle forms of emotional abuse. Signs of emotional abuse may include the lack of eye contact, trembling, agitation, evasiveness, or hypervigilance.

Negative communications are devastating because they can attack the older person's mind and emotions. These messages can be so subtle and routine that people may not even recognize them as abusive. Emotional abuse is insidious in that it can damage the older adult's sense of self-esteem and can even destroy the will to live without leaving any obvious signs.

Financial Abuse

Financial abuse exists when the resources of an older person are stolen or misused by a person whom the older adult trusts. Such incidents are reported frequently in the news. Children and grandchildren may take money from the older family member, rationalizing that money is owed to them for providing care or that it will eventually be theirs anyway. People who expect to benefit from the older person's estate may be afraid that the needs of the older adult will consume all of the money and leave them with nothing, so they decide to take it while they can. Regardless of the caregivers' rationalizations in these situations, it is financial abuse if the older person's money is taken and spent by others for their own purposes. On the other hand, it is not abusive to use the older adult's resources to provide for his or her personal needs.

Many older adults are overly trusting of family members, often refusing to believe that their children would steal from them. This state of denial often continues, despite clear evidence to the contrary. Often, all of the savings have been spent, the house has been sold, and any objects of value have disappeared before they will accept the truth. Even then, some older adults make excuses to try to cope with the harsh reality. Abusive caregivers often abandon the older person once all of his or her assets are gone. In such cases, older adults are left homeless, penniless, and in despair. Signs of financial abuse include unusual banking activity such as large or frequent withdrawals, missing bank statements, missing personal belongings, particularly those of value, and signatures on checks or documents that do not match the elderly person.

Some actions that senior citizens can take to protect their financial assets include (1) arranging for direct deposit of Social Security, pension, and any other benefit checks; (2) taking great care in the selection of anyone appointed as the power of attorney or giving advice regarding a will; (3) keeping ATM pin numbers secure—do not write them in a location where others may see them, and do not give the number to anyone; (4) having written agreements regarding expectations and fees for any services; (5) keeping valuables out of site in a secure location such as a safe deposit box; and (6) remembering that home helpers or attendants are employees not friends—pay the fair and agreed wage, and keep tips and gifts for special occasions.

Abandonment

Abandonment occurs when dependent older persons are deserted by the person or persons responsible for their custody or care under circumstances in which a reasonable person would continue to provide care. Abandonment usually leaves the older person physically, emotionally, and financially defenseless. Older adults who have been abandoned by their families usually become wards of the state.

Responses to Abuse

It is natural to think that an older person suffering from one or more forms of abuse would complain, but this is rarely the case. Fear of being treated even worse or fear of being institutionalized or abandoned may prevent the victim from seeking help.

Clinical Situation

Trends and Issues

An 84-year-old woman was admitted to the hospital for dehydration and malnutrition. Six months earlier, she had suffered a mild stroke. Since then, her 86-year-old husband had been caring for her at home. On admission, the woman weighed 91 pounds. Stage 2 pressure ulcers were present on both buttocks. Her clothing and undergarments were soiled, and she was in serious need of a bath. She reported episodes of incontinence of bladder and bowel. Her only reported activity consisted of sitting in a lounge chair watching TV. She was wearing a wig, which covered hair that was matted tightly on her scalp. After several days of carefully combing out the snarls, the nurse realized the woman's shoulder-length hair had not been washed in months. The patient's husband explained, "I tried to do my best, but since she had always done all of the cooking, I didn't know what to do." He made sure she took her prescribed medicines, and he tried to see to it that she had enough to eat and drink, but he said that she was "picky." He also stated that he was unsure just how to take care of his wife's hygiene needs: "I tried to wash her up, but she said she wanted to be left alone." He explained that he shopped for groceries when she was asleep. He was afraid that if he called anyone for help, they would place his wife in an institution, and he could not cope with this idea. She had not complained to anyone for the same reason. Their children all lived out of state and had not visited since she had the stroke. The patient and her husband had assured their children by phone that everything was all right. It was only when she complained of chest pain that they sought medical attention.

Older people who manifest signs of abuse must be assessed carefully (Box 1-6). They may try to protect and defend the abuser, deny that abuse is occurring, or seem resigned to the situation, believing that there is no better alternative.

All questioning about and assessment of abuse must be done with great tact and sensitivity. It is best to question the elderly person alone so they can speak freely and without intimidation from the potential abuser. The rights of older people to determine their own affairs to the full extent of their abilities must be respected. Information obtained must be kept

Box 1-6 Signs That May Indicate Elder Abuse

- The older person demonstrates excessive agreement or compliance with the caregiver.
- The older person shows signs of poor hygiene such as body odor, uncleanliness, or soiled clothing or undergarments.
- The older person has malnutrition or dehydration.
- The older person has burns or pressure sores.
- The older person has bruises, particularly clustered on trunk or upper arms.
- The older person has bruises in various stages of healing that may indicate repeated injury.
- The older person lacks adequate clothing or footwear.
- The older person has had inadequate medical attention.
- The older person verbalizes a lack of food, medication, or care.
- The older person verbalizes being left alone or isolated in some way.
- The older person verbalizes fear of the caregiver.
- The older person verbalizes a lack of control in personal activities or finances.

confidential and shared only with agencies as authorized by the patient or necessitated by law. All observations, both objective and subjective, must be carefully documented in case legal action is required. Detailed records should be kept regardless of whether legal action is anticipated. Data may become significant only at a later date when they are impossible to reconstruct if not appropriately recorded. Photographs may be necessary to provide proof of neglect or abuse. These may include pictures of wounds, injuries, or living conditions. It is wise to avoid using the term *abuse* when working with older adults, because they may become defensive and will probably deny it. Using words such as *problems* or *concerns* is more likely to yield truthful information.

When there is any question of abuse, an experienced professional who is skilled in dealing with elder abuse should oversee the case. Physical abuse and financial abuse are criminal offenses. Nurses have a moral, legal, and ethical responsibility to report any suspected cases of abuse (see Critical Thinking box for more information). Nurses who provide care to at-risk groups, particularly the young and the older adult population, must be aware of their legal obligations with regard to suspected abuse. Nurses must know the state laws pertaining to abuse, as well as the proper authorities to contact and how to contact them. Once the responsible authorities are notified, they are obligated by law to investigate and pursue any legal action necessary to protect the safety of the abused and to protect them from further harm.

[?] Critical Thinking

Your Knowledge of Elder Abuse

- Is elder abuse increasing today? If so, why?
- What would you do if you thought a close friend or relative was an elder abuser?
- What do you think is the best way to reduce the incidence of elder abuse? Why?
- What would you do if you suspected that a nursing assistant was abusing patients?
- What can you as a student nurse do to prevent elder abuse?
- What resources are available in your community to help prevent elder abuse?

ABUSE BY UNRELATED CAREGIVERS

Understandably, we would like to think that all persons seeking employment as caregivers to older adults are responsible, caring individuals, but, unfortunately, this is not the case. People who are hired to provide for the safety and well-being of older adults can sometimes become their greatest threat. Increased use of unrelated caregivers exposes older adults to additional risks.

As the number of older adults increases and as more frail older people remain in their homes, the demand for nursing assistants, home health aides, and housekeepers increases. Most people who work as nursing assistants or housekeepers are decent, caring individuals who provide difficult services for little reward. The salaries paid to nursing assistants and housekeepers are generally low, the hours are long, and the work is emotionally and physically demanding. Under these conditions, it is difficult to find caring, responsible people who are willing to provide these types of services. When the demand for caregivers exceeds the supply of desirable workers, employers may be forced to hire people who are willing to take these jobs only because they cannot find other employment.

[icon] Coordinated Care

Collaboration

Elder Abuse in Institutions

Abuse in institutional settings is most likely to occur when the nursing assistants are forced to work under stressful conditions and have the poor ability to deal with that stress. The risk for abuse increases when caregivers perceive that they are not valued, supported, or acknowledged.

The following are ways that may help decrease stress and the likelihood of abuse:

- Improve staff training to identify and defuse potential abuse situations.
- Initiate a stress-reduction program, including staff support groups, a "time out" room for use when the staff's stress level is high, and other stress-relieving interventions.
- Recognize the value of nursing assistants to the team's effort by involving them in care planning and consulting with them regarding potential problems and possible solutions.
- Increase recognition of good, compassionate caregiving through verbal praise, employee-of-the-month recognition, bonuses, or other rewards.
- Provide an institutional mechanism for dealing with nursing assistants' complaints and concerns in a proactive rather than punitive manner.

Specific federal and state laws designed to prevent undesirable persons from contact with vulnerable people, such as the young and the older adult population, are in force today; however, sometimes people with criminal records, inadequate training, or other serious shortcomings manage to gain employment, despite safeguards such as state registries, employment histories, and reference checks. Undesirable individuals may unwittingly be hired to provide care for older adults by families, home health agencies, and even health care institutions.

In home settings, unscrupulous caregivers have been known to take money and personal belongings from defenseless older people under their care. They may physically abuse older persons and threaten them with physical harm if the abuse is reported. They may threaten to quit, leaving the older person in fear of being placed in an institution. Using threats enables these individuals to remain undetected until they have caused serious harm. When they are discovered, they often disappear, only to reappear somewhere else and repeat their pattern of abuse.

Even health care institutions are not immune to problems of elder abuse. Most people assume that because hospitals and nursing homes are licensed and regulated, this type of behavior does not occur. Unfortunately, this is wishful thinking. Many institutions have difficulty hiring enough people to meet the required staffing levels. Although most health care institutions and agencies screen applicants in an attempt to find the most qualified individuals and to avoid hiring anyone with a history of abusive or criminal behavior, some unscrupulous people manage to avoid detection and are employed as caregivers to older adults. These unsuitable caregivers may victimize older adults before they can be detected. Nurses who supervise other caregivers must constantly be on the lookout for abusive behaviors (Box 1-7). Any indication of abuse in an institutional setting must be reported as soon as it is suspected so that appropriate action can be taken and the abusive person removed. The importance of this nursing responsibility cannot be stressed enough.

To reduce abuse and to meet the emotional and physical needs of older adults and their caregivers, a wide variety of services have evolved. The types of services available vary from area to area, with some far-sighted cities offering many services. Nurses who work with older adults should become knowledgeable about the services that are available in their communities. Resources may include education programs designed to improve an awareness of the problem of elder abuse, support groups for caregivers of older adults, respite care programs, and senior day care centers. Many hospitals and health care agencies (e.g., American Red Cross) provide educational programs in nutrition, medication administration, bedside care, and other aspects of caring for older adults. The need for these programs is growing as the older adult population increases.

SUPPORT GROUPS

Caregivers to older adults are often isolated from other people. The demands of providing care prevent them from getting the rest, encouragement, and support they need. Caregivers who want or need to share their experiences and frustrations have started forming support groups to help one another cope with stress. These support groups may be specialized (e.g., for caregivers of people with Alzheimer's disease) or more general in nature. Support groups allow caregivers to share their feelings and to learn new strategies for improving their coping skills. Some groups schedule speakers to discuss topics of common interest or offer social activities to promote stress reduction.

RESPITE CARE

Respite care allows the primary caregiver to have time away from the constant demands of caregiving, thereby decreasing caregiver stress and the risk for abuse. Many caregivers are unable to lead normal lives because they cannot leave their responsibilities for more than a few minutes without fear of some disaster occurring. Respite care gives the primary caregiver the opportunity to attend church, go shopping, conduct personal business, obtain medical care, and participate in other activities that most people take for granted. Respite care may be provided by family members, volunteers, or one of the many service agencies that have proliferated within the past few years. Caregivers may be reluctant to use respite care out of guilt, fear, or other misguided emotions. Nurses should encourage caregivers to protect their own health and well-being by regularly taking advantage of respite care.

Box 1-7	Abusive Behaviors in Health Care Settings

- Use of sedative or hypnotic drugs that are not medically necessary
- Use of restraints when they are not medically indicated
- Use of derogatory language, angry verbal interactions, or ethnic slurs
- Withholding of privileges such as snacks or cigarettes
- Excessive roughness in handling during care or during transfers
- Delay in taking a resident to the bathroom or allowing a resident to lie in body waste
- Consumption of a resident's food
- Theft of money or personal belongings
- Physical striking or any other assaultive behavior / toward a resident
- Violation of a resident's right to make decisions
- Failure to provide privacy

Get Ready for the NCLEX® Examination!

Key Points

- Chronologic age is not always the most reliable way to measure aging because the number of years a person has lived provides little information about his or her physiologic or functional ability.
- A large segment of today's aging population lives a more dynamic, positive lifestyle than ever before.
- Stereotyping and negative perceptions of aging and older persons appear to be on the decline, yet subtle forms of ageism still exist and need to be addressed.
- The United States will face significant challenges to meet the costs of providing adequate health care to an aging population.
- As older adults become an increasingly larger segment of the population, they are having a significant impact on politics, economics, housing, and social family dynamics.
- Providing quality care for an increasingly large aging population places increased demands on both family and professional caregivers.
- Although many positive changes have occurred, the frailest older adults remain vulnerable to physical, emotional, and financial abuse.

Additional Learning Resources

SG Go to the Study Guide on pp. 379–397 for additional learning activities to help you master the chapter content.

evolve Go to your Evolve website (http://evolve.elsevier.com/Wold/geriatric) for the following FREE learning resources:
- Animations
- Answer Guidelines for Nursing Care Plan Critical Thinking Questions
- Answers and Rationales for Review Questions for the NCLEX® Examination
- Glossary with pronunciations in English and Spanish
- Video Clips

Review Questions for the NCLEX® Examination

1. Myths related to aging include that most elderly: (Select all that apply.)
   1. Live in institutional settings
   2. Suffer from a significant loss of intellectual function
   3. Have frequent interaction with family and friends
   4. Experience significant personality changes
   5. Are seriously depressed
   6. Are sick, frail, and dependent on others

2. The Baby Boom generation:
   1. Was born between 1940 and 1960
   2. Is better off financially than previous generations
   3. Shares many social goals and political values with each other
   4. Often provides care to aging parents and grandchildren

3. Medicare legislation was established in the:
   1. 1940s
   2. 1950s
   3. 1960s
   4. 1970s

4. The percentage of senior citizens who live independently in a family setting is approximately:
   1. 70%
   2. 50%
   3. 30%
   4. 10%

5. Durable Power of Attorney for health care enables the health care agent to:
   1. Decide whether the elderly person should be resuscitated
   2. Act only when the elderly person is unable to act for himself or herself
   3. Determine when the elderly person should be hospitalized
   4. Change care decisions if he or she thinks these will benefit the elderly person

6. One of the most significant changes that impact the elderly person and his or her family is:
   1. Loss of independence
   2. Change in physical appearance
   3. Decreased financial resources
   4. Sensory and cognitive decline

7. When assessing an alert for an elderly woman who was admitted to the emergency room accompanied by her daughter with whom she resides, the nurse would become suspicious of abuse if: (Select all that apply.)
   1. Bruises are observed on the arms and upper body.
   2. The daughter answers all questions for her mother.
   3. She has body odor and soiled clothing.
   4. The woman states that she does not like to see the doctor.
   5. The daughter states her mother does not get along with the grandchildren.
   6. Skin is intact with good turgor.

8. A student nurse observes caregivers in a long-term care facility where she is employed. Which of the following observations might indicate abusive behavior? (Select all that apply.)
   1. Failing to close bedside curtains during care activities
   2. Use of physical restraints to decrease wandering behavior
   3. Providing extra snacks as a reward for good behavior
   4. Laughing and talking with co-workers while providing care
   5. Speaking negatively about an elderly client while in the break room
   6. Responding slowly to the call light of a demanding elderly person

2

Theories of Aging

evolve

Objectives

1. Discuss how a theory is different from a fact.
2. Describe the most common biologic theories of aging.
3. Describe the most common psychosocial theories of aging.
4. Discuss the relevance of these theories to nursing practice.

Key Terms

antioxidants (ăn-tē-ŎK-sĬ-dănts) (p. 29)
biologic (bĪ-ō-LŎJ-Ĭk) (p. 28)
free radical (p. 29)

immunologic (Ĭm-ū-nō-LŎJ-Ĭk) (p. 29)
psychosocial (sĪ-kō-SŌ-shŭl) (p. 28)
theory (p. 28)

There is no single universally accepted definition of *aging*. Aging is best looked at as a series of changes that occur over time, contribute to loss of function, and ultimately result in the death of a living organism. Like other living organisms, humans age and then die. The maximal life expectancy for humans today appears to be 110 years, but why is this the case? Theories of aging have been considered throughout recorded history as mankind has sought to find ways to avoid aging. The quest for a "fountain of youth" has motivated explorers such as Ponce de Leon. The search for the extension of youth has led some people to seek the potions of conjurers, which were often more poisonous than beneficial.

To date no one has identified a single unified rationale for why we age and why different people live different length lives. Theories abound to help explain and give some logical order to our observations. Observations, including physical and behavioral data, are collected and studied to scientifically prove or disprove their effects on aging.

Studies of families and identical twins show that there is a strong correlation in the life expectancies of genetically related people. If your grandparents and parents live to be 60, 70, 80, or 90 years of age, you are likely to have a similar life span. This is not always the case, however. Some individuals fail to meet genetic expectations, whereas others significantly exceed expectations. **Biologic** and environmental factors are being studied to explain these variations.

Although there is no question that aging is a biologic process, sociologic and psychological components play a significant role. All of these areas—genetic, biologic, environmental, and **psychosocial**—have produced theories that attempt to explain the changes seen with aging. Despite extensive interest in this topic, the specific causes and processes involved in aging are not yet completely understood. Because we do not have

definitive and reproducible evidence indicating exactly why we age, all of the following remain theories.

BIOLOGIC THEORIES

Biologic theories of aging attempt to explain why the physical changes of aging occur. Researchers try to identify which biologic factors have the greatest influence on longevity. It is known that all members of a species suffer a gradual, progressive loss of function over time because of their biologic structure. Many of the biologic theories of aging overlap because most assume that the changes that cause aging occur at a cellular level. Each **theory** attempts to describe the processes of aging by examining various changes in cell structures or function.

Some biologic theories look at aging from a genetic perspective. The *programmed theory* proposes that every person has a "biologic clock" that starts ticking at the time of conception. In this theory, each individual has a genetic "program" specifying an unknown but predetermined number of cell divisions. As the program plays out, the person experiences predictable changes such as atrophy of the thymus, menopause, skin changes, and graying of the hair. A closely related theory is the *run-out-of-program theory*, which proposes that every person has a limited amount of genetic material that will run out over time, and the *rate of living theory,* which proposes that individuals have a finite number of breaths or heartbeats that are used up over time. The *gene theory* proposes the existence of one or more harmful genes that activate over time, resulting in the typical changes seen with aging and limiting the life span of the individual.

The molecular theories propose that aging is controlled by genetic materials that are encoded to predetermine growth and decline. The *error theory* proposes that errors in ribonucleic acid protein synthesis cause errors to occur in cells in the body, resulting in a progressive decline in biologic function. The *somatic mutation theory* is similar but proposes that aging results from deoxyribonucleic acid (DNA) damage caused by exposure to chemicals or radiation and that this damage causes chromosomal abnormalities that lead to disease or loss of function later in life.

Cellular theories propose that aging is a process that occurs because of cell damage. When enough cells are damaged, overall functioning of the body is decreased. The **free radical** *theory* provides one explanation for cell damage. Free radicals are unstable molecules produced by the body during the normal processes of respiration and metabolism or following exposure to radiation and pollution. These free radicals are suspected to cause damage to the cells, DNA, and the immune system. Excessive accumulation of free radicals in the body is purported to cause or contribute to the physiologic changes of aging and a variety of diseases such as arthritis, circulatory diseases, diabetes, and atherosclerosis. One free radical, named *lipofuscin*, has been identified to cause a buildup of fatty pigment granules that cause age spots in older adults. Individuals who support this theory propose that the number of free radicals can be reduced by the use of **antioxidants** such as vitamins A, C, and E, carotenoids, zinc, selenium, and phytochemicals.

One variation of this theory is the *crosslink* or *connective tissue theory*, which proposes that cell molecules from DNA and connective tissue interact with free radicals to cause bonds that decrease the ability of tissue to replace itself. This results in the skin changes typically attributed to aging such as dryness, wrinkles, and loss of elasticity. Another variation, the *Clinker theory*, combines the somatic mutation, free radical, and crosslink theories to suggest that chemicals produced by metabolism accumulate in normal cells and cause damage to body organs such as the muscles, heart, nerves, and brain.

The *wear-and-tear theory* presumes that the body is similar to a machine, which loses function when its parts wear out. As people age, their cells, tissues, and organs are damaged by internal or external stressors. When enough damage occurs to the body's parts, overall functioning decreases. This theory also proposes that good health maintenance practices will reduce the rate of wear and tear, resulting in longer and better body function.

The *neuroendocrine theory* focuses on the complicated chemical interactions set off by the hypothalamus of the brain. Stimulation or inhibition of various endocrine glands by the hypothalamus initiates the release of the various hormones from the pituitary and other glands, which, in turn, regulate bodily functions, including growth, reproduction, and metabolism. With age, the hypothalamus appears to be less precise in regulating endocrine function, leading to age-related changes such as decreased muscle mass, increased body fat, and changes in reproductive function. It is proposed that hormone supplements may be designed to delay or control age-related changes.

Complementary and Alternative Therapies

Alternative and Complementary Therapies to Slow or Reverse Aging

ANTIOXIDANT THERAPY
- Proposed as a method of neutralizing free radicals, which may contribute to aging and disease processes
- Includes a number of vitamins and minerals, including vitamins A, B_6, B_{12}, C, and E; beta carotene; folic acid; and selenium
- Generally safe when consumed as fruits and vegetables as part of the overall diet
- High doses of some antioxidants may cause more harm than benefits
- No proof that antioxidants are effective
- Discuss with physician before starting use

HORMONE THERAPY
- Proposed to replace a reduction in hormones, which naturally decrease with aging
- Includes hormones such as dehydroepiandrosterone (DHEA), estrogen, testosterone, melatonin, and human growth hormone (HGH)
- Little evidence to support claims made by advocates
- May actually cause more harm than provide benefits
- Usually requires prescription or supervised medical administration

SUPPLEMENTS
- Proposed to replace or enhance nutritional status; often marketed as "natural" remedies
- Include substances such as ginseng, coral calcium, Echinacea, and other herbal preparations
- No proof of effectiveness
- Not regulated by the Food and Drug Administration, so there is no control regarding amount of active ingredients
- High risk for interaction with prescription medications; physician must be notified if these products are used

CALORIE-RESTRICTED DIET
- Proposes that significant calorie reduction can extend life; based on studies in rats, mice, fish, and worms; not proven in humans
- Severe calorie restriction can result in inadequate consumption of necessary nutrients
- Studies show that severely underweight persons have a higher risk for some diseases and even death
- Dietary changes should be discussed with a physician or nutritionist to ensure that adequate nutrition is maintained

---

The **immunologic** *theory* proposes that aging is a function of changes in the immune system. According to this theory, the immune system—an important defense mechanism of the body—weakens over time, making an aging person more susceptible to disease. The immunologic theory also proposes that the increase in autoimmune diseases and allergies seen with aging is caused by changes in the immune system.

A fairly new theory of aging correlates aging to calorie intake. Animal research has shown that a point of metabolic efficiency can be achieved by consuming a high-nutrient but low-calorie diet. It is hypothesized that this diet, when combined with regular exercise, may extend optimal health and life span.

PSYCHOSOCIAL THEORIES

Psychosocial theories of aging do not explain why the physical changes of aging occur; rather they attempt to explain why older adults have different responses to the aging process. Some of the most prominent psychosocial theories of aging are the disengagement theory, the activity theory, life-course or developmental theories, and a variety of other personality theories.

The highly controversial *disengagement theory* was developed to explain why aging persons separate from the mainstream of society. This theory proposes that older people are systematically separated, excluded, or disengaged from society because they are not perceived to be of benefit to the society as a whole. This theory further proposes that older adults desire to withdraw from society as they age, so the disengagement is mutually beneficial. Critics of this theory believe that it attempts to justify ageism, oversimplifies the psychosocial adjustment to aging, and fails to address the diversity and complexity of older adults.

The *activity theory* proposes that activity is necessary for successful aging. Active participation in physical and mental activities helps maintain functioning well into old age. Purposeful activities and interactions that promote self-esteem improve overall satisfaction with life, even at an older age. "Busy work" activities and casual interaction with others were not shown to improve the self-esteem of older adults.

Life-course theories are perhaps the theories best known to nursing. These theories trace personality and personal adjustment throughout a person's life. Many of these theories are specific in identifying life-oriented tasks for the aging person. Four of the most common theories—Erikson's, Havighurst's, Newman's, and Jung's—are worth exploring.

Erikson's theory identifies eight stages of developmental tasks that an individual must confront throughout the life span: (1) trust versus mistrust, (2) autonomy versus shame and doubt, (3) initiative versus guilt, (4) industry versus inferiority, (5) identity versus identity confusion, (6) intimacy versus isolation, (7) generativity versus stagnation, and (8) integrity versus despair. The last of these stages is the domain of late adulthood, but failure to achieve success in tasks earlier in life can cause problems later in life. Late adulthood is the time when people normally review their lives and determine whether they have been negative or positive overall. The most positive outcomes of this life review are wisdom, understanding, and acceptance; the most negative outcomes are doubt, gloom, and despair.

Havighurst's theory details the process of aging and defines specific tasks for late life, including (1) adjusting to decreased physical strength and health, (2) adjusting to retirement and decreased income, (3) adjusting to the loss of a spouse, (4) establishing a relationship with one's age group, (5) adapting to social roles in a flexible way, and (6) establishing satisfactory living arrangements.

Newman's theory identifies the tasks of aging as (1) coping with the physical changes of aging; (2) redirecting energy to new activities and roles, including retirement, grandparenting, and widowhood; (3) accepting one's own life; and (4) developing a point of view about death.

Jung's theory proposes that development continues throughout life by a process of searching, questioning, and setting goals that are consistent with the individual's personality. Thus, life becomes an ongoing search for the "true self." As individuals age, they go through a reevaluation stage at midlife, at which point they realize there are many things they have not done. At this stage, they begin to question whether the decisions and choices they have made were the right choices for them. This is the so-called *midlife crisis*, which can lead to radical career or lifestyle changes or to the acceptance of the self as is. As aging continues, Jung proposes that the individual is likely to shift from an outward focus (with concerns about success and social position) to a more inward focus. Successful aging, according to Jung, includes acceptance and valuing of the self without regard to the view of others.

IMPLICATIONS FOR NURSING

Physical theories of aging indicate that, although biology places some limitations on life and life expectancy, other factors are subject to behavior and life choices. Nursing can help individuals achieve the longest, healthiest lives possible by promoting good health maintenance practices and a healthy environment.

Psychosocial theories help explain the variety of behaviors seen in the aging population. Understanding all of these theories can help nurses recognize problems and provide nursing interventions that will help aging individuals successfully meet the developmental tasks of aging.

Get Ready for the NCLEX® Examination!

Key Points

- Many biologic, environmental, and psychosocial theories have been proposed to explain why we age.
- These theories remain theories because the exact processes that cause the changes seen with aging are not completely understood.
- Further research and study are needed to determine which theory or combination of theories is most accurate.
- Once this is determined, we will be able to institute measures to slow aging and prolong the human life span.
- To date, hormone replacement therapy appears to have more risks than benefits.

Additional Learning Resources

SG Go to the Study Guide on pp. 379–397 for additional learning activities to help you master the chapter content.

evolve Go to your Evolve website (http://evolve.elsevier.com/Wold/geriatric) for the following FREE learning resources:
- Animations
- Answer Guidelines for Nursing Care Plan Critical Thinking Questions
- Answers and Rationales for Review Questions for the NCLEX® Examination
- Glossary with pronunciations in English and Spanish
- Video Clips

Review Questions for the NCLEX® Examination

1. A friend asks the nurse what could be done to improve the chance of a long life. Using current theories of aging, the nurse recommended that her friend discuss this first with her physician, but the one approach more likely to cause harm than good was:

    1. Antioxidant foods such as vitamins A, B_6, B_{12}, C, and E
    2. Hormones such as HGH, DHEA, and estrogen
    3. Calorie-restricted diet
    4. Herbal and nutritional supplements

2. The same friend asks how long humans can live. The nurse would reply that currently the maximum life expectancy of humans appears to be:

    1. 100 years
    2. 105 years
    3. 110 years
    4. 120 years

3. According to Erikson, the primary developmental task of the elderly population is:

    1. Generativity versus stagnation
    2. Trust versus mistrust
    3. Intimacy versus isolation
    4. Integrity versus despair

Objectives

1. Describe the most common structural changes observed in the normal aging process.
2. Discuss the impact of normal structural changes on the older adult's self-image and lifestyle.
3. Describe the most commonly observed functional changes that are part of the normal aging process.
4. Discuss the impact of normal functional changes on the older adult's self-image and lifestyle.
5. Identify the most common diseases related to aging in each of the body systems.
6. Differentiate between normal changes of aging and disease processes.
7. Discuss the impact of age-related changes on nursing care.

Key Terms

carcinoma (kăr-sĬ-NŌ-mă) (p. 35)
cardiomegaly (kăhr-dē-ō-MĔG-ă-lē) (p. 47)
cataracts (KĂT-ă-răkts) (p. 64)
dementia (dĕ-MĔN-shē-ă) (p. 58)
diverticulosis (dĬ-vĕr-tĬk-ū-LŌ-sĬs) (p. 53)
glaucoma (glă-KŌ-mă) (p. 64)
hypothyroidism (hĬ-pōTHĬ-royd-Ĭzm) (p. 60)
ischemic (Ĭs-KĒ-mĬk) (p. 46)
nystagmus (nĬs-TĂG-mŭs) (p. 66)

orthostatic hypotension (ŏr-thō-STĂT-Ĭk hĬ-pō-TĔN-shŭn) (p. 45)
osteoporosis (ŏs-tē-ō-pă-RŌ-sĬs) (p. 39)
seborrheic dermatitis (sĕb-ō-RĒ-Ĭk dĕr-mă-TĬ-tĬs) (p. 36)
seborrheic keratosis (sĕb-ō-RĒ-Ĭk kĕr-ă-TŌ-sĬs) (p. 33)
senile lentigo (SĒ-nĬl lĕn-TĬ-gō) (p. 33)
senile purpura (SĒ-nĬl PŪR-pū-ră) (p. 34)
xerosis (zĕr-Ō-sĬs) (p. 34)

The changes in body function that occur with aging are not random and do not develop suddenly or without warning. Rather, they are part of a continuum that begins the moment life begins. From the moment of conception, tissues and organs develop in an orderly manner. When fully developed, these organs and tissues perform specific functions and interact together in a predictable way. Throughout life, human growth and development occur methodically.

Early in life, the physical changes are dramatic. In only 9 months of gestation, the human organism develops from two almost invisible cells into a unique, functioning individual measuring approximately 20 inches in height and usually weighing between 6 and 9 pounds. For the next 13 to 15 years, rapid physical growth continues. By approximately age 18, the human body reaches full anatomic and physiologic maturity.

The peak years of physiologic function last from the late teens through the thirties—the so-called prime of life. Physiologic changes are still occurring during this time, but they are subtle and not easily recognized. Because these changes do not happen as rapidly or as dramatically as do those that occur early in life, they are more likely to be ignored.

As a person moves into his or her fifth and sixth decades of life, these physiologic changes become more apparent. In the seventh and eighth decades and beyond, they are significant and no longer deniable.

It is important to recognize that although age-related changes are predictable, the exact time at which they occur is not. Just as no two individuals grow and develop at exactly the same rate, no two individuals show the signs of aging at the same time. There is wide person-to-person variation in when—and to what degree—these changes occur. Heredity, environment, and health maintenance significantly affect the timing and magnitude of age-related changes. Some people are chronologically quite young but appear old. The most severe cases of this occur in a rare condition called **progeria.** When they are only 8 or 9 years of age, children with progeria have the physiology and appearance of 70-year-olds. At the other extreme, there are persons in their sixties, seventies, and even older who are vigorous and appear much younger than their chronologic age. Most people show the signs of aging at a rate somewhere between these two extremes.

We can observe many normal changes in the body's physical structure and function during the aging process. There are also changes that indicate the onset of disease or illness. Nurses are expected to be able to tell the difference between normal changes and abnormal changes that signify a need for medical or nursing intervention. To identify these differences, nurses must have a good understanding of the normal structures and functions of the body. This knowledge should help nurses understand how normal and abnormal changes affect the day-to-day functional abilities of older adults. As nurses, we must be aware of the physical changes that are likely to occur, assess each individual to determine the extent to which these changes have occurred, and then make our care plans in response to that specific person's needs.

Some diseases are more commonly seen with advanced age. Most older adults experience one or more chronic conditions. The leading causes of disability over age 65 are heart disease, stroke, arthritis, hypertension, accidents, diabetes mellitus (DM), cancer, and diseases of the ears and eyes. Currently, the five leading causes of death among older adults are (1) heart disease, (2) cancer, (3) cardiovascular disease (primarily stroke), (4) pneumonia, and (5) chronic obstructive pulmonary disease.

It is essential for nurses to learn that each aging person, just like each younger person, is unique. The type and extent of changes seen with aging are specific and unique to each person. Nurses must avoid falling into the trap of stereotyping older adults. Stereotyping is dangerous because it leads us to accept as inevitable some changes that are not inevitable. Stereotyping can also cause us to mistake early signs of disease as a part of aging.

THE INTEGUMENTARY SYSTEM

The integumentary system, which includes the skin, hair, and nails, undergoes significant changes with aging. Because many of these structures are visible, changes in this system are probably the most obvious and are evident to both the aging individual and others.

The **epidermis,** the outermost layer of the skin, is an important structure that provides protection for internal structures, keeps out dangerous chemicals and microorganisms, functions as part of the body's fluid regulation system, and helps regulate body temperature and eliminate waste products. It also contains melanocytes that produce the pigment **melanin,** which provides protection from ultraviolet radiation.

The **dermis** contains **collagen** and elastin fibers, which give strength and elasticity to the tissues. The **sebaceous** (oil-producing) and eccrine (sweat-producing) glands are located in the subcutaneous tissue, as are the hair and nail follicles and the **sensory nerve receptors.** Hair and nails are composed of dead **keratinized** cells. Hair pigment, or color, is related to the amount of melanin produced by the follicle and, like skin pigmentation, is hereditary. Nails are rigid structures that protect the sensitive, nerve-rich tissue

at the tips of the fingers and toes. Nails also aid dexterity in fine finger manipulation.

Subcutaneous tissue consists of **areolar connective tissue,** which connects the skin to the muscles, and **adipose tissue,** which provides a cushion over tissue and bone. Subcutaneous tissue provides insulation to regulate body temperature. It is here that **white blood cells** (WBCs) are available to protect the body from microbial invasion through the skin. Blood vessels in the subcutaneous tissue supply the tissue with nourishment and assist in the process of heat exchange. These superficial blood vessels dilate or constrict as needed to release heat or to conserve heat lost through convection.

EXPECTED AGE-RELATED CHANGES

With aging, the epidermis becomes more fragile, increasing the risk for skin damage such as tears, maceration, and infection. Rashes caused by contact with chemicals, such as detergents or cosmetics, are increasingly common in older individuals. Skin repairs more slowly in older than in younger individuals, increasing the risk for infection.

Melanocyte activity declines with age, and in light-skinned individuals, the skin may become very pale, making older individuals more susceptible to the effects of the sun. Clusters of melanocytes can form areas of deepened pigmentation, a condition called senile lentigo; these areas are often referred to as *age spots* or *liver spots* and are most often seen on areas of the body that are most exposed to sunlight. In a condition called seborrheic keratosis, slightly raised, wartlike macules with distinct edges appear (Figure 3-1). These lesions, which can range in color from light tan to black, are most often observed on the upper half of the body, and they may cause discomfort and itching. Skin tags, or **cutaneous papilloma,** are small, brown or flesh-colored projections of skin that are most often observed on the necks of older adults.

Aging results in decreased elastin fibers and a thinner dermal layer (Table 3-1). With the loss of elasticity, the skin starts to become less supple. "Crow's feet," or wrinkles, develop. Skin that is very dry or that has had excessive exposure to sunlight or harsh chemicals is more likely to wrinkle at a younger age. Hair color tends to fade or "gray" because of pigment loss, and hair distribution patterns change. Color changes, and hair loss patterns tend to be hereditary. The hair on the scalp, pubis, and axilla tends to thin in both men and women. Hairs in the nose and ears often become thicker and more noticeable. Some women experience the growth of facial hair, particularly after menopause. Fingernails grow more slowly, may become thick and more brittle, and ridges or lines are commonly observed. Toenails may become so thick that they require special equipment for trimming.

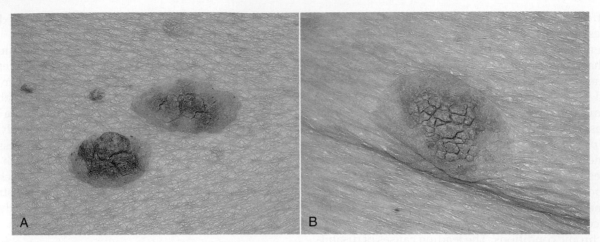

FIGURE 3-1 Seborrheic keratoses usually appear at approximately the fifth decade of life and gradually increase in number with age. These superficial, benign growths can enlarge to 20 mm in diameter and have a convoluted surface.

Table 3-1	Integumentary Changes Associated With Aging

PHYSIOLOGIC CHANGE	RESULTS
Decreased vascularity of dermis	Increased pallor in white skin
Decreased amount of melanin	Decreased hair color (graying)
Decreased sebaceous and sweat gland function	Increased dry skin; decreased perspiration
Decreased subcutaneous fat	Increased wrinkling
Decreased thickness of epidermis	Increased susceptibility to trauma
Increased localized pigmentation	Increased incidence of brown spots (senile lentigo)
Increased capillary fragility	Increased purple patches (senile purpura)
Decreased density of hair growth	Decreased amount and thickness of hair on head and body
Decreased rate of nail growth	Increased brittleness of nails
Decreased peripheral circulation	Increased longitudinal ridges of nails; increased thickening and yellowing of nails
Increased androgen/estrogen ratio	Increased facial hair in women

NURSING ASSESSMENTS AND CARE STRATEGIES RELATED TO INTEGUMENTARY CHANGES	
NURSING ASSESSMENTS	CARE STRATEGIES
Monitor skin temperature.	Adjust room temperature and provide adequate clothing or covers to prevent chilling.
Assess skin turgor over sternum or forehead, not forearm. Check tongue for furrows.	Provide adequate fluid to prevent dehydration.
Assess for skin breakdown or changes in color or pigmentation.	Institute measures to reduce pressure over bony prominences; possible dermatology referral.
Assess areas where skin surfaces touch and trap moisture (under breasts, adipose rolls, etc.) for signs of maceration or yeast infection.	Keep skin dry. Pad surfaces to reduce friction. Report abnormal observations for treatment.
Determine adequacy of hygiene and need for toenail trimming.	Modify skin care to reduce drying. Refer to podiatrist.

Sweat gland function decreases, and thus the amount of perspiration decreases. This results in heat intolerance because the body's cooling system through the process of evaporation is less efficient.

A decrease in the function of sebaceous and sweat gland secretion increases the likelihood of dry skin, or **xerosis** (Figure 3-2). Dry skin is probably the most common skin-related complaint among older adults, particularly when it is accompanied by itching, or **pruritus.** This problem is often more severe on the lower extremities because of diminished circulation.

The walls of the capillaries become increasingly fragile with age and may hemorrhage, leading to senile purpura, the red, purple, or brown areas commonly

FIGURE 3-2 Xerosis.

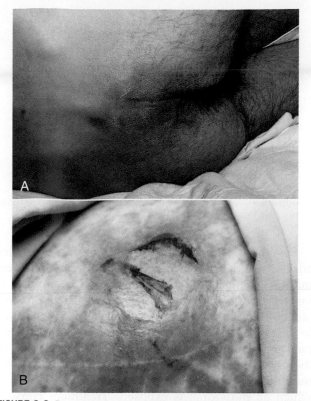

FIGURE 3-3 Pressure ulcers. A, Early-stage pressure ulcers, or stage I lesions, are commonly dismissed as minor abrasions because their primary attribute is nonblanchable erythema. B, Stage II ulcer, which is characterized by some skin loss, may be difficult to identify accurately because of its resemblance to a blister or abrasion.

seen on the legs and arms. By 70 years of age, the body has approximately 30% fewer cells than at age 40. The remaining cells enlarge, so body mass appears approximately the same. Total body fluid decreases with age. Plasma and extracellular volume remain somewhat constant, but intracellular fluid decreases. This loss of intracellular fluid increases the risk for dehydration. Tissue changes include a decrease in subcutaneous tissue that is visible in the eye orbits, hollows in the supraclavicular space, and sagging of breasts and neck tissue.

COMMON DISORDERS SEEN WITH AGING

Basal Cell Carcinoma and Melanoma

It is important to distinguish normally occurring changes in the skin from lesions that may be precancerous or cancerous. Cases of basal cell carcinoma are commonly observed in older adults who have spent significant amounts of time in the sun. By age 70 approximately 20% of white, non-Hispanic men have developed a non-melanoma cancer. Male senior citizens are also most at risk for melanoma, a potentially deadly form of skin cancer due to its ability to metastasize. In 2009 more than 8,000 deaths were attributed to melanoma.

The unusual appearance of moles should be suspected to be melanoma. Irregular shapes, irregular borders, changes in color, changes in size or symptoms, such as itchiness or bleeding, are all considered to be abnormal. Elderly men, in particular, should be taught to self-screen for changes in the skin. Suspicious changes should be documented and reported so that it can be examined promptly by a physician. Early diagnosis and treatment is effective at prolonging life.

Pressure Ulcers

Shrinkage in the cushion provided by subcutaneous tissue along with vascular changes places the older adult at increased risk for pressure ulcers (i.e., breakdown of the skin and tissues located over bony prominences) (see Figure 3-3). This is a significant problem for immobilized people such as those who are

bedridden or confined to wheelchairs. Special precautions to prevent this type of problem are discussed in Chapter 17.

Inflammation and Infection

Changes in the integumentary system increase the older adult's risk for skin inflammation and infection. Skin inflammation and infection often occur on visible surfaces of the body such as the face, scalp, and arms, making the conditions distressing to the older adult.

Common types of inflammation include rosacea and various forms of dermatitis. **Rosacea** appears as redness, dilated superficial blood vessels, and small "pimples" on the nose and center of the face (Figure 3-4). It may spread to cover the cheeks and chin. Left untreated, it can lead to swelling and the enlargement of the nose or to conjunctivitis. There is no known cause for this disorder, but it is most common in postmenopausal women, people who flush easily, and individuals taking vasodilating medications. Treatment of vasodilation includes lifestyle modification such as avoidance of triggers such as stressful situations, extreme heat, sun exposure, spicy foods, and alcoholic beverages. In addition oral and topical medications or light and laser treatments may provide some benefits.

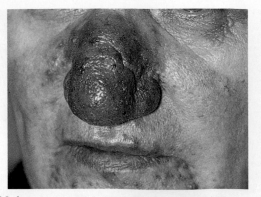

FIGURE 3-4 Rosacea pustules and papules. Note the bulbous red nose of rhinophyma.

Several forms of dermatitis are common in older adults, including contact, allergic, and **seborrheic dermatitis**. **Contact** and **allergic dermatitis** appear as rashes or inflammation that is either localized to certain areas of the body or generalized (Figure 3-5). Clues to the causative substance are gained from the unique pattern presented on each individual. Identification of the particular irritant may be difficult because of the number of chemicals, drugs, and other substances to which an individual is exposed. Treatment consists of avoiding the offending substance.

Seborrheic dermatitis is an unsightly skin condition characterized by yellow, waxy crusts that can be either dry or moist (Figure 3-6). Caused by excessive sebum production, seborrheic dermatitis can occur on the scalp, eyebrows, eyelids, ears, axilla, breasts, groin, and gluteal folds. There is no known cure, but treatment with special shampoos and lotions helps control the problem.

Infectious diseases of the skin and nails commonly seen in older adults include herpes zoster (also called *shingles*); fungal, yeast, and bacterial infections; and infestation with scabies (mites). Each of these diseases has a unique cause, characteristic appearance, and specific treatment that are beyond the scope of this text.

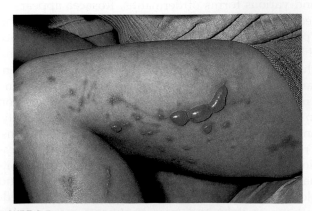

FIGURE 3-5 *Rhus* dermatitis. Linear bullae are characteristic of an allergic contact dermatitis.

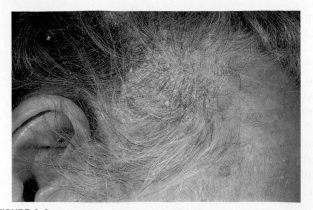

FIGURE 3-6 Seborrheic dermatitis is characterized by itching and patches of scales that exfoliate. The most common sites are on the scalp, behind the ears, and on the midface, including the eyebrows and lashes.

Hypothermia

The decrease in the amount of subcutaneous tissue reduces the older adult's ability to regulate body temperature. Very thin older adults lose the insulation provided by subcutaneous and adipose tissue. This loss of insulation is most likely to result in hypothermia if the person is exposed to an environment that is too cold.

THE MUSCULOSKELETAL SYSTEM

The musculoskeletal system performs many functions. The bones of the skeleton provide a rigid structure that gives the body its shape. The red bone marrow in the cavities of spongy bones produces red blood cells (RBCs), platelets, and WBCs. Structures such as the ribs and pelvis protect easily damaged internal organs. The muscles provide a power source to move the bones. The combined functions of bones and muscles allow free movement and participation in the activities necessary to maintain a normal life.

BONES

Bone consists of protein and the minerals calcium and phosphorus. Calcium is necessary for bone strength, muscle contraction, myocardial contraction, blood clotting, and neuronal activity. It is normally obtained by eating dairy products and dark-green leafy vegetables. Vitamin D is needed for the absorption of calcium and phosphate through the small intestine; vitamins A and C are needed for **ossification,** or bone matrix formation.

For the long bones to remain strong, adequate dietary intake of these nutrients is important. However, the dietary intake of minerals alone does not maintain bone strength. It is also necessary to apply stress to the long bones to keep the minerals in the bones. This needed stress is best provided by weight-bearing activities such as standing and walking. The calcium that is needed for clotting and nerve and muscle functions is constantly being withdrawn from the bone and moved into the bloodstream to maintain consistent blood levels. Calcium is normally redeposited in the bone at an equal rate, replacing the calcium that is lost. As long as this movement of calcium is in balance, the bone remains strong.

Hormones also play an important role in bone maintenance. **Calcitonin,** which is produced by the thyroid gland, slows the movement of calcium from the bones to the blood and lowers the blood calcium level. Parathyroid hormone (PTH) increases the movement of calcium from the bones to the blood and increases the blood calcium level. PTH also increases the absorption of calcium from the small intestine and kidneys, thus further increasing the blood calcium level. Insulin and thyroxine aid in the protein synthesis and energy production needed for bone maintenance. Estrogen and testosterone, produced by the ovaries and testes, respectively, help retain calcium in the bone matrix.

VERTEBRAE

The spinal column consists of a series of small bones, called **vertebrae,** that stack up to form a strong, flexible structure. The spinal column supports the head and allows for flexible movement of the back. The segments of the spinal column consist of cervical, thoracic, lumbar, and sacral vertebrae. The muscles that move the back connect at bony processes that protrude from each vertebra. The **spinal cord,** the nerve tissue that extends downward from the brain, passes through the **vertebral canal,** which runs through an opening in each vertebra. The bones of the spinal column protect this nerve tissue from injury.

Fibrous pads, called **intervertebral disks,** are located between the vertebrae and cushion the impact of walking and other activities.

JOINTS

Joints are the places where bones meet. The freely moving synovial joints are lined with **cartilage,** which allows free movement of the joint surfaces. Many of these joints contain a **bursa,** which is a fluid sac that provides lubrication to enhance joint mobility (Figure 3-7).

TENDONS AND LIGAMENTS

Tendons are structures that connect the muscles to the bone, and **ligaments** are structures that connect bones to other bones.

MUSCLES

There are three types of muscle tissue in the body: cardiac muscle, smooth muscle, and skeletal muscle. **Cardiac muscle,** located in the heart only, is responsible for the pumping action of the heart that maintains the blood circulation. **Smooth muscle** is found in the walls of hollow organs such as the blood vessels, stomach, intestines, and urinary bladder. Because cardiac and smooth muscle normally cannot be stimulated by conscious effort, they are called **involuntary muscles.**

Skeletal muscle accounts for the largest amount of muscle tissue in the body. The major function of skeletal muscle is to move the bones of the skeleton.

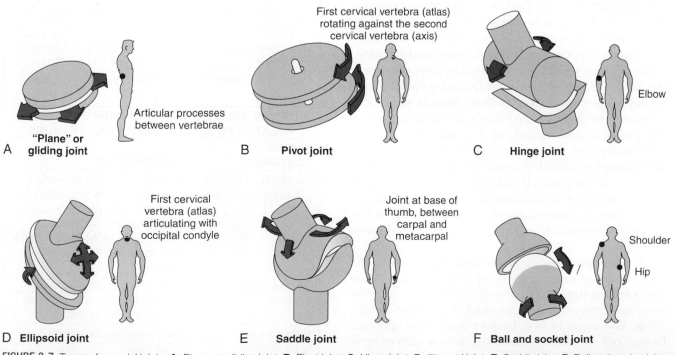

FIGURE 3-7 Types of synovial joints. **A,** Plane, or gliding joint. **B,** Pivot joint. **C,** Hinge joint. **D,** Ellipsoid joint. **E,** Saddle joint. **F,** Ball and socket joint.

Because their actions can be controlled by conscious effort, skeletal muscles are considered **voluntary muscles.** Muscles are connected to bones by tendons. Contraction or relaxation of muscles causes the bones to move. Controlled and coordinated movement of bones and muscles allows us to perform the variety of movements required for activities of daily living. Special effort and practice allow us to perform special activities such as dancing, playing sports, and playing the piano.

The amount of muscle mass and the type of muscle development differ greatly among individuals. Men normally have larger muscles, or more muscle mass, than do women, particularly in the muscles of the upper body. The male hormone testosterone stimulates muscle development. In both men and women, the largest and strongest skeletal muscles are found in the legs and upper arms; the smallest and weakest are located in the lower back.

Muscle tissue is normally in a state of slight contraction. This muscle tone is necessary to support the head, to keep the spine erect, and to perform any controlled movement. Muscle mass is built and muscle tone is maintained by means of exercise. There are two general types of exercise: **isometric exercise,** which involves muscle contraction without body movement, and **isotonic exercise,** which involves muscle contraction with body movement. Isometric exercise helps maintain muscle tone and strength but does little to increase muscle size. Isotonic exercise maintains muscle tone and strength and increases muscle mass if it is done repetitively. **Aerobic exercise** is isotonic exercise that occurs for 30 minutes or longer. Aerobic exercise strengthens the skeletal, cardiac, and respiratory muscles. People who lead inactive or sedentary lifestyles suffer from the lack of isotonic exercise. Regardless of age, unless people undertake an exercise program, they manifest poor muscle development and strength.

Muscle movement is controlled by impulses from the parietal lobes of the cerebrum and is coordinated by impulses from the cerebellum. **Muscle sense** is a term used to describe the brain's ability to recognize the position and action of the muscles without conscious effort. Receptor cells in the muscles, called **proprioceptors,** send information to the brain that enables it to integrate all body movements. This coordinative function of the brain allows us to walk, bend, or eat without consciously thinking about all of the separate movements and feeling all of the different positions.

Muscles need energy to function. The most abundant source of muscular energy is glycogen. **Adenosine triphosphate** (ATP), the direct energy source for muscular contraction, is a product of glycogen metabolism. Glycogen is first broken down into glucose. During cell metabolism, glucose interacts with oxygen transported in the bloodstream by hemoglobin or oxygen stored in the muscle fibers as myoglobin. This reaction involves the production of ATP, heat, water, and carbon dioxide. If muscle fibers do not receive enough oxygen, glucose may not be oxidized completely, and a chemical intermediate, **lactic acid,** is produced. Elevated levels of lactic acid may result in muscle fatigue and soreness.

EXPECTED AGE-RELATED CHANGES

The major bone-associated change related to aging is the loss of calcium (Table 3-2). This change begins between 30 and 40 years of age. With each successive decade, the skeletal bones become thinner and relatively weaker. Women lose approximately 8% of skeletal mass each decade, whereas men lose approximately 3%. Decalcification of various parts of the skeleton, including the epiphyses, vertebrae, and jaw bones, can result in increased risk for fracture, loss of height, and loss of teeth.

The intervertebral disks shrink as the thoracic vertebrae slowly change with aging. This results in a condition called **kyphosis,** which gives the older adult a stooped or hunchback appearance, with the head dropping forward toward the chest. The combination

Table 3-2	Musculoskeletal Changes Associated With Aging
PHYSIOLOGIC CHANGE	**RESULTS**
Decreased bone calcium	Increased osteoporosis; increased curvature of the spine (kyphosis)
Decreased fluid in intervertebral disks	Decreased height
Decreased blood supply to muscles	Decreased muscle strength
Decreased tissue elasticity	Decreased mobility and flexibility of ligaments and tendons
Decreased muscle mass	Decreased strength; increased risk for falls
NURSING ASSESSMENTS AND CARE STRATEGIES RELATED TO MUSCULOSKELETAL CHANGES	
NURSING ASSESSMENTS	**CARE STRATEGIES**
Assess strength and functional mobility.	Provide assistance as needed, modify physical environment, initiate safety precautions to decrease risk for falls, encourage ROM exercise, refer to physical or occupational therapy.
Assess nutritional intake.	Educate regarding importance of calcium intake, administer supplements as ordered.
Determine activity patterns.	Encourage regular low-impact exercise.

of disk shrinkage and kyphosis results in loss of overall height. A person can lose as much as 2 inches of height by age 70. People who are concerned about their appearance find these changes disturbing because clothing no longer fits properly, and it is increasingly difficult to find flattering styles.

Connective tissues tend to lose elasticity, leading to restriction of joint mobility. Loss of flexibility and joint mobility begins as early as the teen years and is common with aging. Regular stretching exercises can help slow or even reverse flexibility problems.

Muscle tone and mass typically decrease with aging, and these decreases are directly related to decreased physical activity and exercise. People of all ages who exercise regularly have better muscle mass and tone. Hormonal changes, particularly the decrease in testosterone level, tend to reduce muscle mass in aging men. Reduction in blood supply to the muscles as a result of aging or disease can lead to changes in muscle function. Less glycogen is stored in aging muscles, thereby decreasing the fuel available for muscle contraction. Any condition that restricts oxygen availability (e.g., anemia and respiratory problems) can lead to an excessive production of waste products such as lactic acid and carbon dioxide. This can increase the incidence of muscle spasms and muscle fatigue with minimal exertion. Decreased endurance and agility may result from a combination of these factors. Neuronal changes in the areas of the brain responsible for muscle control can result in alterations of muscle sense, which may be observed in older adults as an unsteady gait and impairment of other activities that require muscular coordination.

As a person ages, muscle mass decreases, and the proportion of body weight resulting from fatty, or **adipose,** tissue increases. This is significant in the administration of medications. Intramuscular injection sites may not be as well muscled, and fatty tissue tends to retain medication differently than does lean tissue. Absorption and metabolism of drugs can be significantly different from those in younger persons.

COMMON DISORDERS SEEN WITH AGING

Osteoporosis

Excessive loss of calcium from bone combined with insufficient replacement results in osteoporosis. Currently, 55% or more of Americans over age 50 have decreased bone density, and more than 10 million have osteoporosis. This disorder is projected to become even more common as the population ages. Osteoporosis is characterized by porous, brittle, fragile bones that are susceptible to breakage. Spontaneous fracture of the vertebrae or other bones can occur in the absence of obvious trauma. In fact, spontaneous hip fractures may lead to a fall, rather than the fall leading to the hip fracture. Simple falls or other traumas are more likely to result in fractures in people who have osteoporosis. Common fracture sites include the hip (usually the neck of the femur), ribs, clavicle, and arm (when trying to break a fall). Factors that increase the risk for osteoporosis include the following:

- Female gender
- Caucasian or Asian race
- Small body frame
- Family history of osteoporosis
- Poor nutrition (diet low in calcium and vitamin D)
- Malabsorption disorders such as celiac disease
- Menopause (low estrogen levels)
- Chemotherapy
- Lack of exercise/immobility
- Excessive alcohol consumption
- Cigarette smoking
- Hormonal imbalances (hyperthyroidism and hyperparathyroidism)
- Long-term use of medications, including phenytoin (Dilantin), heparin, and oral corticosteroids

Osteoporosis is best prevented and treated by lifestyle modifications and medications. Lifestyle modifications include a well-balanced diet with adequate amounts of calcium and vitamin D, regular exercise, smoking cessation, and restriction of alcohol intake. Calcium and vitamin D supplements are commonly necessary for individuals who do not consume adequate amounts of these nutrients. Medications that increase bone strength and density are often prescribed. These include alendronate (Fosamax), risedronate (Actonel), ibandronate (Boniva), raloxifene (Evista), and calcitonin (Calcimar). Hormone replacement therapy (HRT) has beneficial effects on bone density but also brings increased risk for heart attack, blood clots, stroke, and breast cancer. Use of hormonal therapy is controversial and requires a candid risk/benefit analysis between the patient and physician.

Degenerative Joint Disease

Osteoarthritis. The incidence of **osteoarthritis,** the most common form of arthritis, increases with age. Osteoarthritis is estimated to affect 43 million adults in the United States and to cost $86 billion annually in treatment costs. By age 70, as many as 70% of adults will experience some degree of disability or discomfort from this disorder. Although common with aging, osteoarthritis is not a normal part of aging. It affects men and women equally, although men are usually affected at a younger age. The cause of osteoarthritis is unknown; however, chemical, nutritional, genetic, hormonal, and mechanical factors are believed to play a role. People employed in jobs that involve placing a high amount of physical stress on certain joints are likely to experience changes in those joints later in life. After years of normal joint use, the cartilage on the bones' articulating surfaces thins and begins to wear out. Bony particles or spurs (osteophytes) may form within the joint, causing pain, swelling, and restriction of movement in affected joints. **Heberden's nodes,** which are caused by abnormal cartilage or bony enlargement, may be seen in the distal joints of the fingers. Pain may occur with activity or exercise of the affected joints and may worsen with emotional stress. Synovial membrane of the bursa may become damaged or inflamed. This is particularly true in the weight-bearing joints of the spine, hips, knees, and ankles. Obesity increases the stress on joints and can aggravate symptoms.

Osteoarthritis is treated by administering nonsteroidal antiinflammatory drugs (NSAIDs), by injecting corticosteroids into the joints, by rest and heat, and by an individualized exercise program. Dietary supplements, including glucosamine, chondroitin sulfate, and various vitamins, have shown benefits for some individuals and are being studied for safety and effectiveness. Intraarticular injection of hyaluronic acid, a joint lubricant, has received mixed reviews. In severe cases, arthroscopic removal of bone fragments or surgical joint replacements may be necessary.

Rheumatoid Arthritis. **Rheumatoid arthritis** is a collagen disease that results from an autoimmune process. This disease causes inflammation of the synovium, damage to the cartilage and bone of joints, and instability of ligaments and tendons that support the joints. The onset is typically earlier in life, occurring at between 30 and 50 years of age, although a significant number of individuals first develop the disease after age 60. This form of arthritis is seen more commonly in women. Rheumatoid arthritis is characterized by periods of exacerbation (sometimes called *flares*), during which the symptoms are severe and cause further damage, and **remission,** during which the progress of the disease halts. Rheumatoid arthritis can also result in muscle atrophy, soft tissue changes, and bone and cartilage changes. Symptoms of rheumatoid arthritis include the following:

- Pain and stiffness, particularly in the morning or after a period of rest
- Warm, tender, painful joints
- Fatigue
- Sense of feeling unwell
- Occasional fevers

The most serious deformities and problems are typically observed when an individual has suffered from this disease for an extended period. Affected individuals are best treated by a **rheumatologist,** a physician who specializes in the disorder.

Treatments for rheumatoid arthritis include lifestyle changes such as stress reduction, balanced rest and exercise, and joint care using splints to support joints. A wide variety of classifications of medications are used to treat this condition, including the following:

- NSAIDs—such as aspirin, acetaminophen, ibuprofen, naproxen
- Corticosteroids—such as methylprednisone
- Disease-modifying antirheumatic drugs (DMARDs)—such as cyclosporine, azathioprine, sulfasalazine, methotrexate
- Tumor necrosis factor inhibitors—such as etanercept, infliximab
- Interleukin-1 inhibitor—such as anakinra

Surgical interventions, including synovectomy, tendon reconstruction, and joint replacement, may be performed to reduce pain, to improve joint function, and to allow the individual to maintain the highest possible level of independent function.

Bursitis. **Bursitis,** inflammation of the bursa and the surrounding fibrous tissue, can result from excessive stress on a joint or from a localized infection. Bursitis commonly results in joint stiffness and pain in the shoulder, knee, and elbow, ultimately leading to restricted or reduced mobility. Although this problem can occur at any age, age-related changes in the musculoskeletal system make it a more common problem in older individuals. Treatment includes resting the joint and administering NSAIDs. Corticosteroid preparations are occasionally injected into the painful areas to reduce inflammation. Mild range-of-motion exercise is encouraged to prevent permanent reduction or the loss of joint function.

Gouty Arthritis. Gouty arthritis is caused by an inborn error of metabolism that results in elevated levels of uric acid in the body. Crystals of these acids deposit within the joints and other tissues, causing episodes of severe, painful joint swelling. Some joints, such as those of the great toe, are more commonly affected. Chills and fever may accompany a severe attack. Attacks of gout become more frequent as a person ages. If left untreated, this disease can result in the destruction of the joints. It is observed more often in men but is also common in women after menopause. Weight reduction and decreased intake of alcohol and foods rich in purines, such as liver or dried beans or peas, are often recommended.

THE RESPIRATORY SYSTEM

The respiratory system provides the body with the oxygen needed for life. Without oxygen, cells quickly die. The brain cells are the most sensitive cells in the body; they will die if deprived of oxygen for as little as 4 minutes. Breathing, the process of inhaling to take in oxygen and exhaling to release carbon dioxide, occurs at a rate of 12 to 20 times per minute for our entire lives. The respiratory system is typically divided into two parts: the upper respiratory tract and the lower respiratory tract. The entire respiratory tract is lined with mucous membranes.

UPPER RESPIRATORY TRACT

On its way to the lungs, air passes through the **upper respiratory tract,** which includes the air passages of the nose, mouth, and throat, all of which are located above the chest cavity. Mucous membranes line the nasal passages and warm and humidify the air that passes through the nose. Cilia and mucus in the nasal passages trap particulate matter (bacteria and debris) and sweep it toward the pharynx, where it is routinely swallowed and destroyed by gastric acid. The cough and sneeze reflexes also help prevent debris and foreign objects from entering the respiratory tract. The **pharynx,** which is located at the back of the oral cavity, has three segments: the oropharynx, nasopharynx, and **laryngopharynx.**

The nasopharynx is connected to the middle ear by the **eustachian tubes,** which help maintain proper air pressure in the middle ear. The **larynx,** or voice box, is composed of cartilage rings and folds of tissue, called **vocal folds.** The **epiglottis,** which is the uppermost cartilage ring, prevents food from entering the airway. During inhalation, the vocal folds move to the sides of the larynx to allow air to pass freely. During exhalation, we can speak and sing by controlling the distance between these folds, which vibrate when air is forced through them and produce sound.

LOWER RESPIRATORY TRACT

The **lower respiratory tract** includes the lower trachea, bronchial passages, and alveoli, all of which lie within the chest cavity. The **trachea** is a cartilaginous passageway that connects the larynx to the bronchial passages of the lungs. The trachea branches into two major **bronchi,** which further divide like the branches of a tree into smaller and smaller **bronchioles.** At the ends of the bronchioles are the **alveoli,** or air sacs, which are the functional units of respiration. A thin layer of fluid lines each tiny air sac, which is surrounded by pulmonary capillaries to allow the efficient exchange of gases by diffusion. It is here that oxygen enters the bloodstream for transport to body tissue, and it is here that carbon dioxide from the body leaves the bloodstream. This gaseous exchange is essential for normal cell function and for the maintenance of the blood's acid-base balance.

Because the alveoli have a moist lining, their surfaces could adhere if they touched when the alveoli were empty. This is prevented by a special protein substance called **surfactant.**

AIR EXCHANGE (RESPIRATION)

The movement of air into and out of the alveoli is called **ventilation.** Ventilation requires the action of muscles, primarily the **diaphragm** and the **intercostal muscles.**

During inhalation, the diaphragm contracts and moves downward while the intercostal muscles pull the ribs upward and outward. These combined activities increase the size of the chest cavity until the air pressure inside the lungs is lower than the atmospheric pressure and air is drawn into the lungs. This process is known as **inhalation** or **inspiration.** When the air pressure inside the lungs equals or exceeds atmospheric pressure, air ceases to enter the lungs. When the diaphragm and intercostal muscles relax, the diaphragm moves upward and the ribs move inward, making the chest cavity smaller. As the chest cavity becomes smaller, the pressure in the lungs becomes greater than the atmospheric pressure. Air is forced out of the lungs until the pressure in the lungs equals the atmospheric pressure. This action is known as **exhalation** or **expiration.** Regulation of respiration is both neurologic and chemical. The respiratory centers in the medulla and pons of the brainstem continuously monitor and control the rate and depth of involuntary respiration. Most breathing is unconscious and involuntary. If we had to think about inhaling and exhaling every breath, we would have little time to do anything else. However, breathing can be conscious and voluntary. When swimming, singing, or engaging in other activities that require breath control, we can temporarily alter our breathing patterns.

EXPECTED AGE-RELATED CHANGES

With aging, changes are seen throughout the respiratory tract (Table 3-3; Box 3-1). Years of exposure to air pollution, cigarette smoke, and other hazardous chemicals may take their toll on the air passageways and lung tissue. Decrease in elastic recoil of the lungs leads to diminished air exchange. Mucous membranes in the nose become drier as the fluid content of body tissue decreases; thus, the incoming air is not humidified as effectively. The number of cilia decreases, diminishing the ability of the cilia to trap and remove debris. Decreased vocal cord elasticity leads to changes in voice pitch and quality, and the voice develops a more tremulous character.

Musculoskeletal system changes that occur with aging alter the size and shape of the chest cavity. Kyphosis contributes to a barrel-chested appearance. Costal cartilage located at the ends of the ribs calcifies and becomes more rigid, thus reducing the mobility of the rib cage. Intercostal muscles atrophy, and the diaphragm flattens and becomes less elastic. All of these changes reduce lung capacity and interfere with respiratory function, resulting in a decreased ability to inhale and exhale deeply.

Several factors increase the possibility of inadequate oxygenation and the risk for respiratory tract infections in older adults. The cilia movement inside the lungs decreases. The airways and alveoli are less elastic, and there is a decrease in the number of

Table 3-3	Respiratory Changes Associated With Aging	
PHYSIOLOGIC CHANGE	**RESULTS**	
Decreased body fluids	Decreased ability to humidify air resulting in drier mucous membranes	
Decreased number of cilia	Decreased ability to trap debris	
Decreased number of macrophages	Increased risk for respiratory infection	
Decreased tissue elasticity in the alveoli and lower lung lobes	Decreased gas exchange; increased pooling of secretions	
Decreased muscle strength and endurance	Decreased ability to breath deeply; diminished strength of cough	
Decreased number of capillaries	Decreased gas exchange	
Increased calcification of cartilage	Increased rigidity of rib cage; decreased lung capacity	
NURSING ASSESSMENTS AND CARE STRATEGIES RELATED TO RESPIRATORY CHANGES		
NURSING ASSESSMENTS	**CARE STRATEGIES**	
Assess breathing depth and effort.	Position to facilitate ease of respiration. Encourage incentive spirometry or nebulizer as ordered.	
Assess cough and sputum production.	Encourage adequate fluid intake. Encourage smoking cessation and avoidance of environmental pollutants.	
Assess for signs and symptoms of respiratory infection.	Teach avoidance of individuals with active infection. Teach careful handwashing and disposal of contaminated secretions. Encourage annual influenza vaccination.	

Box 3-1	Pulmonary Function Changes Commonly Observed With Aging

- Diminished breath sounds
- Lower maximum expiratory volume
- Increased residual volume
- Reduced vital capacity

capillaries surrounding the alveoli, which interferes with gas exchange. The lung tissue itself has decreased physical mobility and elasticity, with can lead to increased pooling of secretions, especially in the lower lobes.

COMMON DISORDERS SEEN WITH AGING

Chronic Obstructive Pulmonary Disease

Chronic obstructive pulmonary disease (COPD) is not a single disease but a group of three commonly occurring respiratory disorders: asthma, emphysema, and chronic bronchitis. Although they may appear independently, these disorders usually occur in a combination. COPD is common in people who have a history of smoking or who have had a high level of exposure to environmental pollutants. In **asthma,** the trachea and bronchioles are extremely sensitive to a variety of physical stimuli and emotional stress that then cause constriction of the bronchial passages and increase mucus production within the airways. This narrows the airways and restricts airflow. Elderly individuals may be less aware of bronchospasms and therefore be slower to seek emergency care. This can result in poor outcomes. **Emphysema** is characterized by changes in the structure of the alveoli. The air sacs lose elasticity, become overinflated, and are ineffective in gas exchange. **Chronic bronchitis** involves inflammation of the trachea and bronchioles. Chronic irritation leads to excessive mucus secretion and a productive cough.

Individuals with COPD manifest symptoms such as productive cough, wheezing, cyanosis, and dyspnea on exertion. They are at higher risk for developing respiratory tract infections; in severe cases, respiratory failure can occur.

Influenza

Influenza, often referred to as the *flu,* is a highly contagious respiratory infection caused by a variety of influenza viruses. Many different strains of influenza have been identified, and new forms are being identified continually. The various forms of influenza, such as the Hong Kong or Beijing flu, are often named for the area where they are first recognized. Epidemics occur at regular intervals and are seen most often in the winter months. The virus is usually spread through airborne droplets and moves quickly through groups of people who live or work in close contact with one another. The incubation period is brief, often only 1 to 3 days from the time of exposure. The onset of symptoms is sudden; symptoms include chills, fever, cough, sore throat, and general malaise and may be dramatic and leave the victim feeling severely ill.

Older adults are at higher risk for serious complications of influenza than are younger people. More than 90% of deaths resulting from influenza occur in the older-than-65 population. Influenza presents a special danger for older adults with a history of respiratory disease or other debilitating conditions. Yearly flu shots are recommended for all persons older than 65 years of age to reduce the chance of contracting the most common forms of influenza. Immunizations should be given in the fall so that the level of immunity is high before the risk for exposure occurs. Immunization should be obtained every year because the vaccine is different from the previous year. Each year the vaccine is customized to protect against the particular strain of the virus that is anticipated to be prevalent in the country.

Some people refuse or are hesitant to take the vaccine because of the mild symptoms that may be experienced after inoculation. It is important to explain to older adults that these symptoms are mild and will protect them from more severe problems later. Individuals who are allergic to eggs should not receive the vaccine. Influenza vaccine is cultured in egg protein and can cause a serious allergic reaction in allergic individuals. Given properly, these vaccines are 70% to 80% effective in preventing illness.

Pneumonia

Pneumonia is acute inflammation of the lungs caused by bacterial, viral, fungal, chemical, or mechanical agents. In response to the agent, the alveoli and bronchioles become clogged with a thick, fibrous substance that decreases the ability of the lung to exchange gases. Pneumonia can progress to a state in which the exudate fills the lung lobes, which then become consolidated or firm. Pneumonia can be detected by radiologic examination. Breath sounds exhibit characteristic changes.

The symptoms of pneumonia differ with the causative organism. Viral pneumonia, sometimes called *walking pneumonia,* is most commonly seen following influenza or another viral disease. Symptoms include headache, fever, aching muscles, and cough with mucopurulent sputum. Treatment for viral pneumonia varies according to the symptoms.

Bacterial pneumonia can be caused by a number of organisms, most commonly *Staphylococcus, Streptococcus, Klebsiella,* and *Legionella.* The symptoms of bacterial pneumonia are abrupt and dramatic in onset. Chills, fever up to 105° F, tachycardia, and tachypnea are common, as is pain with respiration, or dyspnea. The associated cough may be dry and unproductive or purulent and productive. The color of the sputum is significant and should be observed carefully. The type of microorganism involved can be determined by Gram stain and sputum culture. Bacterial pneumonia is treated with bacteria-specific antibiotics and supportive medical and nursing care.

Aspiration pneumonia is an inflammatory process of the bronchi and lungs caused by inhalation of foreign substances such as food or acidic gastric contents. The risk for aspiration is highest in older adults with a poor gag reflex and in those who must remain supine, because these individuals can easily inhale or regurgitate food during oral or tube feeding.

Aspiration of highly acidic gastric secretions can lead to cell membrane damage with exudation and, ultimately, to respiratory distress. Aspiration of large amounts of feeding solution is likely to trigger coughing or choking episodes and dyspnea. If these fluids are not removed immediately by suction, respiratory distress and death may result. Aspiration of small amounts of liquid can result in continued and progressive inflammation of the lungs. The person suffering from aspiration pneumonia typically has a rapid pulse and respiratory rate. Sputum is frothy but free of bacteria; however, a superimposed bacterial infection may develop.

Tuberculosis

Tuberculosis is an infectious disease caused by the bacillus *Mycobacterium tuberculosis,* which spreads by means of airborne droplets. When an infected person coughs or sneezes, contaminated droplets are released into the air. These droplets are inhaled by other people, the bacillus lodges in their lungs, and the disease spreads. Malnutrition, weakening of the immune system, crowded living conditions, poor sanitation, and the presence of systemic diseases such as diabetes and cancer increase the older adult's risk for contracting tuberculosis.

The symptoms of tuberculosis include cough, night sweats, fever, dyspnea, chest pain, anorexia, and weight loss. The cough may be nonproductive or productive. Sputum may be green or yellow; with hemoptysis, the presence of blood may impart a rusty color.

Because skin tests for tuberculosis are not reliable in older adults, diagnosis is based on chest radiography or sputum cultures of acid-fast bacilli. Early detection is important to prevent further spread of the disease.

Treatment today consists of drug therapy using a variety of antimicrobial agents such as isoniazid, rifampin, ethambutol, and streptomycin. A combination of these drugs is usually administered and continued for many months. Many of these drugs are associated with numerous adverse effects, particularly in older adults. Nursing care of the older adult with tuberculosis focuses on maintaining good nutrition, monitoring compliance with the medication administration schedule, and detecting side effects.

Lung Cancer

Lung cancer, or bronchogenic cancer, is one of the most deadly forms of cancer in the United States. The age range at which diagnosis of lung cancer peaks is 55 to 65 years. Although lung cancer is more common in men, it has become increasingly common in women and has recently passed breast cancer as a leading cause of death. The survival rate after diagnosis of lung cancer is poor, rarely exceeding 5 years.

Lung cancer results from exposure to **carcinogenic,** or cancer-causing, agents, particularly tobacco smoke, air pollution, asbestos, and other hazardous industrial substances. Cough, chest pain, and blood-tinged sputum are typical symptoms, which can easily be missed because they resemble those of pneumonia and other common respiratory conditions of older adults.

The treatment of choice is surgical resection of the lungs. This procedure is associated with a high mortality rate in older adults. Radiation and chemotherapy are used in some patients, with varying amounts of success.

THE CARDIOVASCULAR SYSTEM

The cardiovascular system moves blood throughout the body. This continuous, closed system is responsible for the transportation of blood with oxygen and nutrients to all body tissue. It also transports waste products to the organs that remove them from the body. Through its action, the cardiovascular system helps maintain homeostasis within the body. The heart pumps the blood, and the blood vessels dilate or constrict to aid in the maintenance of blood pressure and exchange of materials between the blood and body tissue.

HEART

The heart is a muscular organ located centrally in the thoracic cavity between the lungs. The **sternum,** or breastbone, protects its anterior surface. The heart's tip, or **apex,** projects toward the left side of the body and extends directly above the diaphragm muscle.

Three **pericardial membranes** form a sac around the heart. The innermost membrane is on the surface of the heart and is called the **epicardium,** or **visceral pericardium.** The middle membrane is the **parietal pericardium,** and the outermost membrane is the **fibrous pericardium.** The space between the epicardium and the parietal pericardium is the **pericardial cavity;** it contains a small amount of **serous fluid** that prevents the membrane surfaces from rubbing together during cardiac activity.

The heart, which is composed of cardiac muscle (called **myocardium**), is a hollow organ with four distinct chambers. The right side of the heart consists of the **right atrium** and **right ventricle,** which are separated by the **tricuspid valve.** The right side of the heart is a low-pressure pump that moves deoxygenated blood through the pulmonary valve and pulmonary artery and out to the lungs. After the blood is oxygenated, it returns to the left side of the heart through the **pulmonary vein.** Because less effort is required to move blood the short distance through the lungs of a healthy individual, the muscle wall of the right side of the heart is relatively thin. The left side of the heart also has two chambers, the **left atrium** and **left ventricle,** which are separated by the **mitral valve.** The pressure within the left side of the heart is higher than that in the right side because the left side is responsible for blood distribution to the entire body. To provide the necessary force, the left ventricle has a thicker muscle wall than does the right ventricle. When blood leaves the left ventricle, it proceeds through the aortic valve into the **aorta** and its branches and out to the rest of the body.

The heart chambers and valves are lined with **endocardial** tissue. **Endothelial** tissue continues out from the heart and lines all of the blood vessels. This smooth layer allows the blood to flow freely and reduces the risk for clot formation.

BLOOD VESSELS

The **arteries** are blood vessels that carry blood away from the heart. With the exception of the pulmonary artery, arteries carry oxygenated blood. The aorta, the largest artery in the body, leaves the heart and branches into a series of progressively smaller arteries and capillaries. These vessels run through the entire body and reach all organs and tissues.

Arterial walls are composed of three layers of tissue. The innermost layer is the **endothelium,** or **tunica intima.** This layer is a continuation of the endocardial tissue that lines the inside of the heart. The middle layer, or **tunica media,** is composed of smooth muscle and connective tissue. This smooth muscle is controlled by the autonomic nervous system and dilates or constricts the artery to maintain the blood pressure. The outermost layer, or **tunica externa,** is composed of strong fibrous tissue that protects the vessels from bursting or rupturing under high pressure. The relative thickness of the tunica media and externa enables the arteries to perform properly.

The **veins** are vessels that carry blood toward the heart. With the exception of the **pulmonary vein,** veins carry deoxygenated blood. **Venules,** the smallest veins, are connected to the smallest capillaries. Veins and venules are composed of the same three layers of tissue seen in arteries. The veins use a system of **valves,** which are created by endothelial tissue folds, to aid in the return of blood to the heart. The valves prevent backflow of blood, which could be a problem when the blood is moving toward the heart against the force of gravity.

The smooth muscle layer of the veins is much thinner than that of the arteries because the veins are not as important in the regulation of blood pressure. The outer fibrous layer is also thinner because blood pressure in the veins is much lower than that in the arteries.

A special set of blood vessels, the **coronary arteries** and **veins,** supplies the heart with blood enriched with oxygen and nutrients. These arteries are the first branches of the ascending aorta. Because the heart muscle works continuously, it has high oxygen demands. Any condition that obstructs the normal supply of blood to the heart can damage the myocardium. If it is severely deprived of oxygen and nutrients, the heart muscle will die. Too much damaged or destroyed tissue results in cardiovascular system failure and death.

CONDUCTION SYSTEM

To function effectively, the cardiovascular system must work in a controlled, organized, and rhythmic manner. The heart's rhythm is established by specialized cells within the heart muscle that make up the electrical system of the heart. The body's natural pacemaker, the **sinoatrial node,** is a group of specialized cells in the right atrium. Impulses generated in the sinoatrial node travel across the atria to the **atrioventricular node** in the lower interatrial septum. From there they are conducted through the bundle of His, through the right and left bundle branches, through the Purkinje fibers, and, finally, to the ventricular myocardium. When the cells of the heart's electrical system **depolarize,** the myocardium depolarizes and the heart contracts (systole), following which the special cells and the myocardium repolarize as the heart relaxes (diastole). This process alternately empties and fills the chambers, which pump blood through the circulatory system.

EXPECTED AGE-RELATED CHANGES

The heart does not atrophy with aging as other muscles do. In fact, the heart muscle mass increases slightly with age, and the thickness of the wall of the left ventricle also increases slightly. The increase in muscle mass may occur to offset some loss of tone. The aging heart may function less effectively even when no pathologic changes are present (Table 3-4). Loss of tone typically leads to the decrease in maximal cardiac output seen in older adults. The normal conduction system, SA node, AV node, the bundle of His, and its branches all lose cells starting fairly early in life (in the twenties). Cardiac response to autonomic stimulation shows decreased response to adrenergic stimulation due to changes in the receptors. Older persons enhance cardiac output by increasing stroke volume, whereas younger persons increase output by increasing heart rate.

The heart valves show some degree of thickening and increased calcification with aging, resulting in mild degrees of mitral valve regurgitation. As in other body tissues, the endocardium and endothelium lose elasticity with aging. When these tissues become increasingly fibrous and sclerotic, venous return from the peripheral areas of the body decreases. **Orthostatic hypotension** occurs because the circulation does not respond quickly to postural changes. Less effective pumping of the heart muscle combined with sclerotic changes in the veins can lead to **dependent edema** and to the appearance of **varicosities** in the lower extremities. Weakness of the valves in the rectal veins can lead to hemorrhoids.

Table 3-4 Cardiovascular Changes Associated With Aging

PHYSIOLOGIC CHANGE	RESULTS
Decreased cardiac muscle tone	Decreased tissue oxygenation related to decreased cardiac output and reserve
Increased heart size, left ventricular enlargement	Compensation for decreased muscle tone
Decreased cardiac output	Increased chance of heart failure; decreased peripheral circulation
Decreased elasticity of heart muscle and blood vessels	Decreased venous return; increased dependent edema; increased incidence of orthostatic hypotension; increased varicosities and hemorrhoids
Decreased pacemaker cells	Heart rate 40–100 beats per minute; increased incidence of ectopic or premature beats; increased risk for conduction abnormalities
Decreased baroreceptor sensitivity	Decreased adaptation to changes in blood pressure
Increased incidence of valvular sclerosis	Increased risk for heart murmurs
Increased atherosclerosis	Increased blood pressure, weaker peripheral pulses

NURSING ASSESSMENTS AND CARE STRATEGIES RELATED TO CARDIOVASCULAR CHANGES	
NURSING ASSESSMENTS	CARE STRATEGIES
Assess apical and peripheral pulses.	Observe closely for abnormal sounds; determine presence and strength of peripheral pulses comparing both sides of the body. When assessing lower extremities, start distally and move toward trunk.
Assess blood pressure lying, sitting, and standing.	Hypotension is likely to occur while changing position; encourage patient to change positions slowly and to seek assistance if dizzy.
Assess ability to tolerate activity.	Instruct patient to rest if short of breath or fatigued.

COMMON DISORDERS SEEN WITH AGING

Cardiovascular disease is the leading cause of morbidity and mortality in the United States, accounting for more than 75% of all deaths in men and women older than 65 years of age.

Coronary Artery Disease

Some degree of coronary artery disease is present in most persons older than age 70. The coronary arteries supply blood to the heart. If these vessels become narrowed or obstructed because of atherosclerosis, the heart may not receive adequate oxygen and nutrients. Many older adults have seriously obstructed coronary arteries, yet they remain essentially asymptomatic. Once circulation to the heart muscle decreases significantly, the amount of oxygen delivered to the heart decreases and ischemia occurs. The pain that may be experienced with ischemia is referred to as **angina pectoris** (literally, chest pain). Although the symptoms of ischemia do include chest pain or pain radiating down the left arm, such pain is not always present or recognized in older adults. Vague gastrointestinal (GI) discomfort or shortness of breath may be reported, or there may be no symptoms at all. People experiencing an angina attack are advised to decrease their activity and rest until the episode passes. Physicians usually prescribe coronary vasodilators, such as nitroglycerin, or β-adrenergic blocking agents for people with ischemic heart disease.

When one or more coronary arteries become totally obstructed by atherosclerosis or embolus, the person is said to have a **myocardial infarction** (MI), or heart attack. The mortality rate from MI is four times higher in those older than 70 years of age than in younger individuals. Symptoms of a heart attack in older adults are more variable than in younger people. Most older adults are likely to have symptoms such as sudden-onset dyspnea or chest discomfort, confusion, syncope, and decreased urine production. Diaphoresis is uncommon. Many older adults who have heart attacks die suddenly (Box 3-2).

If severe atherosclerotic occlusion of the coronary arteries is detected before MI, angioplasty, stent placement, or coronary bypass surgery may be performed. The age and overall health of the individual are considered before any of these surgical procedures are

| Box **3-2** | Signs and Symptoms of Myocardial Infarction (Heart Attack) in Older Adults |

1. Sudden-onset dyspnea
2. Chest discomfort (not crushing pain)
3. Anxiety and confusion
4. Syncope
5. Decreased urine production
6. Diaphoresis (uncommon)

attempted. MI caused by an embolus that is detected quickly can be treated using thrombolytic agents such as streptokinase or tissue plasminogen activator, but the use of these drugs may increase the risk for stroke.

Occlusion of the coronary arteries decreases the flow of nutrients and oxygen to the myocardium. Total oxygen deprivation results in myocardial tissue necrosis. Cardiac tissue necrosis is irreversible. The types of problems experienced after an MI depend on the location and extent of the damage to the heart muscle. Mild damage may not be associated with symptoms and may be detectable on the electrocardiogram only. This type of infarction is often referred to as a *silent* heart attack. Moderate damage may limit a person's physical activity. Extensive damage or damage to a critical area of the heart may result in death.

Coronary Valve Disease

The valves of the heart become less pliant over time. In addition, calcium deposits may develop on the valves, preventing them from sealing completely. This can result in mitral valve prolapse, mitral regurgitation, and, ultimately, congestive heart failure (CHF). Symptoms of mitral valve prolapse include chest pain, palpitations, fatigue, and dyspnea. Calcium deposits on the valves roughen the lining and increase the risk for clot formation in the chambers of the heart and in the blood vessels.

Cardiac Arrhythmias

Cardiac arrhythmias, including ventricular arrhythmias, atrial fibrillation, and conduction disturbances, are increasingly common with aging. Heart block is a common conduction disturbance caused by disruption of the electrical conduction system of the heart. This disruption can be caused by fibrotic tissue infiltration or MI. Sinus node dysfunction, sometimes called *sick sinus syndrome*, is the primary conduction disorder seen in older adults. This condition causes a disturbance in the rate and rhythm of heart contraction, resulting in symptoms such as lightheadedness, fatigue, palpitations, and syncope. When the disturbance is severe, an artificial pacemaker may be used to regulate cardiac activity.

Congestive Heart Failure

CHF is primarily a problem of the aging population. It is estimated that more than two million people suffer from this disorder, resulting in almost one million hospitalizations each year. The term *congestive heart failure* is descriptive of the disease process: The patient's lungs are often congested, and edema appears because the heart's pumping action is ineffective. CHF is not a single disease but rather a syndrome that accompanies and results from many other disorders. A variety of cardiovascular diseases can contribute to the development of CHF. Coronary artery disease, MI, hypertension, valve disease, and cardiac infection or inflammation may increase the risk for CHF. Diseases of other body systems, including bronchitis, emphysema, asthma, hyperthyroidism, liver disease, kidney disease, and anemia, can also lead to CHF. Metabolic changes and fluid and electrolyte imbalances seen with malnutrition can lead to CHF. Excessive sodium intake with fluid retention increases the risk for CHF. The effects of alcohol, digoxin, hormones, some antineoplastics, corticosteroids, and NSAIDs can directly or indirectly lead to CHF.

CHF is associated with a wide range of symptoms, depending on the type and severity of the underlying disease. Mild **chronic CHF** tends to have a slow, insidious onset. Older adults who experience mild symptoms such as dyspnea, orthopnea, or paroxysmal nocturnal dyspnea often decrease their activity spontaneously. They may not recognize these symptoms as serious and may attribute them to "slowing down" with aging. Many older adults do not seek medical attention until they have serious problems and are unable to perform even minimal activities (Box 3-3). **Acute CHF** can result in severe pulmonary congestion or cardiogenic shock and is often fatal in older adults. Chronic CHF can become acute CHF with increased physical or emotional stress. People with CHF are more susceptible to fluid and electrolyte imbalances, infections, and renal or liver failure.

Medical management of CHF includes dietary restriction of sodium to decrease fluid retention, administration of diuretics (e.g., furosemide) to reduce fluid overload, administration of cardiotonic medications (e.g., digoxin) to increase the pumping efficiency of the heart, and planned levels of activity designed to reduce cardiac workload. Use of medical devices, including pacemakers, left ventricle assist devices, and implanted sensors, is increasingly common.

Cardiomegaly

Although aging does not routinely affect the size of the heart, many older adults do develop cardiomegaly, or enlargement of the heart, which is often related to

CHF. As we age, the muscular wall of the left ventricle thickens. Because arteries and veins lose elasticity with age, the heart must pump harder to move blood through the vessels. The muscles of the left ventricle hypertrophy in an attempt to improve the output of blood from the heart to meet the body's tissue demands for oxygenated blood.

The right side of the heart may also hypertrophy. Right-sided enlargement is a result of increased resistance in the pulmonary circulation. When one side of the heart is weakened, the other side is soon affected.

Peripheral Vascular Disease

Vessel changes with aging can lead to mild or severe problems. In arteriosclerosis, the walls of the arteries become less elastic and plaque forms in the lumen, further restricting blood flow. Excessive plaque is often related to lifestyle factors or to other disease conditions, most commonly obesity, high cholesterol intake, cigarette smoking, and DM. If the lumen becomes too narrow, blood flow to peripheral sites, particularly the lower extremities, may be restricted. This decreased blood flow deprives the tissue of oxygen and nutrients and causes ischemia. If the lumen is completely obstructed, tissue death may result.

An early symptom of arterial occlusive disease is pain. **Intermittent claudication,** which manifests as a cramping pain in the legs during or after walking, is common with diminished peripheral circulation. Severe circulatory impairment can result in tissue necrosis that requires amputation.

Acute occlusion may occur if a thrombus or embolus obstructs the blood vessel. Sudden pain, pallor, pulselessness, loss of sensation, or a change in body temperature should be assessed and reported promptly.

Occlusive Peripheral Vascular Problems

Thrombus formation (clotting) in the lumen of a vein is a common problem, particularly in older adults who are immobile. These clots can form quickly because of sluggish blood flow within the vessels. Increasing the patient's activity and using antiembolism stockings help prevent problems related to venous stasis or pooling.

Thrombi form most often in the veins of the lower extremities, where they irritate and inflame the vessel and cause thrombophlebitis. Signs of thrombophlebitis include edema, swelling, warmth over the affected area, aching, cyanosis or pallor, and a positive Homans' sign (pain induced by dorsiflexing the foot of the affected leg).

Medical management of thrombophlebitis typically includes rest, elevation of the affected leg, application of elastic stockings or wraps, administration of analgesics, anticoagulant therapy, and sometimes application of heat.

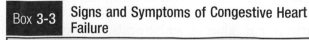

Box 3-3	Signs and Symptoms of Congestive Heart Failure

1. Dyspnea (shortness of breath) with exertion
2. Orthopnea (dyspnea at rest when recumbent)
3. Coughing or wheezing with exertion or at rest
4. Fatigue, weakness, or generalized muscle weakness with minimal exertion
5. Peripheral edema
6. Weight gain without an increase in food intake (as a result of fluid retention)
7. Nausea, vomiting, or anorexia
8. Paroxysmal nocturnal dyspnea (extreme orthopnea during sleep)

If a thrombus breaks loose from the vein and travels in the circulatory system, it is referred to as an **embolus.** Emboli can be life-threatening. They are particularly dangerous if they reach small blood vessels in the lungs or brain, where they can occlude the blood supply to vital tissues.

Varicose Veins

Varicose veins are seen when blood pools in the veins and dilates or stretches them. The decrease in vascular muscle tone that occurs with aging increases the risk for this. Varicosities are most often seen as a twisting discoloration in the superficial veins of the lower extremities. Older adults who are obese, are inactive, or spend a great deal of time standing are more likely to have varicosities. The risk for inflamed varicosities increases with age.

Varicosities can result in leg cramps or a dull, aching pain in the legs. Patients can reduce or prevent related problems by avoiding constricting garments such as garters or rolled stockings, by refraining from sitting with crossed legs, by increasing activity, by resting with the legs elevated, and by wearing elastic stockings that promote venous return.

Aneurysm

Aneurysm, the pouching or ballooning of arteries, is common in older adults who suffer from arteriosclerotic blood vessel changes. Older adults with a history of angina, MI, or CHF are at increased risk for developing aneurysms. As parts of the muscular walls of the arteries develop plaque and become rigid, other areas of the vessels stretch, dilate, and weaken. The walls of the dilated areas become thin and prone to rupture.

Aneurysms of the abdominal aorta are most common in older adults. These are sometimes observed as a pulsating mass near the umbilicus, or navel. Patients may have abdominal pain and GI complaints. Aneurysms can also develop in peripheral and cerebral blood vessels. Thrombi can form in aneurysms and block the flow of blood. Rupture of an aneurysm results in massive, life-threatening hemorrhage. Early detection and surgical repair of the damaged area provide the best chance for survival.

Hypertensive Disease

Hypertension is prevalent in the older-adult population. It is estimated that more than 50% of persons older than 65 years of age have some form of hypertensive disorder. Hypertension is categorized as **essential** (primary) or **secondary.** Essential hypertension, the more common form, has no known cause. Many factors, including heredity, diet, obesity, stress, smoking, increased serum cholesterol levels, and abnormal sodium transport, are known to contribute to essential hypertension. Secondary hypertension occurs as a result of a coexisting disease process or other known cause. Renal, vascular, and endocrine pathologic conditions are among the most common causes of secondary hypertension.

Essential hypertension tends to have a gradual onset and is often asymptomatic until complications arise. Most often, hypertension is discovered during a routine physical examination. It is diagnosed based on two elevated blood pressure determinations on three separate days. A reading of 140/90 mm Hg is considered the upper limit of normal in adults, but some physicians consider slightly higher readings normal in adults older than 60 years of age.

Essential hypertension cannot be cured, but it can be treated. Treatment includes nonpharmacologic approaches such as rest, smoking cessation, use of stress-reduction techniques, weight loss, and dietary-sodium restriction. Pharmacologic approaches typically include administration of oral diuretics and β-blockers. The person experiencing hypertension must be monitored continuously to determine the effectiveness of therapy. Treatment of secondary hypertension is directed at the underlying pathologic condition.

THE HEMATOPOIETIC AND LYMPHATIC SYSTEMS

Body fluids distribute essential protective factors, nutrients, oxygen, and electrolytes throughout the body. The two major fluids of the body are blood and lymph. These fluids flow through the body within two parallel circulatory systems.

BLOOD

Blood flows within the heart and vessels of the cardiovascular system. The general functions of blood include **transportation** of nutrients, waste products, blood gases, and hormones; regulation of fluid-electrolyte balance, acid-base balance, and body temperature; and **protection** against pathogenic attack by the WBCs and against excessive blood loss through clotting mechanisms.

Blood is 91% to 92% liquid; the remaining 8% to 9% is solid. The liquid of the blood is called **plasma.** As a liquid, plasma is a substance in which many other substances can dissolve and be transported, including nutrients (e.g., glucose, amino acids, and lipids), electrolytes (e.g., sodium, potassium, calcium, and chloride), hormones, vitamins, antibodies, and waste products. Carbon dioxide is carried in the plasma as bicarbonate ion. Plasma contains a variety of proteins. **Albumin,** the most abundant plasma protein, is important in the maintenance of **osmotic pressure** needed to regulate blood pressure and volume. In the **fibrinogen** component are prothrombin, fibrinogen itself, and other clotting factors that circulate until they are required by the body. **Globulins** function as transport agents for lipids and fat-soluble vitamins;

the γ-globulin fraction is composed of antibodies that provide immunity from pathogens. The solid portion of the blood is composed of three types of blood cells: RBCs, WBCs, and platelets.

Erythrocytes

Erythrocytes, or RBCs, live for approximately 120 days; therefore, the body produces new RBCs throughout life. They are formed in the red bone marrow by **stem cells,** which undergo mitosis. For mitosis to occur, and thus for RBCs to form, vitamin B_{12} and folic acid are necessary for deoxyribonucleic acid (DNA) synthesis. For maturation, the RBCs need adequate amounts of protein and iron.

When RBCs become old and fragile, they are removed from the circulation by the **reticuloendothelial cells** of the spleen, liver, and red bone marrow. Their iron is reused in new RBCs formed by the red marrow. Excess iron is stored in the liver for later use. The **heme** portion of the RBC is converted to bilirubin in the reticuloendothelial system and is then processed by the liver. The liver secretes the bilirubin, or **bile pigment,** with the other components of bile, into the duodenum for use in digestion. This bile pigment helps give stool its characteristic brown color. If excessive numbers of RBCs are destroyed or if the liver does not function adequately, excessive amounts of bilirubin remain in the circulation. High bilirubin levels result in jaundice, a yellow discoloration of the sclera of the eyes and of the skin of light-skinned individuals.

Leukocytes

Leukocytes, or WBCs, have protective functions: They destroy dead or damaged tissue, detoxify foreign proteins, protect from infectious disease, and function in the immune response. WBCs are produced in the lymphatic tissue of the spleen, lymph nodes, thymus, and red bone marrow. The five types of WBCs are **neutrophils, eosinophils, basophils, lymphocytes,** and **monocytes.**

Platelets

Platelets, more properly called **thrombocytes,** are not whole cells but pieces of cells. They are produced when large cells called **megakaryocytes** fragment and enter the circulation. Platelets, which remain in circulation for approximately 10 days, play an important role in the blood's clotting mechanism.

LYMPH SYSTEM

The lymph and circulatory systems are parallel and interdependent. In fact, the lymph system is sometimes considered part of the circulatory system because it is responsible for returning fluids from the tissues to the circulation. The major components of the immune system—lymphocytes and antibodies— are formed by the lymph system to protect the body from pathogenic microorganisms, malignant cells, and foreign proteins. The lymph system consists of the lymph vessels, fluid, nodes, and nodules; the spleen; and the thymus gland.

Lymph Vessels, Fluid, and Nodes

Lymph vessels are located in most tissue spaces. These permeable vessels absorb fluid and proteins from the tissues. Muscular compression on the vessels moves this fluid through a series of lymph nodes and nodules that trap and phagocytize foreign materials before the fluid enters the circulatory system at the subclavian veins. Lymph nodes and nodules also produce lymphocytes and monocytes and phagocytize pathogens.

Spleen and Thymus

The spleen is responsible for producing lymphocytes and monocytes, which enter the bloodstream. It also contains fixed **plasma cells,** which produce antibodies to foreign antigens, and fixed macrophages, which phagocytize pathogens and other foreign substances in the blood. Although people can survive without a spleen, they may be more susceptible to certain bacterial infections, including pneumonia.

The thymus, which is located behind the thyroid gland, is large in fetuses and infants. The embryonic bone marrow and the spleen produce the initial **T lymphocytes,** or T cells, which are responsible for recognition of foreign antigens and for cell-mediated immunity. The thymus shrinks with age, but once the T cells are established in the spleen and lymph nodes, they are self-perpetuating.

Lymphocytes and Immunity

B lymphocytes, or B cells, are also produced in the embryonic bone marrow. These cells are responsible for the recognition of antigens located on a foreign cell and for humoral immunity. In humoral immunity, T cells and B cells often cooperate: Sensitized **helper T cells** detect antigens and induce the B cells to produce antibodies, which are then found in the globulin portion of plasma. When the antigen has been destroyed, **suppressor T cells** reduce helper T-cell activity and stop the immune process. Conversely, in cell-mediated immunity, antibodies are not produced. Instead, activated T cells divide into memory T-cells (which recognize the pathogen) and killer T cells (which destroy bacteria by disrupting their cell membranes).

EXPECTED AGE-RELATED CHANGES

The characteristics of blood change somewhat as a person ages (see Table 3-5). Plasma viscosity increases slightly and is most often related to a general decrease in total body fluid. Blood cell production in the bone

Table 3-5 Hematopoietic and Lymphatic Changes Associated With Aging

PHYSIOLOGIC CHANGE	RESULTS
Increased plasma viscosity	Increased risk for vascular occlusion
Decreased red blood cell production	Increased incidence of anemia
Decreased mobilization of neutrophils	Less effective phagocytosis
Increased immature T cells response	Decreased immune response

NURSING ASSESSMENTS AND CARE STRATEGIES RELATED TO HEMATOPOIETIC AND LYMPHATIC CHANGES	
NURSING ASSESSMENTS	CARE STRATEGIES
Monitor laboratory tests, including Hgb, Hct, WBC, and differential.	Report abnormal findings promptly to physician.
Assess nutritional intake for adequacy of protein, iron and vitamins	Administer nutritional supplements as ordered.

marrow decreases slightly, resulting in a small decrease in total RBCs and WBCs. Unless extreme physiologic stress or disease is present, blood levels of RBCs, WBCs, and platelets remain within normal limits.

The number of T cells in the body does not appear to decrease with aging, but more of the cells are immature. The ratio of helper cells to suppressor cells is increased. These T-cell changes lead to a diminished immune response. Consequently, older adults are at greater risk for developing infections, particularly respiratory and urinary tract infections (UTIs). Older adults are also at increased risk for acquiring nosocomial infections. Studies have shown that women older than 55 years of age have limited antibody titers to tetanus toxoid, raising questions about changes in humoral immunity with aging. If the ability to produce antibodies is affected by aging, changes in immunization practices for the aging population may be necessary.

Changes in the immune response may modify the usual signs and symptoms of infection. Such changes may be difficult to recognize in older adults: Body temperature may not become significantly elevated until the infection is severe, and pain may not be present to indicate infection. Some examples include the following: (1) Older adults with pneumonia may not have a fever or chills; (2) dysuria is often absent in older adults with UTIs; (3) pain may be absent with peritonitis or appendicitis, even though the individual is obviously ill; and (4) the physiologic response of older adults to tuberculosis skin testing may be delayed or less intense than that of younger individuals.

COMMON DISORDERS SEEN WITH AGING

Anemia

Anemia is defined as inadequate levels of RBCs or insufficient hemoglobin. The most commonly observed anemias in older adults are iron-deficiency anemia, pernicious anemia, and folic acid–deficiency anemia.

Iron-deficiency anemia results from inadequate nutritional intake, blood loss, malabsorption, or increased physiologic demand. Pernicious anemia is associated with decreased intake or absorption of vitamin B_{12}. Folic acid–deficiency anemia is usually caused by poor nutrition, chronic alcohol abuse, or malabsorption syndromes such as Crohn's disease. Anemia is common in the older adult population, and these problems are explored further in other chapters.

Leukemia

Leukemia is the result of excessive production of immature WBCs. There are both acute and chronic varieties, and leukemia is also classified by the type of abnormal cells present. Other blood disorders (e.g., anemia) and hemorrhage (related to a decrease in the number or function of platelets) are commonly seen with leukemia. **Chronic lymphocytic leukemia** is the form most often seen in older adults. Approximately 75% of those diagnosed with chronic lymphocytic leukemia are older than age 60. Depending on the stage of the disease and the patient's overall health, life expectancy may vary from a few to as many as 20 years after diagnosis.

THE GASTROINTESTINAL SYSTEM

Food and fluids containing the nutrients needed for survival normally enter the body through the GI tract. Although it is possible to live without food for several days, the cells require a regular supply of nutrients to support their normal physiologic activities.

As appealing as a banana split, turkey dinner, or bowl of strawberries may be to us, these foods are useless to our cells until they are broken down into simple, usable forms by the GI system. The GI tract prepares food for digestion. It then digests, processes, and absorbs the nutrients, which are used by the cells of the body. The GI system also stores and discards wastes and plays a major role in maintaining fluid balance by absorbing water. After we chew and swallow food, we do not need to think about its further processing, because the GI system takes care of removing the nutrients and discarding the waste. However, in unusual situations, the GI tract can be bypassed by administering specially prepared nutrients directly into the bloodstream (parenteral nutrition, or hyperalimentation).

The GI tract begins at the mouth and ends at the anus. Each part of the GI tract performs its own distinct functions.

ORAL CAVITY

Food normally enters the body through the mouth and is prepared for digestion in the **oral cavity.** The teeth mechanically process food by biting, tearing, grinding, and chewing it, a process called **mastication.** The normal adult has 28 to 32 permanent teeth with shapes and sizes that vary depending on their function. The incisors are used to bite, the **canines** to tear, and the **premolars** and **molars** to chew and grind. Each tooth is composed of a crown, which is the part visible above the gingiva (gum), and a **root,** which is imbedded in a socket in either the mandible or maxilla of the jaw. The periodontal membrane lines the tooth socket and holds the teeth in place. The crown of the tooth is protected by an extremely hard casing called **enamel.** The **pulp cavity** of the tooth contains blood vessels and nerve endings.

TONGUE

The tongue is a highly flexible structure controlled by and composed primarily of skeletal muscle. **Papillae,** which contain the taste buds, are located on the upper surface of the tongue. Cranial nerves control the movement of the tongue and carry the impulses for the perception of taste. The tongue aids in mechanical digestion by positioning food between the teeth and mixing it with saliva in the oral cavity.

SALIVARY GLANDS

Three pairs of **salivary glands** excrete saliva into the oral cavity. Saliva is composed primarily of water but also contains the enzyme **amylase,** which begins the digestion of starch. Saliva production normally increases in response to the sight or smell of food. Inadequate amounts of saliva result in a dry mouth and in difficult swallowing. When adequately mixed with saliva, food reaches a consistency that makes it more suitable for chemical digestion. The tongue lifts against the hard palate, pushing the bolus of food to the pharynx at the back of the oral cavity. From here, the bolus of food enters the esophagus.

ESOPHAGUS

Once in the **esophagus,** food is moved by a process called *peristalsis,* a wavelike motion of the smooth musculature that propels material through the entire GI tract. The esophagus is a hollow muscular tube that passes from the pharynx through the flat layer of diaphragm muscle and to the stomach. The esophagus is located above the diaphragm, and the stomach is located immediately below the diaphragm. The lower esophageal sphincter, also called the *cardiac sphincter,* is at approximately the same level as the diaphragm, where the esophagus meets the stomach. It allows food to enter the stomach but prevents the stomach contents from moving backward (refluxing) into the esophagus.

STOMACH

The **stomach** is a muscular sac in which both mechanical and chemical digestion take place. The stomach is lined with mucous membrane, which helps prevent damage to the muscle walls. Special stomach glands secrete mucus; others secrete enzymes, intrinsic factor, and hydrochloric acid. This mixture of enzymes and acids is called **gastric juice,** or **digestive juice.** The pyloric sphincter at the distal end of the stomach retains the bolus of food and the digestive juices within the stomach, where they can be churned, mixed, and further broken down for later digestion and absorption. Once the food has been processed in the stomach, it is referred to as **chyme.** After adequate mixing, small amounts of chyme are released through the pyloric sphincter into the small intestine.

SMALL INTESTINE

The **small intestine** is more than 20 feet long and is divided into three segments called the **duodenum,** the **jejunum,** and the **ileum** (in order of progression away from the stomach). Additional substances are added to chyme in the small intestine to complete digestion. Intestinal digestive glands secrete intestinal juice, which is alkaline and contains many enzymes. The common bile duct and pancreatic duct converge and enter the duodenum at the sphincter of Oddi. **Bile,** which is produced in the liver and stored in the gallbladder, breaks down fat by **emulsifying** it. **Pancreatic juice** contains enzymes that break down proteins. The pancreas also produces sodium bicarbonate; when released into the duodenum, it neutralizes the hydrochloric acid from the stomach. After all of these chemicals have acted on the material in the GI tract, the process of digestion is completed, and the nutrients are in elementary forms (e.g., glucose and amino acids) that can be used by the cells of the body.

Absorption of nutrients occurs primarily in the small intestine. Special **villi,** projections of the lining of the small intestine that are rich in capillaries and lymphatic vessels, increase the surface area of the lining. As the digested nutrients pass over these villi, they are absorbed into the blood and lymph by the capillary network and lymphatics.

Once the nutrients have been absorbed, undigested material and water are propelled into the large intestine by peristalsis. A structure called the **ileocecal valve** is located between the ileum of the small intestine and the cecum of the large intestine. This structure prevents waste products from moving backward into the small intestine.

LARGE INTESTINE

The **large intestine** is approximately 5 feet long and is divided into segments called the **ascending, transverse, descending,** and **sigmoid colon** and the rectum.

The major functions of the large intestine are absorption of water, minerals, and vitamins, and storage and elimination of indigestible wastes.

As the **effluent,** or discharge of waste products, moves through the large intestine, water is absorbed and the mass becomes increasingly solid in consistency. It is stored in the sigmoid and descending colon. When peristalsis causes the effluent to enter the rectum, its presence there triggers the defecation reflex, in which strong peristaltic movements propel the mass from the rectum and through the anus. Another reflex-like action occurs when the stomach is distended with food, stimulating vigorous peristalsis of the rectum and a desire to defecate. The internal anal sphincter is an involuntary muscle that relaxes when the rectum is full. The external anal sphincter, which is usually under voluntary control after 2 to 3 years of age, may be contracted to prevent defecation. When the external sphincter relaxes, wastes are eliminated from the large intestine.

EXPECTED AGE-RELATED CHANGES

Over time, changes in the GI tract can interfere with normal digestion (Table 3-6). In the oral cavity, gingival tissue may recede and the periodontal bonds that hold the teeth in place may loosen. If the teeth are not structurally sound, the ability to bite and chew can be impaired. Good oral hygiene can slow these changes. It is no longer considered normal for older adults to lose some or all of their teeth, which was common in the past.

Dental caries (cavities) can soften the enamel and expose nerves in the tooth pulp. The resulting pain can decrease the ability and the desire to eat.

Esophageal dilation and problems related to swallowing may be observed with aging. Commonly, the **gag reflex** is depressed in older adults, even in those without neurologic problems. This can lead to episodes of choking and to aspiration. The tone of sphincter muscles, particularly the lower esophageal sphincter, may decrease, increasing the incidence of esophageal reflux or heartburn.

In the stomach, atrophy of the gastric glands may result in a decreased production of intrinsic factor and hydrochloric acid; this, in turn, can interfere with normal digestion and absorption of nutrients. These changes can contribute to anemia and other malabsorptive problems. A decrease in gastric mucus production leads to risk for injury and bacterial penetration into the systemic circulation. Decreases in gut-associated lymphoid tissue can have an effect on immune response. Peristalsis of the intestine slows with aging, increasing the likelihood of constipation and the incomplete elimination of feces during a single bowel movement.

Table 3-6	Gastrointestinal Changes Associated With Aging
PHYSIOLOGIC CHANGE	**RESULTS**
Increased dental caries and tooth loss	Decreased ability to chew normally; decreased nutritional status
Decreased thirst perception	Increased risk for dehydration and constipation
Decreased gag reflex	Increased incidence of choking and aspiration
Decreased muscle tone at sphincters	Increased incidence of heartburn (esophageal reflux)
Decreased saliva and gastric secretions	Decreased digestion and absorption of nutrients
Decreased gastric motility and peristalsis	Increased flatulence, constipation, and bowel impaction
Decreased liver size and enzyme production	Decreased ability to metabolize drugs leading to increased risk for toxicity
NURSING ASSESSMENTS AND CARE STRATEGIES RELATED TO GASTROINTESTINAL CHANGES	
NURSING ASSESSMENTS	**CARE STRATEGIES**
Assess oral cavity for dentition, condition of mucous membranes and hygiene.	Educate regarding importance of good oral hygiene; stress need for adequate fluid intake. Dental referral as necessary.
Assess swallow and gag reflexes.	Encourage posture that facilitates swallowing. Consult with speech therapy for swallow studies and safe dietary regimen.
Monitor weight changes.	Weigh at least one time per month, more often if fluid balance issues present.
Assess intake of nutrients and fluid.	Educate regarding recommended dietary intake. Establish calorie count and intake and output if problems are suspected.
Assess bowel sounds and bowel elimination patterns.	Establish bowel routines. Teach importance of adequate fluid, fiber, and activity. Administer laxatives, stool softeners, suppositories, or enemas as needed to prevent constipation and impaction.

COMMON DISORDERS SEEN WITH AGING

Hiatal Hernia

A **hiatal hernia** is the protrusion of the stomach into the thoracic cavity through the esophageal opening in the diaphragm (see Figure 3-8). Men older than 50 years of age are most likely to experience problems with hiatal hernias, and as many as 40% to 60% of those 60 years of age or older may be affected. Some demonstrate no symptoms; others complain of severe distress that may be intermittent or continuous. Reflux episodes usually occur after meals, especially when the person lies down to rest immediately after eating. Complaints may include sour stomach, heartburn, or generalized epigastric distress. Sometimes the symptoms can resemble an angina attack. As mentioned, hiatal problems are most likely to occur after meals or when the person is at rest; in contrast, angina attacks are most likely to occur with physical exertion. Vital signs do not normally change in response to problems with hiatal hernias.

Gastroesophageal reflux disease is a major problem that can occur with hiatal hernias. With gastroesophageal reflux disease, the gastric contents move backward into the esophagus, where they increase the risk for aspiration. This can present serious concerns in older adults who have diminished gag or cough reflexes. Occasionally, the hernia through the diaphragm is reduced surgically, but typical treatment involves the use of antacids, histamine₂ antagonists, proton pump inhibitors, and dietary modifications. Fatty foods, carbonated beverages, alcohol, and foods that contain caffeine or caffeine-like substances (e.g., coffee, cola, and chocolate) should be avoided to reduce problems with reflux. Smaller, more frequent meals are often beneficial because overeating is likely to enlarge the stomach and cause it to bulge into the diaphragm. It is recommended that food and fluids be restricted after the normal evening meal, and affected persons should avoid lying down too soon after eating. In severe cases, the head of the bed may need to be elevated during sleep to reduce the risk for aspiration.

Gastritis and Ulcers

Chronic atrophic gastritis is an inflammatory change in the mucous membranes of the stomach in which the mucosa becomes thin and abnormally smooth and may develop hemorrhagic patches. All or parts of the stomach may be involved.

Both **gastric** and **duodenal ulcers** can occur with aging, but gastric ulcers are more common. Many factors contribute to the development of gastric ulcers. Behaviors such as smoking or alcohol ingestion, physical trauma such as surgery or fractures, disease processes such as pneumonia, and psychological stress resulting from hospitalization or nursing home placement can increase the risk for ulcers. A bacterium, *Helicobacter pylori,* has been implicated as the cause of some gastric ulcers. Drug-induced ulcers related to the use of iron supplements, aspirin, and NSAIDs are particularly common in older adults.

Peptic ulcers in older adults do not cause the classic epigastric pain that is seen in younger people. Older adults suffering from ulcers are more likely to complain of generalized pain and to exhibit a decreased activity level, decreased appetite, and weight loss. Vomiting, melena, and generalized signs of anemia may result from gastric bleeding. If a gastric ulcer progresses to the point of perforation, severe hemorrhage can result. If the person has already been weakened by occult bleeding, hemorrhage may be serious enough to result in death.

Early recognition and reporting of symptoms by the nurse is important so that treatment can be started before serious problems occur. Medical treatment of ulcers in older adults is generally preferred to surgical correction (Box 3-4).

Diverticulosis and Diverticulitis

Diverticula are small pouches or sacs that develop because of weaknesses in the intestinal mucosa. Between 30% and 40% of persons older than age 50 have some diverticula, and the incidence of diverticulosis increases with each decade of life. Most people with diverticula experience no symptoms, and there is no specific treatment unless symptoms occur. The patient

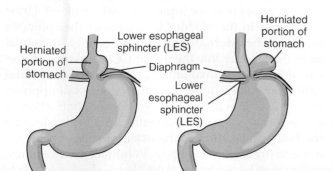

FIGURE 3-8 Hiatal hernia. A, Sliding hernia. B, Paraesophageal hernia.

Box 3-4	Medical Treatment of Ulcers

- Dietary modifications, including avoidance of alcohol, caffeine, and other suspect foods that tend to irritate the problem or increase hydrochloric acid production
- Avoidance of tobacco, which stimulates acid release
- Administration of antacids to reduce acidity
- Administration of histamine H₂-blocking agents, such as famotidine, cimetidine and ranitidine, to prevent ulcer formation or to promote ulcer healing
- Stress-reduction programs
- Administration of proton pump inhibitors such as omeprazole and lansoprazole

should continue to eat a normal diet with adequate fluids and roughage. If rectal bleeding occurs, medical intervention is necessary to determine the source.

Diverticulitis involves inflammation of one or more diverticula. This inflammation may result in bowel obstruction, perforation, or abscess formation. In cases of severe diverticulitis, the patient may need to be hospitalized. Oral intake of food is restricted and intravenous fluids are administered to give the diseased area an opportunity to "rest." Surgical correction, including bowel resection or colostomy, may be required if conservative medical treatment is unsuccessful. As many as 25% of elderly people who have diverticulitis require surgery.

Cancer

The incidence of **colon cancer** begins to increase at 40 years of age and peaks between the ages of 60 and 75. Carcinoma of the colon is more common in women, whereas carcinoma of the rectum is more common in men. Any changes in bowel elimination should be viewed with suspicion, especially signs of obstruction or bleeding. Routine screening for rectal cancer is recommended for those older than 40 years of age.

Hemorrhoids

Hemorrhoids, sometimes called **piles** by older adults, are common at all ages but may be particularly troublesome to older patients. People with chronic constipation and obese people are most likely to have problems with hemorrhoids. Pain and small amounts of bright red blood at the rectum are common complaints. Most patients with hemorrhoids do not require surgery. Diet changes, stool softeners, or bulk laxatives are usually effective in reducing problems related to constipation and hemorrhoids.

Rectal Prolapse

Bulging of the rectum through the anus is most likely to occur in women older than age 60, especially those who have given birth to many children. Some form of medical intervention may be needed if this condition causes distress. Surgery may be performed to strengthen the musculature. Insertion of a wire loop at the anal sphincter may be attempted in very old people.

THE URINARY SYSTEM

The urinary system consists of two kidneys, two ureters, the urinary bladder, and the urethra. The urinary system supports homeostasis by eliminating wastes and excessive fluid from the body. The kidneys continuously filter the blood and selectively save or eliminate water, electrolytes, and wastes. Those substances not reabsorbed by the kidneys are eliminated from the body as urine.

KIDNEYS

The kidneys are two bean-shaped organs located on each side of the spine behind the peritoneal lining of the abdomen and at the lower edge of the rib cage. The left kidney is usually located slightly higher than the right kidney. Each kidney is surrounded by an adipose tissue pad and is further protected from trauma by the muscles of the back. Within each kidney is a maze of nearly a million **nephrons,** the functional portion of the kidney. Blood is filtered in the glomerulus of the nephron, and this filtrate is destined to become urine. This highly vascular organ receives blood from the renal artery, which branches off the abdominal aorta. Blood returns to the circulation through the renal vein, which connects to the inferior vena cava. Adequate blood flow to the kidneys is very important; any condition that decreases renal blood flow interferes with normal kidney function.

The kidneys play an important role in fluid and electrolyte balance and acid-base balance in the body. They remove nitrogenous wastes, excess glucose, and drug metabolites from the bloodstream. They also help regulate blood pressure. The kidneys typically produce between 1 and 2 L of urine every 24 hours. If excessive fluid is lost elsewhere (e.g., in perspiration or diarrhea), urine output normally decreases. Excessive fluid or alcohol intake tends to increase urine production. A single kidney can meet the needs of the entire body.

URETERS AND BLADDER

The **ureters** are tubes of smooth muscle that allow urine to drain from each kidney into the bladder. When the body is upright, urine drains by means of gravity. Pressure of the enlarging bladder against the lower portion of the ureter keeps the ureter closed and prevents urine from flowing back toward the kidneys.

The **bladder** is a hollow muscular sac located below the peritoneum and normally entirely within the pelvic cavity. The bones of the pelvis protect the bladder from trauma. In women, the bladder is located anterior to the uterus; in men, it is superior to the prostate gland.

The muscular wall of the bladder is lined with a mucous membrane and is capable of stretching to hold large volumes of urine (up to 1000 mL or more). Urine is retained in the bladder by means of the sphincter muscles. The **internal sphincter** is located at the outlet from the bladder into the urethra. Control of the internal sphincter is involuntary. The **external urethral sphincter** comes under voluntary control at approximately 2 to 3 years of age. Voluntary contraction of the external sphincter prevents urine from leaving the body. Relaxation of the external sphincter allows urine to drain from the body. Voluntary control of urination may be overcome if the bladder becomes overly enlarged with urine. In adults, the urge to urinate typically occurs when urine volume in the bladder reaches approximately 200 to 400 mL.

The urethra is a tubelike passage that leads from the bladder to the outside of the body. At the point of exit, it is referred to as the *urinary meatus*. The female urethra is 1 to 1.5 inches long; the male urethra is 7 to 8 inches long. The urethra is part of the reproductive system in men and is used to transport semen as well as urine; however, ejaculation and urination cannot take place at the same time. The prostate gland surrounds the urethra. Although this normally causes no problems, an enlarged prostate can interfere with urination.

CHARACTERISTICS OF URINE

Urine is approximately 95% water, with the remainder composed of waste products and salts. The specific gravity (which measures the amount of solids dissolved in water) of urine is normally maintained within close limits. A specific gravity of 1.010 to 1.025 is considered normal. Dilute urine has a low specific gravity, and concentrated urine has a high specific gravity. Urine is normally clear, and its color ranges from pale yellow to dark amber. It may be alkaline or acidic, depending on the diet of the individual. High-protein diets tend to make the urine more acidic; vegetarian diets tend to lead to alkaline urine. Acidic urine is less compatible with bacterial growth than is alkaline urine and may help reduce the risk for a UTI.

EXPECTED AGE-RELATED CHANGES

The kidneys decrease in size from approximately 400 g at age 40 to only 250 g by age 80. By age 70, they lose approximately one-third of their efficiency and they lack functional reserve. Despite this, the kidneys usually are able to remove wastes adequately to maintain normal blood levels. As a person ages (Table 3-7), the number of functional units or nephrons decreases. In addition, the kidneys lose mass and decrease in size. Vascular changes, such as those that occur with atherosclerosis or arteriosclerosis, lead to decreased blood supply to the kidneys. Decreased blood flow results in an altered **glomerular filtration rate.** At 90 years of age, the glomerular filtration rate can be as little as half of what it was at age 20. The **blood urea nitrogen** remaining in the blood increases significantly with age, from a normal of 10 to 15 mg/dL in young adulthood to 21 mg/dL by age 70.

The nephrons and collecting system of the aging body are less sensitive to the effects of antidiuretic hormone. Less sodium and water are reabsorbed and more potassium is lost, resulting in the production of a less concentrated urine with aging.

Aging results in reduced urinary bladder size, which leads to decreased **bladder capacity** (i.e., the volume of urine the bladder can hold before a person experiences the urge to void). Many older people need

Table **3-7** Urinary Changes Associated With Aging

PHYSIOLOGIC CHANGE	RESULTS
Decreased number of functional nephrons	Decreased filtration rate with decrease in drug clearance
Decreased blood supply	Decreased removal of body wastes; increased concentration of urine
Decreased muscle tone	Increased volume of residual urine
Decreased tissue elasticity	Decreased bladder capacity
Delayed or decreased perception of need to void	Increased incidence of incontinence
Increased nocturnal urine production	Increased need to awaken to void or episodes of nocturnal incontinence
Increased size of prostate (male)	Increased risk for infection; decreased stream of urine; increased hesitancy and frequency of urination

NURSING ASSESSMENTS AND CARE STRATEGIES RELATED TO URINARY CHANGES	
NURSING ASSESSMENTS	**CARE STRATEGIES**
Monitor for signs of drug toxicity.	Promptly notify physician of relevant observations.
Assess for urinary frequency.	Palpate bladder after voiding or use Doppler to determine whether bladder is emptying completely.
Assess for signs and symptoms of urinary tract infection.	Obtain a urine specimen for analysis.
Assess frequency and timing of episodes of incontinence.	Establish a toileting schedule based on assessment data.

to void when only 100 mL of urine is present. In addition, overactivity of the detrusor muscle can result in contraction of the bladder before the bladder is full. Either or both of these factors can lead to the urinary urgency and frequency that is common in older adults. To further aggravate the situation, loss of muscle tone can impair voluntary control of the external sphincter muscle. Atonic muscular changes may also occur in the wall of the bladder. Loss of tone may result in reduced urinary stream, incomplete or unsuccessful voiding, continuous dribbling of urine, or urinary retention with overflow voiding (a condition in which the person voids frequently but never completely empties the bladder). Urinary retention contributes to the risk for UTIs, especially in older adults, because retained urine is a good medium for bacterial growth.

The prostate gland enlarges with age. Most men older than 60 years of age experience some degree of prostate gland enlargement as a result of **benign prostatic hyperplasia** or cancer. Because it surrounds the urethra, an enlarged prostate gland can compress and narrow the passageway, which, in turn, causes problems with voiding. Hesitancy, frequency, the inability to maintain a steady stream of urine, and urinary retention are common indicators of prostatic hypertrophy.

COMMON DISORDERS SEEN WITH AGING

Urinary Incontinence

Urinary incontinence, the involuntary loss of urine, is not a routine or normal occurrence with aging. Incontinence may occur as a result of physiologic changes, other medical problems such as UTIs, neurologic problems, or changes in the ability to function. Several classifications of medication can contribute to incontinence. Urinary incontinence is discussed in greater detail in Chapter 18.

Urinary Tract Infection

The incidence of UTIs increases significantly with age. Only 3% of women in their forties experience UTIs, whereas close to 15% experience UTIs by age 60. Men also develop UTIs, but they are less common in men and develop at an older age. Both the normal changes of aging and the increased incidence of health problems contribute to this increased incidence of UTIs (Box 3-5).

Chronic Renal Failure

An increasing number of people older than 70 years of age are being treated with dialysis for chronic renal failure. This was an age-restricted treatment in the past; however, today many older adults receive life-prolonging hemodialysis or peritoneal dialysis, depending on their needs and their physician's judgment.

Box **3-5**	Risk Factors for Urinary Tract Infections

- Inadequate or improper hygiene related to difficulty in cleansing after toileting
- Urinary stasis and incomplete emptying of bladder resulting from physiologic changes and decreased mobility
- Coexisting diseases such as diabetes, hypertension, stroke, and dementia
- Medical interventions, including catheterization and repeated use of antibiotics (which can lead to resistant strains of bacteria)
- Increased exposure to microorganisms in hospitals or extended-care facilities

Chronic renal failure may be a result of other chronic health conditions such as hypertension, DM, chronic UTIs, or urinary tract obstructions. It may also result from acute renal failure caused by hypovolemia, hypotension, or antibiotic toxicity.

The symptoms of chronic renal failure are extensive and often mimic those of other conditions. These symptoms include changes in urine output, muscle weakness, edema, nausea and vomiting, itchy and dry skin, and numerous neurologic symptoms. Blood tests reveal significant changes, particularly elevated levels of blood urea nitrogen and creatinine.

THE NERVOUS SYSTEM

The nervous system processes and controls body functions and links us with the outside world. Through the nervous system, we perceive sensations and detect changes in our environment. We store information about the world within the nervous system and use this information to respond to the world. A functioning nervous system is necessary for survival. Internally, the nervous system and the endocrine system maintain homeostasis.

Many of the functions of the nervous system (e.g., regulation of heartbeat and body temperature) occur at an unconscious level. Other activities, such as writing, working with tools, or singing, can be done with conscious thought and effort only. Some activities, such as breathing, occur unconsciously but can also be controlled consciously. The nervous system functions at an unconscious or reflex level at birth; neurologic control is gained with maturation. With advanced age, the nervous system becomes prone to deterioration and is susceptible to many types of injury and illness. Because of the serious consequences of age-related neurologic problems, it is important to examine this system in greater detail.

The nervous system is composed of highly specialized cells called **neurons.** Each neuron consists of a **cell body,** which contains the cell nucleus; multiple **dendrites,** which are fibers that transmit impulses (messages) to the cell body; and one **axon,** which carries impulses away from the cell body.

Nerve impulses are electrochemical in nature. An impulse travels through the neuron by fast-moving ion shifts across progressive segments of the cell membrane until it reaches the end of the axon. Axons and dendrites do not touch each other. A small gap called a **synapse** separates these structures. Special chemicals called **neurotransmitters** are released by the axon to stimulate a **receptor site** on another nerve cell. This allows the nerve impulse to move from one nerve cell to another. When the receptor has been stimulated, the neurotransmitter activity is halted by an inactivating chemical that stops prolonged transmission of impulses. In the peripheral nervous system, the most common neurotransmitters are **acetylcholine** and norepinephrine. In the central nervous system, dopamine, serotonin, and **norepinephrine** are important. Each neurotransmitter has a specific inactivator.

The nervous system consists of two major divisions: the central nervous system and the peripheral nervous system.

CENTRAL NERVOUS SYSTEM

The **central nervous system** is composed of the **brain** and the spinal cord. The brain is the master integrator of the nervous system. Thought, decision making, behavior, and all life processes are controlled by the various segments of the brain.

Medulla

The **medulla oblongata** extends from the spinal column to the pons of the brain. This area controls many vital functions, including heart rate, constriction of blood vessels (which affects blood pressure), and respiration. Reflex centers for coughing, vomiting, swallowing, and sneezing are also located in this area. Severe trauma to this area of the brain is life threatening.

Pons and Midbrain

The **pons** also exerts control over respiratory patterns and works with the medulla to regulate breathing rhythm. The **midbrain** integrates visual and auditory reflexes and helps maintain balance and equilibrium.

Cerebellum

The **cerebellum** works to coordinate body movement at an unconscious level. It allows excitation of muscles by neurons higher in the brain while it inhibits unnecessary impulses; thus, it enables smooth movements without jerkiness. Picking up a cup of coffee and bringing it to your mouth in a coordinated way is an example of the activity of the cerebellum. If you had to think consciously of all of the individual movements to accomplish this activity, the coffee would be cold before you could drink it.

Hypothalamus

The **hypothalamus,** a small area of the brain above the pituitary gland, is the coordinating center for the autonomic nervous system. It also secretes releasing and inhibiting hormones that affect the secretions of the pituitary gland (such as growth-hormone-releasing factor) and thus results in various effects on the endocrine system. Other hormones are produced in the hypothalamus, move to the pituitary, and are released by that gland, including antidiuretic hormone and oxytocin. The hypothalamus regulates body temperature, controls food intake, and is involved with visceral responses such as the increased heart rate that occurs with anger.

Cerebrum

The **cerebrum** is the largest part of the human brain. It is divided into lobes, which are named according to the cranial bones under which they lie. Because of the manner in which nerve impulses are routed in the central nervous system, the left lobes control the right side of the body and the right lobes control the left side of the body—they function **contralaterally.** The **frontal lobes** control voluntary motor activity, judgment, planning, organization, problem solving, and behavior regulation. **Broca's area,** which controls the movements related to speech, is found on the left frontal lobe in right-handed individuals. The **parietal lobes** interpret impulses and sensations from the skin and muscles. In addition, they are responsible for facial, shape, and color recognition. Taste sensation overlaps both the parietal and temporal lobes of the brain. The **temporal lobes** receive auditory (hearing) and olfactory (smelling) impulses and are devoted to new memory, learning, music, and emotions. The occipital lobes deal with vision, depth perception, and three-dimensional perception.

PERIPHERAL NERVOUS SYSTEM

The **peripheral nervous system** consists of the cranial and the spinal nerves and includes the **somatic nervous system** and the **autonomic nervous system.** The peripheral nervous system is a relay system that detects changes in both the internal and external environments and relays this information to the central nervous system. It also transmits impulses from the brain and spinal cord to the appropriate end organs. To prevent messages from short-circuiting each other in the peripheral nervous system and to speed impulse conduction, the axons of many types of nerves are surrounded by **Schwann cells,** which form the protective **myelin sheath.** Probably because of the myelin sheath, injured peripheral nerves can be surgically repaired or they may even regenerate spontaneously if the damage is not too severe. Neurons in the central nervous system lack this guiding sheath; if damaged, they usually die.

EXPECTED AGE-RELATED CHANGES

Many cellular changes have been observed in the aging brain, including a reduction in its size and weight resulting from a decrease in the volume of the cerebral cortex. There is approximately a 3% reduction in brain tissue in each decade from age 50 to 90. Brain shrinkage has been linked to a decrease in the number of functional cortical neurons (Table 3-8). Mental function is often changed as these cells are lost or undergo functional changes. Cerebral blood flow decreases with aging because of the gradual accumulation of fatty deposits (i.e., **arteriosclerosis**). Decreased blood flow also results in a slower rate of cerebral metabolism. A progressive decrease in the

Table 3-8	Neurologic Changes Associated With Aging
PHYSIOLOGIC CHANGE	**RESULTS**
Decreased number of brain cells	Slowed thought processes, decreased ability to respond to multiple stimuli and tasks
Decreased number of nerve fibers	Decreased reflexes, decreased coordination, decreased proprioception
Decreased amounts of neuroreceptors	Decreased perception of stimuli
Decreased peripheral nerve function	Decreased motor responses, increased risk for ischemic paresthesia in extremities
NURSING ASSESSMENTS AND CARE STRATEGIES RELATED TO NEUROLOGIC CHANGES	
NURSING ASSESSMENTS	**CARE STRATEGIES**
Assess alertness level, cognition, and functional abilities.	Report abnormal findings to physician. Refer for neurologic evaluation.
Assess balance and reflexes.	Educate regarding safety precautions and use of assistive devices. Structure tasks to reduce confusion; allow adequate time to perform tasks.

number of branches and the connections between dendrites occurs over time. Studies of neurotransmitters show that serotonin levels increase with aging, and norepinephrine levels decrease. Levels of monoamine oxidase, which metabolizes catecholamines, increase. In the peripheral nervous system, the velocity of nerve conduction decreases as much as 30% between 20 and 90 years of age.

Because of these physiologic changes, motor responses take longer in older individuals. Simple actions such as walking and talking often become slower with age. Reflex movements become sluggish, and reactions are slowed. Some loss of coordination is common. Tasks that require quick perception of stimuli and highly coordinated responses (e.g., driving in rush-hour traffic) may pose a risk to those with significant neurologic loss. Many aging people recognize these changes and modify their lifestyles to avoid potentially dangerous situations.

COMMON DISORDERS SEEN WITH AGING

Parkinson's disease

Parkinson's disease, also called **paralysis agitans,** is a progressive, degenerative disorder of the central nervous system. The cause of Parkinson's disease is unknown. Specific neurons in the brain that produce the neurotransmitter dopamine are lost. Symptoms usually begin after age 40 years and appear gradually.

The incidence of Parkinson's disease increases in older age groups.

People suffering from Parkinson's disease may manifest a variety of symptoms. The initial signs of the disease tend to be unilateral and include slight tremors on one side, in addition to a more general weakness and slowing down. As the disease progresses, these tremors become typical and obvious when the person is at rest, decrease with conscious movement, and are totally absent during sleep. Emotional stress or fatigue often worsens the tremors. Later in the course of the disease, both sides of the body become affected. Tremor increases, the body becomes more rigid, and movements become slower. The face takes on a flat, open-mouthed, masklike expression, and eye blinking decreases in frequency. Speech slows and may be unclear. Swallowing may be affected. Many have trouble either starting to walk or stopping once they have begun. Gait changes, and the affected individual appears to lean forward and walk with short, shuffling steps that occur faster and faster until the person almost runs in an attempt to avoid falling. It is common for people with Parkinson's disease to fall both forward and backward, because with increasing rigidity they lose the ability to compensate for shifts in their center of gravity. In severe cases, the affected person may become extremely rigid and unable to move.

Changes in mental processes may accompany physical changes. Although intelligence is not consistently affected by the disease, as many as 50% of persons suffering from parkinsonism experience some form of **dementia** late in the disease. Personality changes, frustration, and depression are common.

Medical treatment aimed at decreasing the symptoms of Parkinson's disease includes medications such as levodopa (combined with carbidopa), amantadine, bromocriptine, and anticholinergic drugs. These medications may allow less severely affected individuals to function almost normally. Unfortunately, the effects of these drugs lessen over time, or the symptoms worsen. Various combinations of medications are often ordered to maximize benefit. Because stress worsens the symptoms, it is particularly important to minimize frustration and emotional upset in these individuals. Neurosurgery may be performed in selected situations to decrease tremors and enhance functional ability.

Dementia

Dementia is a general term for a permanent or progressive organic mental disorder. Dementia is characterized by personality changes; confusion; disorientation; deterioration of intellectual functioning; and impaired control of memory, judgment, and impulses. Dementia can be a result of drug intoxication, trauma, disease processes, hormonal imbalances, and vitamin deficiencies. Some forms are treatable and reversible, particularly when an early diagnosis is made. Other forms do not respond to any known form of treatment. The most common form of dementia is Alzheimer's disease. Other forms include the following:

- **Vascular dementia,** or multi-infarct dementia, is the second most common form of dementia. It results from hemorrhage or ischemic brain lesions, is more common in men than in women, and is most common after age 70. Signs of depression are common, and sufferers may be suicidal. Onset of vascular dementia is sudden, as opposed to the gradual onset of Alzheimer's disease, and usually follows an episode of reduced blood flow to the brain tissue. Persons with hypertension or other types of cerebrovascular disease are most likely to develop this form of dementia. Risk for vascular dementia can be reduced by identifying and treating factors that contribute to the development of vascular disease, including high lipid (cholesterol) levels, elevated homocysteine levels, high blood pressure, smoking, and obesity.
- **Dementia with Lewy bodies** (DLB) is caused by microscopic deposits in the brain (Lewy bodies) that cause damage to nerve cells. In addition to classic symptoms of dementia, visual hallucinations are characteristic of this form of dementia. Many individuals with this form of dementia develop Parkinson-like symptoms, including slowness, limb and facial stiffness, and tremors.
- **Frontotemporal dementia,** formerly called *Pick's disease,* is a fairly uncommon form of dementia caused by the degeneration of the frontal and temporal lobes of the brain. This form of dementia is more likely to affect individuals under age 65.

Alzheimer's Disease

Alzheimer's disease (or **senile dementia, Alzheimer's type**), is the most common form of dementia and is typically seen in individuals older than 60 years of age. From age 65 onward, the incidence of Alzheimer's disease doubles approximately every 5 years. By age 85 as many as 50% of the population is affected. It is estimated that 4.5 million elderly men and women are affected in the United States and 24 million people worldwide. Researchers estimate that 81 million people worldwide will be affected by Alzheimer's disease or another form of dementia by 2040.

🌐 Cultural Considerations

Alzheimer's Disease

- Alzheimer's symptoms begin, on average, 7 years earlier in U.S. Latinos than in non-Latino whites. The incidence of Alzheimer's disease and related dementias in the Latino community is expected to increase dramatically during the first half of this century, rising from 200,000 today to over 1.3 million by 2050.
- A disproportionate number of African Americans suffer from Alzheimer's disease. African Americans were found to be three times more likely to develop Alzheimer's disease than Americans of European extraction. More accurate testing that is adapted to cultural differences provides better assessment of cognitive changes.
- Japanese-American men have a higher prevalence of Alzheimer's disease than do similar groups of men living in Japan. Among the Americans of Japanese descent, 9.3% were suffering from dementia of all causes and 5.4% had Alzheimer's disease.

Alzheimer's is a chronic, progressive, degenerative disease in which large numbers of brain cells and tissues are affected by atrophy, beta-amyloid plaques, and neurofibrillary tangles. The brain level of the neurotransmitter acetylcholine decreases, leading to a disturbed ability to reason and retain new information. Levels of norepinephrine and dopamine are also decreased in Alzheimer's disease.

The disease progresses from mild forgetfulness to a total loss of function. It is suspected that changes in the brain may begin up to 20 years before obvious symptoms are noticed. The disease follows a somewhat predictable course with increased severity of symptoms (see Box 10-5). The time from diagnosis to death ranges from the average of 8 years to more than 20 years (Figure 3-9). The financial and social costs of Alzheimer's disease are staggering, as evidenced by the following:

- The Alzheimer's Association and the National Institute on Aging estimate that the current cost of caring for individuals who suffer from Alzheimer's disease is at least $100 billion.
- An additional $65 billion is spent by businesses to cover the direct cost of health care, lost productivity, absenteeism, and worker replacement.
- The average lifetime cost of care for an individual with Alzheimer's disease is $174,000, although this may be higher in some parts of the country.

The cause of Alzheimer's disease is unknown. Some even question whether it is a single disease or whether varied forms exist. Extensive research is taking place

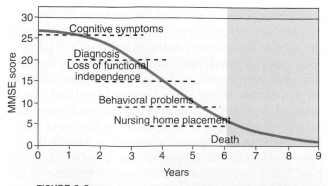

FIGURE 3-9 Typical Progression of Alzheimer's disease.

worldwide to identify a cause so that a cure can then be found. Genetics is believed to be a risk factor for the development of Alzheimer's disease. Children of people with Alzheimer's disease have four times the risk for developing the disease. The apolipoprotein E (ApoE) gene has been implicated as a risk factor; however, everyone has apolipoprotein E. It is estimated that about 15% of the population has the genetic form of ApoE, which increases the risk for Alzheimer's disease. The fact that a person has the affected gene does not mean that person will develop the disease, but the risk is greater.

Other factors implicated in Alzheimer's include inflammatory processes, immunologic changes, elevated glucose levels such as those found with diabetes, severe hypertension, and traumatic head injuries. In addition to physiologic factors, scientists are studying diet, exercise, educational level, social activity patterns, and environmental factors to determine whether any identifiable lifestyle factors may contribute to the problems or help reduce the incidence or severity of the disease.

Physical examination and laboratory tests are typically performed to rule out reversible causes of dementia such as **hypothyroidism** or vitamin B_{12} deficiency. Empirical diagnosis is made based on the evaluation of behavioral changes; psychometric testing to measure memory, attention, and problem solving; and brain scans such as CT or PET.

Until very recently, no definitive diagnostic test for Alzheimer's disease existed. The only way to confirm the diagnosis was a postmortem examination of the brain tissues. In 2010 researchers in Belgium identified specific proteins that could not only be used diagnostically, but also had a high predictive significance for the development of this form of dementia. Spinal fluid levels that are low in beta amyloid proteins and high in tau proteins are highly indicative of Alzheimer's. Identified changes in these protein levels may precede the first classic symptoms of the disease by a decade. These tests are still in the research stage and are not available to the public. Much more work needs to be done. These studies and others offer promise of earlier detection, better treatment, and hope for a cure for this devastating illness.

Currently, older adults suffering from Alzheimer's disease are treated with several classifications of drugs. Cholinesterase inhibitors are used for patients with mild-to-moderate disease. These drugs are designed to prevent the breakdown of acetylcholine, the neurotransmitter that plays an important role in memory and thinking skills. Drugs in the class include donepezil (Aricept), rivastigmine (Exelon), and galantamine (Razadyne, formerly known as Reminyl). Tacrine hydrochloride (Cognex) was prescribed in the past but is no longer recommended because it can cause liver damage.

Another drug, memantine (Namenda), has been approved to treat moderate-to-severe Alzheimer's disease. This drug is believed to work by regulating the level of glutamate, a neurotransmitter that helps the brain process, store, and retrieve information. Drugs specific to Alzheimer's treatment are often supplemented with antidepressants, anxiolytics, and antipsychotics, which are prescribed based on behavioral or psychotic symptoms that frequently coexist with Alzheimer's symptoms.

Alternative Treatments for Alzheimer's Disease. Vitamins C and E, coenzyme Q10, selenium, ginkgo biloba, hyperazine A, and coral calcium have been recommended as "natural" remedies for the treatment of Alzheimer's disease. Doses are varied and have not been evaluated by the Food and Drug Administration for effectiveness or safety. Additionally many of the elderly, particularly those diagnosed with Alzheimer's disease have lower than normal levels of melatonin. Melatonin, a hormone secreted by the pineal gland, plays a role in sleep rhythms. There is potential but limited evidence that melatonin, which is available over the counter, or possibly new drugs that have more targeted responses might provide some benefits by improving sleep patterns and decreasing the incidence of the behavioral changes seen at the end of the day called "sundowning." Since "natural" remedies can interact with prescription medication these substances should only be used under the direction of the physician.

Clinical trials are being conducted to determine the benefits of a passive vaccine containing manufactured antibodies designed to change blood levels of beta-amyloid. Other research is focused on a vaccine designed to use antibodies to directly attack beta-amyloid plaques. Yet another group of researchers have identified a compound called *AF267B* that they believe will affect both the plaque and tangles classically observed in Alzheimer's disease. Perhaps one of these research projects or some other scientific breakthrough will bring an end to the scourge of Alzheimer's disease.

Transient Ischemic Attack

Transient ischemic attacks (TIAs) are brief episodes of cerebrovascular insufficiency that are usually the result of obstruction of the cerebral blood vessels. Such obstruction is usually caused by an embolus or atherosclerotic plaque. TIAs occur most commonly in middle-aged and older people.

TIAs occur without warning. Most episodes last a few minutes only, but some may persist as long as 24 hours. A person may have several attacks within a day or may go for months without experiencing another attack. A variety of symptoms may indicate a TIA. Common symptoms include blurred, tunnel, or double vision; blindness; vertigo; transient numbness and weakness; aphasia or slurred speech; and gait disturbances. The person generally remains conscious throughout the attack. The symptoms of TIAs disappear spontaneously and do not cause permanent neurologic damage.

TIAs may be warnings of an impending stroke, but this is not necessarily the case. Some individuals who suffer from TIAs never have a stroke.

Cerebrovascular Accident

A cerebrovascular accident (CVA), commonly called a *stroke*, is a disturbance of the blood supply to the brain. Most CVAs are related to atherosclerosis, hypertension, diabetes, or a combination of these. They can occur at any age, but they most commonly affect individuals older than age 65. CVAs are often fatal and are a leading natural cause of death in the United States. The likelihood of CVA fatality increases with advanced age. CVAs occur slightly more often in men than in women. African Americans are affected more often than other groups, possibly because there is a higher incidence of hypertension in the African-American population. Even when they are not fatal, CVAs are a leading cause of disability.

Several specific types of CVAs exist, categorized by the process that disturbs the blood flow: (1) cerebral infarction, caused by either an embolus or a thrombus, (2) cerebral insufficiency, resulting from atherosclerotic changes that restrict blood flow, or (3) cerebral hemorrhage, caused by weakened vessels or aneurysms that rupture spontaneously or as a result of hypertension.

If a CVA is suspected, care is directed at supporting essential life functions—maintaining an open airway, providing adequate oxygenation, and preventing trauma. Hospitalization is necessary during the acute post-CVA phase. The need for rehabilitation or extended care is determined by the physician and is based on the individual's particular situation. The onset of a CVA may be sudden, or symptoms may progress gradually. The nature of symptoms varies with the type of CVA, the area of the brain that is affected, and the extent of the damage (Boxes 3-6 and 3-7). Because the two sides of the brain serve very different functions, the symptoms depend on which side is affected. Effects of CVAs are contralateral: Damage to the right hemisphere affects the left side of the body; damage to the left hemisphere affects the right side of the body. Some individuals manifest mild symptoms, whereas in others the symptoms are more severe. A few victims of CVA recover completely, but most have some lingering deficits. Most improvement occurs within the first 6 months after a CVA. Any deficit lasting longer than 6 months is likely to be permanent. Recurrence of CVAs is common, and each occurrence is likely to cause additional problems.

Box 3-6 | Signs and Symptoms of Right Brain Hemisphere Damage

- Left hemiparesis (weakness of the left arm and/or leg)
- Impaired sense of humor
- Disorientation to time, place, and person
- Difficulty recognizing people
- Visual/spatial problems, including loss of depth perception
- Neglect of the left visual field (may not see objects or hazards on the left side of body)
- Loss of impulse control (may strike out, cry, or shout if upset)
- Unaware of neurologic function loss (may try to stand or walk despite hemiparesis)
- Poor judgment (may deny illness or problems or tend to overestimate the ability to perform activities)
- Inappropriate responses (may smile continually or demonstrate euphoric behavior even in serious or tragic situations)
- Confabulation (may make up detailed but inaccurate explanations to compensate for memory losses, which can be very believable to persons who are not aware of the facts)

Box 3-7 | Signs and Symptoms of Left Brain Hemisphere Damage

- Right hemiparesis (weakness of the right arm and/or leg)
- Language disturbances:
  Aphasia—defective or absent language skills that may be expressive (motor), in which words cannot be formed; receptive (sensory), in which language is not understood; or mixed, in which both processes are affected
  Agraphia—loss of the ability to write
  Alexia—inability to comprehend written words; reading problems
- Neglect of the right visual field (may not see objects or hazards on the right side of body)
- Behavior changes (slow, cautious, and anxious when attempting new activities)
- Mood changes (tendency toward worry or depression; verbalization of feelings of worthlessness or guilt; anger and frustration)

THE SPECIAL SENSES

The special senses, including sight, hearing, balance, smell, and taste, are integrally connected to the central nervous system by the cranial nerves. The other senses include touch, pressure, and proprioception, which is the awareness of body movement and position in space. These senses are the means by which we gather information from the world around us and about our relationship to this world. The special senses provide our first line of protection against hazards in the environment. Unless all of these senses function properly and provide us with good information, we are at risk for suffering from these hazards.

It is important to understand the visual and auditory changes that occur with aging, because these changes may have serious implications for safety. A great deal of the information in the world that we receive and respond to comes to us through our senses of sight and hearing. We may think older adults are confused or senile, when actually their sensory perceptions are merely impaired because of the changes associated with aging.

THE EYES

The **eyes** are two globe-shaped structures located in the orbits of the skull on each side of the nose. Because the eyes are so important, they have surrounding structures designed to protect them from both physical and biologic hazards.

The **eyelids** are controlled by skeletal muscle and are lined with a smooth mucous membrane called the **conjunctiva.** The eyelids can close; thus, they and the eyelashes located on their margins provide protection from dust and flying debris. Tears are produced by the **lacrimal glands** located at the upper and outer corners of the eye. These glands lubricate the eye, prevent particles of debris from scraping the surface, and inhibit the growth of bacteria by means of the enzyme **lysozyme.** Tears leave the eye at the medial corner through the **lacrimal sac** and the nasolacrimal duct that drains into the nose.

The eye itself is composed of three layers. The outermost layer, the **sclera** (commonly called the *white of the eye*), is composed of fibrous connective tissue and supports the inner structures of the eye. The anterior part of the sclera is the **cornea,** a transparent structure that **refracts,** or bends, light rays. The sclera contains small capillaries that are sometimes visible on its surface. The cornea does not contain any capillaries or nerves.

The middle layer of the eye, the **choroid,** contains pigments that absorb light and keep the interior of the eye dark. The choroid is highly vascular and supplies nourishment to the surrounding tissue. Located in the anterior portion of the choroid are the **iris** (the colored portion), the **pupil** (an opening in the iris through which light enters the eye), the **lens** (a transparent oval disk), and the **ciliary body** (muscles that change the shape of the lens to refract light waves). The lens does not contain any capillaries or nerves.

The innermost layer of the eye is the **retina.** This structure covers the posterior two-thirds of the eye and contains the visual receptors, highly specialized structures called **rods** and **cones.** These receptors use chemical changes in their pigments to detect light. Cones are most abundant near the center of the retina. They detect color and discriminate among different colors based on the wavelength of the incoming light. Rods are more abundant near the periphery of the retina and detect the presence or absence of light. Vitamin

A is essential to the formation of the pigment in the rods that enables their response. Rods are important for vision when there is limited light. Nerves in the retina transmit messages from the rods and cones to the optic nerve, which sends the information to the vision centers of the brain. The macula lutea (yellow spot) is a small area, less than 2 mm in size, located near the center of the retina that provides us with sharp central vision.

The greatest part of the eye mass is made up of two fluid-filled cavities. The small **anterior cavity** is located between the cornea and the lens, and it contains **aqueous humor,** a fluid formed by capillaries in the choroid. This fluid passes from the **posterior chamber** through the pupil to the **anterior chamber,** and it supplies the nourishment for the lens and cornea, which do not have a blood supply. Because aqueous humor is produced continuously, some must be absorbed or the amount of fluid becomes excessive. Normally, absorption takes place through small veins located at the juncture of the iris and cornea. The presence of excess fluid increases the pressure within the anterior chamber. The posterior cavity of the eye, the **vitreous,** is much larger and contains a gelatinous substance called the **vitreous humor.** Vitreous humor holds the retina in contact with the choroid of the eye.

REFRACTION

The eye functions much like a camera. Light waves enter the eye through the cornea and then pass through the aqueous humor, lens, and vitreous humor to the retina. When light waves strike the retina, they stimulate the receptors in the cones and rods. The rods react chemically to the amount of light and regulate nerve impulses to the brain based on this information. Different cones respond to different wavelengths of light rays (different colors) and thus determine the perceived color of objects. Based on information gathered from the rods and cones, the image projected on the retina is translated into nerve impulses by the retina, which then sends the information through the optic nerves to the visual centers of the cerebral cortex in the **occipital region.** The optic nerves from both eyes meet at the **optic chiasm** just under the pituitary gland. At the optic chiasm, the medial fibers (from the image on the part of the retina closest to the nose) cross to the opposite side of the brain, whereas the lateral fibers (from the outside part of the retina) do not cross. This allows visual centers on both sides of the brain to process messages from both eyes and is important for binocular vision. Because of position, each eye "sees" things somewhat differently from the other and sends slightly different messages to the brain. The brain receives messages from both eyes, correlates the information, and makes sense of it. Binocular vision is also important for **depth perception,** the sense of how far you are from another person or object.

For information to be received accurately, all of the eye's structures must function together to focus the light rays. The shape of the lens is controlled by the ciliary body, whose muscles relax or contract to change the shape of the lens so that it can bend the light waves correctly and bring an object into clear focus. This change in lens shape is called **accommodation.**

EXPECTED AGE-RELATED CHANGES

Refractive errors, or errors in focusing ability, occur when the cornea is misshapen or when the lens cannot appropriately change shape to focus images.

With aging, many structural and functional changes may occur in the eye (see Table 3-9). The eyelids become less elastic and sag. Eyelashes tend to be shorter, thinner, and in some cases, absent. A grayish haze of the peripheral cornea, **arcus senilis** (Figure 3-10),

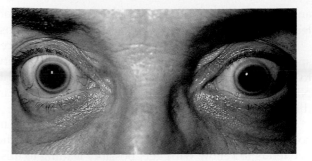

FIGURE 3-10 Arcus senilis.

develops with aging and is more common in dark-skinned persons.

Legal blindness is defined as visual acuity of 20/200 or less in the worse eye, even with the best correction or a visual field extent of less than 20 degrees in diameter. Vision impairment is defined as having vision worse than 20/40 with correction. The rate of legal blindness and visual impairment increases significantly in later years of life, particularly after age 75. According to research done by the National Eye Institute, blindness affects blacks more than whites or Hispanics, whereas Hispanics have higher rates of visual impairment than people of other races.

Refractive errors are the most common visual problem in the United States. Most people older than 50 years of age experience some degree of farsightedness, also called *hyperopia* or *presbyopia*, which literally means "elderly eye." Refractive errors become increasingly common as the ciliary muscles lose their ability to contract easily, and progressive rigidity of the lens restricts accommodation. A combination of these changes makes it increasingly difficult to focus on close objects, perform detailed close work, or read. Presbyopia is usually corrected by the use of contact lenses or eye glasses that help the aging person focus on close objects. Laser surgery is also an option for some individuals.

Astigmatism, a malformation of the cornea, causes blurring of images at all distances. People of all ages can have astigmatism, but younger people compensate for it by quickly refocusing the blurred and unblurred images. When this ability decreases with aging, astigmatism appears to worsen. Corrective lenses help with this.

A decrease in tear production is common in older adults because the volume of body fluids and secretions decreases with age. An 80-year-old person produces only 25% of the tears he or she produced during the teenage years. Environmental factors such as central heating, dry climate, and wind or air pollution can further aggravate the problem. Many older adults complain of dry, burning, or itching eyes caused by friction from the lids or from small particles of debris. The decline in tear production also reduces the

Table 3-9	Vision Changes Associated With Aging
PHYSIOLOGIC CHANGE	**RESULTS**
Decreased number of eyelashes	Increased risk for eye injury
Decreased tear production	Increased risk for eye irritation
Increased discoloration of lens	Decreased color perception
Decreased tissue elasticity	Increased blurring
Decreased muscle tone	Decreased diameter of pupil; increased refractive errors; decreased night vision; increased sensitivity to glare, decreased peripheral vision

NURSING ASSESSMENTS AND CARE STRATEGIES RELATED TO VISUAL CHANGES	
NURSING ASSESSMENTS	**CARE STRATEGIES**
Assess for signs of irritation, inflammation, and dryness.	Encourage regular use of synthetic tear preparations to help reduce irritation due to inadequate tear production.
Assess visual acuity.	Encourage or schedule regular professional eye examinations. Educate regarding importance of adequate light with minimum glare. Explain importance of using eye glasses appropriately for reading or distance, particularly when driving.
Assess ability to detect objects within the environment.	Provide adequate lighting and contrast in colors to highlight important structures such as the edge of stairs, light fixtures, faucets, etc.

antibacterial protection provided by enzymes and can lead to decreased resistance to bacterial eye infections.

Older adults may have poor **dark adaptation** responses and may experience a decrease in the ability to adjust from light to darkness and darkness to light. **Night blindness,** the inability to see well at night or in dim light, grows increasingly common with aging.

Color vision and the ability to detect changes in color contrast are affected by aging. The lens of the eye tends to yellow with age, possibly leading to misperception of colors. All dark colors may be perceived as black, and subtle differences in shades may not be detectable. Younger people who find "blue-haired women" amusing should look at them through a lens that is slightly tinted yellow. Amazingly, the hair looks clean and white.

Peripheral vision and depth perception often decrease with aging. It is important to recognize these changes because they significantly increase the risk for accidents and injuries.

Another common occurrence with aging is **floaters.** Many older adults report seeing flecks, spots, cobwebs, or brilliant crystals within their eyes. These are harmless but can be frustrating because they interfere with many visual activities such as reading, sewing, or doing other detailed work.

COMMON DISORDERS SEEN WITH AGING

Blepharitis

Blepharitis, a chronic inflammation of the eyelids, is one of the most common disorders of the eye. Symptoms of blepharitis include burning, itching, and sensitivity to light. Discomfort is often worse on awakening. Blepharitis can be caused by *Staphylococcus* bacteria, by sebaceous gland dysfunction, or in conjunction with skin conditions such as seborrhea or rosacea. There is no definitive cure for this disorder, but treatment can reduce the severity of the problem. Common treatment includes the use of warm compresses, eyelid massage, lid scrubs, and the use of antibiotic ointments. Dietary intake of antioxidants has been proposed as being of some benefit.

Diplopia

Diplopia, or double vision, is not normal and indicates some disturbance of the nervous system that requires further investigation by a physician.

Cataracts

Cataracts, which cause a clouding of the lens of the eye, are increasingly common with aging. Studies done in the United States show that 5% of people between 52 and 62 years of age develop cataracts. By age 75 to 85, the incidence of cataracts increases to 46%. Factors that increase the risk for cataracts include (1) female gender, (2) sunlight exposure, (3) myopia, (4) steroid use, (5) tobacco exposure, (6) eye trauma, and (7)

diabetes. Cataracts develop over time and result in progressive, painless loss of vision. The amount of vision loss depends on the degree of lens opacity and the area of the lens that is affected. Vision in bright light or glare may be particularly difficult with certain types of cataracts. Individuals with cataracts require frequent changes in eyeglass prescriptions while the cataract matures. When vision is severely affected, surgical removal of the cataract or the lens is the medical treatment of choice. Today, this surgery is common and, in most cases, can be performed on an outpatient basis. Once the cataract is removed, vision is corrected by means of surgically implanted lenses, contact lenses, or cataract glasses.

Glaucoma

Glaucoma is a disease characterized in most cases by increased fluid pressure (intraocular pressure) within the eye that may result in damage to the retina. Initially, peripheral vision is affected. Tunnel vision and, eventually, permanent blindness may result. The incidence of glaucoma increases with age. Additional risk factors include family history, diabetes, African-American ancestry, hypertension, and steroid use.

Persons with glaucoma seldom experience obvious symptoms, so serious damage usually occurs before the disease is even recognized. However, a test for increased intraocular pressure can be performed easily. The test for glaucoma is simple, painless, and takes only minutes. It is normally part of a routine ophthalmic examination, and everyone older than 40 years of age should be tested routinely for glaucoma. Early detection and treatment can delay progression of the disease. Medications, surgery, and laser therapy can be used to treat glaucoma, but any damage already done cannot be reversed.

Age-Related Macular Degeneration and Retinal Detachment

The **macula,** the small area in the center of the retina where visual acuity is best, is susceptible to damage and destruction. **Age-related macular degeneration** (AMD) occurs most often in people over age 50. The incidence of this disorder increases significantly after age 75 and is more common in women. It is more common in fair-haired, blue-eyed individuals and those who smoked or had excessive exposure to sunlight. The exact cause of macular degeneration remains unknown, but two types of the disorder have been identified. The atrophic form, also called *dry AMD,* is a result of inadequate nutrient supply or waste removal resulting from vascular changes. When cells atrophy or die, the macula is damaged and central vision is significantly diminished. Vision is restricted but not totally lost, because noncentral vision remains. Although not scientifically proven, antioxidants such as vitamins C and E, beta carotene, lycopene, and zinc supplements appear to have some protective, if not therapeutic, benefits. Use of these substances, particularly in megadoses, should be done under the direction of a physician only.

The neovascular form of macular degeneration, also called *wet AMD*, results from abnormal growth of tiny blood vessels under the retina. These vessels ruin vision by leaking fluid and blood, which cause the retina to become swollen and distorted. This form is more likely to cause severe vision loss. Laser surgery or microsurgery may be attempted to seal leaking vessels, slow their growth, and prevent further vision loss.

Circulatory changes in the blood vessels of the eyes are common with DM, resulting in a condition called **diabetic retinopathy.** This condition is characterized by the hemorrhaging of small blood vessels into the vitreous humor and has effects similar to neovascular macular degeneration (i.e., loss of vision). Patients with diabetes are two to three times more likely to develop blindness resulting from retinopathy. Retinopathy is related not to age but rather to the severity and duration of hyperglycemia. More diabetic retinopathy is seen in older adults because of the higher incidence of diabetes with aging.

Normal shrinkage of the eye and changes in the consistency of the vitreous humor are common with aging and may result in **retinal detachment,** which is the separation of the retina from the choroid. Any or all of these changes can result in the loss of central vision.

THE EARS

The ear is composed of three distinct portions: **outer ear, middle ear,** and **inner ear.** The two main functions of the ear are the detection of sound and the maintenance of balance.

The outer ear consists of the visible curved structure, called the **pinna,** or **auricle,** and the **external ear canal.** The pliable auricle is made of cartilage. The size or shape of the external ear has little influence on hearing.

The middle ear begins at the **eardrum,** or **tympanic membrane.** This transparent membrane stretches across the end of the ear canal and separates it from an air-filled chamber called the **middle ear.** Air pressure in the middle ear is controlled through the **Eustachian tube,** which connects the middle ear to the nasopharynx. Attached to the tympanic membrane is a series of three small bones, the **malleus** (hammer), **incus** (anvil), and **stapes** (stirrup). Sound waves enter the ear through the external ear canal and cause the tympanic membrane to vibrate. This, in turn, causes movement of the three small bones, which then transmit the vibrations to the **oval window,** the opening into the inner ear.

The inner ear is a complex, fluid-filled structure that has several functions. A portion called the **cochlea** contains the hearing receptors, which consist of hair cells with fine movable projections that are set in motion when sound waves reach their fluid surroundings. When these hairs move, impulses are carried through the auditory nerve (a cranial nerve) to the midbrain and then to the temporal lobe of the brain, where the sound is heard.

Other specialized hair cells are found elsewhere in the inner ear: the vestibule and the **semicircular canals.** Hair cells from these structures transmit information in response to gravity, change of position, and motion through the cranial nerves. The central nervous system processes this information and maintains equilibrium.

EXPECTED AGE-RELATED CHANGES

Just as other body tissues become thinner with age, so does the tympanic membrane (Table 3-10). The small muscles that support the membrane show signs of atrophy with advanced age. Arthritic changes affect the joints between the small bones of the middle ear, and hair cells in the inner ear often deteriorate.

Table 3-10 Auditory Changes Associated With Aging	
PHYSIOLOGIC CHANGE	**RESULTS**
Decreased tissue elasticity	Decreased ability to distinguish high-frequency sounds
Decreased joint mobility	Decreased hearing ability
Decreased ceruminous cells in external ear canal	Increased risk for cerumen impaction causing conductive hearing loss
Atrophy of vestibular structures and in the inner ear	Increased problems with balance; decreased number of hair cells
NURSING ASSESSMENTS AND CARE STRATEGIES RELATED TO AUDITORY CHANGES	
NURSING ASSESSMENTS	**CARE STRATEGIES**
Assess hearing and balance.	Refer for audiometric testing as needed.
Inspect ear canal for cerumen impaction.	Administration of prophylactic drops may reduce likelihood of impaction formation. Irrigation may be needed if impaction is present.
Assess functioning of hearing aid if used.	Check that batteries are working and that device is not plugged with cerumen. Keep an amplifying device on each patient care unit to use with hard of hearing individuals who do not have a functional hearing aid.
Assess for social isolation or behavioral background noise.	Encourage socialization in areas without excessive changes.

Presbycusis, defined as an alteration in the hearing capacity related to aging, affects an estimated 13% of people older than 65 years of age. Men appear to be more affected by this problem than women. The aging person with presbycusis loses the ability to perceive tones of higher frequencies. Speech sounds such as *s, sh, ch,* and soft *t* may not be audible, so the aging person may hear only parts of spoken words. Simple words such as *cat, hat, sat,* and *that* may all sound the same. If other noises are present in the environment, sounds become even less distinct. The aging individual may have difficulty sorting out words and making sense of what is being said.

COMMON DISORDERS SEEN WITH AGING

Otosclerosis

Otosclerosis, a hardening or fixing of the stapes to the oval window, interferes with sound wave transmission into the inner ear. This condition occurs slightly more often in women than in men. Surgical correction is possible.

Tinnitus

Tinnitus, or ringing in the ears, is commonly reported by aging people. Tinnitus may be a result of trauma to the ear, pressure from cerumen against the eardrum, otosclerosis, presbycusis, or Ménière's disease. Tinnitus can also be caused by certain medications.

Deafness

Deafness, the inability to hear sounds fully, may be temporary or permanent, depending on the cause. Deafness can be unilateral, affecting one ear only, or bilateral, affecting both ears.

Conductive hearing loss occurs when something interferes with transmission of the sound waves. A plug of **cerumen** (earwax) in the external canal, rupture or scarring of the eardrum, the presence of fluid or an infection in the middle ear, or any condition that interferes with movement of the small bones of the middle ear may result in conductive hearing loss or deafness.

Nerve or sensorineural deafness occurs when either the receptors in the inner ear or the cranial nerves are damaged or destroyed. Some antibiotics and viral infections can cause nerve deafness. Chronic exposure to loud noise can speed up the degeneration of the hair cells. Many young people today are experiencing significant hearing loss from excessive exposure to extremely loud music, and this will have serious implications as they age. Work-related noise has also been shown to have negative effects on hearing. Many aging individuals who worked in foundries or other noisy places may have suffered employment-related hearing loss. The Occupational Safety and Health Administration now requires employers to protect employees from excessive exposure to loud noise on the job.

Central deafness is caused by trauma or disease in the temporal lobes of the brain. This may be a result of tumors, CVA, or injury. Central deafness is not common.

Ménière's Disease

Ménière's disease is a fairly common chronic disorder of the inner ear observed in people older than 40 or 50 years of age. Persons suffering from this disorder experience severe vertigo (not simple dizziness) to the point that they may be unable to stand or walk. They may also report nausea, tinnitus, hearing loss, and a sensation of pressure in the ear. Diaphoresis, vomiting, and nystagmus (rapid, involuntary eye movement) may also be observed. Episodes generally appear suddenly and may last for minutes or hours. The frequency of attacks is unpredictable. Ménière's disease tends to affect one ear, and it can result in nerve deafness that sometimes persists even if treatment relieves the other symptoms.

TASTE AND SMELL

The receptors for our sense of taste are located in the papillae, or taste buds, on the superior surface of the tongue. In these papillae are chemical receptor cells that are sensitive to salty, sweet, sour, and bitter chemicals. When mixed with moisture such as saliva or water, food releases chemicals that are detected by these receptors. Foods get their subtle flavors by their unique interaction with various receptors. The detection of odors occurs when the olfactory receptors in the upper nasal cavities respond to airborne chemicals. When vapors escape from food or other volatile substances, they enter the nose and stimulate the receptors.

Information from both taste and smell receptors is then transported to the nervous system through the cranial nerves. When these senses are intact and functioning well, many people salivate and can "taste" a meal while it is being prepared. Without a sense of smell, food has little flavor. Most of us have had severe nasal congestion from colds or allergies, and have found that without smell, food has either a strange taste or no taste at all. Some individuals with chronic nasal congestion report ongoing problems with appetite because food has little flavor or appeal. People with permanent damage to the olfactory senses report a permanent change in taste (hypogeusia) that often results in a loss of appetite. Alterations in taste sensation may also be a side effect of brain tumors, gingival disease, periodontitis, systemic disorders such as DM or hypothyroidism, and medications. Research is being conducted to determine the correlation between loss of smell and the onset of Alzheimer's disease.

Table 3-11	Olfactory Changes Associated With Aging
PHYSIOLOGIC CHANGE	**RESULTS**
Decreased number of papillae on tongue	Decreased ability to taste
Decreased number of nasal sensory	Decreased ability to receptors and to detect smells
NURSING ASSESSMENTS AND CARE STRATEGIES RELATED TO OLFACTORY CHANGES	
NURSING ASSESSMENTS	**CARE STRATEGIES**
Assess ability to smell and taste.	Teach importance of storing food properly. Keep drugs and chemicals separated from foods.

EXPECTED AGE-RELATED CHANGES

With aging, there is a decrease in the number of functional receptors in both the nasal cavities and papillae on the tongue (Table 3-11). By age 60 it is estimated that half of adults will experience some alteration in smell and taste. The changes in taste particularly affect the receptors for sweet and salty tastes. Because salt enhances the flavor of food, older adults often add salt in an attempt to add flavor. Complaints of flavorless food are common even if the food seems well seasoned and tasty to younger individuals. Good oral hygiene, better food preparation, and flavor enhancers are sometimes helpful in improving taste.

The term **burning mouth syndrome** is used to describe the oral sensation of burning or tingling. This may be associated with a vitamin B deficiency, inadequate saliva production, allergies, GERD, trauma, and diabetes.

THE ENDOCRINE SYSTEM

The endocrine system and the nervous system perform the major integrating and regulating functions of the body. The endocrine glands secrete chemical substances called **hormones** to regulate body processes. Hormones are secreted directly into the capillaries of the bloodstream, where they circulate until they reach their target organs and cause specific effects. Some endocrine glands produce a single hormone; others produce several different hormones. Some hormones have one target organ only; others target multiple organs. The production of hormones is regulated by a negative feedback process in which the endocrine glands constantly monitor the effects of hormones circulating in the system. If the effect is adequate, the gland decreases production. If it is inadequate, the gland increases production. The process of regulation is similar to a system consisting of a thermostat and a furnace in a home. When the temperature reaches that for which the thermostat is set, the thermostat signals the furnace to stop producing heat. If the temperature drops below the preset level, the thermostat signals the furnace to produce more heat. In a highly complex manner, the endocrine glands constantly monitor the effects and the levels of the many hormones circulating in the body and increase or decrease production as needed to meet body demands.

PITUITARY GLAND

The pituitary gland is often referred to as the *master gland* of the body because of the many functions it regulates. It is located within the skull cavity and is connected directly to the hypothalamus. There are two major segments of the pituitary gland: the **anterior pituitary** and the **posterior pituitary.** The posterior pituitary is the site of connection between the nervous system and the endocrine system. The posterior pituitary hormones are actually produced in the hypothalamus of the brain and are stored in the posterior pituitary until needed. The major secretion of the posterior pituitary gland is the **antidiuretic hormone.** This hormone maintains fluid balance in the body by causing the kidneys to reabsorb fluid; in the absence of the antidiuretic hormone, the kidneys excrete more fluid. By controlling fluid balance, the antidiuretic hormone aids in the maintenance of blood pressure. Oxytocin, another hormone of the posterior pituitary gland, stimulates the contraction of the uterus during childbirth and ejection of milk from the breast during lactation.

The anterior pituitary produces many hormones. **Growth hormone** increases the rate of protein synthesis and aids in the transport of amino acids to cells. In adults, this hormone also participates in fat release from adipose tissue and the use of this fat as an energy source. **Thyroid-stimulating hormone** stimulates the normal growth and activity of the thyroid gland. Adrenocorticotropic hormone (corticotropin) stimulates the activity of the adrenal cortex. **Gonadotropic hormones** include follicle-stimulating hormone and **luteinizing hormone,** which are responsible for the maturation and function of the gonads, and **prolactin,** which supports lactation.

THYROID GLAND

The **thyroid gland** surrounds the trachea and is located just below the larynx (voice box). The major hormones produced by the thyroid gland are **thyroxin,** triiodothyronine, and **calcitonin.** The thyroid hormones triiodothyronine and thyroxin increase the rate of metabolism; regulate the metabolism of fat, carbohydrates, and protein in the cells; and increase body temperature. They also affect cardiac, neurologic, and musculoskeletal functions. The function of calcitonin is to keep calcium and phosphate within the bone matrix.

PARATHYROID GLANDS

The **parathyroid glands** are located on the posterior surface of the lobes of the thyroid gland. **PTH,** an antagonist of calcitonin, stimulates the movement of calcium and phosphorus from the bones into the blood.

PANCREAS

The **pancreas** is both an exocrine and an endocrine gland. It functions as an exocrine gland during digestion. The endocrine secretions of the pancreas are produced by α cells and β cells in the islets of Langerhans. The α cells produce glucagon, which stimulates the liver to convert glycogen to glucose. The β cells produce insulin, which increases the permeability of cell membranes and enables the cells to use glucose, amino acids, and fatty acids.

ADRENAL GLANDS

The **adrenal glands** are located on the top of each kidney. The **adrenal medulla** is the inner portion of the gland, and the **adrenal cortex** is the outer portion. The adrenal medulla secretes **epinephrine** and norepinephrine, which are the major neurotransmitters of the sympathetic portion of the autonomic nervous system. Thus, hormone release from the adrenal medulla has effects similar to those of the sympathetic nervous system. These hormones help the body cope with stressors by decreasing functions that are not required for the fight-or-flight response and by increasing cardiac activity, blood pressure, release of energy reserves, and other functions necessary for survival when faced with danger.

The adrenal cortex releases **mineralocorticoids, glucocorticoids,** and small amounts of sex hormones. The mineralocorticoid aldosterone is important in the regulation of fluid and electrolyte balance and the maintenance of blood pressure. The glucocorticoid **cortisol** is involved in the conversion of glycogen to glucose and in antiinflammatory activities. DHEA, dehydroepiandrosterone, is a hormone that the body can convert into estrogen and testosterone. Production of this hormone increases dramatically at puberty and peaks in the mid twenties. Levels then decrease over the years so only about 20% remains by age 70. Use of this hormone and its analog DHEA-S, dehydroepiandrosterone sulfate, has been evaluated as possible treatment for aging or at least for some of the negative consequences of aging. Most scientific studies have shown no significant benefits.

OVARIES AND TESTES

The **testes** and **ovaries** secrete the hormones involved in sexual maturation and function. The primary hormones secreted by the ovaries are **estrogen** and progesterone. These hormones are responsible for maturation of the ova, stimulation of the uterine endometrium, and the development of the secondary female sexual characteristics. The testes secrete the major male sex hormone, **testosterone,** which is responsible for the maturation of sperm and for the development of the secondary male sexual characteristics.

EXPECTED AGE-RELATED CHANGES

With aging, a variety of changes occurs in the endocrine function (Table 3-12). The pituitary gland continues to produce adequate levels of critical hormones throughout life. It produces less growth hormone as we age, leading to a decrease in muscle mass. In recent studies, the growth hormone was administered to older men, who then showed significant increases in muscle mass. Growth hormone is expensive, may have undesirable side effects, and is currently an investigational drug.

A decrease in the production of thyroid-stimulating hormone is seen in some older adults. Basal metabolic rate begins to decrease in young adulthood and continues to decrease gradually throughout the remainder of life. Because lean body mass also decreases, the overall metabolic rate does not change significantly. In response to a decreased thyroid function, some older people become more sensitive to cooler temperatures.

Table 3-12	Endocrine Changes Associated With Aging
PHYSIOLOGIC CHANGE	**RESULTS**
Decreased pituitary secretions (growth hormone)	Decreased muscle mass
Decreased production of thyroid-stimulating hormone	Decreased metabolic rate
Decreased insulin production or increased insulin resistance	Increased risk for type 2 diabetes mellitus
Decreased production of parathyroid hormone	Increased blood calcium levels (seen with osteoporosis)
NURSING ASSESSMENTS AND CARE STRATEGIES RELATED TO ENDOCRINE CHANGES	
NURSING ASSESSMENTS	**CARE STRATEGIES**
Monitor laboratory values, paying special attention to minerals such as calcium and sodium levels and blood glucose.	Educate patient regarding dietary needs and self-testing of blood glucose.
Assess for body temperature, weight, hair distribution or behavioral changes which may indicate endocrine imbalance.	Notify physician of assessment findings.

Studies of parathyroid function reveal conflicting information. PTH appears to decrease with age, except in cases of osteoporosis, where it appears to increase. Elevated levels of PTH may lead to increased blood calcium levels. This is of concern particularly for older women, who may manifest symptoms of confusion, kidney stones, and osteoporosis.

Pancreatic function appears to decrease with aging; however, barring the onset of some form of DM, its function remains adequate to meet normal body functioning.

Adrenal function is not altered significantly with advancing age. Adequate hormone levels are produced to meet bodily needs.

The levels of gonadotropic hormones decrease more significantly in women than in men. After menopause, estrogen and progesterone production drops significantly. As the production of female sex hormones decreases with aging, some changes in secondary sexual characteristics may be observed, such as the development of facial hair and genital atrophy. Studies indicate that estrogen depletion in postmenopausal women has negative effects on bone density, cardiovascular function, memory, and cognition (see the Complementary and Alternative Therapies box). Because production of the male hormone testosterone decreases gradually with aging, changes are gradual and often indistinguishable.

Complementary and Alternative Therapies

Hormone Replacement Therapy and Human Growth Hormone

Research is being done to determine the safety and effectiveness of various hormone replacement therapies (HRTs) in slowing or reversing common physiologic changes seen with aging. Estrogen replacement therapy, long thought to prevent cardiac problems and osteoporosis, vaginal discomfort, and skin changes in women, has recently come under scrutiny. Research shows that HRT does not protect the heart as once believed (American College of Obstetricians and Gynecologists, 2002). In fact, it has been shown to increase the risk for many problems, including the following:

- Cardiac disease
- Blood clots
- Liver and gallbladder disease
- Hypertension
- Cancer

Human growth-hormone therapy, which can cost up to $15,000 per year, has been marketed as a "cure" for aging. Proponents say that it is a veritable "fountain of youth" that provides the following benefits:

- Increased muscle mass
- Increased bone mass
- Improved energy by expanding cardiac and pulmonary function
- Extended life span

In fact, some propose that growth-hormone replacement therapy should start earlier in life to produce maximal benefits. Opponents state that this therapy is not a panacea. They believe it is essential to consider the risks and side effects of growth-hormone therapy, which include the following:

- Fluid retention
- Increased blood pressure
- Increased incidence of cancer

Use of hypothalamic hormones is now under study, but no conclusive information is available.

Supplementary use of DHEA and DHEA-S has shown little or no conclusive evidence of anti-aging benefits. Short-term use has not shown significant adverse effects but long-term use has not been proven safe. A physician should be consulted before use.

COMMON DISORDERS SEEN WITH AGING

Diabetes Mellitus

The incidence of DM increases with age. The likelihood of acquiring diabetes doubles with each decade of life. The American Diabetes Association cites that in 2009 about 23% of persons older than 60 years of age have diabetes, primarily type 2. Other studies indicate that 43% of those diagnosed with diabetes were older than age 85.

DM is a disease with multiple causes that is characterized by abnormal metabolism of carbohydrates, protein, and fats, resulting in elevated plasma glucose levels. Long-term complications include retinopathy (resulting in a loss of vision), nephropathy (resulting in renal failure), peripheral neuropathy (resulting in foot ulcers and amputation), autonomic neuropathy (resulting in GI, genitourinary, and cardiovascular symptoms and sexual dysfunction), atherosclerotic vascular problems (resulting in an increased incidence of cardiovascular, cerebrovascular, and peripheral vascular disease), hypertension, cognitive changes, and periodontal disease.

The most current classification system categorizes DM according to its etiology, or cause. The first category, **type 1** diabetes mellitus, is defined as being a result of either autoimmune destruction of the β cells of the pancreas or unknown idiopathic causes. The second category, **type 2** diabetes mellitus, results from a combination of resistance to insulin action and inadequate compensatory insulin secretion. In the third category, **other specific types** of DM are identified by their unique etiologies, including genetic defects or syndromes, exocrine diseases of the pancreas, diseases of the endocrine system, drugs or chemicals, infections, or other uncommon immune-mediated disorders. A fourth category, **gestational** diabetes mellitus, exists only during pregnancy. This classification system replaces the older system (insulin-dependent diabetes mellitus, or IDDM, and noninsulin-dependent diabetes mellitus, or NIDDM), which was based on the treatment method used.

Diagnosis of DM is made based on symptoms and on the determination of elevated plasma glucose levels. A casual (no specific relation to meals) plasma glucose level of 200 mg/dl or higher, particularly when symptoms are present, warrants further testing. This can be done using the oral glucose tolerance test or the fasting plasma glucose (FPG) level (no calorie intake for at least 8 hours). The FPG level is the more commonly accepted test because it is less costly and less time-consuming. FPG levels less than 110 mg/dl are classified as normal. FPG levels between 110 and 126 mg/dl are classified as impaired fasting glucose. FPG levels of 126 mg/dl or higher warrant a provisional diagnosis of diabetes. Abnormal results must be confirmed on a subsequent day to make the diagnosis.

Type 1 Diabetes Mellitus. Type 1 DM can occur at any age, but its onset is usually before age 25. Approximately 10% to 15% of people with diabetes have type 1 DM. Type 1 DM typically has a sudden onset, but it may occur slowly, depending on the rate at which the pancreatic β cells are destroyed. People suffering from type 1 DM produce little or no insulin because of β-cell destruction. Absolute lack of insulin production results in excessively high levels of glucose in the blood (hyperglycemia) and leads to the classic symptoms of diabetes. Symptoms include **polyuria** (excessive and frequent urination), **polydipsia** (excessive thirst), and **polyphagia** (excessive appetite). Even with increased food and fluid intake, the person with type 1 DM may lose weight.

The patient with type 1 DM is prone to further metabolic problems. When the body is unable to use glucose because of inadequate insulin production, starvation at the cellular level occurs. The body may attempt to meet cell needs by using fat or muscle as a source of fuel. This results in an accumulation of **ketones** (by-products of incomplete metabolism of fatty acids) in the bloodstream. As the blood ketone level increases, the acid-base balance is altered, the blood becomes too acidic, and a condition called **ketoacidosis** occurs. The body attempts to maintain acid-base balance through the compensatory systems of the kidneys and lungs. When a severe imbalance occurs, **ketonuria** may occur, and acetone (or "apple pie") breath may be detected. Severe acidemia can result in a deep and rapid pattern of breathing called **Kussmaul's respirations.** If not recognized and treated, type 1 DM results in death.

Type 1 DM requires continuous, careful monitoring and medical supervision. Treatment involves a careful balance of diet, insulin therapy, exercise, and stress management. Each patient requires an individualized program that meets his or her particular needs.

Changes in diet or activity, infections, and stress can easily cause problems for the patient with type 1 diabetes. The plasma glucose levels of a patient receiving insulin therapy must be monitored closely. Plasma glucose levels may be determined by the laboratory or by a variety of self-testing devices. Any significant changes in plasma glucose levels should be reported promptly to the physician.

Patients with type 1 diabetes who live independently must be taught the importance of following the prescribed balance of diet, insulin, and exercise. They should be strongly urged to call the doctor immediately if they have any signs of infection, particularly any infection that results in vomiting. Special medical identification bracelets or necklaces are advisable. Such devices can help ensure that proper care is provided in emergencies.

Type 2 Diabetes Mellitus. The form of DM that is most often observed in older adults is type 2 DM, which accounts for 85% to 90% of all persons with diabetes. This form of DM is more commonly observed in individuals who are older than 40 years of age, who are obese, or whose family history includes type 2 DM. The symptoms of type 2 DM are usually mild and unrecognized by an aging person. Diagnosis often occurs during routine medical visits or when the person seeks medical attention for visual disturbances, delayed wound healing, or recurrent vaginal or yeast infections.

With type 2 DM, the individual may have normal or even elevated levels of insulin. Despite these normal levels, glucose does not enter the cells normally. It is suspected that a problem with the receptor sites on the cells prevents normal cellular functioning in these individuals.

Physicians prefer to control type 2 DM by dietary means. Weight loss is encouraged because it often results in a spontaneous decrease in plasma blood glucose levels. If diet alone is not successful, oral hypoglycemic agents may be prescribed. When under physical stress resulting from infection or surgery, persons with type 2 DM may experience abnormally high plasma glucose levels. In these cases, the classic symptoms of DM may occur, and the person may require insulin administration to maintain normal plasma glucose levels. Once these levels are normal and the stressor is removed, insulin administration is typically discontinued. Plasma glucose levels should be monitored frequently to ensure that they remain within normal limits.

Long-term glycemic control is monitored using the glycated hemoglobin A1C. An A1C of 7% or less is desirable. Good glucose control has been shown to reduce the risk of vascular complications.

Hypoglycemia

Hypoglycemia is a potentially serious problem for people receiving insulin or oral hypoglycemic agents. Classic signs of hypoglycemia include headache, nausea, weakness, tremors or trembling sensations, pallor, anxiety, irritability, tachycardia, sweating, and hunger. Many of these symptoms can be easily missed or misinterpreted in the older adult population. If hypoglycemia is suspected, the plasma glucose level should be measured promptly. Treatment is based on the specific plasma glucose level. Those with levels of

40 to 60 mg/dl respond best to foods such as milk and crackers, and those with levels of 20 to 40 mg/dl respond best to refined carbohydrates such as honey, juice, or sugar. If unconscious, the patient is treated with an intramuscular injection of glucagon or an intravenous infusion of 50% glucose. Individuals who are prone to hypoglycemia should be taught to carry a carbohydrate source, such as hard candy or glucose tablets.

Hypothyroidism

Reduced function of the thyroid gland, called *primary hypothyroidism,* is more common in older than in younger persons. The symptoms of hypothyroidism include cold intolerance, dry skin, dry and thin body hair, constipation, depression, and lack of energy. Because many of these changes are commonly observed with aging, the changes may not be recognized as signs of hypothyroidism. Diagnosis is made by means of blood tests. Treatment of hypothyroidism with very high levels of thyroid hormone has been shown to reduce bone density in older women but not in older men.

THE REPRODUCTIVE AND GENITOURINARY SYSTEMS

In both men and women, the genital and urinary systems are located close to each other. As mentioned previously, many structures in men are used for both the sexual and elimination functions. In women, the structures of elimination are completely separate from those of reproduction.

FEMALE REPRODUCTIVE ORGANS

The primary female sexual organs include the **ovaries, fallopian tubes, uterus,** and **vagina.** These structures, which are necessary for normal human reproduction, are located in the pelvic cavity between the bladder and the bowels. It is important to visualize their location to understand the symptoms that may occur if the size, shape, or position of these organs changes. During the reproductive years, the ovaries produce the hormones estrogen and progesterone. Under the influence of these hormones, the ova mature in the ovaries, and the endometrium of the uterus changes in vascularity to support a possible pregnancy. When a woman reaches menopause (sometime between 45 and 60 years of age), the hormonal function of the ovaries decreases and then ceases. This physiologic timing of the end of reproduction probably developed because it increased the likelihood that the mother would live to see her children reach maturity. Recent technology and extensive medical intervention can allow pregnancies to occur after menopause, but the number of women who choose to become pregnant this late in life is probably not significant. Most women who reach menopause are either resigned or delighted to reach the end of the reproductive stage.

MALE REPRODUCTIVE ORGANS

The male organs of reproduction consist of the **testes,** a series of ducts and glands, and the **penis,** which contains the passageway by which **sperm,** the male sex cells, leave the body in the **ejaculate.** The testes are suspended in a tissue sac called the **scrotum,** which hangs between the thighs. The testes produce the hormone **testosterone,** which is responsible for the production and maturation of sperm. Testosterone is also responsible for the secondary sex changes in men, including body hair patterns, voice changes, and muscle development. A series of ducts and glands provides additional fluid volume to the ejaculate and adds nutrients needed for sperm maturation and development. The **prostate gland** is located just below the urinary bladder. The prostate produces an alkaline secretion that increases sperm motility, and it contracts to aid in the ejaculation of sperm.

EXPECTED AGE-RELATED CHANGES

Changes in Women

Several significant changes occur with menopause (Table 3-13). Production of progesterone and estrogen diminishes. There is no longer the need to produce ova to be fertilized, and there is no need to prepare a site to support a pregnancy. Other changes related to the decline in hormones are not as desirable. Along with other body tissue, the tissues of the external female reproductive organs atrophy as a result of vascular changes. The tissues of the reproductive organs become less elastic, and the amount of subcutaneous tissue decreases. This results in a flattening of the tissue of the external genitalia, or labia, and often the amount and distribution of pubic hair decreases. Vaginal epithelial tissue becomes thinner and less vascular. The tissue of the vagina is drier and more alkaline, and fewer **rugae** (folds) are present within the vagina. The uterus, cervix, ovaries, and fallopian tubes decrease in size and may be difficult to palpate on examination. The decrease in hormone production and resulting tissue changes may lead to more fragile, more easily irritated vaginal tissue. Decreased vaginal secretions may lead to **vaginitis,** which can cause vulvar soreness and pruritus or painful intercourse (called **dyspareunia**). Once menopause has occurred, vaginal bleeding is considered abnormal. Older women who receive estrogen supplements may experience fewer reproductive tissue changes, and, in some cases, the lining of the uterus responds to these supplemental hormones. Vaginal bleeding may occasionally be observed in these women.

The breasts are part of the secondary female sexual organs. Because of the decrease in hormones with aging, breast tissue atrophies. As supporting muscle tissue atrophies, the breasts tend to sag and decrease in size.

Table 3-13	Reproductive Changes Associated With Aging	
PHYSIOLOGIC CHANGE	**RESULTS**	
Female		
Decreased estrogen levels	Decreased vaginal secretions	
Decreased tissue elasticity	Decreased pubic hair; increased vaginal tissue fragility; increased tissue irritation; decreased size of uterus; decreased vaginal length and width; decreased size of vaginal opening; increased pain with intercourse (dyspareunia); decreased breast tissue mass	
Increased vaginal alkalinity	Increased risk for infection	
Male		
Decreased testosterone levels	Decreased amount of facial and pubic hair	
Decreased circulation	Decreased rate and force of ejaculation; decreased speed gaining an erection	
NURSING ASSESSMENTS AND CARE STRATEGIES RELATED TO REPRODUCTIVE CHARGES		
NURSING ASSESSMENTS	**CARE STRATEGIES**	
Assess for signs and symptoms of infection or inflammation.	Report unusual vaginal discharge to physician. Administer treatment as prescribed.	
Assess factors that may interfere with sexual activity.	Discuss normal physiologic changes and the possible effects of medications on sexual function. Educate females regarding use of artificial lubrication. Possible referral of males to physician for pharmacologic treatment of erectile dysfunction.	

Changes in Men

Male age-related changes in the reproductive system are less noticeable because testosterone continues to be produced into old age, although the amount tends to decrease. Men even in their late eighties have successfully fathered children.

With aging, there is some change in the size and firmness of the testes. The penis retains the ability to become erect, although it may take longer and require more stimulation. Once achieved, erection may last longer than at a younger age. Ejaculations tend to be slower and less forceful in aging men and may not occur during each sexual encounter, particularly if intercourse is frequent.

Enlargement of the scrotum may indicate problems with the testes or part of the duct system. The penis should remain free from any tissue changes, and the presence of ulcers, nodules, or other changes is abnormal. The prostate gland commonly enlarges with age. Most aging men experience some degree of prostate enlargement. The signs and symptoms most often experienced include urinary frequency, hesitancy, dysuria, decreased force when voiding, dribbling, nocturia, increased incidence of UTIs, and decreased force during ejaculation. In cases of **benign prostatic hyperplasia,** surgical intervention such as a **transurethral prostatectomy** may help reduce the symptoms.

COMMON DISORDERS SEEN WITH AGING

Uterine Prolapse

Prolapse of the uterus (into the vagina) is commonly observed in older women. This is particularly a problem for those who have had many pregnancies or for those who delivered children with little medical assistance. Most often, the first signs of uterine prolapse involve changes in either urine or bowel elimination. Urinary frequency, urinary retention, recurrent UTIs, back pain, and constipation may be symptoms. In some cases, the cervix and uterus may prolapse through the vagina and be observed protruding outside of the vulva. Surgical correction of this condition may be required.

Vaginal Infection

Change in vaginal pH may lead to increased incidence of vaginal infections, particularly **yeast infections.** This is most often manifested by increased vaginal discharge, irritation, odor, and itching.

Breast Cancer

The risk for **breast cancer** does not disappear with increased age. Breast cancer continues to be a major cause of cancer deaths in women, and the incidence of this form of cancer continues to increase with age. It is important that regular breast examinations (including mammography) continue as a woman ages. Any sign of dimpling; masses; nipple retraction; or breast drainage, discharge, or bleeding is suspicious and requires further medical attention.

Prostate cancer

There are no obvious changes in function to indicate the presence of **prostate cancer.** Therefore, it is important for aging men to have regular medical examinations. A skilled physician who palpates the prostate may detect changes that indicate malignancy. Prostatic cancer is a major cause of death in aging men.

Get Ready for the NCLEX® Examination!

Key Points

- Nurses must possess knowledge about the normal structures and functions of all of the body systems so that deviations from the norm can be detected.
- All of the body systems are affected to a greater or lesser degree by aging. Although these changes are normal and should be expected, they can have a significant impact on the older person's functional ability, self-image, and lifestyle.
- In addition to normal, age-related changes, a variety of diseases is increasingly common in the aging population.
- Nurses must be careful to distinguish between normal physiologic changes and abnormal alterations that indicate the need for prompt medical attention.

Additional Learning Resources

SG Go to the Study Guide on pp. 379–397 for additional learning activities to help you master the chapter content.

evolve Go to your Evolve website (http://evolve.elsevier.com/Wold/geriatric) for the following FREE learning resources:

- Animations
- Answer Guidelines for Nursing Care Plan Critical Thinking Questions
- Answers and Rationales for Review Questions for the NCLEX® Examination
- Glossary with pronunciations in English and Spanish
- Video Clips

Review Questions for the NCLEX® Examination

1. The normal physiologic change of aging that places an elderly client at an increased risk for digitalis toxicity is decreased:
   1. Gastrointestinal motility
   2. Bone density
   3. Vital capacity
   4. Glomerular filtration

2. Which are normal age-related changes? (Select all that apply.)
   1. Decreased visual acuity
   2. Increased heart rate
   3. Decreased long-term memory
   4. Increased motor responses
   5. Increased muscle mass
   6. Decreased depth of respiratory
   7. Increased calorie requirements
   8. Decreased bladder capacity
   9. Increased subcutaneous tissue
   10. Decreased rate of peristalsis

3. Older patients with Parkinson's disease are likely to exhibit:
   1. Rigidity and tremors when at rest
   2. Hemiparesis and aphasia
   3. Exaggerated reflexes and dementia
   4. Tremors with movement and weakness

4. The nurse observes that there is no hair on the legs of an 80-year-old man. This is most likely related to physiologic changes affecting the:
   1. Integumentary system
   2. Circulatory system
   3. Endocrine system
   4. Nervous system

5. When discussing expected changes in the female reproductive system to an older adult, the nurse should explain that:
   1. Increased pubic hair is expected
   2. Uterine enlargement is normal
   3. Vaginal tissues become more vascular
   4. Production of vaginal secretions decreases

6. The nurse performs an assessment of the skin of an elderly person. The abnormal finding that needs to be reported is:
   1. Increased patches of dark pigmentation on exposed skin
   2. A dark, elevated patch that bleeds when touched
   3. Deep wrinkles and frown lines around the mouth and eyes
   4. Numerous brown or flesh-colored skin tags around the neck

7. The nurse encourages the client to maintain a steady weight in the recommended range to decrease risk of the most common endocrine disease observed in the elderly, which is:
   1. Hypothyroidism
   2. Hyperthyroidism
   3. Diabetes mellitus
   4. Diabetes insipidus

chapter

4

evolve

Health Promotion, Health Maintenance, and Home Health Considerations

http://evolve.elsevier.com/Wold/geriatric

Objectives

1. Describe recommended health-maintenance practices, and explain how they change with aging.
2. Discuss the relationship of culture and religion to health practices.
3. Identify how perceptions of aging affect health practices.
4. Describe how health maintenance is affected by cognitive and sensory changes.
5. Discuss the impact of decreased accessibility on health-maintenance practices.
6. Describe methods of assessing health-maintenance practices.
7. Identify older adults who are most at risk for experiencing health-maintenance problems.
8. Identify selected nursing diagnoses related to health-maintenance problems.
9. Describe nursing interventions that are appropriate for older adults experiencing alterations in health maintenance.
10. Discuss the role of home health as it relates to health promotion and health maintenance in the elderly.
11. Differentiate between unpaid and paid home health care providers.
12. Identify the factors to consider when seeking home health care assistance.

Key Terms

health maintenance (p. 75)
health promotion (p. 75)

noncompliance (p. 85)
prophylactic (prō-fĭ-LĂK-tĭk) (p. 77)

As people live longer and the percentage of older adults in the population increases, society faces several major challenges. One of the most significant of these challenges involves meeting the health care needs of the aging population.

Today's older adults are generally healthier than were the older adults of previous generations. Improvements in sanitation, public health, and occupational safety implemented during the twentieth century have helped raise the age at which a person can expect to experience a life-threatening disease.

Older adults can and do experience acute, life-threatening medical conditions just as younger persons do, but acute episodes in older adults are more likely to be associated with chronic conditions. Either an acute condition is caused by a chronic problem, or a chronic problem persists after an acute episode. It is estimated that 80% of older adults live with chronic conditions such as arthritis, hypertension, diabetes, heart disease, and vision or hearing disorders. Most of those with a chronic illness are able to meet their own needs; only approximately 25% require any special type of care. Both acute health care and chronic health care are expensive.

Although older adults make up only approximately 12% of today's population, they account for more than one-third of all health care expenditures. For the most part, today's older adult population has benefited from improvements in medical care. Advances in surgery, technology, and pharmacology have enabled us to prolong life in situations that even a few years ago would have been impossible.

This level of care is not without substantial cost. Because a significant portion of older adults' health care expenses is covered by Medicare and Medicaid, the burden on the younger members of society is becoming overwhelming. Despite steady increases in payroll taxes on the working population, Medicare has operated at a deficit since the start of the twenty-first century. Because there is a limit to how much taxpayer money is available, society must identify appropriate and acceptable ways to control health care costs.

One way of dealing with a steady increase in demand for health care services involves rationing the type and amount of care provided to older adults. This approach would prohibit or severely limit the type of care provided, particularly in cases in which the potential for significant improvement in health status is limited. For example, some of the more costly treatments and procedures (e.g., renal dialysis and bypass surgery) could be refused if the person were older than a predetermined age. This method has been adopted in some countries but is unpopular in the United States. To avoid rationing health care, we must find ways to maximize the effectiveness of our health care expenditures. In 2009 a health care reform legislation was passed, but it is very complex and the legality of some proposed changes is being challenged. Time will tell whether this is truly an effective reform or not.

Most studies reveal that it is more cost-effective to prevent problems than it is to attempt to cure or treat them. Therefore, more health care providers and the public (including older adults) are beginning to recognize the need to devote more attention to **health promotion** and **health maintenance**.

Health promotion is not a new concept. For decades, health care providers have stressed the importance of good nutrition, exercise, and regular medical care. Although most of this information was directed toward younger people, many older people who desired to live longer, healthier lives also paid attention. As the benefits of healthy lifestyle choices became obvious, television, radio, and other media joined health care providers in promoting health awareness. Awareness of the importance of good health-maintenance practices increased. Many individuals have modified their lifestyle and health care practices to improve their overall health and quality of life (Box 4-1). Those who are unaware or are unwilling to heed this advice persist in risky, health-threatening behavior. Nurses need to be aware of the health promotion and maintenance practices that will most benefit older adults. Nurses also need to understand why some older adults choose to adopt positive health behaviors, whereas others persist in seemingly self-destructive behavior.

RECOMMENDED HEALTH PRACTICES FOR OLDER ADULTS

DIET

Older adults should consume a well-balanced diet based on the food pyramid and recommended daily allowances of nutrients. Some changes in caloric intake and protein and vitamin needs appear to be desirable with aging (see Chapter 6).

When special diets are indicated, older adults need to learn how to read and interpret the information provided on packaging labels. This is particularly important with sodium-restricted diets because sodium is common in foods that do not necessarily taste salty. Because food labels are often printed in very small type, older adults should be sure to bring their eyeglasses or a magnifying glass when they shop. If someone else shops for them, that individual needs to know how to shop wisely.

EXERCISE

Regular exercise should be a part of any daily plan for older adults (Figure 4-1). Exercise can help keep the joints flexible, maintain muscle mass, control blood glucose levels and weight, and promote a sense of well-being. Exercise does not need to be aerobic to benefit older adults. Walking, swimming, golfing, housekeeping, and active lawn work or gardening are all considered exercise. To be of most benefit, exercise should consist of at least 30 minutes of continuous activity. The type, level, and amount of exercise that is most beneficial differ for each person and should be based on physician recommendations.

TOBACCO AND ALCOHOL

It is never too late to stop smoking. Even the body of an older person can repair damage once smoking is discontinued. Cessation may be difficult when smoking has been a long-standing habit, but various aids are

Box 4-1	Advice for the Young and Not-So-Young Adult

- Accept that you are getting older—adjust to the changes, and plan for possibilities.
- Explore options for the future—look for things you want to accomplish in your life.
- Find work or creative outlets that make you happy—look for ways to grow throughout your life.
- Modify your lifestyle to promote health—exercise, watch your diet, and manage stress.
- Develop and maintain relationships—bonds formed with friends and loved ones provide support as we age; we can never have too many.

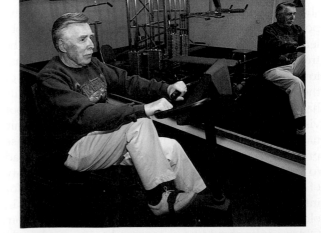

FIGURE 4-1 An older adult in exercise class practices health promotion.

now available to help smokers quit. Before using any of these aids, older adults should seek guidance from their physicians because they may need to follow some special precautions related to existing health problems.

Excessive consumption of alcoholic beverages is never recommended. Alcoholism is an all too common problem in the older adult population—both men and women—because alcohol may be used as a means of coping with depression, sleep disorders, or other problems. Occasional or moderate alcohol consumption by older adults usually is not prohibited or restricted unless some medical condition or medication precludes its use. Some physicians even recommend a glass of wine or beer as an appetite enhancer in certain situations.

PHYSICAL EXAMINATIONS AND PREVENTIVE OVERALL CARE

Older adults should be examined at least once a year by their physicians—more often if known health problems exist. Some older adults resist this because of the cost or fear about what the physician may find. Cost is a real concern to many older adults, but inadequate health maintenance should be of more concern. A delay in the recognition of problems may make them more difficult and more costly to treat. Physical examinations provide an opportunity for the physician to detect problems before they become more serious, to monitor and treat chronic conditions, and to prevent some health problems.

Physical examinations in older adults should include evaluations of height and weight, blood pressure, and blood cholesterol levels if this has been a concern, as well as a rectal examination. In addition, women should have a pelvic examination, mammogram, and Papanicolaou (Pap) test to rule out cervical cancer. Older men need a prostate examination and blood tests to rule out prostate cancer. Persons with identified risk factors for colon cancer require occult blood screening and, possibly, a colonoscopy.

Evaluation of joints, feet, and gait should be part of the physical examination. Problems with the knees and shoulder joints can cause pain, limitation of activity, poor sleep, and decreased overall function. Some problems require surgical correction, whereas others can be treated more simply using analgesics, antiinflammatory medications, or physical therapy. Inspection of the feet often reveals problems. Many older adults have difficulty caring for their toenails because of poor vision, an inability to reach the feet, or hypertrophic nail changes. Bunions, calluses, and corns also cause problems for older adults. Neglecting the feet can lead to discomfort, restricted mobility, and a poorer quality of life. If the feet are not properly cared for, the risks for infection and even amputation increase, particularly in older individuals with compromised circulation. Older adults should be encouraged to wear properly fitted shoes that provide good support. Regular visits to a podiatrist can significantly reduce foot problems. Joint or foot problems, illness, pain, and other conditions commonly seen with aging can contribute to gait changes that are likely to result in imbalance or falls. When gait problems are identified, physical therapy for gait retraining and strengthening exercises, use of assistive devices, and environmental modification are appropriate (see Chapter 9).

Vision should be checked yearly to monitor for glaucoma or other eye problems. Refractive examinations can detect the need for a change in eyeglass prescription. Hearing examinations need not be done on a yearly basis unless a problem is suspected. When signs of diminished hearing are present, audiometric testing is appropriate.

Blood tests for hypothyroidism, diabetes, or cholesterol levels; electrocardiograms; and other diagnostic tests are not routinely part of the physical examination. Older adults should be aware of the need to communicate any symptoms they experience so that their physicians can determine the need for additional testing.

In addition to regular physical examinations, older adults should be sure to obtain immunization against diseases such as pneumonia and influenza that are more common in older adults than in younger adults. Because the immune system is less responsive than that of younger persons, it is important that they receive vaccinations in a timely manner.

The pneumonia vaccine is given starting at 65 or 70 years of age; repeating the vaccination every 10 years is recommended. The influenza vaccine must be obtained on a yearly basis, usually in the fall, because the strain of the virus changes frequently. Flu shots can be obtained from private physicians or from clinics that are available in most communities. Even with immunization a larger percentage of elderly contract influenza.

Although tetanus infection is rare in the United States, approximately half of the cases of tetanus affect the elderly. Persons who were never immunized against tetanus should receive a three-dose series of injections. Those who have been immunized at an earlier age should receive a tetanus booster every 10 years after age 65. Specific injuries may require a booster even if 10 years have not elapsed.

The risk of developing shingles, a herpes zoster infection that causes a classic rash and painful neuralgia, increases with age. The shingles vaccine has been available since 2006. This vaccination is recommended for people over age 60, provided they have a normal immune system. Benefits of this vaccine should be determined based on individual risks, preferences, and the physician's recommendations. It is very expensive and is effective approximately 50% of the time.

The need for the hepatitis B immunization is based on individual risk factors and should be discussed with a physician.

Prophylactic use of medications such as aspirin (to prevent cardiovascular disease) and vitamin E (thought to decrease risk for stroke, heart attack, and Alzheimer's disease) is gaining increased acceptance in the medical community. Older adults should be encouraged to discuss the possible benefits of this type of therapy with their physicians and then follow the recommendations.

Use of prescription and over-the-counter medications is common in the aging population. Older people with medical conditions must understand the reasons for and the importance of their treatment plans. They should keep a record card listing all of their medications and the names of the physicians who prescribed them. This card should be shown to all licensed professionals they see so that serious drug interactions are prevented. Older adults must know how and when to take prescribed medications, how to use over-the-counter medications safely, how to store their medications, and when to report side effects. Sharing prescription medications with friends or neighbors is dangerous and should be avoided. Medications can be confusing and even overwhelming to many people. Additional precautions regarding medications are discussed in Chapter 7.

To keep track of medical appointments, older adults should have a calendar or datebook where they can record all appointments or reminders for things such as immunizations. They also should be aware of signs and symptoms that indicate a need to seek medical attention that exceeds routine yearly examinations. Signs and symptoms indicating the need for prompt medical attention are listed in Box 4-2.

Older adults who have health problems or allergies, those taking medications such as heparin, and those with implanted medical devices such as pacemakers are advised to wear a Medic Alert bracelet or necklace. If they do not wish to wear such a warning device, these individuals should at least carry a card in their wallets or purses to provide the necessary health information.

Box 4-2 Signs and Symptoms Indicating a Need for Prompt Medical Attention

- Severe pain; radiating or crushing chest, neck, or jaw pain; severe unremitting headache
- Difficulty breathing
- Loss of consciousness
- Loss of movement or sensation in any body part(s)
- Sudden vision changes
- Unusual drainage or discharge from any body cavity
- Wounds that do not heal
- Nausea or vomiting that persists for 24 hours or longer
- Elevated body temperature
- Inability to urinate
- Swelling of the lower extremities
- Excessive (greater than 10%) weight gain or loss
- Sudden or dramatic behavior changes
- Sudden changes in speech or ability to follow directions.

🏃 Health Promotion

Medications

- Take prescription medications only as ordered.
- Store medication as directed.
- Report any suspected side effects to your physician.
- Keep a card with names of all medications, dose, and name of physician with you at all times.
- Keep the card up to date.
- Show the card to all health care providers.
- Wear a medical alert bracelet, listing serious diseases and allergies.
- Do not use OTC medication without consulting physician or pharmacist.
- Do not take anyone else's medication or share your medication with anyone.

DENTAL EXAMINATIONS AND PREVENTIVE ORAL CARE

Dental examinations should be obtained and an inspection of the oral cavity performed on a regular basis (at least once a year). Today's older adults are keeping their natural teeth longer than previous generations were able to, probably because of better nutrition and improved prophylactic dental care. Gum disease and tooth decay are major causes of tooth loss. To prevent or slow the progress of these dental problems, older adults should brush their natural teeth at least daily using a fluoride toothpaste and should floss carefully between the teeth. Mouthwash may help refresh the breath, but it cannot replace regular brushing.

It is recommended that older adults use soft-bristle brushes to clean all tooth surfaces, particularly those individuals suffering from arthritis, because they may have difficulty holding and brushing with a standard toothbrush. Enlarging the brush handle using tape, wide rubber bands, sponges, or polystyrene or lengthening the brush by attaching a wood or plastic strip may make it easier to hold. Some older adults prefer an electric toothbrush that provides the proper movement.

Circular or short back-and-forth brushing works best to clean the teeth. Close attention should be paid to removing all plaque from along the gumline. Red, swollen, or bleeding gums indicate the need to see a dentist. People should have their teeth professionally cleaned at least once a year to remove stains and other debris missed by routine brushing.

Older adults who wear dentures still need regular oral examinations because people older than 65 years of age account for more than half of the new cases of oral cancer each year. Good oral hygiene is also necessary. Dentures must be brushed or cleaned at least once a day to remove food debris, bacteria, and stains and to prevent gum irritation or bad breath. Some denture wearers prefer to brush the dentures using a special dentifrice, whereas others prefer to use a soaking solution that works overnight. Either cleansing method is appropriate, but the chemicals should be rinsed thoroughly from the dentures before they are put back into the mouth.

An older person wearing dentures for the first time needs to become adept at inserting and removing them. Eating with dentures is often awkward, necessitating some relearning so that the wearer can chew effectively. Taking smaller pieces of soft, nonsticky foods and chewing more slowly are recommended. Because dentures make the mouth less sensitive to heat, cold, and foreign objects such as bone fragments, special care is required when eating.

Poor fit is a major reason that some older adults fail to wear their dentures regularly. This contributes to problems with nutrition and digestion. A few extra appointments with the dentist are often necessary to help fit the dentures properly. These adjustments are important because poorly fitting dentures can cause irritation to the gums or mucous membranes of the mouth. Additional adjustments may be needed if the denture wearer gains or loses weight.

Other changes in the oral cavity (e.g., dryness) are also common with aging. Although saliva production does not decrease in all older adults, a variety of medical conditions, medications, and treatments can cause or contribute to dry mouth. Dry mouth can best be relieved by drinking more water. Excessive use of hard candy, caffeine beverages, alcohol, or tobacco increases dryness of the mouth.

MAINTAINING HEALTHY ATTITUDES

Strong connections exist between the mind and body. Older adults who maintain a positive outlook on life tend to follow good health practices and remain healthier longer.

Regular interaction with other people of all age groups helps maintain a positive attitude toward life. It is recommended that older adults get out of the house as often as possible, even if only for shopping or dinner. Keeping in touch with family and friends is important. When spouses or friends are lost through death or relocation, older adults benefit from attempting to establish new relationships by joining church or community social groups. Volunteering in hospitals, schools, literacy centers, or other community agencies is a popular and desirable activity because it helps promote a sense of value and self-worth (Figure 4-2). As noted earlier in this text, many elderly continue to remain active in the workforce. This may be out of financial necessity or as a way to remain a productive, contributing member of society. A decrease in social interaction can contribute to the deterioration of cognitive and adaptive skills. Nurses cannot force an individual to participate beyond his or her wishes, but a little encouragement and information about options can help stimulate the older person's interests.

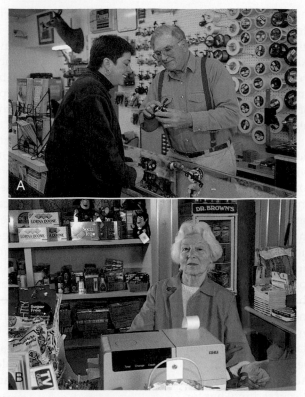

FIGURE 4-2 Many older people continue to work and learn after the traditional retirement age.

FACTORS THAT AFFECT HEALTH PROMOTION AND MAINTENANCE

The actions taken to promote, maintain, or improve health are based on that individual's perception of his or her health. Health perceptions influence day-to-day choices regarding hygiene practices; nutrition; exercise; use of alcohol, drugs, and tobacco; accessing health care; and many other activities. Health-maintenance practices include safety precautions taken to prevent injury from automobile accidents, falls, poisoning, and other hazards. Health perceptions and health-maintenance practices in older adults are influenced by personal beliefs, religious and cultural beliefs, socioeconomic status, education, and life experiences.

As people mature, they establish a set of beliefs, perceptions, and values related to health. These perceptions include basic ideas regarding what health is and how to best maintain it. These beliefs form the foundation for each person's health practices. Based on their unique beliefs, most people perform activities that they perceive to be helpful in maintaining their health and avoid activities they perceive as harmful. It is difficult to change a person's lifetime health practices. Only those who are highly motivated to change are likely to be successful.

RELIGIOUS BELIEFS

Religious beliefs contribute to an individual's perceptions. These beliefs can promote health maintenance or interfere with good health practices and result in increased health risks. For example, some religions teach that the body is a temple, stressing the importance of avoiding alcohol, tobacco, and other behaviors that are harmful to health. Individuals with these religious beliefs tend to live longer, healthier lives than do people who do not share these values. Other persons, whose religions teach that illness is a punishment for sins, may feel that they are not worthy of health and must endure illness as atonement for things they have done wrong in their lives.

CULTURAL BELIEFS

Cultural beliefs and practices also play a significant role in health perception and health maintenance. For example, reliance on home health remedies is common in many cultures. Some home remedies are harmless, whereas others are quite dangerous. Problems can occur when home remedies are used in place of conventional medical care or when their use results in delayed care, which can be serious or even fatal if the illness is a serious one. Culture also plays a significant role in the selection of food and the methods used for food preparation. These preferences and practices play a significant role in health promotion and maintenance. Diets that consist mainly of fruit, vegetables, and grains are common in some cultures, whereas diets high in fat and sodium are prevalent in others. These variations can contribute to the good health of some ethnic populations or to the health problems seen in others.

🌐 Cultural Considerations

Biocultural Differences

Considerable evidence still exists that race and ethnicity contribute to disparities in health throughout the United States. The following are some of these disparities:

- Higher incidence of hypertension in the African-American population
- Higher incidence of diabetes in the American-Indian and Hispanic populations
- Higher incidence of stomach and cervical cancer in the Hispanic population
- Higher incidence of obesity among African-American and Hispanic women

As our society becomes increasingly diverse, nurses need to become more aware of the religious and cultural factors that affect the health-maintenance practices of all persons (Figure 4-3). Information about the beliefs and practices of organized religions and major cultural groups is available through sources such as textbooks on transcultural nursing. Although nurses can gain valuable insight from such sources, we must be careful not to generalize. It is common for two individuals from similar religious and cultural backgrounds to have widely disparate perceptions and

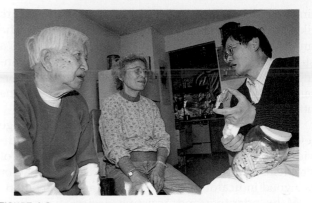

FIGURE 4-3 While providing information in a home care setting, this nurse compares traditional and Western remedies. Culture influences how health, illness, and pain are perceived. The nurse must take cultural variations into account to communicate effectively with patients and their families.

practices. Although a general understanding of cultural factors is important, the best source of accurate information about a person's beliefs and practices is that individual. An overview of common health practices helps nurses understand the underlying values and beliefs that motivate each individual.

KNOWLEDGE AND MOTIVATION

Factors other than religious and cultural beliefs also play a part in health perceptions and health-maintenance practices. Knowledge plays a key role in maintaining health and promoting safety; knowledge of recommended health practices is essential to make good choices. Health and safety teaching must start early and be reinforced throughout life. Whenever there is a significant change in a person's health status, additional teaching is necessary to ensure the safety and highest possible level of wellness of that individual. People cannot make informed decisions regarding their health and safety unless they know the ramifications of various behaviors. Individuals experiencing cognitive changes resulting from disease processes or chemical dependence may not be able to understand the need for safety or health-maintenance practices despite repeated teaching. People with severe cognitive or perceptual problems are likely to experience injuries and alterations in health-maintenance practices.

Health maintenance requires motivation in addition to knowledge. People experiencing grief, depression, hopelessness, or low self-esteem may not be motivated to maintain good health practices. Motivating individuals to maintain health is often difficult. All of the teaching in the world will not replace the desire to live a healthy life.

MOBILITY

Even people who are knowledgeable and motivated to maintain their health may have trouble if they cannot obtain the goods or services they need. People with limited physical mobility, transportation, or money are likely to experience difficulty. A person who knows the importance of nutritious food but who cannot get to a store or afford the food will have difficulty maintaining good health. A person who knows that it is important to see a physician but who can neither get to the office nor pay for medical care is similarly at risk.

Assessment of the values, perceptions, knowledge level, motivations, and lifelong health practices of individuals provides an understanding of the likelihood of problems with health maintenance. Previous behavior is a good indicator of future practice and motivation.

Many adaptive and assistive devices have been developed to promote safe mobility for older adults and others experiencing difficulty moving about or performing many of the activities of daily living. The Department of Education has a website (www. abledata.com) and telephone line (1-800-227-0216) to provide information on thousands of products designed to assist people with physical limitations to help themselves.

PERCEPTIONS OF AGING

Many beliefs about health and health maintenance are formed early in life. The longer a belief is held, the harder it is to change that belief. Therefore, it is often difficult to change the health behaviors of older adults.

Perceptions of good health and good health practices vary widely among the aging population. Older adults have their own beliefs about what is normal and expected with aging. Some are willing to accept declining health as a normal part of aging, whereas others are not. Those who perceive a decline in health as normal and expected with aging may do little to prevent loss of function, simply accepting the changes. It is common to hear these older adults say, "Why should I bother to see the doctor? It's just old age." Some older adults often ignore early signs of illness or attribute them to aging. This often results in a delay before seeking medical care. Others, particularly those who have followed good health practices throughout their lives, believe that old age is not synonymous with disease or loss of function. They continue to follow high-level health-maintenance practices in all aspects of their lives, including diet, exercise, rest, and medical attention.

Perceptions regarding aging greatly affect a person's motivation and willingness to participate in health-maintenance activities. A person who feels capable and in control of his or her life is more likely to be willing to change behaviors and to work at maintaining health. Older adults who feel useless, helpless, or without purpose, particularly the newly widowed or those who are estranged from their families, are less likely to be motivated to maintain their health.

IMPACT OF COGNITIVE AND SENSORY CHANGES

Cognitive and sensory changes related to aging or disease can lead to problems with health maintenance. Even the normal sensory changes of aging can increase the risks for personal neglect or injury. When significant cognitive or perceptual problems occur, the risks are even greater.

An older person with changes in vision and smell may have body odor or wear soiled clothing because he or she cannot see or smell soiling. Changes in vision, hearing, smell, sensation, taste, and memory can also lead to decreased awareness of normal environmental hazards. Sensory changes increase the risk for injuries from falls, poisoning, fire, and other traumatic events. Vision changes can cause the older person to miss the edge of a step or a curb, resulting in a fall. Changes in smell and taste can result in consumption of spoiled, unsafe food. Changes in sensation can lead to the use of overly hot bath water, resulting in burns. Changes in the sense of smell can cause the older adult to not perceive a burning odor, leading to the increased likelihood of injury from fire.

Older adults who are seriously impaired either perceptually or cognitively commonly lack awareness of their own needs. They may ignore parts of their hygiene or may completely forget to perform routine health-maintenance activities such as bathing, eating, or taking medication. Common health practices may be neglected, even though the person is physically capable of performing the activities.

Cognitively impaired older adults are at serious risk for injury because they are unable to recognize the danger of their actions or lack of actions. They may forget to turn off the burner on the stove, forget to put on a coat when going outside in winter, turn up the furnace instead of turning it off, or walk into a busy street without looking for traffic. Severely impaired persons are at great risk for experiencing problems related to safety and health maintenance, often requiring some form of supervised living or institutional care for their own protection.

IMPACT OF CHANGES RELATED TO ACCESSIBILITY

Aging persons are likely to experience more problems accessing goods and services than are younger people. Access may be limited by decreased physical mobility, lack of transportation, or limited finances. If more than one of these factors is present, the risk for ineffective health maintenance increases dramatically.

Physical limitations, including loss of motor skills, decreased strength and endurance, and the presence of disease, make health-maintenance activities more difficult. Decreased physical strength and agility can interfere with normal health-maintenance practices. Simple acts such as bathing, cooking, and cleaning can be too physically demanding for some older adults, who may be too fatigued to even attempt normal self-care activities. This lack of strength or energy often results in poor health-maintenance practices.

Transportation difficulties present many problems for older adults. Simply getting to the grocery store, pharmacy, or physician's office when necessary can be a major impediment to health maintenance. Even if older adults desire to practice good health maintenance, they may be hindered by a lack of transportation.

Finances cannot be ignored when discussing health maintenance. Although Social security, Medicare, and Medicaid offset some financial concerns, they do not cover the entire cost of health care prescriptions or meals. The lack of these resources may cause older adults to limit medical care. Many older adults persist in trying to treat themselves before seeking medical attention. They may try to stretch the time between medical visits or take less than the prescribed amount of medications to conserve money. Financial constraints can also affect the ability of the older person to purchase special foods and equipment necessary to promote or maintain health.

Finances can also affect safety. Many older adults live in older housing, which is more likely to contain safety hazards such as poor electric wiring, steep stairwells, and inadequate lighting. High crime rates in poorer areas make older adults who live there particularly vulnerable to rape, mugging, and theft. Even if these factors are not a problem, simple home maintenance can increase the risk for injury. Because it is costly to hire people to do even routine home-maintenance chores, many older adults attempt these tasks alone. Some fall from chairs or ladders while trying to paint walls, clean windows, or hang pictures. Many injure themselves trying to shovel snow or mow the lawn.

HOME HEALTH

As already discussed, most older adults wish to remain at home for as long as possible. For them to do so, additional assistance is likely to be needed. Some of this assistance does not require professional training and can be provided by family members. More complex interventions require the expertise of specialized caregivers. As the number of older adults has increased, the demand for home care services has also increased and promises to continue to grow for the foreseeable future. Home health interventions can both promote health and help the elderly person maintain the highest level of function possible for the longest period of time. Assistance in the home can help overcome problems related to noncompliance by providing motivation, verifying that care is completed, and providing better access to health care services.

According to the National Association for Home Care, more than 7.6 million people in the United States require some form of home care. Almost 70% of these are over age 65. Medicare spending for home health care has fluctuated over the past 15 years from a low of $8 billion in 2001 to a high of $18.3 billion in 2009. If the legislation stands, changes proposed under health care reform are projected to decrease spending for home health care by 13% over the next 10 years. Money saved will be used to offset the cost of providing coverage for younger uninsured individuals. These numbers do not include unpaid care provided by family members, friends, or volunteers. Researchers estimate that in the year 2000 unpaid caregivers provided services that had an economic value of **$257 billion**. Without the dedicated help of all of these individuals, the health care delivery system would be overwhelmed, and many older adults would experience a poorer quality of life.

UNPAID CAREGIVERS

Most unpaid caregivers are family or friends of the elderly person, although they may be volunteers from a church or other charitable organizations. Caregivers can be divided into primary and secondary classifications. Primary caregivers provide for most of the day-to-day needs of the elderly. These are usually close family members such as spouses or children, but they may be paid employees. Secondary caregivers help intermittently with things like shopping, transportation, and home maintenance. Usually, those family members who reside closest to the elderly person provide the most direct assistance, whereas those who live farther away are less involved. This can be a source of interfamily strife. One family member may be resentful of doing everything while others do little or nothing. Of course, this is not always the case; some families develop a good balance and distribution of effort. Even family members who live at great distances from an elderly relative can provide high-level long-distance support, usually through an intermediary agency.

Most caregivers are women. They are of all ages, with the average being in the mid- to late forties. They come from all ethnic, racial, and religious backgrounds. Most are providing care to the elderly in spite of multiple other responsibilities, including their children, homes, and jobs. Many caregivers experience exhaustion, anxiety, and burnout as a result of multiple demands, particularly when they feel that their assistance is not appreciated. Often they will require teaching, guidance, and assistance while learning how to perform new skills and effective ways to respond to the needs of the older adult. This teaching needs to be done in a kind and courteous manner. According to interviews with unpaid caregivers, overly judgmental nurses and other professionals made them feel inept, inadequate, and anxious. Nurses should be careful not to denigrate the services or capabilities of these caregivers. Unpaid caregivers should not be criticized or made to feel guilty that they are not doing enough. Instead, the nurse should work to develop a partnership with family caregivers that includes ongoing assessment, teaching, coaching, psychological support, and guidance. Nurses and other professionals need to be kind to unpaid caregivers, to recognize the value of their service, and to provide positive feedback. Box 4-3 lists agencies that provide assistance and information to elder caregivers.

PAID CAREGIVERS

Almost any kind of home help can be arranged, from the simplest to the most complex. Agencies that provide home health services have proliferated in recent years. Many of these are highly ethical organizations that provide a valuable service to the elderly. Others are less scrupulous and may even increase the risks for a vulnerable older person. Informal referrals from friends, senior citizen centers, churches, or volunteer organizations may be helpful in locating a reliable caregiver. Additional help with identifying qualified help can be obtained from the local Area Agency on Aging offices, state or local social service agencies, or tribal councils. Although some assistance may be provided free of charge by volunteer organizations and some may be covered by insurance or Medicare, the services of most independent contractors or private agencies require considerable out-of-pocket expense. It is wise to verify the cost of services before making any commitments. Home care is usually less expensive

---

| Box 4-3 | Elder-Related Information and Services |

- Administration on Aging (www.aoa.gov)—202-619-0724
- Eldercare Locator (www.eldercare.gov)—800-677-1161
- Medicare benefits (www.medicare.gov)—800-633-4227
- National Institute of Medicine (www.medlineplus.gov) 202-334-2352
- National Institute on Aging Information Center (www.nia.gov)—800-222-2225
- National Council on Aging (www.benefitscheckup.org) 202-479-1200
- Federal, state, or local government benefits (www.govbenefits.gov)—800-333-4636
- Department of Veterans Affairs (www.va.gov)—877-222-8387
- USA.gov (USA.gov/Topics/Seniors.shtml) 800-333-4636
- Department of Housing and Urban Development (www.hud.gov)—202-708-1112
- Low-Income Home Energy Assistance Program (www.ncat.org)—866-674-6327
- National Resource Center on Supportive Housing and Home Modification (www.homemods.org)—213-740-1364
- American Association of Homes and Services for the Aging (www.aahsa.org) 202-783-2242

| Box 4-4 | Questions to Ask When Selecting a Home Health Agency |

- How long has the agency been in business in this community?
- What services does the agency provide?
- What do these services cost? Is financial aid available? How are charges billed?
- Is the agency certified by Medicare? Is it accredited by any organization such as The Joint Commission Long Term Care accreditation program ?
- Does the agency have a Bill of Rights for the elderly?
- Does the agency have a specific written plan of care for the older adult that is developed with patient and family input?
- What kind of screening is done when hiring employees? Are references available to the family?
- How are caregivers trained and supervised?
- What level of professional supervision is provided?
- Is there an RN on-call 24 hours a day?
- How and when is information communicated between the agency and the family?
- What is done to protect confidentiality?
- How are conflicts or complaints resolved?

Modified from the U.S. Department of Health and Human Services Administration on Aging Fact Sheet, "Home Health Care: A Guide for Families."

---

than care in an institutional setting, but this is not always the case. Much will depend on the extent and complexity of the care needed. Cost is always an issue, whether providers admit it or not. Even wealthy people need to be cautious that they spend their money wisely; those with average incomes need to pay even more attention to costs.

It is always wise to check references before hiring anyone to work with the elderly. Because the caregiver is often alone and unsupervised with the older adult, any signs of unscrupulous or abusive behavior must be investigated. Ideally, paid caregivers will have a history of punctuality and reliability because an elder often becomes anxious if the caregiver is unreliable. These caregivers should provide certification that they are free of communicable diseases, including tuberculosis. A background check should be conducted to ensure that they have committed no serious criminal acts. Reputable home care agencies often provide these checks as part of their service and may also bond their employees to protect the patient against loss due to thefts or damage to property. It is also advisable to plan an introductory visit and trial sessions to determine the compatibility of the caregiver and the elderly person. Box 4-4 provides a list of important questions to ask when selecting a home health agency.

TYPES OF HOME SERVICES

Elderly people require different levels of home assistance. The level of care needed is likely to change as the person's health status changes over time.

An elderly person who is generally healthy may require only transportation to appointments and assistance with household chores such as mopping, vacuuming, laundry, grocery shopping, and meal preparation—all considered unskilled interventions.

An infirm elderly person may need additional help with hygiene and dressing. Elderly persons with altered cognition may also need ongoing supervision for safety and help with medication preparation and administration. More compromised older adults may require assistance with dressing changes, management of wounds, pain management, or other skilled interventions. Even end-of-life hospice care may be provided in the home.

A thorough assessment by a trained professional, usually a registered nurse (RN) or social worker, can best determine how much and what kind of help will most benefit each older adult. Working in conjunction with the patient's physician, the case manager (typically an RN) assesses, plans, supervises, and coordinates services. Services are best delivered by a team that includes RNs, licensed practical nurses (LPNs)/licensed vocational nurses (LVNs), health aides, housekeepers, dietitians, and social workers, as well as occupational, physical, and speech therapists. Nursing supervision of unlicensed personnel is critical for safe home care. Aides must have adequate training to perform safely in the care setting, and they need to know the limits within which they must work. For example, aides are not permitted in most cases to measure and dispense medications, although they may be permitted to give medications to the elderly person if the nurse or a family member first sets these up in prelabeled and timed packaging. Social workers help manage the financial aspects of care, as well as interaction, with other agencies or facilities, particularly if the patient needs to be admitted to a hospital or other health care facility. Social workers also are responsible for the assessment of family dynamics and possible intervention in suspected cases of neglect or abuse. A chaplain may or may not be part of the team. Home hospice is more likely to have chaplains available for end-of-life issues. In addition, the case manager may have responsibility for arranging that all necessary equipment and supplies (such as oxygen, wheelchairs, and hospital beds) are available and remain in good operating condition.

❖ NURSING PROCESS FOR INEFFECTIVE HEALTH MAINTENANCE AND INEFFECTIVE SELF HEALTH MANAGEMENT

Elderly individuals who are unable to identify or seek out help and those who are unable to follow through with a therapeutic regime are at risk for serious health-related problems (Nursing Care Plan 4-1). Assessment of health perceptions and health-maintenance practices is necessary to take into account the unique problems, beliefs, and perceptions of each aging person. It is important to assess both past and current health-management practices because these are good predictors of future health practices.

■ Assessment/Data Collection

- How does the person rate his or her current health?
- Does the person feel in control of the conditions that affect his or her health?
- What does the person routinely do to maintain his or her health?
- How does the person manage illnesses?
- What are the person's religious or cultural beliefs regarding health and health practices?
- How do the person's health practices compare with recommended health practices?
- How often does the person see a physician, dentist, or other health professional?
- Does the person undertake high-risk behaviors such as smoking, excessive alcohol intake, or drug consumption?
- Does the person have adequate financial resources to maintain his or her health?
- Does the person have access to the goods and services necessary to maintain health?
- Is the person's knowledge adequate to make informed decisions regarding his or her health?

See Box 4-5 for a list of the characteristics of older persons who are at risk for alterations in health maintenance.

■ Nursing Diagnoses

Ineffective self health management
Ineffective health maintenance

■ Nursing Goals/Outcomes Identification

The nursing goals for an older person demonstrating ineffective health maintenance are to verbalize appropriate health-maintenance practices, demonstrate adequate health-maintenance practices, and identify community resources that can assist in health maintenance.

Box 4-5 | **Characteristics of Older Adults Who Are Likely to Experience Ineffectiveness in Health Maintenance**

- Lack of adequate knowledge about recommended health practices
- Physical limitations
- Limited financial resources
- Altered cognitive or perceptual function
- Difficulty accessing health-related goods or services
- Loss of motivation because of grief, hopelessness, or powerlessness

★ Nursing Care Plan 4-1 | Health Maintenance

Mrs. Fisher is an alert, well-groomed 82-year-old who lives alone in an apartment. She has a history of type 2 diabetes mellitus. Her blood glucose levels, which you test weekly, are consistently 200 mg/dl or higher. Her physician has prescribed a 1200-calorie diabetic diet and an oral hypoglycemic medication.

When you arrive at Mrs. Fisher's apartment early for a home visit, you find an open box of ginger snaps next to the chair where she was sitting. She says, "I like to sit around most of the day and read or watch TV." You ask about the cookies and she replies, "They're not very sweet; I need to have some food that I enjoy. I won't live forever, you know." You check the bottle of oral hypoglycemic medication and find that she has taken only two tablets in the past week. She states, "I forget to take them. They don't help anyway, and they cost too much."

Nursing Diagnosis
Noncompliance

Defining Characteristics
- Consistently elevated blood glucose levels
- Failure to take prescribed medications
- Failure to follow prescribed diet
- Complaints of lifestyle changes in conflict with personal values

Patient Goals/Outcomes Identification
Mrs. Fisher will do the following:
- Follow her prescribed diet
- Increase her activity level
- Take her prescribed medications
- Achieve blood glucose levels of less than 120 mg/dL

Nursing Interventions/Implementation
1. Assess Mrs. Fisher for any signs of tissue breakdown or other problems related to hyperglycemia.
2. Allow her to verbalize feelings and problems experienced with activity, diet, and medications.
3. Review her daily food intake.
4. Explain the importance of following her prescribed diet.
5. Set up a reminder system for daily medications.
6. Explore ways of increasing her physical activity.
7. Encourage her to comply with the plan of care.
8. Praise positive health care behaviors.
9. Continue to monitor her blood glucose level and notify the physician if it remains elevated.
10. Arrange a consultation with the dietitian at her next physician's office visit.

Evaluation
At the next home visit a week later, you find that Mrs. Fisher's blood glucose level is 174 mg/dl. She states proudly that with the new medication system, she has remembered to take six of her oral hypoglycemic tablets and forgot one day only. She further states that she has taken four short walks with her neighbor. After providing positive feedback on these signs of improved health maintenance, you discuss diet with her. Mrs. Fisher states that she has tried to be more careful, but, because she still likes an occasional cookie, she will limit herself to one or two at most a day. Improvement is demonstrated, but Mrs. Fisher's goals are met partially only. You will continue with the plan of care and reassess her again in 1 week.

Critical Thinking Questions
1. What additional approaches could be implemented to improve compliance with the medication regimen?
2. How could you help Mrs. Fisher decrease her snack intake? Can you suggest ways to motivate her to increase her activity?

■ Nursing Interventions/Implementation

The following nursing interventions for ineffective health maintenance should take place in hospitals or extended-care facilities:

1. **Assess the person's ability to resume normal health-maintenance practices.** After hospitalization or rehabilitation in an extended-care facility, older adults must be assessed carefully to determine whether they are capable of returning home and resuming normal health-maintenance practices. Ideally, discharge from the facility should be delayed until the nurse can be reasonably sure that the patient is ready to take responsibility for his or her own health care needs. If possible, an assessment of the home environment should also be made before discharge. If necessary, the environment should be modified to promote health maintenance and safety. A referral for a follow-up visit after discharge helps ensure that the older person is safe and able to meet his or her health-maintenance needs.

2. **Teach the skills required to monitor health status if and when the patient returns home.**

Before discharge from a health care institution, older adults should have a thorough explanation of what they need to do to maintain health, including when to call or see the physician; what medications are required and when they should be taken; how to perform home screening procedures (e.g., blood glucose monitoring and daily weights); and how to keep records and monitor their health condition.

3. **Consult with the social worker or with agencies that can assist with health-maintenance practices.** The community social worker or social agencies may be able to help older adults meet their health-maintenance needs by providing transportation, delivering food or groceries, assisting with home maintenance, or offering other services.

The following interventions should take place in the home:

1. **Assess the existing health-maintenance practices.** The nurse should assess the older person's knowledge of the factors that promote health. Any problem areas should be examined in greater detail. The nurse should also determine what motivates the person to maintain his or her health because these motivators may be valuable if modifications in health care practices become necessary.

2. **Explain and reinforce positive health-maintenance behaviors.** The nurse should review health practices regarding diet, safety, stress management, exercise, elimination, and sleep. It is important to review when and how to contact a physician, particularly in cases of a serious illness or emergency. If older adults are receiving treatment for any health problems, they should know what health care behaviors are recommended to maintain the highest level of wellness (Box 4-6). They should know what medications to take and when to take them, as well as how to perform any special care or treatments.

3. **Assist in identifying family or community resources that promote health maintenance.** Individuals living in their homes may be unaware of services that are available to provide help. Often, a little assistance is all that is needed to enable an older person to live a healthy, independent lifestyle. If assistance is delayed, health maintenance may deteriorate to a point at which hospitalization or institutional placement is required. These services should be identified before they are required to avoid delays or waiting lists for the services.

4. **Use any appropriate interventions that are used in the institutional setting.**

❖ NURSING PROCESS FOR NONCOMPLIANCE

A person is different than the previous diagnoses in that a person should only be considered to be noncompliant when he or she fails to follow through with recommended health practices in spite of adequate teaching and resources. Failing to take prescribed medications, failing to attend scheduled medical appointments, and failing to follow prescribed diets are examples of noncompliant behaviors. Many factors may be related to noncompliance: cognitive impairment, inadequate knowledge, inadequate resources, lack of transportation, fear, anger, decreased self-esteem, substance abuse, and conflict of beliefs or values. Noncompliance should be suspected when a person does not show the expected amount of progress toward wellness, when a person gets worse instead of better, or when a person develops repeated or unexpected complications.

■ Assessment/Data Collection

- Does the person verbalize unwillingness or inability to follow through with the necessary health maintenance or medical care recommendations?
- Does the person verbalize a conflict between personal beliefs or values and the treatment plan?
- Are there unexpected relapses, or do the health problems appear to be getting worse instead of better?
- Does the person often miss medical appointments? What reasons does he or she give?
- Is there more medication left in the bottle than would be expected if it were taken properly?
- Are there signs of the presence of prohibited foods (e.g., candy for persons with diabetes and salt shaker for persons with sodium restriction)?

Box 4-7 lists the characteristics of older persons who are at risk for noncompliance.

■ Nursing Diagnosis

Noncompliance

Box 4-6	Recommended Health Practices to Maintain Wellness

- Eat a well-balanced diet.
- Establish a regular exercise program.
- Quit smoking.
- Consume alcohol in moderation.
- Get routine immunizations as recommended.
- Stay involved in activities and with others.
- Keep a healthy attitude.
- See the dentist and physician regularly.

Box 4-7	Characteristics of Older Adults Who Are Likely to Be at Risk for Noncompliance

- Cognitive or perceptual problems
- Lack of adequate financial resources
- Poor self-esteem or altered body image
- Lack of a support system of friends and family
- Substance abuse problems
- Negative past experiences with the health care system
- Differing cultural or religious beliefs

Patient Goals/Outcomes

The patient goals for an older person demonstrating noncompliance are to identify factors that contribute to noncompliant behavior and demonstrate the acceptance of treatment.

Nursing Interventions

The following nursing interventions for noncompliance should take place in hospitals or extended-care facilities:

1. **Identify the reasons for noncompliant behavior.** A person might not comply with recommended health-maintenance practices for many reasons. Unless the nurse can determine the specific reasons why the person is not following the recommended practices, interventions are likely to be inappropriate and unsuccessful. If the person does not take medication because of forgetfulness, more teaching will not help. If the person refuses medication because he or she feels unworthy of living, no amount of reminders will help. Interventions must address the root problem. Forgetful people need a system of reminders; persons with poor self-esteem need to feel valued before care is accepted. Individuals who exhibit self-neglect may require treatments for depression, dementia, or any physical problems that are hampering their ability to care for themselves. The individual may need to be monitored so that any excessive deterioration in their health or levels of self-care can be observed and acted upon. Treatment should include home health care that is provided in a way that does not reduce autonomy any more than is essential. Self-neglect may be an indicator that a person would benefit from assisted living or some other form of residential care. These individuals might improve if they have more opportunities for social interaction. If persons are legally determined to be incompetent of making decisions about their own care, they may have a legal guardian appointed and be compelled to accept help. If they are in possession of their mental faculties, they have a right to refuse treatment.

2. **Provide care in a nonjudgmental manner.** The values and beliefs of older adults are often different from those of their caregivers. If the nurse indicates verbally or nonverbally that the older person's beliefs and practices are in some way inferior, the nurse is not likely to be able to convince the person to comply with the desired health practices.

3. **Actively include the patient in planning care, and adapt or modify the care plan so that it is more acceptable to the patient.** Develop all plans with, not for, the older person. Each individual can then incorporate his or her unique culture, beliefs, and values into the plan that is developed. This enables older adults to retain control and responsibility for their own health care. When they "own" the plan and determine the goals, they are more likely to be compliant.

4. **Emphasize the benefits of compliant behavior.** Many aging persons do not comply with recommended health care practices because they do not really believe that compliance will help. If the person has the opportunity to benefit when he or she is compliant, active involvement in care is more likely. For example, if a person with diabetes continually sneaks extra food and therefore frequently has high blood glucose levels, the nurse can demonstrate how much lower the blood glucose level is when the person follows the prescribed diet. If less insulin or fewer injections would be required when the blood glucose level is controlled, these benefits should be stressed. Unfortunately, it is not always possible to see any obvious immediate benefits from compliant behavior.

5. **Acknowledge the aging person's right not to comply with the plan of care.** If an alert older person chooses not to comply with the plan of care despite explanations, teaching, and reminders, the nurse must recognize that this is, in fact, a right of the individual.

The following interventions should take place in the home:

1. **Assess the support system.** In the home setting, it is particularly important to identify the strengths of older adults and the amount of support they receive from friends and family. The likelihood of achieving compliance is far greater when patients are willing to learn and to modify their behavior and when they have others who are willing to help. Individuals who resist intervention and receive little support are likely to continue to have problems with compliance.

2. **Help structure the environment to promote compliance.** Many individuals are noncompliant simply because they are confused or forgetful. Memory devices can catch their attention and verify that critical actions take place. For example, if the person forgets to eat meals, a checklist for the days of the week and the three basic meals can be posted on the refrigerator door. Each time the person fixes a meal, the box is checked. Likewise, special divided containers are available for people who have trouble remembering to take their medication. Medication for an entire week can be prepared by a responsible assistant or nurse. A simple glance in the box lets the person know whether he or she has taken the right medication at the right time. Bold markings on a calendar, preferably one with large print, can be used to mark special events. Signs in bold letters can be posted in appropriate places. For example, "take a drink" can be posted over the sink of a person whose fluid intake is inadequate.

3. **Enlist the help of family, friends, and neighbors to provide reminders.** Reminder phone calls from friends or family are useful for less frequent occasions such as doctor visits. It is wise for the friend or family member to call the person the day before the appointment and then again on the day of the appointment to ensure that he or she has not forgotten. It is even better for a responsible friend or family member to transport the person to the medical appointment. Responsible friends and family members can also provide help in setting up the weekly pillbox and preparing other reminders around the home.

4. **Involve social service agencies in promoting compliance.** If the person is noncompliant because of financial or transportation problems, a social worker or social service agency may be able to provide assistance that enables the person to comply with the care plan.

5. **Use any appropriate interventions that are used in the institutional setting.** (See Nursing Care Plan 4-1.)

Get Ready for the NCLEX® Examination!

Key Points

- A large percentage of today's aging population continues to live independently, despite a variety of chronic health problems.
- Health maintenance is an ongoing challenge for these people, their families, and health care providers.
- Careful assessment of the aging person's perception of his or her health, health practices, and knowledge of safety factors is an important part of nursing care in all settings.
- Early detection of problems and early intervention can prevent more serious complications and enable older adults to maintain the highest possible level of wellness and function.
- Home health assistance—both unpaid and paid—can help older adults remain independent for a longer period of time.
- Nurses play an important role in case management and in providing services to older adults in their homes.
- Caution should be used when selecting home care providers for older adults.

Additional Learning Resources

SG Go to the Study Guide on pp. 379–397 for additional learning activities to help you master the chapter content.

evolve Go to your Evolve website (http://evolve.elsevier.com/Wold/geriatric) for the following FREE learning resources:
- Animations
- Answer Guidelines for Nursing Care Plan Critical Thinking Questions
- Answers and Rationales for Review Questions for the NCLEX® Examination
- Glossary with pronunciations in English and Spanish
- Video Clips

Review Questions for the NCLEX® Examination

1. The activity that best promotes health maintenance for the typical senior citizen is:
   1. One hour of low-impact tai chi per week
   2. Thirty-minute walk 3–5 times a week
   3. Twenty minutes of step aerobics 2 times a week
   4. Five to 10 minutes of stationary bike riding done daily

2. The nurse recognizes that regular dental visits are:
   1. Necessary for only those elderly people who still have their natural teeth
   2. Recommended on a yearly basis for all elderly people, even those with dentures
   3. Not necessary if the person brushes and flosses properly three times a day
   4. Desirable, but not necessary unless pain or another problem occurs

3. An older person does not follow through with health recommendations from the physician. The person does not take prescribed medications or keep medical appointments. The nurse formulates a care plan for the nursing diagnosis:
   1. Noncompliance
   2. Knowledge deficit
   3. Disturbed thought processes
   4. Impaired health seeking behavior

4. Immunizations that the elderly need to receive on a yearly basis include the following: (Select all that apply.)
   1. Pneumonia vaccine
   2. Influenza vaccine
   3. Tetanus vaccine
   4. Polio vaccine
   5. Hepatitis B vaccine

5. When attempting to help an elderly person improve his or her health-maintenance practices, the nurse will need to assess which factors? (Select all that apply.)
   1. Physical strength and endurance
   2. Availability of transportation
   3. Cultural beliefs
   4. Cognitive and sensory changes
   5. Socioeconomic status
   6. Religious beliefs
   7. Social support system
   8. Educational level

Communicating with Older Adults

Objectives

1. Identify communication techniques that are effective with older adults.
2. Define *empathetic listening*.
3. Identify the significance of nonverbal communication with older adults.
4. Discuss the verbal communication techniques used when sending and receiving messages.
5. Differentiate between social and therapeutic communication.
6. Discuss ways communication is affected by culture.

Key Terms

confrontation (KŎN-frăn-tā-shŭn) (p. 97)
empathy (ĔM-pă-thē) (p. 93)
proxemics (prŏk-SĒ-mĭks) (p. 91)

rapport (ră-PŎR) (p. 86)
symbols (SĬM-băls) (p. 90)

Communication is the process of exchanging information (i.e., sending messages back and forth between individuals or groups of people). Problems between individuals, families, or groups, as well as difficulties on the job or in society, are often the result of poor communication. Each of us who participates in communication is a unique individual with our own personal values, beliefs, perceptions, culture, and understanding of how the world operates. This is particularly important to remember when working with older adults. Oldest adults of today formed their opinions, values, and beliefs in a very different society from ours today. Most of today's oldest adults grew up during the Great Depression, when men sold apples on street corners and searched for pieces of coal in railroad yards to survive. They lived through a major world war and witnessed the beginning of the Nuclear Age when the first atomic bomb was dropped. They grew up in a world without many of today's conveniences, including televisions and private telephone lines. The upcoming generation of elderly is very different. The Baby Boomers who came of age during the Vietnam war, grew up in a world challenged by drugs, protests, and "free love." They grew up with stereos, television, and astronauts walking on the moon. Most Baby Boomers have adapted to the use of cell phones and computers. Technology was, and will continue to be, a part of their lives.

Whatever their background, older adults have had time to encounter many situations, both good and bad. It is often difficult for a younger person to understand the experiences that have made older adults whom they are today. The most effective way to bridge the gulf between the generations is good communication (Table 5-1).

Effective communication is not easy, even among people of the same age group and background. Communication among people from different age groups and backgrounds is even more challenging. This is particularly true when one of the parties is elderly; however, effective communication can occur even when people hold significantly different values, beliefs, and perspectives. Effective communication does not mean that we will like or agree with everything that another person says, but rather that we respect the person's right to think and say it. This atmosphere of mutual respect and understanding helps build trust and rapport. Conscious, ongoing effort is required to become an effective communicator.

Effective communication requires the following:
1. The need or desire to share information
2. Acceptance that there is value and merit in what the other person has to say, demonstrated by a willingness to treat the other person with genuine dignity and respect
3. Understanding of factors that may interfere with or become barriers to communication
4. Development of the skills and techniques that facilitate effective interchange of information

INFORMATION SHARING (FRAMING THE MESSAGE)

Verbal communication involves sending and receiving messages by means of words. Some verbal communication is formal, structured, and precise; some is informal, unstructured, and flexible. Formal or therapeutic communications have a specific intent and purpose. Informal or social conversations are less specific and are used for socialization. Both have a place in nursing. Nurses must be effective in both formal and informal

Table 5-1	Communication Dos and Don'ts When Working with Older Adults	
DO	**DON'T**
Identify yourself.	Assume that the person knows who you are.
Address the person using the name he or she desires (e.g., Mrs. Smith and Bill).	Use "baby talk" or patronizing names such as "sweetie" or "honey."
Speak clearly and slowly in a low tone of voice.	Shout.
Get to know the person.	Make generalizations about older people.
Listen empathetically.	Pay too much attention to tasks and forget the person.
Pay attention to body language—yours and theirs.	Ignore non-verbal messages as insignificant.
Use touch appropriately and frequently.	Be afraid to use touch as a method of communication.

communication and must know how and when to use each type.

Nonverbal communication takes place without words. We are communicating all the time, whether we are aware of it or not. Research has shown that only 7% of communication comes from the actual words we use; the other 93% is nonverbal. Approximately 38% of communication is transmitted by paralinguistic cues (i.e., tone, pitch and volume of voice), and 55% is transmitted by body cues. The importance of understanding nonverbal communication can be summed up in the statement, "What you are saying (nonverbally) is so loud I can't hear you."

FORMAL OR THERAPEUTIC COMMUNICATION

Therapeutic communication is a conscious and deliberate process used to gather information related to a patient's overall health status (physical, psychosocial, spiritual, etc.) and to respond with verbal and nonverbal approaches that promote the patient's well-being or improve the patient's understanding of ongoing care. This type of communication looks easy and natural when performed by an experienced health professional, but it is a skill that requires time, effort, and practice to develop. Careful use of words and language is an art. Knowledge of the individual's educational background and interests provides nurses with a starting point for conversation. Social discussions often center around past employment, family, or other interests. Increased knowledge of the individual enhances

the nurse's ability to respond empathetically. Effective verbal communication requires the ability to use a variety of techniques when sending and receiving messages.

When communicating verbally, whether in a formal or an informal situation, nurses should know as much as possible about the other person involved. A person's age, marital status, cultural or ethnic orientation, educational background, interests, and the ability to hear and see influence the communication techniques used and the words chosen. As nurses, we need to be careful to choose words that the patient can understand—not so simple that we are "talking down" to the patient, but also not so technical or "medical" that the meaning is unclear. Avoid acronyms such as *TURP* or *CBC* unless you are sure that the person understands them. Careful listening to the patient's speech can give clues about the appropriate level of language.

Cultural Considerations

Communication Styles

- Americans tend to be bold and ask direct questions, particularly in a crisis. We expect the answers to be similarly clear and direct.
- Members of other cultures may prefer to proceed less directly and need to establish a relationship through "small talk" before addressing more serious concerns. Although this may seem less productive, the nurse's awareness that the patient and his or her family may be more comfortable with this type of communication can contribute to greater success in the long-term relationship.

Some home health nurses had a good laugh at the office when one nurse recounted the following experience during a home visit:

Her elderly patient reported that he was recently hospitalized. When she explored the reason for this hospitalization, he told her, "I was castrated." She asked whether he knew why this was necessary. He replied, "Because of my prostitute." At this point, she pulled things together in her mind (and restrained the unprofessional urge to break out in laughter), realizing that what her patient meant to say was that he was *catheterized* because of problems with his *prostate* gland. This is an example of medical terminology gone awry.

Also remember that different words can have different meanings to persons of different generations or cultures. *Gay* may mean happy and lighthearted or an alternative lifestyle. *Cool* may be a temperature or something really good. *Bread* may be something you eat or something you spend. Consider the culture, ethnicity, experiences, and perspective of the older patient when choosing your words.

INFORMAL OR SOCIAL COMMUNICATION

Simple chitchat has a place in nurse-patient communications. If nurses talked only about things related to health treatment, they would know little about their patients. Small talk; pleasantries; and conversations about the weather, a favorite television show, or the latest news can demonstrate that the nurse thinks of the patient as a real person, not just a patient. This also goes the other way. Older patients often like to know something about the nurses who care for them; they may ask about the nurse's family, hobbies, vacations, and so forth. This is particularly true in extended-care facilities because the nursing staff often becomes a new family for the aging person. Do not be afraid to be "human" when communicating with elderly patients.

Be honest with your older patients. When you do not have time to visit, explain why so that patients do not personalize and think they have done something wrong. Do not be afraid to use humor appropriately. It has been said that "laughter is the best medicine," a medicine that is too often in short supply around the elderly. Pick the right time and place. Make sure that the humor is culturally sensitive. Remember that it is okay to laugh at yourself but never at the other person. Aging does not cause people to lose their sense of humor. A humorous story or cartoon may help brighten their day.

NONVERBAL COMMUNICATION

Because so much of our communication is nonverbal, it is essential that we examine each aspect of nonverbal communication to see its effect on our interactions with the older adult (Figure 5-1).

> If two people entered a room—one wearing a white laboratory coat with a stethoscope around her neck and the other wearing a clerical collar and a cross—what message would you receive? Would these people have to say anything for communication to take place? What is being communicated? The items we wear or carry (e.g., clothing, jewelry, stethoscopes, masks, gowns, and gloves) send messages; we use these symbols to communicate something about who we are. Distinctive uniforms are worn to make people identifiable. Police officers, flight attendants, clergy, and nurses wear uniforms so that they can be recognized even in a crowd.

SYMBOLS

In the health care setting, uniform styles and colors help patients distinguish the various caregivers. Many patients, particularly older adults, were unhappy when nurses stopped wearing caps. The white uniform and cap were **symbols** that helped older adults distinguish nurses from other caregivers. For this reason,

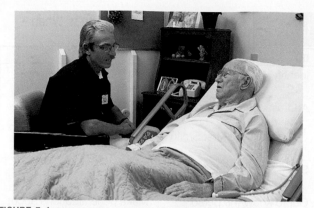

FIGURE 5-1 Nonverbal communication signals that the nurse is interested in the patient and in what he is saying.

nurses in some nursing homes continue to wear white uniforms and caps. In other settings, nurses may not wear any distinguishing uniform, or they may wear scrub suits. Street clothes, such as a navy blue outfit with an identifying name tag, are preferred in some agencies, particularly in home care or public health. This can be confusing to older adults because such clothing is not distinctive enough to identify the individual as a nurse and because many older adults cannot read the small print on name tags. Older adults have been heard to say to caregivers, "Who are you? What are you going to do to me?" Although nurses may not place much importance on wearing a uniform, it does play a role in communication.

Cultural Considerations

Nonverbal Communication

- Culture and nonverbal communication play important roles in patient perceptions. For example, Russian immigrants new to the United States may perceive that they are being treated incompetently and without adequate respect, based on cultural misunderstandings.
- In Russia, illness is viewed as a serious matter, and patients expect to be treated by stern, authoritarian care providers who give directions and do not seek input from the patients. Care providers wear appropriate uniforms, indicating their role and status.
- By contrast, in the United States, the patient is likely to be attended to by smiling, friendly, nonauthoritarian care providers who seek to involve the patient in decision making.
- These caregivers are normally dressed in scrubs or casual clothing that does little to identify their role or status. This contrast can lead to the mistaken interpretation that the caregivers are inexperienced and do not take the patient's concerns seriously.

TONE OF VOICE

Think of the sound of a whisper, shout, or whine. Try saying, "I don't want to do that," first in a whisper, shout, and whine, and then in a normal speaking voice. Was your understanding of the message the same in each situation? Probably not. To survive we learn early in life to understand that tone of voice is a fairly reliable way of judging a person's emotions. Because the nonverbal message is so strong, we typically respond to the emotion we perceive from the tone of voice and may not even hear the words. When a person shouts at us, we normally shout back. Shouting is often associated with anger or displeasure, yet many people shout in an attempt to communicate with someone who is hard of hearing. Shouting is not an appropriate way to deal with hearing problems because our tone of voice may lead the hearing-impaired person to think we are angry with him or her when this is not the case. Speaking in a low tone of voice close to the person's good ear is much more effective. Use of other nonverbal methods of communication, such as communication boards or gestures, can also help.

BODY LANGUAGE

You walk past a room and observe a nurse standing in the doorway, with his or her head sticking into the room and body still in the hallway. The nurse's mouth is saying, "Can I help you?" but the body is saying, "I'm in a hurry. You really don't want anything, do you?" We communicate many things by how we move, stand, sit, and position our bodies. In dealing with all patients, but particularly older adults, it is important that we be aware of what we are communicating through our body language.

In situations in which the words and body language are conveying two different messages, most people respond to the body language. Standing at the door, hurrying down the hallway, sitting behind the nurses' station, and working in the medication or treatment room all communicate that the nurse is busy and does not want to be interrupted. Many older adults and their families are intimidated by this body language and may hesitate to interrupt, even to report serious concerns. Nurses must be careful not to create barriers between themselves and their patients. Going *into* the rooms to talk with patients, sitting down at eye level with residents, and spending time in the lounge with visitors are all ways of nonverbally communicating that you are truly interested and concerned.

Another part of nonverbal communication involves watching for the messages that patients are communicating to us through their body language. For example, patients who slump down or slouch in their chairs may be communicating fatigue or physical weakness, or they may be communicating a lack of interest, sadness, defiance, or a number of other things. Turning away from the nurse could indicate anger, fear, or lack of interest. When body language says something different from the words, believe the body language. Explore the situation using techniques such as reflective or open-ended statements. (These techniques are clarified later in the chapter.)

SPACE, DISTANCE, AND POSITION

Physical space, distance, and position are other ways we communicate. The study of the use of personal space in communication is referred to as proxemics. *Personal space* refers to how close we allow someone to get to us before we feel uncomfortable. The amount of space that separates two individuals when they communicate is significant. In the traditional American culture, most people are comfortable when strangers are 12 feet or more away. This is considered **public space;** at this distance, there is no real positive or negative connection with the other person. Between 4 and 12 feet is considered **social space.** This is a comfortable distance for a casual relationship; in which communication is at an impersonal level. If a nurse stays this far away from his or her patients, the message being communicated is indifference. A distance of 18 inches to 4 feet is considered **personal space.** This is the optimal distance for close interpersonal communication with another person. A nurse who communicates from within this space is usually viewed as concerned and interested. The space within 18 inches of the body is considered intimate space. Most people allow only trusted individuals to get this close. Entering the intimate space without permission is usually perceived as a threat.

A nurse or other caregiver may approach an older adult to provide care or treatment and, without thinking, enter this intimate space too quickly. (Because of the nature of their work, nurses and other caregivers are used to entering a person's intimate space, and they take this for granted.) An older adult who has poor vision or hearing, who has been sleeping, or who is not totally alert may be startled by the nurse's approach. He or she may not be able to recognize the nurse as a trusted person at first and may strike out verbally or physically. This response results from fear of physical attack. It is essential that nurses recognize the importance of personal space and attempt to get the older adult's attention and (if possible) permission before attempting to perform any physical care.

GESTURES

Gestures are a specific type of nonverbal communication intended to convey ideas. Gestures are highly cultural and generational; those that are acceptable in one culture may be considered offensive in another. Some gestures that are accepted today as commonplace were once considered crude or insulting. Gestures that have a certain meaning in one culture may have a different meaning in another. For example, nodding the head up and down means *yes* in most cultures, but to some Eskimo tribes it means *no*. Before using gestures, it is wise to determine that both parties have the same understanding of just what a particular gesture means.

Gestures are helpful for people who cannot use words. After a stroke, many individuals suffer from a condition called **aphasia.** Because of brain damage, these individuals may not be able to recognize words or to "find" the words they want to use. This inability to communicate wants, needs, and feelings is often frustrating to the affected person, and the use of gestures and other nonverbal forms of communication can be effective.

🌐 Cultural Considerations

Preventing Cultural Bias in Caregiving

Culture, language, and communication are closely connected. Failure to recognize the impact of culture on communication can be a barrier to effective health care.

Health care providers, like others, often base their evaluation of a patient's words or behavior on their own culture and ethnic assumptions. To minimize cultural misunderstanding, health care providers need to do the following:

- Recognize their own cultural biases and assumptions.
- Increase their knowledge and understanding of the attitudes, beliefs, and communication styles of cultures other than their own.
- Recruit, retain, and promote health care providers from diverse ethnic and cultural backgrounds.
- Provide skilled interpreters, visual aids, and educational materials for predominant language groups.
- Address complaints or grievances that arise from cross-cultural misunderstandings so that care becomes more culturally sensitive.

FACIAL EXPRESSIONS

Facial expressions are yet another form of communication. The human face is most expressive, and facial expressions have been shown to communicate across cultural and age barriers. Smiles, frowns, and grimaces appear to have the same meaning whether you are in the outback of Australia or in a boardroom on Wall Street. Humans respond to facial expressions from the time they are born. We tend to mirror the expressions of the person with whom we are communicating: Smiles tend to elicit smiles, and frowns elicit frowns. Fear, anger, joy, and a variety of other emotions can be conveyed by a simple change in facial expression. Nurses need to be aware of this fact and ensure that their expressions communicate what is intended. Too often, nurses are preoccupied while interacting with an older adult. A frown may lead the individual to think that he or she has done something wrong. A wrinkled nose, particularly when cleaning up an episode of incontinence, could be viewed as a lack of acceptance. A smile when listening to serious concerns may make the person wonder whether the nurse really cares about what is being said.

EYE CONTACT

"Look me in the eye" is a phrase many white Americans have heard. Looking someone in the eye is perceived in our culture and other cultures as a measure of honesty. Yet in some cultures (e.g., African Americans and some groups from Southeast Asia), averting the eyes communicates respect. When dealing with older adults, it is important to be sensitive to the meaning of eye contact for them. Face-to-face, eye-to-eye contact can be helpful when communicating with older adults, providing this does not frighten or intimidate them. Eye contact is often interpreted to be a sign of attentiveness and acceptance. Face-to-face contact also maximizes the chance that an older adult with hearing problems can read lips if necessary. Sitting at the bedside may facilitate eye contact.

PACE OR SPEED OF COMMUNICATION

Nurses tend to be substantially younger than the aging people they serve. The resulting difference in rate of speech and movement can be overwhelming and frustrating to older adults. Many choose not to respond or interact with younger nurses because they feel they are being hurried. Do not become impatient or uneasy with silence; give the older person enough time to think and organize a response. Provide encouragement and reassurance that they will have all of the time they need. Nurses have too often been observed completing sentences for older adults when they should have the patience to wait for the individuals to organize their thoughts and speak. Many times, nurses complete the communication according to their own way of thinking rather than waiting to hear what the older adult wants to say. This is disrespectful and demoralizing. Patience and active listening are greatly needed skills when working with older adults. "Slower is better" should be the motto impressed in the mind of anyone who chooses to work with older adults.

TIME AND TIMING

Timing is related to the pace of communication, but it has other distinct implications as well. The amount of time a person must wait after seeking attention is important. Delays in response to a call light or direct request from a person may be interpreted as a lack of concern, even if this is not intended. The response to this perception may manifest in anger, displeasure, anxiety, fear, and many other feelings. Studies have shown that nurses take longer to respond to terminally ill patients. Nurses also tend to give delayed responses to demanding individuals. This can set up a vicious cycle, because the longer a person waits for a response, the greater his or her anger, fear, and anxiety becomes. This only increases the demanding behaviors, which often occur in an attempt to reduce fear. If the older adult's needs are dealt with promptly, the number of demands tends to decrease not increase. Making older adults wait unnecessarily constitutes a subtle form of abuse.

Many older individuals have an altered sense of time. A message that is communicated too early may lead to either forgetfulness or to repeated questions of "Is it time yet?" A message that is communicated too late may lead to distress and frustration. Older adults often need more preparation time than younger individuals need to get ready for an activity such as going to the bathroom or getting necessary items together. Communicating an exciting message late in the evening (whether it is good or bad news) may disturb older adults to the point that they are unable to sleep. Nurses need to be aware of these issues so that they can choose the proper time to communicate.

TOUCH

Touch is a form of communication. No words are required, and there is no need for high-level sensory or cognitive functioning. When all else fails, touch is left. Caring touch is a basic need of all humans, and many older adults suffer from touch deprivation. Many older people, particularly those who have lost their spouses and have little contact with children or other family, have no one to meet this need. Research shows that psychotic patients and older adults are touched the least by caregivers. Those who most need physical contact and the comfort provided by touch receive the least.

Use of touch as a method of communication is often difficult and uncomfortable, particularly for young or inexperienced nurses. Touching is a very personal form of communication. Affection, understanding, trust, hope, and concern can be communicated by a hand placed on a shoulder, a stroke of the forehead, or a frail hand held by another stronger one. Touch is a common method of expressing concern and caring. People who are emotionally close hold hands and touch and hug one another. High on the list of things lonely older people say they miss are hugs and touching. Empathetic use of touch is a much-needed skill when working with older adults. When words do not work, touch often does (Figure 5-2). If there is any doubt whether the patient wants to be touched, the nurse can ask or watch how the person responds to the touch. Touching should be done with caution when a person is experiencing pain so as not to cause further discomfort.

Whereas appropriate use of touch is of great benefit to older adults, inappropriate touching can be destructive. Touch is inappropriate when it is used to communicate anger or frustration. Rough handling, slapping, pushing, or otherwise communicating displeasure constitutes patient abuse and is out of place at all times. Cultural beliefs may dictate when, who, and how people may touch. If there is any question regarding the appropriateness of touch, clarification should be obtained beforehand.

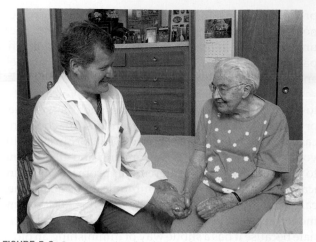

FIGURE 5-2 Comfort and well-being can be promoted with eye contact and gentle touch.

SILENCE

Saying nothing is also saying something. Being with another person and remaining silent is difficult for many people, including nurses. At times, words can be intrusive; they can interfere with true communication. Many times, older adults require more time to compose their thoughts. Silence permits them to focus on the point of discussion while continuous talking is distracting. At times, no words are necessary. During intense grief, pain, or anxiety, simply *being there* without saying or doing anything may be the most appropriate form of communication nurses can give. The simple presence of another human expresses true concern and can be worth more than all of the words in the world.

ACCEPTANCE, DIGNITY, AND RESPECT IN COMMUNICATION

Empathy is defined as the willingness to attempt to understand the unique world of another person. It is the ability to put oneself in another person's place and to understand what he or she is feeling and thinking in various situations. Empathetic listening involves actively trying to understand the other person, not just knowing many facts about that person.

Effective communication starts with proper introductions. Nurses should determine how each older adult wishes to be addressed. It is presumptuous for nurses to become too familiar with older adults by addressing them by their first names. It is better to start by using the older adult's proper title and name (e.g., Mrs. Quinn and Dr. Jones) and then clarifying which form of address the person prefers. If someone wishes to be called by a first name or a nickname, the person will usually say so. In special situations, such as when a patient has dementia or other alterations in cognition, first names may be most appropriate because that may be the only name the person can remember. Use of the pronoun *we*—as in "Are we ready to get dressed now?"—is inappropriate and should not be used unless the nurse plans to get dressed along with the patient. Use the term *I* when speaking about yourself and *you* when referring to the patient.

Often younger persons use a sing-song voice or refer to older adults by "baby talk" names such as "sweetie" or "honey," thinking that this conveys affection and caring. This type of speech may be appropriate with young children, but it is patronizing and demeaning to older adults and considered inappropriate in a clinical setting. This type of communication, sometimes called *Elderspeak,* is a form of ageism. It is far too commonly heard in health care settings, which is unfortunate because it has a subtle way of diminishing an older person's self-esteem. Use a normal conversational tone of voice whenever possible. When communicating with older patients, nurses must avoid language that stereotypes or dehumanizes them. Such language may be overheard by the older patient or family members, who may interpret it as disrespectful. It is best to first speak in terms of the *person*; for example, the nurse should refer to "Ms. Todd, who has diabetes"—not the "diabetic in bed 14B." The nurse should also pay attention to the possible negative connotation that words can have to older adults or their family and substitute more positive terms when possible. For example:

- Instead of *diapers*, say *briefs, pads,* or use a trade name such as *Depend.*
- Instead of *blind* or *deaf*, say *visually* or *hearing-impaired.*
- Instead of *senile* or *dementia,* say *cognitively challenged.*
- Instead of *nursing home,* say *care facility.*

There is a reason we have two ears and only one mouth. We are supposed to listen twice as much as we talk!

To communicate effectively, we must first learn to listen actively and empathetically. Listening is more than simply hearing. Hearing involves the ability of the ears to detect sound, whereas listening involves interpretation (i.e., figuring out what the sounds mean). We have not really listened until we understand for certain what was intended by the speaker. We cannot simply listen to the words; we must listen for the meaning of the words.

Active listening skills are needed in all areas of nursing, but particularly in dealing with older adults. Empathetic listening requires sensitivity to the strengths and limitations of the aging individual (e.g., hearing changes, vision changes, fatigue and pain). Empathetic listening involves patience when an older adult needs extra time to voice a response, or repeats the same thing many times. It includes a willingness to spend time getting to know the older adult better as a human being—not just as another

body in need of skilled physical care. Listening to an older person reminisce about his or her life can help the nurse gain better understanding of the person's values, perceptions, strengths, needs, and concerns (see Chapter 11).

Too often, nurses provide excellent physical care to people they have not taken the time to know. Nurses need to stop talking "over" patients while they do procedures, put away their clipboards, and sit down and really talk with older patients more often. Empathetic listening requires the ability to focus on the aging person, not simply on the tasks at hand. If we do not really listen, our older patients are likely to stop talking and we will all be poorer for the loss.

BARRIERS TO COMMUNICATION

For effective communication, we must learn to identify the barriers that can interfere with an exchange and the methods that help overcome these barriers. Effective communication is not easy (Figure 5-3). More than just the ability to talk to someone, communication involves all of the ways that we send messages to someone else, including nonverbal ways. Different physical problems require different communication approaches. Communication makes use of all of the senses. Hearing and vision are the senses used most often in communication, but touch, smell, and even taste also play a part in the relay of messages. It is important to remember this when communicating with older adults because their perceptions may be altered by normal physiologic changes that occur with aging. Pain or extreme fatigue may make communication difficult. It is best to limit conversation to essential topics during these times. A variety of disease processes, such as cerebrovascular accidents and dementia, significantly affects

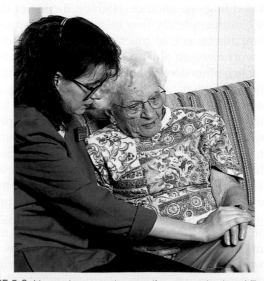

FIGURE 5-3 Nurses integrate therapeutic communication skills into all aspects of care.

communication processes and requires specific approaches. Diverse social and cultural backgrounds of older adults also make the area of communication a challenge for nurses.

Coordinated Care
Communication Skills

Supervision

When it is necessary to correct a subordinate for unsatisfactory performance, try to avoid "You" messages, such as "You never complete your assignments." Instead use assertive "I" messages—for example, "I am upset and disappointed when patients' needs are not thoroughly met." This is less likely to result in an argument and will more likely lead to problem solving. Also, be sure to praise people in public but correct them in private.

HEARING IMPAIRMENT

If the person wears a hearing aid, make sure it is clean, that the batteries are working, and that the device is in the correct ear. Try to minimize background noise because this can distort sounds and make hearing more difficult. Many people who are hearing-impaired spontaneously begin to read lips. In addition to the basic strategies, the following actions are likely to be beneficial:

1. Stand in front of the person.
2. Do not eat or drink while you are having a conversation.
3. Keep your hands away from your face when speaking.
4. Try different ways (words) of saying the same thing.
5. Speak more slowly and slightly louder while modulating the voice to a lower pitch.
6. Avoid exaggerated mouth motions during speech.
7. Use visual cues or written materials that support the spoken words.

Box 5-1 provides additional strategies for communicating with impaired older adults.

APHASIA

Individuals who have had a cerebrovascular accident or other head injuries may experience aphasia, which is a partial or total loss of the ability to use or understand words. It affects the ability to understand and express oneself through words, gestures, and writing but does not necessarily affect intellectual function. Consultation with a speech therapist can help the nurse devise approaches that will optimize function. In addition to the basic strategies, some commonly recommended approaches include the following:

1. Keep messages simple but adult.
2. Use nonverbal modes of communication such as picture boards, gestures, yes/no responses, and facial expressions.
3. Use visual aids to support.

| Box 5-1 | **Basic Strategies for Communicating With Impaired Elderly Adults** |

- Try not to startle the person when starting a communication.
- Approach from the front, knock, or announce your presence by calling the person's name.
- Identify yourself.
- Communicate when the person is most alert.
- Eliminate or reduce noise and distractions.
- Make sure you have the person's attention before speaking.
- Focus on abilities, not disabilities.
- Select topics of interest to the person.
- Try to use a variety of words or descriptions until meanings are clear.
- Ask clear, specific questions.
- Ask only one question at a time.
- Pay attention to the emotional context of conversation.
- Use pictures and gestures in addition to words.
- Have the person sit up for conversation whenever possible. Keep messages simple and repeat as needed.
- Be patient and do not interrupt. Slow down the pace of communication.
- Treat the person as normally as possible.

---

4. Try increasingly specific guesses or questions to determine concerns (e.g., Something's wrong with your meal? The coffee? It's too hot? You want milk?).
5. Praise attempts to speak, and avoid correcting or criticizing errors.
6. Reassure the person that it is okay to be frustrated, but avoid empty platitudes such as "You'll be fine."

DEMENTIA

Dementia causes both cognitive and language deficits. The elderly person suffering from dementia has no control over these changes, so the responsibility for effective communication rests with the nurse. Depending on the severity of the dementia, the individual may demonstrate different levels of function. The abilities and limitations of each individual suffering from dementia must be evaluated so that the most effective interactions can be planned. Some characteristics of dementia include a limited attention span, inability to focus on more than one thought at a time, confusion of fact and fantasy, and the inability to follow complex instruction. According to the Alzheimer's Association, "For persons with dementia, behavior is frequently a form of communication." Problems with communication can result in agitation, restlessness, abusive language, or combativeness. Repetitive vocalizations, urgency, and change in tone or pace of speech can indicate an unmet need, even when the sounds are meaningless. Caregivers should try to determine the meaning of the behavior, not ignore it as meaningless.

In addition to the basic strategies, some recommended approaches include the following:

1. Talk about one thing or ask only one question at a time.
2. Limit choices; too many options are confusing.
3. Keep the conversation in the here and now.
4. Ask simple yes/no questions.
5. Try "filling in" or "repairing" thoughts. Rather than letting a person get upset trying to find the right words, you may offer some likely choices. However, be careful not to get in the habit of finishing the thoughts and sentences of patients who are not cognitively impaired.
6. Avoid asking questions that require information, such as "How was your day?"
7. Use gestures or demonstrate an action so that the person can mimic your behavior.
8. Avoid the use of an intercom, which may confuse the person.
9. Avoid arguing if the person does not accept your reality.
10. Redirect the person who is acting out to a more appropriate activity.
11. Share activities such as looking at a magazine, viewing family photos, or listening to music.
12. Avoid trying too hard to communicate. If words do not work, try gentle touch.
13. Watch your tone of voice because patients with dementia are often very sensitive to nonverbal cues and may sense your frustration and become more agitated or upset.

CULTURAL DIFFERENCES

A Chinese guide in Beijing asked his tour group (in very clear English), "What do you call a person who speaks more than one language?" The group replied, "multilingual." He then asked, "What do you call a person who speaks only one language?" The group was not sure how to reply, so he provided the answer: "Americans." Although this is rather a strong generalization, the majority of Americans still speak only one language—English. We tend to expect everyone else, no matter where we are in the world, to understand us. If others do not speak English, Americans' typical response is to talk more loudly, as if volume will make a difference. Fortunately (or, some would say, unfortunately), most other countries have a significant number of people with some knowledge of English in addition to their native language.

Many community colleges and multicultural centers offer special courses in languages for health care providers. Often, these courses are specifically designed to meet the needs of the local community. This benefits the minority communities as well as the nurses, who have the opportunity to become particularly desirable employees.

Immigrants from many European, Central American, African, and Asian countries bring varied levels of English proficiency, which presents increased challenges to health care providers. To communicate effectively, we need to know what language a person speaks. We also need to know what level the person is most comfortable using because, during times of stress, a person may revert to his or her first language. It is most advantageous if caregivers from similar cultural and ethnic backgrounds are available to act as translators. Many facilities actively try to recruit individuals who are trained and qualified to work with the needs of the dominant cultural groups in a community. In an increasingly diverse world, this is not always possible. In these cases, other interpreters are needed. To be an effective interpreter, a person needs to be proficient in both languages and ideally trained regarding the ethics of the job. Interpreters should also have some understanding of the clinical concepts they will be expected to explain. A study done in a pediatric setting revealed that even official translators made many serious errors that were potentially dangerous. The same problem is likely to hold true when dealing with the elderly. Family and friends of the patient do not have this training and frequently bring personal and emotional connections that may influence the communication or make the patient reluctant to share information. Although family members are not the most appropriate persons to interpret sensitive or technical medical information, they may be helpful in translating simple questions or requests.

Some basic rules to keep in mind when working with an interpreter include the following:

- Ask short questions and provide brief units of information so that the interpreter does not lose the main idea in translation.
- Avoid excessively technical language.
- Avoid slang, idioms, or colloquial expressions.
- Encourage the interpreter to give you the response using the patient's own words, without input or paraphrasing, whenever possible.
- Focus on the patient, not the interpreter.
- Listen for emotional tone and nonverbal clues when the patient responds, even if you do not understand the words.
- Allow enough time.
- Make sure that there is mutuality by encouraging the patient to ask questions of the staff through the interpreter.

In addition to making adaptations for language, the nurse should pay close attention to nonverbal communications. Ignorance of cultural beliefs and practices can lead to mistakes that damage rapport. When in doubt, ask the elderly person or family if there are any special actions or behaviors that should be avoided.

Culture, Ethnicity, and Communication

- Of which cultural or ethnic group(s) do you consider yourself to be part?
- List all of the cultural or ethnic groups with whom you occasionally or regularly have contact.
- Consider the cultural or ethnic group with which you identify:
  - Identify any gestures you consider acceptable.
  - Is direct eye contact typical? Are there times when direct eye contact is not considered appropriate?
  - How close do people stand when talking to each other?
  - Do people touch frequently? Whom do they touch? Where or how do they touch? What type of touch is not allowed? Are there gender differences related to touching?
- Do you live primarily in the "here and now," or do you think it is essential to plan for the future?
- How important is it in your culture to be on time and keep appointments?
- Do you feel comfortable or ill at ease when communicating with individuals from diverse cultures? Does your comfort level change when the interaction is one-on-one or when you are in a group? Does it change if you are the only member of a specific culture or ethnicity in a group dominated by another culture or ethnicity?
- Identify two or three situations in which you felt that a person from another age, cultural, or ethnic group did not understand you or misinterpreted your nonverbal communication.
- Identify two or three situations in which you felt that you did not accurately understand the communication sent by a person from another age, cultural, or ethnic group.
- Can you think of any specific cultural beliefs or practices that you would want a nurse caring for you to understand?

SKILLS AND TECHNIQUES

INFORMING

Informing uses direct statements regarding facts. A good information statement is clear, concise, and expressed in words the patient can understand. When the nurse is informing, the nurse is active and the patient is passive. Informing is the least effective form of communication because the patient is not actively involved. When nurses give information, they should ask their patients to restate what they understand using their own words. A message may need to be repeated and rephrased to ensure understanding. This should be done tactfully and with care that the nurse does not show signs of annoyance or frustration.

DIRECT QUESTIONING

It is best to keep communication conversational and not too aggressive. Too many direct questions can overwhelm an older person and may block rather than expand communication. Direct questioning is helpful when nurses need to obtain specific information or in emergency situations when time is precious. Direct questions tend to include the words *who, what, when, where, do you,* and *don't you.* Direct questioning is appropriate when information must be obtained quickly; however, if it is overused, patients may become defensive. Many students and new nurses approach patient assessment with a list of 50 questions that must be answered. After the first 10 questions, patients begin to feel as though they are on trial and communicate only the bare minimum of information. Direct questions tend to yield brief answers and often a *yes* or *no* only.

USING OPEN-ENDED TECHNIQUES

Open-ended communication techniques include open-ended questions, reflective statements, clarifying statements, and paraphrasing. These techniques allow the patient more leeway to respond, thus establishing a more empathetic climate. The patient is more likely to feel that the nurse is interested in him or her personally and not just trying to fill out a stack of forms. Examples of open-ended techniques include the following: "And after you moved to the nursing home, what happened?"; "And then?"; "That must have been frightening!"; "What I heard you say is . . ."; "It sounds like you think (feel). . . ." Open-ended techniques allow patients to express more about their feelings and perceptions. They also allow nurses to verify that the information being relayed is accurate.

CONFRONTING

Confronting is used when there are inconsistencies in information or when verbal and nonverbal messages appear contradictory. **Confrontation** is one of the most difficult communication techniques to use and should be used only after good rapport has been established. It is never advisable to confront a highly agitated or confused person because conflict and a breakdown in communication will result. Confrontation should be used only when there is adequate time to explore the problem and come to some form of resolution.

COMMUNICATING WITH VISITORS AND FAMILIES

Nurses must be prepared to interact with their patients' friends, families, and other visitors. These people make up the older adult's social network and support system. Families and friends are interested and concerned about what is happening to their loved ones. Not only do they turn to nurses for information and reassurance, but also they can be a good source of information for the nurse.

These *significant others,* as they are often called, can help in many ways if nurses are responsive to them. Many of the older adult's significant others are themselves senior citizens. Nurses must be aware that communication with these individuals may also require special attention and the use of special techniques. It is important to take the time to develop good rapport with your patients' significant others. Good communication with these important people can do a great deal to facilitate care. Because they have known the patient longer and better than the nursing staff has, they are often able to detect subtle changes before trained nurses can. Many times, nurses need to rely on the significant others to interpret the behaviors and communications of older adults. Listen to what they have to say.

? Critical Thinking

Communication Skills

- Look at the people on each side of you in class. What is their body language communicating?
- Think of a person (e.g., friend, instructor, TV personality, and politician) you consider to be a good communicator. Next, think of a person you consider to be a poor communicator. Fold a piece of paper in half. Write the name of the effective communicator on one side and the ineffective communicator on the other side. Below each name, list the characteristics that make that communicator effective or ineffective. Compare and contrast your findings.
- Compare your own communication skills to those of the people whose names you wrote down. Are you more like the effective or ineffective communicator? How? What can you do to become more effective in your communication ability?

DELIVERING BAD NEWS

No one likes to get bad news, and no one likes to be the one who has to tell someone else bad news. Most people try to avoid this daunting task. Ideally, this task should be performed by the most experienced and knowledgeable person, such as the physician, but, occasionally, the nurse must be the one to break bad news to an elderly person. This could be information regarding the patient's health or about someone near and dear to the patient—for instance, the death of a spouse or other loved one. The EPEC Project, funded by the Robert Wood Johnson Foundation, has developed guidelines for physicians that have relevance for nursing practice. Important concepts include the following:

- Prepare yourself. Make sure you have all of the information and that it is accurate.
- Think through what you want to say so that the message is compassionate and culturally sensitive.
- Establish an environment that respects the patient's privacy.
- Determine whether anyone else (chaplain, family members, etc.) should be present when the news is delivered.
- Make sure there is adequate time, free from interruptions, to deal with the expected emotional response.

- Determine what the person already knows and, if possible, how much they want to know.
- Recognize that ethical and cultural variations may influence the way information is delivered.
- Use simple, direct, but sensitive language to begin the message, such as, "I'm afraid I have bad news for you."
- Respond to the person's emotional reaction—for example, "I'll try to help you. Is there anything I can do?" or "Do you want to talk about how you're feeling?"
- Develop a plan for follow-up. Help the older person and significant others with appointments, referrals, transportation, and so forth.
- Communicate significant information to other caregivers as part of a plan of care.

HAVING DIFFICULT CONVERSATIONS

Emotionally loaded topics are likely to generate strong emotions and often lead to conflict. Conflict is a normal and routine part of human interaction; it can occur between elderly parents and adult children, nurses and elderly patients, nurses and patient families, nurses and other nurses, or nurses and physicians. Difficult conversations may occur in clinical areas or in home settings involving friends and family members.

Some people prefer to avoid conflict entirely and pretend it does not exist, but avoidance just delays solving problems that need to be addressed. The following guidelines are suggestions based on conflict resolution research:

- Pick a place that is private and a time when you will be free from distractions.
- Try to focus on a single topic; do not bring up old grievances that get in the way.
- If a conversation is not going well, take a look at your own feelings and motivations. Are you reacting to this issue or to another issue that was problematic in the past?
- Express your feelings using "I" statements, such as "I get upset when . . . doesn't get done" rather than "You" statements, such as "You always ignore what I ask you to do."
- Respect the right of the other person to agree or disagree.
- Keep a balance between talking and listening. Try not to dominate the conversation.
- View each communication as a new opportunity to learn something about the other person and about his or her unique feelings, beliefs, and perspectives. Listen to the other person and seek clarification as to his or her reasons and feelings.
- Do not prejudge or assume that you already know what the person is going to say. You may be wrong.
- Be aware of your own feelings regarding the issue under discussion. Keep feelings separate from facts. The fact that someone does not do what you want

does not mean that the person does not like you or that he or she is doing it to upset you.

- Avoid blaming the other person. Look for ways to solve disagreements.
- Accept that difficult conversations are part of life and that things do not always go right.
- Learn from both negative and positive interactions, and try to improve the communication next time.
- Try to achieve a win-win solution.

IMPROVING COMMUNICATION BETWEEN ELDERLY PATIENT AND PHYSICIAN

Clear communication between the elderly patient and their physician is essential. Most physicians are aware of effective communication protocols, but, because of time constraints or other factors, they may not always use these techniques. Ineffective communication can result in frustration for both parties and can contribute to a lack of compliance by the patient. Also, it is not uncommon for an elderly person to become passive, evasive, or tentative when talking with the physician.

The nurse can often help minimize these problems by (1) suggesting that the patient keep a written list of concerns and questions so time is not wasted while the patient tries to remember them, (2) asking the physician to repeat and summarize directions to the patient, (3) identifying printed materials that support the physician recommendation, (4) suggesting that a trusted friend or family member be present to take notes and help the elderly person express his or her concerns, or (5) acting as a patient advocate by asking the physician to clarify questions or concerns the patient has verbalized to you.

COMMUNICATING WITH PHYSICIANS

The quality of communication between nurses and physicians can have a significant impact on the quality of care elderly patients receive. Communication problems between nurses and physicians can lead to job frustration, blame, and distrust, all of which diminish the level of care provided and increase the risk for problems or errors. Conversely, good communications tend to improve job satisfaction, decrease errors, and promote quality care of the elderly. Physicians and nurses are busy. No one has time to waste on unnecessary or nonproductive interactions. Mutual respect and a willingness to collaborate for the good of the elderly patient can form a strong basis for good interactions. The nurse can use a number of strategies to decrease frustrations and optimize the efficiency and effectiveness of communication (Box 5-2).

When you call a physician, start by identifying who you are (name and title), the patient or patients you are calling about, and the specific reason for the contact. Plan ahead and have a focus for the communication. Know what you want to report or find out. Be organized, clear, precise, and complete. Provide

---

Box 5-2	Additional Tips for Improving Nurse-Physician Communication

- Work at developing professional relationships based on trust and respect.
- At some point, try to meet face to face with physicians you speak with on the phone.
- Assume that you are both on the same team.
- Report good news, not just problems and bad news.
- Be prepared for conflict.

Adapted from Burke M, Boal J, Mitchell R: Communicating for better care: improving nurse-physician communication, *Am J Nurs* 104:40, 2004.

---

background information. Remember, the physician is not looking at the chart and may see the elderly patient once a month only, or even less frequently in the case of an independent elderly adult. Provide all necessary and relevant information that the physician might need. Identify the patient by name, major diagnoses, and any medications related to currently presenting symptoms or concerns. Be prepared to clarify any data or information that the physician may request.

Keep a list or log of issues to be reported or discussed with each physician so that all issues can be covered in one interaction. This will prevent repetitive interruptions for both the physician and the nurse. Identifying parameters (or guidelines) when the physician wishes to be contacted (e.g., patient's blood sugar over 200 and blood pressure under 120 systolic) can minimize problems related to under or over notification.

Emergency situations need to be handled immediately, but these make up a small portion of nurse-physician interaction. Most communications involve either routine or somewhat urgent information that can be handled in a more methodical, planned manner. It is helpful to determine whether there is a best time and method to use when contacting the physician regarding nonemergency situations. Today there are many ways to transmit information, including standard telephone, cell phone, Fax, e-mail, Blackberry, and others. Planning ahead to identify the best time and methods will optimize communication and enhance care of the patient while minimizing frustration.

PATIENT TEACHING

Education plays an important role in promoting and maintaining the health of older adults. Teaching may be a one-on-one session or a group experience. The ability to teach, explain, and motivate is increasingly part of the role of today's nurse. To perform this role successfully, the nurse needs to know basic principles and techniques of adult education and adaptations specific to older adults.

It has been said that "you can't teach an old dog new tricks." Research has shown that this is not true. Elderly people can learn new things. It has been established that mental abilities such as numeric tasks, word fluency, inductive reasoning, and spatial orientation develop through the first four decades of life and then hold fairly stable until the seventies in most individuals—even longer in others. Although younger individuals tend to do better at learning information that requires memorization, older individuals compensate by using the verbal skills, experience, and judgment they have acquired over time. Learning is maximized when it can draw on the previous experiences of older adults.

Adult learners are oriented toward problem solving, and they view learning as most desirable when it is relevant to their own lives. Teaching will be most effective when the patient recognizes and accepts the importance of learning new information or techniques. Older adults will be more willing to learn when the topic is important to them. For this reason, the nurse should try to determine ahead of time those things the elderly patient thinks are most important. The nurse can prioritize teaching by starting with the area that the *patient* perceives to be most important, then linking that information to the other things the *nurse* thinks are necessary or important. Work in small, discrete blocks of information, proceeding from simple, more familiar concepts to more complex or difficult ones. Remember that success breeds success. When older adults realize that they have mastered one skill or piece of information, they are more likely to have a positive attitude toward additional learning.

It is important to pick the right place and time for teaching. The right place depends on the material the session will cover. Information that is viewed as personal or private is best taught in a quiet space away from others. More general information (such as nutrition teaching, stress reduction, or similar topics) may be best taught in a group, where older adults are free to share personal experiences and solutions with one another. Wherever teaching takes place, the space should be adjusted for the older adult. The temperature should be set appropriately, chairs should be supportive and comfortable, lighting should be adequate and free of glare, and bathrooms should be readily accessible. Snacks and beverages are appreciated by most elderly adults and can make a group learning session a positive social interaction.

When selecting a teaching time, avoid times when the patient is stressed, fatigued, or in pain; all of these situations interfere with the patient's ability to process information accurately. Also, avoid times when older adults may be distracted by things of higher priority to them, such as a favorite television show or anticipated visit from friends or family. When selecting a time for teaching, make sure there is adequate time to discuss the important information. Remember that older individuals will need more time to process information. Avoid trying to teach too much at one

---

Box 5-3 Modification in Preparing or Selecting Printed Materials for Older Adults

- Limit the amount of material on a single page.
- Allow enough white space so that material is clear and distinct.
- Use at least a 12-point font for printed materials. Overhead transparencies should use at least a 20- to 24-point font.
- Thicker letters are easier to read than fine print.
- Avoid elaborate fonts; stick with simple, basic lettering.
- Stick to one style of font per document.
- Use a normal mixture of capital and small letters.
- Select paper and ink of strongly contrasting colors.

---

time. Break teaching into manageable blocks so that the older adult has time to think about a limited number of concepts. Whenever possible, provide printed materials to supplement and reinforce the content that was covered (Box 5-3). Practical examples or illustrations related to the topic may be more effective than a quick recitation of factual information. If the teaching involves a psychomotor skill, such as drawing up insulin or changing a dressing, the older adult should receive one or more demonstrations of the skill and then be given ample opportunities to practice and perform the skill with supervision. The nurse should be patient and supportive, regardless of the amount of time needed. Remember, the goal is learning, not speed.

Modifications may be needed to compensate for common sensory changes experienced with aging. Be sure to face older individuals when speaking. Speak clearly. Try to avoid microphones or amplifiers that might distort sounds or cause interference with hearing aids. Repeat information, and use visual cues or materials to reinforce a verbal message. Support verbal information with printed material and audiovisual aids such as videos. Encourage hands-on practice. Use as many senses as possible, but not necessarily all at once. Too much sensory input may confuse the older adult.

Clinical Situation

Communicating With Older Adults

A physician and a clergyman happened to arrive in an elderly patient's room at the same time. The patient became very anxious and started to cry. The physician and the clergyman were taken aback because the patient was doing well and was ready for discharge. After much time was spent calming the patient and listening carefully, they realized that the patient responded as she did because she thought the doctor was going to tell her that she was dying and that the clergyman was there to console her.

Get Ready for the NCLEX® Examination!

Key Points

- Keys to effective communication include knowledge about the other person and respect for his or her uniqueness.
- To develop rapport and communicate effectively with older adults, nurses must identify sensory changes that can interfere with the transmission of messages and cultural or age-related values that can result in misunderstandings.
- Nurses must accurately recognize and interpret both verbal and nonverbal messages being sent by older adults, their families, and their friends. Nurses also must be aware of the messages they themselves are sending.
- The desire to interact effectively with others, patience, acceptance, respect, empathy, and the use of appropriate communication techniques are essential parts of effective nursing practice (see Table 5-1).
- Specific approaches and adaptations are needed to promote effective communications with older individuals experiencing sensory and cognitive changes.
- Effective communications with physicians are important for quality patient care.
- Communication through teaching is increasingly part of the nurse's role in health promotion and management.

Additional Learning Resources

SG Go to the Study Guide on pp. 379–397 for additional learning activities to help you master the chapter content.

evolve Go to your Evolve website (http://evolve.elsevier.com/Wold/geriatric) for the following FREE learning resources:
- Animations
- Answer Guidelines for Nursing Care Plan Critical Thinking Questions
- Answers and Rationales for Review Questions for the NCLEX® Examination
- Glossary with pronunciations in English and Spanish
- Video Clips

Review Questions for the NCLEX® Examination

1. Which interventions would be appropriate to use when teaching a client who has presbycusis? (Select all that apply.)
   1. Stand on the affected side.
   2. Speak much more loudly.
   3. Use simple statements.
   4. Provide audiovisual tapes.
   5. Repeat information.
   6. Face the client when talking.
   7. Ensure adequate lighting.

2. The actions most likely to enhance the nurse's communication with an elderly person include: (Select all that apply.)
   1. Identify yourself.
   2. Ask many questions to find out about the person.
   3. Play music or turn on the TV to help the person relax.
   4. Use friendly terms like *Dearie.*
   5. Stay in the living area where other people are around.
   6. Use pictures and gestures in addition to words.
   7. Be patient and avoid interrupting.

3. The nurse tries to use communication techniques that are most effective at establishing an empathetic climate. The most effective method is to use:
   1. Open-ended responses
   2. Direct questioning
   3. Informing
   4. Confrontational responses

4. The nurse should remember that older adults are most responsive to teaching when the information is:
   1. Interesting
   2. New
   3. Relevant to their lives
   4. Presented well

Maintaining Fluid Balance and Meeting Nutrition Needs

Objectives

1. Identify the various types of nutrients.
2. Identify the components of a healthy diet for older adults.
3. Describe age-related changes in nutritional and fluid requirements.
4. Identify age-related changes that affect nutrition, digestion, and hydration.
5. Describe methods of assessing the nutritional status and practices of older adults.
6. Identify the older adults who are most at risk for problems related to nutrition and hydration.
7. Identify selected nursing diagnoses related to nutritional or metabolic problems.
8. Identify interventions that will help older persons meet their nutrition and hydration needs.

Key Terms

anemia (ă-NĒ-mē-ă) (p. 107)
basal metabolic rate (BĀ-săl mĕt-ă-BŎL-ĭk rāt) (p. 103)
blood urea nitrogen (blŭd ū-RĒ-ă NĬ-trō-jĕn) (p. 113)
calories (KĂL-ŏ-rēs) (p. 102)
carbohydrates (kăr-bō-HĪ-drāts) (p. 104)
creatinine (krē-ĂT-Ĭ-nēn) (p. 113)
edema (ě-DĒ-mă) (p. 121)
electrolyte (ē-LĔK-trō-līt) (p. 113)
hematocrit (hē-MĂT-ŏ-krĭt) (p. 113)
hemoglobin (HĒ-mō-glō-bĭn) (p. 113)

interstitial (ĭn-tĕr-STĬSH-ăl) (p. 121)
intracellular (ĭn-tră-SĔL-ū-lăr) (p. 121)
intravascular (ĭn-tră-VĂS-cū-lăr) (p. 121)
malnutrition (măl-nū-TRĬSH-ŭn) (p. 110)
minerals (MĬN-ĕr-ălz) (p. 108)
nasogastric (nā-zō-GĂS-trĭk) (p. 120)
proteins (PRŌ-tēnz) (p. 104)
supplement (SŬP-lĕ-mĕnt) (p. 120)
trace element (p. 109)
vitamins (VĪ-tă-mĭnz) (p. 106)

Nutrition plays an important role in health maintenance, rehabilitation, and prevention and control of disease. When dealing with nutritional issues, nurses who work with older adults must consider the following: (1) the basic components of a well-balanced diet for older adults; (2) how the normal physiologic changes of aging change nutritional needs; (3) how the normal physiologic changes of aging may interfere with the purchase, preparation, and consumption of nutrients; and (4) how cognitive, psychosocial, and pathologic changes commonly seen in aging impact the aging individual's nutritional status.

NUTRITION AND AGING

Nutritional needs do not remain static throughout life. As with other needs, the nutritional needs of older adults are not exactly the same as those of younger individuals. An understanding of the nutritional needs of older adults is essential to providing good nursing care. To assess nutritional adequacy and select interventions that promote good nutrition, nurses must be knowledgeable about basic nutrition and diet therapy. Good nutrition practices play a vital role in health maintenance and health promotion. Good eating habits throughout life promote physical wellness and mental well-being. Inadequate nutrition and fluid intake can result in serious problems such as malnutrition and dehydration. Poor nutrition practices can contribute to the development of osteoporosis and skin ulcers and can complicate existing conditions such as cardiovascular disease and diabetes mellitus.

CALORIC INTAKE

Calories are units of heat that are used to measure the available energy in consumed food. Because people's energy requirements differ widely, the number of calories they require also differs significantly. Many factors influence how many calories will be used by a person: activity patterns, gender, body size, age, body temperature, emotional status, and the temperature of the climate in which the person lives. Both acute and chronic illnesses also have an impact on caloric needs. In general, when a person's caloric intake is in balance with the energy needs of the body, his or her weight remains constant. When caloric intake exceeds energy needs, the excess is converted into adipose (fat) tissue for storage, and the individual gains weight.

Table 6-1	Average Weight of Older Adults Per Height					
	WEIGHT (LB)					
HEIGHT (INCHES)	AGE 65–69	AGE 70–74	AGE 75–79	AGE 80–84	AGE 85–89	AGE 90–94
Women						
58	133	125	123	—	—	—
59	134	127	124	116	110	—
60	135	129	126	118	113	—
61	137	131	128	121	116	—
62	139	134	131	124	120	119
63	141	137	134	128	124	119
64	144	140	137	132	133	120
65	147	144	140	136	138	124
66	151	147	143	140	142	129
67	155	151	146	144	—	—
68	159	155	—	—	—	—
69	164	160	—	—	—	—
Men						
61	142	139	137	—	—	—
62	144	141	139	135	—	—
63	146	143	141	136	133	—
64	149	146	143	138	135	—
65	151	149	145	141	139	130
66	154	152	148	144	142	133
67	156	155	151	147	145	136
68	159	158	154	150	148	140
69	163	162	158	154	152	144
70	167	165	162	159	156	149
71	172	169	166	164	160	154
72	177	173	171	170	165	—
73	182	178	175	—	—	—

When caloric intake is less than the energy needs, the person loses weight (Table 6-1).

Various nutrients provide different amounts of calories. Fats, which can come from either plant sources (e.g., oleomargarine) or animal sources (e.g., butter), yield 9 calories/g. Proteins and carbohydrates yield 4 calories/g. Vitamins, minerals, and water yield no calories. Alcohol yields 7 calories/g without contributing any nutritional value.

Studies have shown that caloric needs in healthy individuals decrease at a rate of approximately 5% for each decade between ages 55 and 75 years and 7% percent for each decade after age 75. The body's muscle and lean tissue masses decrease with aging, and adipose tissue increases. As the proportion of muscle and fat changes, the **basal metabolic rate** (the rate at which the body uses calories) decreases. The normal decrease in physical activity commonly seen with aging further slows the rate at which the body burns calories. Healthy individuals who maintain an active lifestyle that includes exercise may see little need to change their caloric intake. Inactive individuals may need to restrict caloric intake significantly. The lowest recommended daily intake to adequately meet nutritional needs is 1200 calories.

When determining the adequacy of caloric intake, disease processes must be considered. Diseases that result in restricted mobility and physical activity (e.g., arthritis and stroke) are likely to decrease caloric needs. Other disease processes (e.g., infections and various forms of cancer) actually increase the body's caloric requirements. Individuals suffering from diabetes mellitus require special diets, which are prescribed by a physician. Diet plays an important role in the medical management of diabetes and is used to control and treat the disease. The diabetic diet normally includes calorie restrictions and is specially balanced with regard to the percentage of fats, proteins, and carbohydrates.

NUTRIENTS

Although caloric needs often decrease with age, the need to include all of the various nutrients does not. Therefore, foods high in nutritional value and relatively low in calories must be selected to maximize the amount of nutrients the body receives while reducing the number of calories.

Vital nutrients needed by all people include carbohydrates, protein, fats, vitamins, minerals, and fluids. Because many foods contain a combination of these nutrients, various methods of determining nutritional balance have been developed. One way to measure the adequacy of a person's diet and nutritional intake is determined by comparing his or her intake to accepted standards. The most common standard for determining the balance of a diet plan is the food pyramid (Figure 6-1). This pyramid has been revised several times through the years to best reflect our understanding of nutritional needs. The current form, MyPlate, was designed by the United States Department of Agriculture (USDA) in 2011. The plate is divided into color-coded food groups, including vegetables, fruits, grains, and protein, with dairy on the side. Regardless of the total amount of food consumed, the proportion of food from each group should remain in balance.

The plan is intended to be simple so that people of all ages and educational background are able to use it. More than just a diet, MyPlate offers a health plan that encourages users to adopt healthier eating habits and increase physical activity. General recommendations from the USDA (2011) for the general population include:

- Enjoying food but eating less of it
- Avoiding oversized portions

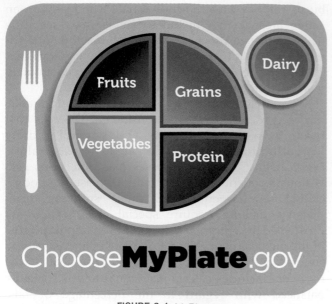

FIGURE 6-1 MyPlate.

- Increasing intake of fruits, vegetables, and whole grains
- Choosing low-fat or fat-free dairy products
- Reducing intake of sodium
- Drinking water instead of sugary beverages
- Making physical activity an everyday occurrence

Additional tips and resources, including recipes and interactive tools are available at www.Choose MyPlate.gov.

Other more detailed standards for measuring the nutritional adequacy of a diet are found in the Dietary Reference Intakes, which include the recommended dietary allowances (RDAs) and the adequate intakes (AIs) (see Appendix C). These references specify the recommendations for the following:

- Calories
- Macronutrients such as protein, carbohydrates, and fats
- Amount of water
- Fiber
- Elemental minerals, including iron, magnesium, manganese, phosphorus, selenium, vanadium, zinc, etc.
- Vitamins
- Electrolytes

Dietary reference intakes are a more complex way of analyzing dietary intake. Use of these standards requires careful weighing and measurement of portions and use of nutritional references or complete nutrition labels that list all of the ingredients in detail. Some older adults may consult these recommendations when selecting vitamins or other nutrients. Nutritional labels are commonly used by physicians, nurses, or dietitians when developing a specific therapeutic diet plan. A more general checklist that older

adults can use to determine their nutritional health is shown in Figure 6-2.

Carbohydrates

Carbohydrates include the familiar sugars and starches that compose approximately half of the standard American diet. A ready source of energy for the body, carbohydrates are usually divided into two categories: simple and complex. Simple carbohydrates are used most readily by the body because their bonds are easily broken. Table sugar, honey, syrup, and candy are examples of simple carbohydrates. Complex carbohydrates must be broken down into simple sugars before they can be used by the body. This breakdown requires time and energy. Foods such as vegetables, whole grains, and fruits contain complex carbohydrates. Foods that contain complex carbohydrates usually also contain other nutrients (e.g., minerals and vitamins), making them more nutritious than foods containing simple carbohydrates only. The American Heart Association recommends that 55% to 60% of calories should come from carbohydrates, with an emphasis on complex carbohydrates. This recommendation appears to be appropriate for the aging population.

In addition to providing essential nutrients, complex carbohydrates usually contain significant amounts of soluble fiber, a substance humans cannot digest, which forms bulk and aids bowel elimination. Fiber is recommended as helpful in preventing constipation, diverticulosis, and diverticulitis. A diet high in complex carbohydrates is recommended as part of the control of many disease processes. The soluble fiber in complex carbohydrates has been shown to reduce blood cholesterol levels, which is helpful for individuals who are at risk for coronary artery disease. Complex carbohydrates also play an important role in the control of diabetes, because they effectively meet energy needs without causing rapid increases in blood glucose levels the way simple sugars do.

Proteins

Proteins are composed of **amino acids,** which are essential for tissue repair and healing. The need for protein remains constant or may increase slightly with aging to compensate for the loss of lean body tissue (Box 6-1). The RDA of protein for women older than 50 years of age is 50 g/day; for men older than age 50 years, the RDA is 65 g/day. Data from the National Health and Nutrition Examination Survey reveal that 10% to 25% of women older than age 55 consume less than half of the recommended daily amount of protein. Protein consumption in older adults can be affected by many factors, including the ability to procure and prepare food, the cost of foods containing protein, and even the ability to chew common high-protein foods.

The Warning Signs of poor nutritional health are often overlooked. Use this checklist to find out if you or someone you know is at nutritional risk.

Read the statements below. Circle the number in the "yes" column for those that apply to you or someone you know. For each "yes" answer, score the number in the box. Total your nutritional score.

DETERMINE YOUR NUTRITIONAL HEALTH

	YES
I have an illness or condition that made me change the kind and/or amount of food I eat.	2
I eat fewer than 2 meals per day.	3
I eat few fruits or vegetables or milk products.	2
I have 3 or more drinks of beer, liquor, or wine almost everyday.	2
I have tooth or mouth problems that make it hard for me to eat.	2
I don't always have enough money to buy the food I need.	4
I eat alone most of the time.	1
I take 3 or more different prescribed or over-the-counter drugs a day.	1
Without wanting to, I have lost or gained 10 pounds in the last 6 months.	2
I am not always physically able to shop, cook, and/or feed myself.	2
TOTAL	

Total Your Nutritional Score. If it's—

0–2   **Good!** Recheck your nutritional score in 6 months.

3–5   **You are at moderate nutritional risk.** See what can be done to improve your eating habits and lifestyle. Your office on aging, senior nutrition program, senior citizens' center, or health department can help. Recheck your nutritional score in 3 months.

6 or more You are at high nutritional risk. Bring this checklist the next time you see your doctor, dietitian, or other qualified health or social service professional. Talk with them about any problems you may have. Ask for help to improve your nutritional health.

Remember that warning signs suggest risk but do not represent diagnosis of any condition.

FIGURE 6-2 Determine your nutritional health. Checklist of warning signs of poor nutrition.

Box 6-1   **Ways to Increase Protein Intake**

- *Add eggs*—Add extra whites to pancakes, omelets, and scrambled eggs; add hard boiled eggs to casseroles and salads.
- *Add cheese*—Sprinkle on salads, melt on sandwiches, serve on crackers, add to casseroles, use to top vegetables, blend in mashed potatoes, use in cheesecake.
- *Add milk, cream, and yogurt*—Add when baking or making pancakes. Use in hot cocoa, sauces, milk shakes, smoothies, on fruit, with cereal, as a desert topping.
- *Add legumes and beans*—Cook these in soups and stews. Use bean curd on salads. Serve ethnic dishes made with chickpeas, such as hummus or falafel.
- *Add peanut butter*—Use in cookies, as a dip for fruit or vegetables, in sauces, and on sandwiches.

Tissue replacement and repair continue throughout life. Any condition in which tissue integrity is altered (e.g., surgery and pressure ulcers) increases the amount of protein needed to aid in tissue repair. Red meats, poultry, fish, eggs, and dairy products are good sources of **complete proteins,** which contain all of the amino acids necessary for making and repairing tissues. Plant foods such as legumes (peas and beans), nuts, and cereals (whole grains and rice) contain smaller amounts of incomplete proteins, which do not individually contain all of the necessary amino acids. Incomplete proteins must be combined carefully to meet protein needs.

Some foods that are high in protein such as steak, ham, organ meats, egg yolks, hard cheese, and whole milk also contain large amounts of fats. Excessive consumption of proteins with a high fat content can contribute to elevated blood levels of cholesterol and triglycerides, which, in turn, contribute to plaque formation and atherosclerotic changes in the blood vessels. Atherosclerosis often results in hypertension and heart disease. For this reason, many physicians and dietitians recommend that high-fat protein foods be restricted. A person who is on a fat-restricted diet should consume low-fat proteins such as fish and lean poultry, as well as protein from plant sources such as peas and beans.

Fats

It is recommended that fats be limited to approximately 25% to 30% of the total daily caloric intake. This recommendation does not change with aging. A certain amount of fat is necessary and desirable in the diet to aid in the absorption of fat-soluble vitamins and to provide adequate amounts of essential fatty acids. Fat is desirable because it adds flavor to food and provides a sense of fullness with a meal. Foods with no fat would be unappealing, poor tasting, and not very satisfying.

When considering fat intake in the diet, it is important to watch the type of fats ingested. The body incorporates fats into substances called **lipoproteins,** which contain cholesterol and proteins. There are three important types of lipoproteins: high-density lipoprotein (HDL), low-density lipoprotein (LDL), and very-low-density lipoprotein (VLDL). LDL is primarily composed of cholesterol and is believed to contribute to blood vessel disease. VLDL is primarily composed of triglycerides and may contribute to vessel disease but not as significantly as does LDL. HDL, the so-called healthy fat, is primarily composed of protein that appears to protect against blood vessel disease.

Some individuals who have been eating high-cholesterol foods for their entire lives may be reluctant to change their eating habits as they age. They may find it difficult or unpleasant to shop for and prepare foods in new ways. Others can successfully alter their dietary intake to avoid foods high in these substances.

Vitamins

Vitamins are organic compounds found naturally in foods. They can also be produced synthetically. Vitamins are needed for a variety of metabolic and physiologic processes. Vitamins are classified as fat-soluble or water-soluble. The fat-soluble vitamins include vitamins A, D, E, and K. The B-complex vitamins and vitamin C are water-soluble (Table 6-2).

The benefits of vitamins for older adults are being closely examined. Some researchers who subscribe to the free radical theory of aging are studying the effects of the so-called antioxidant vitamins. It is theorized that antioxidant vitamins can block or neutralize free radicals and prevent cell damage, thereby slowing the effects of aging and preventing a number of diseases such as cancer and heart disease. Although research into this area is promising, many experts are not yet convinced of the effectiveness of antioxidant vitamins or satisfied that we have an adequate understanding of their method of action, therapeutic dosage, and long-term effects. Vitamins A, C, and E are considered antioxidants.

Vitamin deficiencies have been connected to a variety of problems experienced by older adults, including the following:

- Inadequate intake of vitamin A may contribute to poor wound healing, dry skin, and night blindness.
- Vitamin B_6 deficiency, also common in older adults, is likely correlated with neurologic and immunologic problems. Clinical manifestations of B_6 deficiency may include nausea, vomiting, loss of appetite, dermatitis, motor weakness, dizziness, depression, and sore tongue. Supplements of vitamin B_6 help reverse these problems.
- Vitamin B_{12} deficiency can be related to inadequate protein consumption or physiologic changes in digestion. Normal aging changes result in the decreased production of gastric acid and pepsin, which are necessary for protein digestion. When less protein is digested, less B_{12} is available for

Table 6-2	Summary of Essential Vitamins
Fat-soluble vitamins	
Vitamin A	Found in milk, butter, cheese, fortified margarine, liver, green and yellow vegetables, and fruits Promotes healthy epithelium, ability to see in dim light, normal mucus formation Many older people may be deficient in vitamin A because of chronic conditions that interfere with fat absorption such as gallbladder disease and colitis
Vitamin D	Found in fortified milk and margarine, cod liver oil, fatty fish, and eggs Promotes absorption of calcium May contribute to skeletal changes with aging
Vitamin E	Found in corn and safflower oils, margarine, seeds, nuts, and leafy green vegetables Promotes integrity of red blood cells
Vitamin K	Found in leafy green vegetables and liver; synthesized by bacteria in the colon Essential for formation of prothrombin, which is necessary for blood clotting
Water-soluble vitamins	
Vitamin B_1 (thiamine hydrochloride)	Found in organ meats, pork, legumes, and whole grains Essential for carbohydrate metabolism
Vitamin B_2 (riboflavin)	Found in milk, cheese, eggs, organ meats, legumes, and leafy green vegetables Essential for normal tissue maintenance and tear production
Niacin	Found in lean meats, liver, whole grains, and legumes Essential for energy release from fats, carbohydrates, and proteins
Vitamin B_6 (hydrochloride)	Found in whole grains, vegetables, legumes, meats, and bananas Acts in the processes of protein synthesis and amino acid metabolism May interact with levodopa taken by patients with Parkinson's disease
Folacin (folic acid)	Found in whole wheat, legumes, and green vegetables Important in hemoglobin synthesis and in metabolism of amino acids Common deficiency in older adults
Vitamin B_{12} (cyanocobalamin)	Found in muscle and organ meats, eggs, shellfish, and dairy products Requires production of intrinsic factor by the stomach for absorption; inadequate absorption can result in pernicious anemia Needed for maturation of red blood cells Deficiency is commonly seen with folacin deficiency
Vitamin C (ascorbic acid)	Found in citrus fruits, tomatoes, cabbage, melons, strawberries, green peppers, and leafy green vegetables Important in the formation and maintenance of collagen structure of connective tissue Promotes healing and elasticity of capillary walls

absorption. Vitamin B_{12} deficiency can result in neurologic changes that affect sensation, balance, and memory. Clinical manifestations of B_{12} deficiency can include vomiting, fatigue, constipation, anemia, decreased memory, and depression. If detected early and treated with supplements, some of the symptoms of vitamin B_{12} deficiency may be reversible.

- Vitamin C deficiency may contribute to weakness, dry mouth, skin changes, and delayed tissue healing.
- Vitamin D deficiency is more common in older adults because of less exposure to the sun, reduced capacity of the skin to synthesize the vitamin, and decreased dietary intake. Because vitamin D is required for calcium absorption, a deficiency can contribute to excessive bone demineralization or osteoporosis. Clinical symptoms of vitamin D deficiency include weakness, gait disturbance, and pain. Adequate intake of vitamin D and calcium

supplements can help prevent or even reverse the severity of this problem. Research in Great Britain showed a 19% to 26% decrease in falls by older individuals taking vitamin D in doses between 700 IU and 1000 IU daily.

- Vitamin E appears to play a role in maintaining immune function in older adults and recently has been connected to delaying the onset of symptoms in Alzheimer's disease. The exact dose required to obtain maximal benefits is under study.
- Vitamin K deficiency has recently been correlated to an increased risk of fractures.

Older adults who consume well-balanced diets may not require supplemental vitamins. Those with increased risk factors such as gastrointestinal (GI) problems or inadequate nutritional intake may benefit from selected vitamin supplements. Supplements should be used with caution and under the direction of a physician or dietitian. Excess amounts of the water-soluble vitamins are quickly eliminated from the body and pose few risks. Excess amounts of the fat-soluble vitamins (A, D, E, and K) are retained in fatty tissue or stored in the liver. Overconsumption of these vitamins can lead to toxic symptoms and even permanent liver damage.

Minerals

Minerals are inorganic chemical elements that are required in many of the body's functions. Minerals make up a small proportion of total body weight, yet a slight mineral imbalance can have serious effects.

Calcium, the most abundant mineral in the body, is necessary for bone and tooth formation, nerve impulse transmission and conduction, muscle contraction (including cardiac function), and blood clotting. The main dietary sources of calcium are milk and dairy products. Calcium is normally retained in bone, with only a small amount (1%) found in the tissues and blood. With aging and with immobility, the bones tend to lose calcium, resulting in osteoporosis. In certain disease states, abnormal amounts of calcium leave the bone, enter the bloodstream, and cause **hypercalcemia,** which is an elevated level of calcium in the blood. Hypercalcemia is seen with hyperparathyroidism, disuse atrophy, metastatic bone tumors, and vitamin D excess.

Individuals experiencing hypercalcemia may manifest symptoms, including confusion, abdominal pain, muscle pain, weakness, and anorexia. These symptoms may be easily missed in older individuals because they are vague and common to many other conditions. Extremely high levels of calcium in the blood can result in shock, kidney failure, and even death. When the kidneys attempt to rid the body of excess calcium, hypercalciuria (increased calcium in the urine) results, and the risk for renal calculi (kidney stone) formation is increased.

Adequate calcium intake is important throughout life, but it is particularly important for those at risk for developing osteoporosis, especially postmenopausal women. Calcium may arrest the progress of osteoporosis. Vitamin D aids in the absorption of calcium. For this reason, vitamin D is added to milk products and fortified margarine.

Phosphorus is needed for normal bone and tooth formation, activation of some B vitamins, normal neuromuscular functioning, metabolism of carbohydrates, regulation of acid-base balance, and other physiologic processes. Inadequate nutritional intake of phosphorus can result in weight loss or anemia. The typical dietary sources of phosphorous compounds are dairy products, meat, egg yolks, peas, beans, nuts, and whole grains. Because of its wide availability, meeting the dietary requirements of this mineral normally is not a problem unless the individual is on a highly restricted diet.

Iron is found in the center of the heme portion of hemoglobin. Hemoglobin in the red blood cells transports oxygen to and removes carbon dioxide from the cells. Without adequate amounts of iron, the body cannot produce enough hemoglobin. When hemoglobin levels fall below the normal range, anemia results. Individuals suffering from anemia may manifest many symptoms, depending on the severity of the condition: fatigue, exertional dyspnea, tachycardia, palpitations, headache, insomnia, vertigo, pallor (particularly of the mucous membranes), and cool extremities. The normal changes of aging or other disease processes may resemble these symptoms and prevent recognition of anemia. Laboratory tests for hemoglobin levels are required to determine whether anemia is present (Table 6-3). Two forms of nutritional anemia are commonly seen in older adults: iron-deficiency anemia and pernicious anemia.

Iron-deficiency anemia results from inadequate intake of dietary iron. Rich sources of dietary iron include red meat, particularly organ meats such as liver; shellfish; egg yolks; leafy green vegetables; and dried fruits. Red meat is expensive and, unless properly prepared, can be difficult for older adults to chew. Many people do not like the taste of liver and organ meats and refuse to eat them. In addition, organ meats and egg yolks are high in cholesterol, which is often restricted from the diet. This can make meal planning difficult. In addition to increased nutritional intake of iron rich foods, folic acid and iron supplements are commonly prescribed.

It should be remembered that a concentrated iron formulation (liquid or solid) administered orally can irritate the GI tract. To reduce GI irritation, iron

Table 6-3	Laboratory Values Used to Assess Nutritional Adequacy in Older Adults
DIAGNOSTIC TEST	**APPROPRIATE RANGE**
Hemoglobin	14–18 g/dL (men) 12–16 g/dL (women)
Hematocrit	42%–52% (men) 37%–47 % (women)
Blood urea nitrogen	10–20 mg/dL may be slightly higher in elderly
Creatinine	0.6–1.2 mg/dL (male) 0.5–1.1 mg/dL (female) slightly decreased in elderly
Albumin	3.5–5.0 g/dL
Calcium	9–10.5 mg/dL
Folic acid	5–25 mg/dL
Glucose (fasting)	Fasting 70–110 mg/dL Increase in normal range after age 50.

Data from Pagana KD and Pagana TJ: Mosby's Manual of Diagnostic and Laboratory Tests, ed 4, St Louis, 2010, Mosby.

supplements should be taken during or after meals. Iron solutions can stain the teeth, so a straw should be used with liquid iron preparations. If iron is given by injection, it is important to use the Z-track method for deep intramuscular administration. Foods rich in vitamin C should be given in conjunction with iron to enhance its absorption. Patients should be told that iron will probably turn the stool a dark green or black color, and nurses should keep this in mind when assessing the stool of individuals receiving iron supplements. Concentrated iron supplements can also cause diarrhea.

Pernicious anemia is caused by a deficiency in intrinsic factor secreted by the stomach. Without this factor, vitamin B$_{12}$, which is required for red blood cell maturation in the bone marrow, is not absorbed. In addition, there are fewer white blood cells and there may be cellular changes in the existing cells. Individuals suffering from pernicious anemia may manifest weakness, numbness, or tingling in the extremities; anorexia; or weight loss. Treatment typically consists of cyanocobalamin injections and possibly oral folic acid and iron supplements.

Sodium is a commonly occurring mineral and is one of the important elements in the body. Sodium ions are involved in acid-base balance, fluid balance, nerve impulse transmission, and muscle contraction. Sodium is mostly found in extracellular fluid. Sodium levels are regulated by the kidneys, which retain or eliminate sodium according to the body's needs. Sodium interacts with potassium as part of the fluid exchange through cell membranes. Sodium is naturally present in many foods. The most common, most familiar concentrated form is sodium chloride, or table salt, which is used to flavor and preserve food. The typical American diet tends to be higher in sodium than is nutritionally required. Prepared foods such as canned soups or vegetables and frozen dinners are common in the diet of many older adults. In addition, older adults may use excessive amounts of salt to compensate for the decreased ability to perceive the taste of foods. Excessive blood levels of sodium, or hypernatremia, can cause fluid retention, which in body tissue is manifested as edema. People with hypertension, renal failure, or cardiac conditions are often placed on sodium-restricted diets, and many (especially older adults) report that food is less appetizing when prepared with reduced amounts of sodium. With less appetite, these individuals may eat less.

Potassium is the major intracellular ion in the body. Potassium ions play an important role in acid-base balance, fluid and electrolyte balance, and (with sodium) normal neuromuscular functioning. Potassium is not as abundant in the diets of older adults as are some of the other minerals. Dietary sources of potassium include citrus fruits, milk, bananas, and apple juice. Potassium deficiency, or hypokalemia, is a common problem in older adults. Many diuretic and antihypertensive medications deplete the body of potassium, as can prolonged or frequent diarrhea. Symptoms of hypokalemia include muscle weakness, anorexia, apprehension, irritability, drowsiness, depression, and disorientation. Severe muscle weakness is the most common observation related to decreased potassium levels. Hypokalemia with digitalis therapy is often a cause of cardiac arrhythmias. Because not all patients who have decreased levels of potassium demonstrate observable symptoms, nurses must check laboratory studies to verify levels of the electrolytes. Supplements are often prescribed to increase low blood potassium levels.

Zinc is a trace mineral that plays a role in protein synthesis. In adults, insufficient zinc may result in delayed wound healing, impaired immune function, lethargy, skin changes, diminished sense of smell and taste, and decreased appetite. Certain conditions, including some that are common in older adults, may result in zinc deficiency (e.g., cirrhosis of the liver, kidney disease, malignant cancers and alcoholism). Supplemental zinc may be administered. Dietary sources of zinc include meat, shellfish, and nuts.

Trace elements such as magnesium, copper, iodine, fluorine, chromium, selenium, nickel, and sulfur are necessary in very small amounts for normal body functioning. Selenium is gaining importance as an antioxidant mineral believed to promote heart health; improve tissue elasticity; and decrease the risk of colorectal, lung, and prostate cancer.

WATER

Water is essential for life. Humans can survive for many days without food but not without water. Water plays a role in many aspects of normal body functioning. Water is necessary for the formation of many of the body's secretions, including tears, perspiration, and saliva. Water aids in digestion and in transportation of electrolytes and nutrients. Water facilitates elimination of waste products and plays an important role in temperature regulation.

Approximately 60% of the average adult body is composed of water, with adult men having slightly more body fluid than do women. Older individuals typically have less body fluid than do younger adults. The total amount of body fluid decreases by approximately 8% to 10% in older adults. The amount of water in the bloodstream remains relatively constant with aging, but older adults tend to have less fluid in the intracellular and interstitial spaces than do younger people. This fluid decrease results in loss of skin turgor and leads to the wrinkled appearance that is common with aging. Decreased fluid increases the risk for fluid imbalances such as dehydration. Inadequate fluid intake can lead to altered absorption of medications, interfere with appetite and digestion, and contribute to problems with constipation.

Severe dehydration can make existing medical conditions worse and can ultimately result in death. Most adults require 2000 to 3000 ml of fluid each day. Most of this is consumed as beverages such as water, tea, coffee, and juice. Solid foods, particularly fruits and vegetables, contain significant amounts of water.

Water is normally lost through urination, perspiration, respiration, and defecation. Abnormal fluid loss occurs with diarrhea, vomiting, diaphoresis, gastric suctioning, and wound drainage; essential minerals are often lost along with the water. The amount of fluid taken into the body should be in balance with the amount eliminated from the body. This is referred to as **fluid balance.**

MALNUTRITION AND THE ELDERLY

In America, where obesity is an increasing problem, undernutrition and malnutrition are significant problems for the elderly. Statistics show that a large number of independent elderly— and even more institutionalized older adults—are at risk for malnutrition. **Malnutrition** is defined as a disorder of nutrition resulting from unbalanced, insufficient, or excessive diet or from impaired absorption, assimilation, or use of food. The risk for developing nutritional deficiencies increases with aging, but determining nutritional status is not always easy. Older adults who appear to be healthy may have unhealthy nutritional practices. An obese elderly person may be malnourished, whereas a thin elderly person may be well nourished. Studies have shown that a majority of older Americans believe that nutrition is important for good health but that they do not always follow good nutritional practices. Information from the National Council on Aging Nutritional Assessment Self-Test reveals that older adults have a disproportionately high risk for poor nutrition, which, in turn, has a negative effect on their health. Poorly nourished older adults are more likely to experience functional impairments, fatigue, loss of muscle strength, poor tissue healing, pressure ulcers, and infections. They are likely to develop more postoperative complications, spend a longer time in the hospital, and are at increased risk for death.

The Nutrition Screening Initiative, a coalition headed by the American Dietetic Association, estimated that in 2002 the number of elderly who was malnourished or at risk for malnutrition was as follows:
- 20% to 60% for home care elderly
- 40% to 60% for hospitalized elderly
- 40% to 85% for elderly residing in nursing homes

Other studies have yielded similar results and also report that an additional 5% to 10% of independent elderly in the community are likely to be inadequately nourished. These statistics reveal the magnitude of the problem that needs to be addressed by health care providers.

Symptoms of nutritional problems include unintentional weight loss, lightheadedness, disorientation, lethargy, and loss of appetite. The same or similar symptoms often occur with a variety of illnesses, making it difficult to determine whether the primary problem is medical or nutritional in origin. The medical diagnosis "failure to thrive" has long been used to describe infants and children who fail to grow at the expected rate. The diagnosis "geriatric failure to thrive" is being used with increasing frequency to describe elderly people who experience a pattern of symptoms, including depression, withdrawal, decreased activity, weight loss, decreased appetite, and malnutrition. This is a complex problem that requires nutritional and psychosocial interventions to stop the downward progression. Nurses working in all health care settings need to assess, plan, and implement strategies to maintain or improve the nutritional status of their elderly patients.

FACTORS AFFECTING NUTRITION IN THE ELDERLY

The nutritional status of older adults living in the community is affected by physiologic, economic, and social factors. Lack of appetite is commonly reported. The reasons for this are multiple and form the basis of risk assessment. The more risk factors present, the greater the likelihood of the older person experiencing nutritional inadequacy. Overall nutritional status will be affected if any of these problems persists for a significant period of time.

Physiologic risk factors include the following:
- **Chronic health factors** such as COPD, CHF, arthritis, dementia, and many others can interfere with obtaining and preparing adequate nutritional food. Shopping requires physical exertion. Acts that a young, healthy person does not think about—such as lifting cans from a top shelf, reaching for something near the floor, or moving groceries into and out of a store cart—can physically exhaust an infirm or older adult. Although store personnel or other shoppers would probably help with these activities (Figure 6-3), older adults are often too embarrassed or proud to ask for help. Once food is purchased and taken home, the task of food preparation remains. Opening cans, unsealing jars, and dealing with the ubiquitous plastic wrappers on food all present daunting obstacles to the aging individual. Think of the problems that a young, healthy person may have with current packaging, and then imagine performing the same tasks with decreased muscle strength, arthritis, or other age-related problems.
- **Alcoholism** is suspected to be a risk factor in a larger percentage of older adults than is commonly recognized. Although small amounts of alcohol may stimulate the appetite, consumption of large amounts of

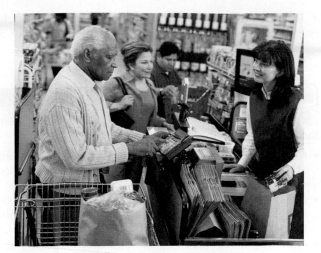

FIGURE 6-3 Shopping for groceries.

alcohol suppresses appetite, interferes with the absorption of essential nutrients, and all too often takes the place of meals.
- **Sensory changes** can cause problems with safe preparation and storage of food. Reading small print on labels can be difficult for an individual with presbyopia, cataracts, or other vision problems seen with aging. This can be problematic for someone on a restricted diet who needs to read the label to choose foods that are permitted. Older adults with altered senses of taste and smell may not be able to detect the changes that indicate spoilage. If spoiled food is eaten, the risk for GI infection or upset is increased.
- **Pain,** whether it is chronic or acute, can interfere with an older person's appetite and desire to procure, prepare, and consume food.
- **Medications** can cause an unpleasant change in the taste of food, suppress appetite, or cause nausea and vomiting. Many elderly complain of a "metallic taste" that interferes with the enjoyment of food. Other medications, such as antihypertensives, drugs used to treat Parkinson's disease, bronchodilators, and antidepressants, can cause a dry mouth, which makes chewing and swallowing more difficult.
- **Problems with chewing, swallowing, or digesting** are common causes of impaired nutrition. Poor oral hygiene, lost teeth, cavities, poorly fitted dentures, and decreased oral secretions affect the taste of food and can interfere with the ability of the older person to chew foods. This is particularly a problem with protein-rich foods, such as meat, unless they are cooked to a very tender consistency or provided in a chopped or ground form.
- **Malabsorption** due to decreased production of digestive enzymes can interfere with protein breakdown and absorption of vitamin B_{12}, calcium, and folate.

Economic risk factors include the following:
- **Cost of food** is a concern for many elderly adults with limited income. Foods rich in protein, such as meats and dairy products, tend to be more expensive than starchy carbohydrates. Fresh vegetables and fruits that are rich in vitamins and minerals may also be costly, depending on the season and locale. Many older adults have limited budgets and may not purchase these more costly items, although they know the nutritional value and importance of these foods. They may skip meals or consume inadequate portions to save money.
- **Difficulty getting transportation** to obtain food is a serious problem for older adults, particularly those who live alone. The simple act of getting to a store may be difficult. Trends toward large chain supermarkets have forced many smaller neighborhood grocery stores to close. These large stores are often located in shopping plazas that are far away from home. Even if there is a nearby neighborhood grocery or convenience store, its prices must be higher for it to stay in business. Either situation presents problems for the older adult. Without a car, a homebound older adult may find it difficult to obtain groceries, medicine, or other necessities. Many times, family members or friends drive the older adult to the store to shop or pick up groceries. As a courtesy to busy or older customers, more stores now offer call-in and delivery services for an added fee. Some communities offer scheduled transportation from senior citizen housing to grocery stores. Others provide volunteers to shop for homebound older adults.
- **Obtaining an appropriate variety and sufficient amount of food** can be difficult for older adults. Most foods are packaged in sizes appropriate for families of four or more. Although some manufacturers are responding to the needs of single adults and older adults by packaging smaller servings, the cost is often higher per serving. Older adults must decide whether thrift or variety is more important.

Social risk factors include the following:
- **Depression** is a common reason for decreased appetite in older adults. Grief, failing health, loss of independence, and many other factors can cause depression. Malnutrition can also be a cause of depression. Often the problem is unrecognized until the person has lost significant weight or develops other health problems.
- **Loneliness** or *social isolation* is one of the more common risk factors for nutritional problems in older adults. Eating is usually more pleasant with company. Widowed or single elderly persons are less likely to prepare and consume nutritious meals than are seniors who have more social contact.
- **Lack of motivation** to cook is commonly an issue for the elderly. Preparing food for one or two people can be more difficult. Most recipes are intended for four,

six, or eight servings. If this much food is prepared, it must be either eaten as leftovers for several days or wasted. Some older adults prepare their favorite meals and then package and freeze individual servings so that they can have variety and avoid waste. Unfortunately, not everyone has a freezer and not all foods can be frozen. Even if packaging problems can be overcome, the food must still be prepared. Because the effort of cooking can be overwhelming to the aging person, meal after meal may consist of sandwiches or cereal. Many communities have established programs designed to help the aging population meet their nutritional needs. Senior citizen meal programs provide both reasonably priced meals and companionship. Meals on Wheels programs deliver a variety of well-balanced meals to the homebound, allowing them to maintain some degree of independence (Figure 6-4).

Problems related to poor nutrition are not limited to older adults residing in the community. Nutritional problems are also an area of concern for seniors who reside in institutional settings. As previously identified, as many as 85% of nursing home residents may be undernourished. Although most institutions maintain well-staffed dietary departments under the supervision of trained dietitians, many older adults do not consume the nutrients that are available to them. This may be related to the physiologic or emotional risk factors discussed previously or to institutional factors outside the control of the elderly person. Some institutional factors that influence nutrition include the following:

- The repetitive nature of institutional meals
- Problems maintaining the temperature and appearance of food while serving many people
- Environmental concerns such as odors or the behavior of others
- Problems related to being fed by others

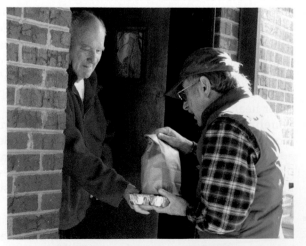

FIGURE 6-4 A Meals-on-Wheels recipient.

- Inability of an institution to meet the specific cultural preferences or general likes and dislikes of a large number of people

Coordinated Care
Collaboration
Nutrition

- Nursing assistants or dietary aides are most likely to be aware of the amount and types of food consumed by older residents.
- Data that are more specific than the typical good/fair/poor ratings or even percentages are important for good care planning.
- Assistants need to report the types of food consumed (e.g., the amount of meat and vegetables versus the amount of applesauce and dessert).

? Critical Thinking
Nutritional Assessment

An 84-year-old woman has been living in a long-term care facility for 6 months. It is noted that she has been losing weight at a rate of approximately 3 to 5 pounds a month. This was not immediately evident because she had been moderately overweight. Now her clothing is loose. She is 66 inches tall and weighs 150 pounds. She never complains about being hungry, and her chart reveals that she eats 50% to 75% of the food at each meal. Her hemoglobin is 9.6 g/dl, and her hematocrit is 32%.

- Is her weight loss desirable?
- What are possible reasons for the weight loss?
- What other information does the nurse need to obtain?

SOCIAL AND CULTURAL ASPECTS OF NUTRITION

Food is more than a means of meeting nutritional needs. Food is also used as part of religious ceremonies, in social interactions, and as a means of cultural expression. Throughout history, food has been linked to the gods. Many major religions such as Islam, Judaism, and Catholicism include some dietary restrictions. These religions may require avoidance of certain foods, fasting, or special methods of food preparation for all members of the faith. Although most religions have more lenient restrictions for older adults and the infirm, many older adults—especially those with great religious faith—want to comply with their religious teachings. Violating dietary rules may deeply upset them. This presents a challenge to caregivers, who are more concerned about adequate nutrition than about religious beliefs. If such a situation arises, it is appropriate for the nurse to consult with a dietitian or with the rabbi, minister, priest, or spiritual leader of the specific religious group to seek clarification and guidance. Many times, the spiritual counselor can provide reassurance to the older adult and guidance to the health care team.

Cultural influences in food are also significant. The foods we eat in our homes from early in life reflect our culture. Some people are happy to eat a variety of foods; others prefer to eat only foods with which they are familiar. Various cultures ascribe certain powers to foods. The culture may dictate what, when, or how foods should be eaten. An older adult from such a cultural background may find it difficult to understand or accept mainstream American nutrition practices. It is important to remember that good nutrition can be achieved within any culture (Table 6-4). Special planning with the dietitian is often necessary to achieve adequate nutrition and meet cultural preferences within an institutional setting. Family members and significant others from the same culture may be willing to provide special foods and assist in meeting the nutritional needs of the institutionalized older adult.

Food is often tied to social events. When people visit friends' homes, they are often served food. Food is served at parties, weddings, and wakes. People on dates go out to eat. Eating alone is often described as one of the worst things about being single or widowed. A common notion is that food eaten alone does not even taste the same. Nurses should remember this when working with older adults.

Many older adults like to go out to eat in restaurants. Eating out has many benefits, including a change of scenery, a wider choice of foods, and the opportunity for social interaction. Most older adults prefer restaurants with table service rather than buffets or fast-food establishments because they tend to be less noisy and do not require a person to balance trays of food. Eating out is an occasional treat for some older adults, but it is a way of life for others. Older adults who eat out regularly should consider their choices and use care to avoid the high-fat, high-sodium items that are common restaurant fare. Many restaurants that cater to older adults offer heart-healthy items and senior portions, often at discounted prices.

Older adults who live in long-term or assisted living settings are usually served one or more meals in a dining room. Independent elderly can obtain low-cost, nutritious meals and participate in social activities at congregate meal centers funded by the Elderly Nutrition Program. Most people tend to eat better when dining with others than when they are left to eat alone in a room or apartment. Nourishing snacks served during group or social activities can supplement an older person's intake and tend to be consumed more readily (Figure 6-5).

❖ NURSING PROCESS FOR RISK FOR IMBALANCED NUTRITION

Changes in weight may be an early indication of actual or potential nutritional problems in older adults. Current weight should be compared with standard height and weight charts that list the desirable weight for various heights (see Table 6-1). The height used should reflect the person's current height, not the height from a younger age that is commonly reported by aging individuals and recorded on their charts. If the individual appears well-proportioned and if his or her weight falls within recommended norms, then the person is probably receiving adequate calories. A slow increase or decrease in weight indicates an imbalance between caloric intake and energy expenditure. A decrease in activity with static caloric intake normally results in gradual weight gain, whereas an increase in activity with consistent caloric intake normally results in weight loss. Nurses should investigate changes in intake or activity that could account for changes in weight.

Adequate caloric intake is not enough. It is also essential that older adults obtain adequate amounts of essential nutrients. To determine whether these nutritional needs are being met, nurses must gather additional information.

Laboratory values may help support other observations. Hemoglobin level, **hematocrit** level, red blood cell (RBC) count, **blood urea nitrogen** (BUN) level, **creatinine** level, albumin level, and other nutritional indices should be reviewed to determine whether specific nutritional deficiencies exist. These laboratory values can be evaluated in the same way for younger and older persons because they do not routinely change with aging.

Hemoglobin is a complex protein-iron molecule that is responsible for the transport of oxygen and carbon dioxide within the bloodstream. If adequate iron is not available, the hemoglobin level and the RBC count will fall below the normal levels. Low hemoglobin levels may result from anemia or blood loss. Common forms of anemia, as discussed in Chapter 3, include iron-deficiency anemia and pernicious anemia. Iron-deficiency anemia may result from blood loss. In older adults, this rarely takes the form of a massive hemorrhage, although a significant amount of blood may be lost from frequent nosebleeds or recent surgery. More common in older adults is subtle blood loss from bleeding gastric or duodenal ulcers, diverticulitis, tumors, or pathologic conditions of the lower gastrointestinal tract.

The blood glucose level of a healthy person changes throughout the day. It is low during periods of fasting, but it rises after a meal and then peaks approximately 30 to 60 minutes after eating. Within 3 hours, it returns to its normal range of 80 to 120 mg/dL. Individuals who have diabetes, are receiving steroid therapy or total parenteral nutrition, or are experiencing high levels of stress are likely to experience problems with control of blood sugar levels.

Electrolyte imbalances may be a result of inadequate electrolyte intake or excessive loss. Abnormal levels of calcium, sodium, and potassium are most commonly

Table 6-4   Characteristic Food Patterns of Selected Cultures

MILK GROUP	PROTEIN GROUP	FRUITS AND VEGETABLES	BREADS AND CEREALS	POSSIBLE DIETARY PROBLEMS
American Indian (Many Tribal Variations; Many "Americanized")				

Fresh milk
Evaporated milk
  for cooking
Ice cream
Cream pie
	Pork, beef, lamb, rabbit
	Fowl, fish, eggs
	Legumes
	Sunflower seeds
	Nuts: walnut, acorn, pine,
	  peanut butter
	Game meat
		Green peas, beans
		Beets, turnips
		Leafy green and
		  other vegetables
		Grapes, bananas,
		  peaches, other
		  fresh fruits
		Roots
			Refined bread
			Whole wheat
			Cornmeal
			Rice
			Dry cereals
			"Fry" bread
			Tortillas
				Obesity, diabetes, alcoholism,
				  nutritional deficiencies expressed
				  in dental problems and iron-
				  deficiency anemia
				Inadequate amounts of all nutrients
				Excessive use of sugar

Middle Eastern* (Armenian, Greek, Syrian, Turkish)				

Yogurt
Little butter
	Lamb
	Nuts
	Dried peas, beans, lentils
	Sesame seeds
		Peppers, tomatoes,
		  cabbage, grape
		  leaves, cucumbers,
		  squash
		Dried apricots,
		  raisins, dates
			Cracked wheat
			  and dark
			  bread
				Fry many meats and vegetables
				Lack of fresh fruits
				Insufficient foods from milk group
				High consumption of sweetenings,
				  lamb fat, and olive oil

African American				

Milk†
Ice cream
Cheese:
  longhorn,
  American
	Pork: all cuts, plus organs,
	  chitterlings
	Beef, lamb
	Chicken, giblets
	Eggs
	Nuts
	Legumes
	Fish, game
		Leafy vegetables
		Green and yellow
		  vegetables
		Potatoes: white,
		  sweet
		Stewed fruit
		Bananas and other
		  fresh fruit
			Cornmeal and
			  hominy grits
			Rice
			Biscuits,
			  pancakes,
			  white breads
			Puddings:
			  bread, rice
				Extensive use of frying, smothering
				  in gravy, or simmering
				Fats: salt pork, bacon drippings, lard,
				  and gravies
				High consumption of sweets
				Insufficient citrus
				Vegetables often boiled for long
				  periods with pork fat and much salt
				Limited amounts from milk group†

Chinese (Cantonese Most Prevalent)				

Milk: water
  buffalo
	Pork sausage‡
	Eggs and pigeon eggs
	Fish
	Lamb, beef, goat
	Fowl: chicken, duck
	Nuts
	Legumes Soybean curd (tofu)
		Many vegetables
		Radish leaves
		Bean, bamboo
		  sprouts
			Rice/rice flour
			  products
			Cereals,
			  noodles
			Wheat, corn,
			  millet seed
				Tendency of some immigrants to
				  use large amounts of grease in
				  cooking
				Limited use of milk and milk products
				Often low in protein, calories, or both
				Soy sauce (high sodium)

Filipino (Spanish-Chinese Influence)				

Flavored milk
Milk in coffee
Cheese: gouda,
  cheddar
	Pork, beef, goat, rabbit
	Chicken
	Fish
	Eggs, nuts, legumes
		Many vegetables
		  and fruits
			Rice, cooked
			  cereals
			Noodles: rice,
			  wheat
				Limited use of milk and milk products
				Tendency to prewash rice
				Tendency to have only small portions
				  of protein foods

Italian				

Cheese
Some ice cream
	Meat
	Eggs
	Dried beans
		Leafy vegetables
		Potatoes
		Eggplant, tomatoes,
		  peppers
		Fruits
			Pasta
			White breads,
			  some whole
			  wheat
			Farina
			Cereals
				Prefer expensive, imported cheese;
				  reluctant to expensive domestic
				  varieties
				Tendency to overcook vegetables
				Limited use of whole grains
				High consumption of sweets
				Extensive use of olive oil
				Insufficient serving from milk group

Japanese (Isei, More Japanese Influence; Nisei, More Westernized)				

Increasing
  amounts
  being used by
  younger
  generations
	Pork, beef, chicken
	Fish
	Eggs
	Legumes: soy, red, lima
	  beans
	Tofu
	Nuts
		Many vegetables
		  and fruits
		Seaweed
			Rice, rice cakes
			Wheat noodles
			Refined bread,
			  noodles
				Excessive sodium; pickles, salty cri
				  seaweed, MSG, and soy sauce
				Insufficient servings from milk group
				May use prewashed rice

Continued

Table 6-4   Characteristic Food Patterns of Selected Cultures—cont'd

MILK GROUP	PROTEIN GROUP	FRUITS AND VEGETABLES	BREADS AND CEREALS	POSSIBLE DIETARY PROBLEMS
Hispanic, Mexican American				
Milk Cheese Flan, ice cream	Beef, pork, lamb, chicken, tripe, hot sausage, beef intestine Fish Eggs Nuts Dry beans: pinto, chickpeas (often eaten more than once daily)	Spinach, wild greens, tomatoes, chilies, corn, cactus leaves, cabbage, avocado, potatoes Pumpkin, zapote, peaches, guava, papaya, citrus	Rice, cornmeal Sweet bread, pastries Tortilla: corn, flour Vermicelli	Limited meats, primarily because of cost Limited use of milk and milk products Large amounts of lard Abundant use of sugar Tendency to boil vegetables for long periods
Polish				
Milk Sour cream Cheese Butter	Pork (preferred) Chicken	Vegetables—limited fresh Cabbage Roots—potatoes Fruits—limited fresh	Dark rye	Sodium in ham, sausage, pickles High consumption of sweets Tendency to overcook vegetables Limited fruits, raw vegetables
Puerto Rican				
Limited use of milk Coffee with milk (café con leche)	Pork Poultry Eggs (Fridays) Dried codfish Beans (habichuelas)	Avocado, okra Eggplant Sweet yams Starchy vegetables and fruits (viandas)	Rice Cornmeal	Small amounts of pork and poultry products Extensive use of fat, lard, salt pork, and olive oil Lack of milk products
Scandinavian (Danish, Finnish, Norwegian, Swedish)				
Cream Butter Cheeses	Wild game Reindeer Fish (fresh or dried) Eggs	Berries Dried fruit Vegetables: cole slaw, roots	Whole wheat, rye, barley, sweets (cookies, sweet breads)	Insufficient fresh fruits and vegetables High consumption of sweets, pickled or salted meats, and fish
Southeast Asian (Vietnamese, Cambodian)				
Generally not taken Coffee with condensed cow's milk Plain yogurt Ice cream (rare) Soybean milk	Fish (daily): fresh, dried, salted Poultry/eggs: duck, chicken Pork Beef (seldom) Dry beans Tofu	Seasonal variety: fresh or preserved Leafy green vegetables Yams Corn	Rice: grains, flour, noodles French bread Cellophane (bean starch) noodles	Fresh milk products generally not consumed Poultry/eggs may be limited Meat considered "unclean" is avoided Preference for a diet high in salt and pepper, as well as rice and pork High intake of MSG and soy sauce
Jewish: Orthodox*				
Milk[†] Cheese[†]	Meat (bloodless; Kosher prepared): beef, lamb, goat, deer, poultry (all types), no pork Fish with fins and scales only No crustaceans	Wide variety	Wide variety	High intake of sodium in meat products

MSG, Monosodium L-glutamate.

*Religious holidays may involve fasting, which is believed to increase the likelihood of preterm labor. Fasting requirement may be waived during pregnancy.

[†]Lactose intolerance relatively common in adults. Milk and milk products not eaten with meat, milk may be taken before the meal or 6 hours after; different sets of dishes and silverware are used to serve milk and meat products.

[‡]Lower in fat content than Western sausage.

From Lowdermilk DL, Perry SE, Bobak IM: *Maternity* and *women's health care*, ed 7, St Louis, 2000, Mosby.

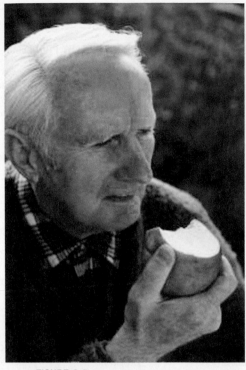

FIGURE 6-5 Good nutrition at any age.

observed. The diet should be assessed to determine whether the patient has adequate intake of the necessary electrolytes. Medications that may cause electrolyte depletion should be considered. Vomiting, diarrhea, and gastric suction are likely to contribute to electrolyte imbalances.

■ Assessment

- Does the person appear noticeably overweight or underweight?
- Does the person's clothing appear abnormally loose or tight?
- What are the person's current height and weight? (Check the chart or weigh the patient if current information is not available.)
- Is the person's weight within normal limits? (See Table 6-1.)
- Has the person's weight significantly increased or decreased in the past 3 to 6 months? If so, how much has it changed?
- How long has this weight change been occurring?

Appetite Changes

- What does the person say about his or her appetite?
- Does the person feel that his or her appetite has changed?
- Why does the person think this is happening?
- How does food taste to the person?
- What does the person like or dislike about the meals he or she eats (or is served)?
- What would the person prefer to eat?

- Does the person have any cultural food preferences that are not being recognized?
- Does the person have any dietary restrictions? Are they understood?
- Does the person complain of nausea or hyperacidity before, during, or after meals?
- Does the person complain of a strange taste in the mouth?
- Does the person have any feeling of chest pain after meals?
- Does the person show an unusual reaction to any foods (e.g., dairy products, nuts, and shellfish)?
- Does the person experience increased eructation or flatulence related to particular foods?
- Is the person depressed?

Nutritional Intake

- Are the person's hemoglobin, hematocrit, and RBC parameters within normal limits?
- Has the person's blood sugar level been taken? Was this a fasting blood sugar? If taken at a nonfasting time, was it before or after a meal? How long before or after?
- Are the person's electrolyte levels (e.g., sodium, potassium and calcium) within normal limits?
- Are serum albumin levels within normal levels?
- Does the person have a history of diabetes mellitus, anemia, or electrolyte imbalances?
- Are there any other observations such as pallor, dizziness, or easy fatigue that may indicate anemia?
- Does the person show any signs of hyperglycemia or hypoglycemia?
- Does the person show any signs of electrolyte imbalance?
- How are the person's electrolyte levels (especially potassium and sodium)?
- Is the person on a prescribed diet that restricts sodium, calorie, sugar, or fluid intake? Does he or she have any other dietary restrictions?
- Does the person receive calcium supplements?
- Does the person drink milk and eat dairy products? (Is the person lactose-intolerant?)
- Does the person receive iron supplements?
- Does the person receive any drugs that can alter electrolyte levels (e.g., diuretics and cardiotonics)?
- Has the person had any recent episodes of vomiting?
- Are there certain foods that the person never consumes? (Look particularly at meats or vegetables that may require more chewing, and compare this information with the person's dental status.)
- What types of foods does the person consume most? First? Not at all?
- What percentage of each type of food does the person actually consume? How much food in general?
- What fluids does the person consume during and between meals?

- Is the person consuming snacks or supplements between meals? If so, are these snacks prescribed?
- Is the person sneaking snacks that are not allowed on a therapeutic diet?
- Does the person receive any medications that could alter the taste of food? If so, when are these medications given?
- Is the person receiving any drugs that require a restricted diet (e.g., monoamine oxidase inhibitors)?

Social and Cultural Factors

- Does the person eat alone in his or her room or in the dining room?
- Does the person socialize with others during meals?
- Does the person's family ever bring favorite foods from home?
- How do these favorite foods meet the individual's nutritional needs?
- Do the favorite foods violate any dietary restrictions (e.g., sodium or calorie restrictions)?

Home Care or Discharge Planning

- Does the person live alone or with others?
- What are the person's health-management and health-maintenance abilities?
- If the person lives at home, does he or she have adequate food in the house?
- Does the person have adequate financial resources to buy food?
- Can the person get to a store to purchase food?
- Does the person have family or friends who will assist with going to the grocery store?
- Can the person prepare the food, or do problems with vision, stamina, or coordination interfere?
- Does the person tire so easily that by the time the food is prepared, he or she is too tired to eat?
- Does the person have adequate equipment for refrigeration and cooking?
- Is the person aware of community resources for nutrition (e.g., Meals on Wheels and senior citizen center meal programs)? Does the person consume alcoholic beverages? How much? How often?

Box 6-2 lists risk factors for imbalanced nutrition.

■ Nursing Diagnoses

Imbalanced nutrition: less than body requirements
Imbalanced nutrition: more than body requirements
Risk for imbalanced nutrition: more than body
   requirements
Readiness for enhanced nutrition

■ Nursing Goals/Outcomes Identification

The nursing goals for older individuals diagnosed with some form of imbalanced nutrition are to (1) maintain body weight within normal limits for height,

---

> **Box 6-2   Risk Factors Related to Imbalanced Nutrition in Older Adults**
>
> - Metabolic disorders (diabetes, thyroid disturbances)
> - Neurologic or musculoskeletal problems that interfere with food preparation, eating, or swallowing
> - Disturbances of the gastrointestinal tract
> - Inadequate resources to obtain food
> - Loss of nutrients as a result of medications, hemorrhage, vomiting, or diarrhea
> - Inadequate or excessive energy because of exercise patterns or disease processes
> - Living alone
> - Selective eating habits related to culture or habit
> - Grief or other emotional difficulties

(2) obtain adequate nutrients to maintain healthy tissue, (3) identify internal and external cues that influence eating patterns, and (4) adhere to a prescribed therapeutic diet.

Nursing Interventions/Implementation

The following nursing interventions should take place in hospitals or extended-care facilities:

1. **Assess the individual carefully to determine the causes of a problem** (e.g., dental problems, depression, cultural factors and activity level). The types of approaches used by nurses vary with the type and extent of the problem.

⊕ Cultural Considerations

Educating the Caregiver

- Because nursing assistants are typically assigned to assist older patients during mealtime, they need to be aware of how their cultural biases may influence what they communicate verbally and nonverbally.
- Home health aides who actually prepare meals for ethnically diverse patients need additional education and training in how to prepare culturally appropriate meals that are acceptable to their aging patients.

2. **Schedule weekly weight checks.** Weight changes related to nutritional intake do not occur rapidly, as they do with fluid imbalance. Daily weight fluctuations often occur. Weighing an older person too often can cause frustration. Weekly weight checks are more reliable indicators of success.
3. **Keep a dietary record of the amount, type, and frequency of food intake.** A careful dietary record helps nurses and older adults determine problem areas, which helps nurses and dietitians develop a dietary plan that is most likely to have the desired outcome. When possible, older adults should be actively involved in this record-keeping.
4. **Explain the importance of nutrition to overall health or disease control.** Many older individuals are already aware of normal nutritional needs.

? Critical Thinking

Culture and Food Preferences

Examine your own cultural food beliefs and practices.
- What are your food preferences?
- What foods should be included in a healthy diet?
- Are there any foods that you must include or avoid in your daily diet?
- Are there foods that cannot be combined or served together?
- Are any foods recommended or prohibited for special age groups across the life span?
- What foods are served for celebrations?
- What is your reaction when you are served foods that are culturally unfamiliar?

If the changes related to aging or disease require dietary modifications, it is important that the modifications and the reasons behind them be explained carefully to the individual. If older adults understand the rationale of dietary changes, they are more likely to cooperate with the new plan.

5. **Determine food likes and dislikes.** People tend to seek the things they like and avoid what they do not like. Knowledge of food preferences can be used when selecting nutritious yet acceptable foods for older adults. Many older individuals are set in their likes and dislikes and are unwilling to change late in life.

6. **Monitor laboratory values.** RBC parameters, hematocrit, and hemoglobin values help in determining whether iron intake is adequate. Electrolyte levels should be monitored to verify that they are within normal limits. Low serum albumin levels may indicate malnutrition.

7. **Assess the condition of the skin, hair, nails, and mucous membranes.** Signs of nutritional inadequacy can be detected by the observation of external surfaces. Cracks at the corner of the mouth, changes in the appearance of the tongue, loss or change in consistency of the hair, and slow tissue healing provide clues to nutritional status.

8. **Consult with the dietitian.** Dietitians are specially trained to assess nutritional needs, and they have in-depth knowledge of the nutritional value of foods. If an aging individual has serious nutritional problems or medical conditions with nutritional implications, it is essential that the dietitian be actively involved in the nutritional plan of care.

9. **Institute measures to increase or decrease nutritional intake.** The following measures can be taken to increase the patient's intake:
   - *Provide a selection of nutritious foods.* Nurses should attempt to provide choices for those who are most in need of nutrients. Many institutions, particularly long-term care facilities, have limited menus for each meal. If the meal served does not appeal to

aging individuals, they may eat very little, if at all. Most institutions have alternatives that do not appear on the menu, usually including simple foods such as eggs, cheese sandwiches, or soup. The older individual may not be aware of these choices or may not wish to cause additional work for the staff. It is the nurse's responsibility to explore these options with the individual.

- *Limit excess intake of fluids during meals.* Too much low nutritional fluid can create a sense of fullness that takes the place of more nutritious food.

- *Supplement food intake with nutritious snacks.* It is often difficult for older adults to consume adequate calories and nutrients within the three routine daily meals. If allowed within the prescribed diet, nutritious snacks that are high in calories and nutrients (e.g., bananas, graham crackers, dried fruits and milkshakes) can be offered between meals. These snacks should be scheduled so that they do not interfere with the person's appetite for regular meals. Many older individuals like to stash snacks in the bedside stand or closet. Nurses can ensure that snacks are not stored where they can spoil or attract insects. Any snacks that are not consumed promptly should be discarded.

- *Ask family members to bring the person's favorite dishes from home.* Family favorites are rarely on the menu in an institutional setting. Special favorites and foods connected with fond memories are most likely to be consumed by older adults. However, before the family brings food, nurses should be sure to discuss the care plan with them to ensure that these foods are permitted. It is frustrating for the family to make a special effort, only to have the meal rejected at the institution.

- *Serve meals in an attractive manner.* Foods that are well prepared and served in an attractive manner are more appealing. Taking plates and cups off the tray or setting a table with place mats and flowers can improve the appearance of a meal. Serving food on fancier dishes, using a special teacup, or making an effort to reduce the institutional character of the meal can help improve a person's appetite (Figure 6-6). Foods should always be served fresh and at the appropriate temperature.

- *Provide a social environment for meals by encouraging older adults to eat in the dining room.* The nature of meals tends to be social (Figure 6-7). Aging individuals often have better appetites when they eat in groups than when isolated in individual rooms. Alert individuals should be grouped with other alert people. Noise and distraction from confused patients can be disturbing and can decrease appetite. Separate seating or rooms can provide the best environment, depending

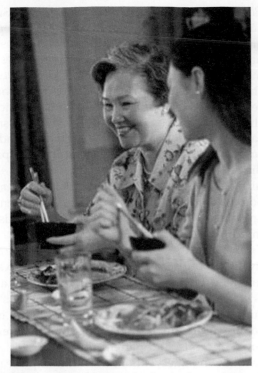

FIGURE 6-6 Chopsticks and Asian food make the meal enjoyable for this older Japanese woman.

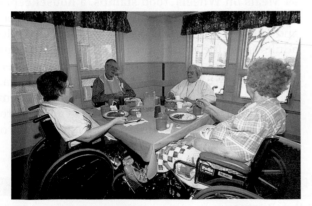

FIGURE 6-7 Nursing home residents enjoy a pleasant meal in the dining room.

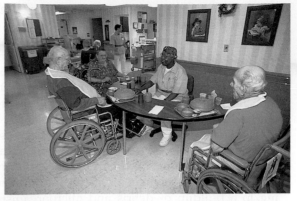

FIGURE 6-8 Special dining tables are used for assistive dining programs. Residents are fed three at a time, in the company of others.

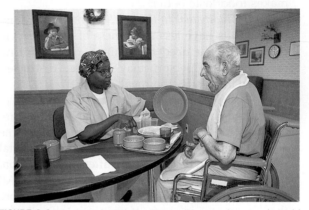

FIGURE 6-9 Nurses open cartons and other containers and provide other assistance at mealtimes.

on the needs of the individual (Figure 6-8). Many older individuals living in institutional settings make friends with whom they prefer to sit. Aging individuals should have the opportunity to seek mutually agreeable seating arrangements in dining rooms without staff interference. If significant others are present at mealtime, they may want to eat with the older individual. Some institutions provide special trays or bag lunches for guests at a nominal charge.

- *Prepare food by opening cartons, buttering toast, or performing other activities that may be difficult for the older person* (Figure 6-9). Problems setting up food and opening cartons may lead older adults to skip or avoid certain foods. Many containers are difficult to open—even healthy young adults can have difficulty. These should be opened with minimal fuss so that the aging person does not feel helpless. Assistance in getting the individual ready to eat by cutting meats or buttering bread should be given unobtrusively.

- *Avoid hurrying the individual during meals.* If an older person eats too rapidly, indigestion, heartburn, or regurgitation may result. If rushed, many older individuals stop eating before they are truly satisfied. A rushed environment should be avoided, and older adults should be allowed adequate time to eat at their own pace.

- *Request a modification in the form of food served if the individual has difficulty chewing.* It may be difficult for older adults to chew some foods, particularly meats and undercooked vegetables. Chopped or ground meat is easier to eat for people with dentures or missing teeth. The dietary department should be notified about these modifications, and the physician should be contacted if an order is required. If the person is alert, pureed foods should be avoided because of their similarity to baby food (unless the individual has severe trouble chewing). If vegetables are routinely a problem, dicing or additional cooking may help. The dietary department should be contacted if problems are detected.

- *Provide assistive devices such as plate sides, gripper spoons, and adaptive cups.* Most older adults prefer to feed themselves whenever possible. An occupational therapist should be consulted regarding utensils that enable aging individuals to eat without undue difficulty.
- *Provide oral hygiene before meals.* Normal decreases in taste and saliva production occur with aging. The decrease in saliva production reduces the normal cleansing mechanism within the mouth, leading to a buildup of debris and microorganisms that alters the taste of food and decreases the appetite. Good oral hygiene freshens the mouth and makes food taste better.
- *Assist the individual to the toilet before meals.* Many older adults have less awareness of their need to eliminate. If the need to eliminate occurs during mealtime, the person may become distracted and lose interest in the meal.
- *Provide supplemental tube feedings, if ordered.* Supplemental gastric or nasogastric tube feedings are ordered for individuals who cannot consume adequate nutrients by eating. These supplemental feedings should be given only after the individual has had adequate opportunity for oral intake. All attempts at oral feeding should be made before the supplement is given. If nasogastric feeding is required, all safety precautions (including checks for tube placement and positioning) should be taken.
- *Time the administration of medications so that they do not interfere with meals.* Some medications leave a bad taste in the mouth or otherwise upset the individual. If possible, these medications should be scheduled away from normal mealtimes.
- *Play relaxing music at mealtime.* Studies have shown that agitated behaviors decrease when quiet, melodic, peaceful music—with a steady tempo yet enough variety for interest—is played during mealtime.
- *Refer individuals for special counseling if emotional difficulties are interfering with appetite.* Individuals with extreme grief and emotional disturbances may require special nutritional approaches. Therapists trained to deal with eating disorders should be consulted to determine the most effective interventions.

The following measures can be taken to decrease intake:

- *Assist in the selection of low-calorie foods.* Decreasing caloric intake helps the person lose weight. Foods high in bulk and low in calories, such as fresh fruits and vegetables, provide a sense of fullness without a sense of deprivation.

- *Plan low-calorie snacks into the daily routine.* Snacks such as diet beverages and unbuttered popcorn are appropriate for older individuals unless they have a medical condition that contraindicates their inclusion. The sodium content of diet beverages should be checked if the person is on a sodium restricted diet. Individuals with diverticulitis should avoid corn with husks. Planned snacks can actually prevent mealtime overeating and consumption of high-calorie snacks if they are part of the aging person's dietary habits.
- *Increase diversional activities to decrease snacking.* Some older and younger people snack when they are bored. Activities that occupy the hands and mind may reduce the urge to eat.
- *Encourage increased activity levels.* Increased activity helps burn calories. Walking is an exercise tolerated well by most older individuals, and it is effective as a means of weight reduction.

10. **Complete a thorough documentation of nutritional status, including assessment, interventions, referrals, and patient response.**

The following interventions should take place in the home:

1. **Assist the individual in obtaining resources such as Meals on Wheels, food stamps, a housekeeper, or shopping services.** Many community agencies and programs have been developed to help older adults meet their nutritional needs. Each community has different services available. Social workers often maintain directories of these agencies and can help older adults establish contact with them. Nurses can clarify and explain the available programs and provide the means for older adults or their families to contact the agencies.

Cultural Considerations

Dietary Practices

Older adults may have distinct preferences based on their heritage. These dietary preferences and practices vary widely across ethnic and cultural groups and are too extensive to publish in this text, but many informational sites are available on the Internet. The following are some website addresses for useful information and teaching materials:
- http://www.nal.usda.gov/fnic/pubs/bibs/gen/ethnic.html
- http://www.nal.usda.gov/fnic/etext/000023.html
- http://multiculturalhealth.org
- http://www.semda.org/info/#pyramid.html
- http://ohioline.osu.edu/htdigsearch/search.php (Enter search terms "eating in America" for fact sheets on many cultures.)

2. **Involve the family in shopping and meal planning.** If the older person is unable to meet his or her nutritional needs without assistance, the family can often provide help. Older individuals are often too proud to ask for help, even from their

own families. With help from a nurse, the older person may be willing to accept this assistance. Family members can provide transportation to the store, read labels, and assist with food preparation. Variety can be provided through meals prepared and then frozen in family members' homes for the older person's use. Family members should be taught about their loved one's relevant dietary restrictions so that meals do not endanger his or her well-being.

3. **Identify senior citizen meal programs available in the community.** Many communities offer meals at churches or senior citizen centers. These meals are prepared by dietitians who are well versed in the nutritional needs of the aging population. These inexpensive meals provide the opportunity for social interaction.

4. **Use any appropriate interventions that are used in the institutional setting.**

❖ NURSING PROCESS FOR RISK FOR IMBALANCED FLUID VOLUME

Fluid balance is not a problem in healthy older adults. However, if there is a sudden change in fluid volume, an older person is more likely to experience significant problems than would a younger person. A seemingly minor problem with fluid balance can quickly become a serious concern in an aging individual. If not detected and treated, dehydration can easily become a significant problem, possibly resulting in death. The very old, African Americans, and men are most likely to experience dehydration.

Older adults have a lower percentage of body fluid (approximately 45% lower) than younger persons have, even when they are well hydrated. Anything that restricts adequate intake of fluids or causes the body to lose water excessively can contribute to the risk for dehydration.

Common risk factors for dehydration include (1) a decreased thirst sensation; (2) decreased effectiveness of the kidney at concentrating urine; (3) hormonal changes, including decreased aldosterone secretion and renin activity; (4) side effects of medications; (5) altered level of mentation; (6) altered levels of functional ability; and (7) fear of incontinence or pain, leading to inappropriate fluid restriction.

As at younger ages, older men have a higher percentage of body fluid than do older women. The decrease in the kidneys' concentrating abilities reduces the body's ability to adapt to changes in fluid volume. The aging body is less able to respond rapidly to fluid volume changes. When the many diseases that affect fluid balance are added to the normal changes of aging, maintaining fluid balance becomes a challenge.

Body fluids are distributed into two major compartments: intracellular and the extracellular compartments. Intracellular fluid is found within the cells and composes approximately two-thirds of the total body fluid. Extracellular fluid (ECF) composes approximately one-third of the total body fluid. ECFs are further classified as intravascular (plasma) and interstitial fluids. ECF is in constant motion throughout the body, carrying nutrients to the cells and removing waste products. The movement of body fluids is affected by the levels of various electrolytes and proteins in the various compartments. Albumin, an important plasma protein responsible for maintaining adequate intravascular fluid levels, is often deficient, contributing to tissue edema and orthostatic hypotension.

Although the intracellular fluid is affected when the body experiences fluid imbalance, the ECF changes more rapidly and significantly. ECF deficit, or fluid volume deficit, can result in hypovolemia or dehydration. ECF excess, or fluid volume excess, can result in hypervolemia (circulatory overload) or edema (excessive fluid in the interstitial spaces).

■ Assessment/Data Collection

- What are the person's vital signs (i.e., blood pressure, pulse, respiration, and temperature)?
- What is the appearance of the skin? Is it moist? Dry?
- What is the skin turgor? Is the tongue dry and/or furrowed? Skin temperature?
- Does the individual complain of thirst? Weakness?
- Does the individual manifest any mood changes, such as restlessness or confusion?
- What is the fluid intake per nursing shift? Per day?
- Is the person receiving fluids through non-oral routes such as nasogastric feeding or intravenous fluid therapy?
- How does this individual's fluid intake compare with the recommended intake?
- Is the person's weight changing rapidly? Is it increasing? Decreasing?
- Is the urine output within normal limits?
- What is the color and consistency of the urine? What is its specific gravity?
- Is there excessive fluid loss through hemorrhage, wound drains, gastric suction, diaphoresis, or mouth breathing?
- Does the person complain about the fit of rings, shoes, or clothing? Are they too loose or too tight?
- Is the person receiving medication that is likely to cause fluid retention or loss?
- Are laboratory values (hemoglobin, hematocrit, electrolytes, BUN, creatinine) within normal limits?

Boxes 6-3 and 6-4 list risks for deficient fluid volume or excess fluid volume in older adults.

Deficient Fluid Volume

Deficient fluid volume occurs when an individual has inadequate intake or excessive loss of fluids. Inadequate fluid intake can easily progress into dehydration which, unless corrected, can result in death. A variety

Box 6-3   **Risk Factors for Deficient Fluid Volume in Older Adults**

- Altered swallow reflex (stroke victims)
- Nausea and an unwillingness to eat or drink
- Acute emotional distress and decreased interest in personal needs
- Inability to obtain adequate fluids without assistance (bedridden patients)
- Altered cognition (Alzheimer's disease or dementia) and lack of awareness of the need for fluids
- Draining wounds, open sores, or ulcers
- Diuretic medications
- Kidney disease
- Tube feedings of low-sodium preparations
- Diaphoresis
- Intermittent or persistent vomiting
- Intermittent or persistent diarrhea

Box 6-4   **Risk Factors for Excess Fluid Volume in Older Adults**

- Increased fluid intake secondary to excess sodium intake, hyperglycemia, or medications
- Compulsive water-drinking
- Decreased urine output secondary to kidney dysfunction
- Heart failure
- Insufficient protein intake or excessive protein loss
- Steroid therapy
- History of alcoholism or liver disease
- Kidney disease

of conditions can contribute to deficient fluid volume in older adults. One author devised an interesting way of identifying older persons who have problems related to fluid intake. They were divided into three groups: (1) people who can drink, but do not—these are persons who are capable of drinking but do not know how much fluid is necessary or have cognitive problems so they forget to drink; (2) people who can drink, but will not—those who report that they never drank much or are afraid of incontinence; and (3) people who cannot drink—those who lack the ability to access fluids independently or have impaired swallow or gag reflexes. Each group will benefit from different nursing approaches. The "don't drink" people need to be offered fluids frequently. The "can't drink" people require special approaches, including positioning, swallowing exercises, thickened fluids, and, if ordered, tube or parenteral feeding. The "won't drink" people need education regarding the importance of fluids and alternative techniques for dealing with incontinence.

Individuals experiencing deficient fluid volume are likely to manifest dry mucous membranes, thirst, decreased skin turgor (assessed over the sternum or on the inner thigh), rapid weight loss (>3% of body weight), sunken eyes, weakness, and decreased volume or increased concentration of urine. Vital signs are likely to be affected. An increase in heart rate and decrease in pulse pressure can indicate a decrease in fluid volume. Hypotension and, particularly, orthostatic hypotension are common. An increase in body temperature may indicate dehydration. Blood studies are likely to change with deficient fluid volume. Hematocrit normally increases as the blood plasma volume decreases. Electrolyte levels, creatinine, and BUN are likely to be altered.

Excess fluid volume. Excess fluid volume can result from excessive intake or inadequate elimination of fluids. A primary indication of excess fluid volume is **edema,** which may manifest as swelling of dependent extremities and increased abdominal girth. Pulmonary edema may result in shortness of breath, dyspnea, cough, gurgling sounds on respiration, and frothy sputum. Because fluid intake exceeds fluid output, weight gain can be sudden and dramatic. The amount of weight gained reflects the amount of fluid being retained. One liter of fluid results in a 1-kg weight gain. Skin over edematous areas may appear shiny and taut. The amount and concentration of urine produced are likely to change with excess fluid volume. Hematocrit normally decreases as the blood plasma volume increases. Electrolyte levels, creatinine, and BUN are also likely to be altered. The individual may experience behavioral changes, including restlessness and anxiety.

■ Nursing Diagnoses

Deficient fluid volume
Excess fluid volume
Risk for deficient fluid volume
Risk for imbalanced fluid volume
Readiness for enhanced fluid balance

■ Nursing Goals/Outcomes Identification

The nursing goals for older individuals with or at risk for deficient fluid volume or excess fluid volume are to (1) manifest vital signs within normal limits or limits specified by the physician; (2) evidence moist oral mucous membranes and good skin turgor without evidence of edema; (3) maintain a stable weight within normal limits; (4) exhibit balanced fluid intake and output; (5) report no problems related to thirst or weakness; (6) exhibit blood studies (hemoglobin, hematocrit, serum electrolytes, BUN, creatinine) within normal limits; (7) verbalize an understanding of the recommended dietary and fluid intake; (8) demonstrate behaviors necessary to maintain appropriate fluid intake; (9) demonstrate a selection of appropriate foods and fluids; (10) verbalize an understanding of prescribed medication(s), including the frequency and any precautions; and (11) verbalize signs and symptoms that should be reported to the physician.

■ **Nursing Interventions/Implementation**

The following nursing interventions should take place in hospitals or extended-care facilities:

1. **Complete a thorough assessment.** A thorough assessment is necessary to determine the presence and severity of any problems related to fluid intake.

2. **Monitor vital signs.** Vital signs can change in response to changes in fluid volume. Orthostatic hypotension is more common in individuals who have inadequate fluid intake than in individuals who have adequate fluid intake.

3. **Monitor intake and output.** Any individual with an actual or potential fluid imbalance should be placed on intake and output (I&O) measurement. Shift and daily totals should be calculated and compared with previous totals. It is essential that all individuals who provide care know how to measure intake and output correctly. All caregivers should be aware that the individual is on I&O so that all fluids are recorded. If family members assist with feeding, they should be taught how to record fluid intake. Keeping intake and output sheets in a convenient place helps ensure prompt recording. Too often, I&O are monitored in a careless manner, and the data collected are meaningless.

4. **Monitor laboratory values.** Shifts in hemoglobin, hematocrit, BUN, creatinine, albumin, or electrolytes may precede or may be a result of fluid imbalance. These changes should be reported promptly.

5. **Weigh the patient daily before breakfast.** Weights measured at a consistent time of day are the most accurate for comparison. The individual should be weighed each day wearing the same clothing. The same scale should be used consistently, and it should be checked for accuracy at regular intervals. Consistency is essential to eliminate errors in readings. Daily weight checks should be recorded promptly on the appropriate record.

6. **Measure changes in girth of body parts such as legs and abdomen.** Measurements should be taken at a consistent spot each day. If the person has no objections, a small ink mark can be made on the skin so that all staff will measure consistently. Retained fluid (edema) increases girth; fluid loss decreases girth.

7. **Maintain adequate fluid intake.** The following measures can be taken to increase intake:
   - *Offer smaller amounts of fluid at more frequent intervals.* Small amounts of fluids taken frequently add up to significant fluid intake. Fluids should be offered, or the individual should be reminded to take a drink, every 30 to 60 minutes throughout the day.
   - *Keep preferred beverages at the bedside.* Many older adults have distinct preferences regarding the type and temperature of beverages they like. Because people are most likely to consume foods and fluids that they like, nurses should determine individual preferences.
   - *Use smaller containers such as medication cups or small juice glasses when offering beverages.* Small beverage containers are less intimidating than are large containers. An older person often can be coaxed into drinking four or five medicine cups of liquid (120 to 150 mL) far more easily than he or she can be persuaded to drink a glassful.
   - *Keep beverages easily available for individuals who are not in their rooms (e.g., in day rooms, activity rooms, lounges, or other common areas).* Low-sodium, low-sugar beverages are ideal because individuals on restricted diets can consume them. Making beverages easily accessible reminds and encourages individuals to drink. Passing a tray of assorted beverages around an area where several older adults are congregated can encourage social interchange and provide mutual encouragement for many to participate even when they might otherwise have refused.
   - *Encourage the intake of foods with a high fluid content such as fruits, vegetables, soups, and cooked cereals.* Significant amounts of fluid are contained in these foods. Individuals who have difficulty drinking liquids can obtain significant amounts of fluid through these alternative sources.
   - *Administer nasogastric, gastric, or parenteral fluids as ordered by the physician.* Individuals who cannot drink adequate fluids may need supplemental fluids administered by other routes. All fluid given by gastric or parenteral route must be counted as fluid intake.

The following measures can be taken to decrease intake:
   - *Avoid keeping fluids at the bedside.* If fluids are easily available, older adults are likely to consume them too freely.
   - *Offer frequent oral hygiene.* When fluids are restricted, saliva production decreases and the mucous membranes feel dry and uncomfortable. Thick, tenacious secretions can build up in the mouth if not removed regularly. Frequent oral hygiene is needed to compensate for the lack of oral fluids and diminished saliva production.
   - *Provide lozenges or hard candy.* Sucking on a hard lozenge stimulates the release of saliva. Candy and lozenges should be given only to those who are alert enough not to swallow or choke on them. Verify that there is no dietary prohibition to additional sugar intake.
   - *Plan a schedule that distributes limited fluids throughout the day.* The total fluid volume intake for the day should be planned within the prescribed limitations. The total can then be divided into appropriate amounts spaced throughout the day. For example, a 600-mL restriction could be divided into

12 servings of 50 mL offered at hourly intervals between 8:00 a.m. and 8:00 p.m. This prevents the person from consuming all of his or her allowance too early in the day and then having to withstand long periods of thirst or to exceed prescribed limits.

- *Limit the quantity of foods that are high in fluid content.* Fluids contained in solid foods can contribute to excess fluid volume and edema. Foods such as fresh fruits and vegetables have a high fluid content, whereas foods such as breads, dried fruits, and cooked meats have a lower fluid content.

8. **Administer medications as ordered by the physician.** Many individuals with fluid imbalances receive medication to prevent or correct this problem. Nurses must ensure that these medications are given on time and that the patient's response to the medications is assessed.

9. **Refer to the dietitian, if appropriate.** Individuals with medical conditions that are likely to cause excessive fluid loss or fluid retention need detailed and specific diet modifications and instructions, which are best provided by a specialist. Nurses should reinforce this teaching.

10. **Provide appropriate skin care.** Persons with excess fluid volume or deficient fluid volume require careful hygiene. Both dry, fragile skin and edematous tissue are highly susceptible to breakdown. The person's physical position should be changed frequently. Care should be taken when moving the patient or handling the skin.

11. **Report and document significant findings promptly.** The signs and symptoms of fluid volume problems rarely occur suddenly. Rather, these problems tend to develop over time. Nurses must be sure that all changes are documented and reported promptly to the nurse in charge and/or to the physician.

The following interventions should take place in the home:

1. **Complete a thorough assessment.** A thorough assessment is necessary to determine the presence and severity of any problems. It may be necessary to bring a scale, measuring tape, and sphygmomanometer to the home to complete a good assessment.

2. **Teach the individual and his or her family members how to monitor fluid intake.** The individual and the family must be aware of methods used to keep track of fluid intake and loss. The family should learn to measure fluid intake using common household containers, and they should be taught to read cartons for fluid content. It is easier for most lay persons to learn to keep track of fluid intake in terms of ounces than in terms of milliliters. A specimen pan or urinal should be provided to measure output.

3. **Promote wellness by reviewing the prescribed dietary and fluid intake with the individual.** It is important that the individual understand the reason for consuming or avoiding certain foods and fluids. The importance of adequate fluid intake, particularly during hot weather, should be stressed. Individuals with no acute problems should be advised to consume a minimum of 64 ounces (2000 mL) of fluid each day. Those who live alone may need reminders to consume this amount. Fluid intake reminders are particularly important during hot weather when increased amounts of fluid are lost through perspiration.

4. **Explain methods of increasing or decreasing fluid intake.** The following measures can be taken to increase intake:
   - *Develop a schedule for fluid intake.* A planned schedule using a time list or clock helps remind older persons, as well as their spouse or caregiver, to consume fluids at regular times. It also helps them keep track of how much fluid is being consumed. They should be encouraged to check off or write amounts next to the times so that they are aware of making progress.
   - *Post signs in the kitchen and other rooms reminding the individual to drink.* Reminders help older adults remember the importance of drinking adequate amounts of fluid.
   - *Encourage friends and family to visit and share a beverage with the individual.* Social contact and sharing are natural over a cup of coffee, soda, juice, or other beverage. This is a pleasant way to promote social interaction and encourage fluid intake at the same time.
   - *Encourage the use of fruit or other foods with high fluid content.*

   The following measures can be taken to decrease intake:
   - Develop a schedule that spreads the limited amount of fluid throughout the day.
   - Encourage the use of hard candy or lozenges to keep the mouth moist.
   - Recommend frequent oral hygiene.
   - Discuss the importance of avoiding foods with high fluid content.

5. **Discuss signs and symptoms that should be reported promptly to the physician.** Fluid imbalance may result in hospitalization and serious complications. This is particularly important for older individuals who are receiving medications that influence fluid balance. The individual should know what signs and symptoms are important. A written list of symptoms should be given to the individual and his or her significant others.

6. **Use any appropriate interventions that are used in the institutional setting.**

❖ NURSING PROCESS FOR IMPAIRED SWALLOWING

Chewing and swallowing are complex processes that involve coordinated movements of the oral cavity, tongue, pharynx, larynx, and esophagus. An individual who is unable to coordinate these movements experiences difficulty swallowing, or **dysphagia.** Dysphagia is often a result of abnormal muscle contraction, infection, scar tissue, cancer, or dental conditions. Problems related to eating, and particularly problems related to swallowing, are serious because they can lead to dehydration, malnutrition, or aspiration. It is reported that as many as 40% of older adults have swallowing problems.

Swallowing problems are commonly a result of neurologic damage, trauma that affects the cranial nerves or facial muscles, or diseases such as Parkinson's or CVA. Recent research indicates that heart failure, diabetes, and general frailty due to age places older adults at risk for impaired swallowing. Older individuals with altered consciousness or severe fatigue are also at risk. Some individuals who are capable of swallowing may be hesitant to do so because of a lack of desire to eat or because of fear after an episode of choking. Older individuals experiencing dysphagia should always be carefully assessed for possible aspiration.

■ Assessment/Data Collection

* Is there any history of stroke or other neurologic disease that could interfere with chewing or swallowing?
* Is the individual alert and able to follow directions?
* Is any facial drooping or difficulty chewing observed?
* Is difficulty swallowing reported by the person or observed by caregivers?
* Does the person complain of something sticking in the throat?
* Does the person cough, choke, or drool when eating?
* Does the person complain of hoarseness or dry throat?
* Does the person store food in the cheek pockets?
* Is the person's gag reflex weak or absent?
* Can the person close his or her lips?
* Does the person experience problems with any particular foods or fluids?

Box 6-5 lists risk factors associated with impaired swallowing in older adults.

Box 6-5	Risk Factors for Impaired Swallowing in Older Adults

* Neurologic problems that result in paralysis or weakness of the face, mouth, or throat
* Altered level of consciousness, awareness, or sensation
* Mechanical devices such as a tracheostomy tube or nasogastric tube
* A narrowing or obstruction of the pharynx or esophagus
* Excessive fatigue

■ Nursing Diagnosis

Impaired swallowing

Nursing Goals/Outcomes Identification

The nursing goals for an older individual diagnosed with impaired swallowing are to (1) pass food from mouth to the stomach without aspiration, (2) maintain adequate nutrition and hydration, and (3) maintain or achieve appropriate body weight.

■ Nursing Interventions/Implementation

The following nursing interventions should take place in hospitals or extended-care facilities:

1. **Assess the individual to determine his or her unique problems and needs.** Not all swallowing disorders are the same. Different approaches must be developed based on the individual's specific problems and needs.

2. **Consult with the speech therapist, occupational therapist, and dietitian to develop a dysphagia program.** These specialists have unique knowledge of the best techniques and methods for dealing with swallowing disorders. It is important for nurses to use their expertise when developing a feeding plan. Special adaptive equipment (e.g., special spoons) is often used to deliver food to the back of the throat, where it is more easily swallowed. Special cups that allow the older individual to drink without tipping the head back are often used. Exercises designed to strengthen the tongue may also improve swallowing ability.

3. **Verify that dentures fit properly and maintain good oral hygiene.** Improperly fitted dentures can slip in the mouth, causing increased problems with swallowing. A dentist should be consulted if this is the problem. Good oral hygiene enhances the appetite and removes any old food or foreign materials that may interfere with swallowing.

4. **Position the person with his or her head upright and the chin flexed slightly forward to facilitate swallowing. Help with head control, if necessary.** Whenever possible, older adults should be seated in a chair for meals. If they must remain in bed, the head of the bed should be raised as high as possible. Malpositioning of the head can interfere with the ability to swallow. Excessive flexion or hyperextension of the neck can interfere with the passage of food through the pharynx and into the esophagus. If a pillow is used for positioning, it should be placed behind the shoulder, not behind the head, which could interfere with swallowing. Individuals with swallowing problems should remain seated upright for at least 30 minutes after a meal to reduce the likelihood of aspiration.

5. **Encourage rest periods before meals.** Eating requires a great deal of effort from individuals

with swallowing disorders. Providing rest before meals helps increase the amount of energy and strength available.

6. **Allow adequate time for meals.** Hurrying a meal increases the risk for aspiration. Older persons with swallowing difficulties are even more likely to have problems if they try to swallow too quickly.

7. **Start with small amounts of food and thickened fluids.** Individuals with swallowing difficulties should be given a moderate amount of food (approximately 15 to 20 mL) at a time. This amount is enough for the individual to detect the presence of food, but it is not so much that it is difficult to swallow. Individuals with swallowing disorders have a great deal of difficulty controlling and swallowing liquids. Therefore, foods that have a high fluid content are necessary to ensure adequate fluid intake. Many facilities add a thickening agent to flavored beverages to turn them into a gelatinous form that is more easily managed by persons with impaired swallowing. Water usually is not given to individuals with swallowing disorders. Because water has no texture or taste, the individual may not be aware of its presence in the mouth and may aspirate it.

8. **Place foods into the unaffected or stronger side of the mouth.** The individual will be able to detect food more easily on the unaffected or stronger side.

9. **Present foods in an appealing manner.** The appearance of food affects the appetite. Even if its consistency is altered (ground or puréed), food should be served as pleasantly as possible. Foods should not be stirred together in an unappealing mixture. Each food should remain identifiable and should be served to the individual in the preferred order.

10. **Select foods based on taste, texture, temperature, and fluid content.** Individuals with swallowing disorders may have altered senses of taste, texture, and temperature. Foods that have distinct flavors and textures, such as applesauce, are accepted more readily than are nondescript, puréed foods. Seasonings and spices can be used to enhance the flavor of many foods. The food should have some consistency; however, foods that require chewing are not advised. Food should be served at a temperature that will not burn the mucous membranes of the mouth. Many individuals with swallowing disorders cannot sense temperature adequately. A variety of temperatures will make the person more aware of the presence of food.

11. **Ensure that the lips are closed by applying slight pressure or stroking.** It is almost impossible to swallow when the lips are open. To prevent aspiration, it may be necessary to close the person's lips mechanically.

12. **Stimulate swallowing by stroking the side of the neck, and support the weakened side if appropriate.** Stroking the neck stimulates the urge to swallow. Supporting the muscles of the affected side of the throat can enhance swallowing.

13. **Give frequent verbal cues.** Individuals with swallowing difficulties may not remember to swallow when food is in the mouth. Some are able to swallow if they are reminded to do so.

14. **Reduce distractions.** The process of eating requires the full attention of the affected individual and the caregiver. Distractions, such as television or visitors, may interfere with concentration and lead to increased problems.

15. **Keep suction equipment available in case of problems.** When giving oral feedings to an individual with a swallowing disorder, it is wise to keep a suction apparatus nearby. Most of these people also have problems with other protective reflexes such as the gag and cough reflexes. They may be unable to clear an airway obstruction. The suction machine should be readily available because delay may lead to aspiration or more serious consequences.

16. **Provide oral hygiene before and after feedings.** Individuals with swallowing disorders are likely to retain food particles in the mouth, leading to altered taste. Good oral hygiene before and after meals removes debris and tenacious saliva and might improve the person's appetite.

17. **Administer tube feedings as ordered by the physician to individuals who are unable to achieve adequate oral intake.** Some individuals with swallowing disorders may not be able to eat enough to meet their nutritional needs. These individuals require feeding through either a nasogastric or a gastric feeding tube. Tube feedings may be used to meet the total nutritional needs of older adults, or they may be given as a supplement for those who need additional fluid or calories. If the feeding is supplemental, it should be given after the individual has had the opportunity to take as much oral nutrition as possible. These feedings are not meant as a time-saving method to replace oral feedings. Care should be used to verify placement and absorption of nutrients before each feeding is given. Medical asepsis should be used when handling all nutrients and feeding equipment to reduce the risk for contamination. Irrigation sets should be replaced every 24 hours. Use of food dyes in feeding solution is not recommended because it may be a source of infection.

18. **Use any appropriate interventions that are used in the institutional setting in the home.**

NURSING PROCESS FOR RISK FOR ASPIRATION

Aspiration, the inhalation of solids or liquids into the upper respiratory tract, is a serious problem for many infirm older adults. Symptoms of aspiration include

(1) a sudden appearance of severe coughing or cyanosis associated with eating or drinking, (2) voice changes, and (3) signs of aspiration pneumonia, including increased respiratory rate, abnormal lung sounds, fever and behavioral changes such as confusion or delirium. Risk for aspiration is increased with dysphagia and with gastroesophageal reflux problems. Symptoms are discussed in Chapter 3.

■ Assessment/Data Collection

- Does the person have cough and gag reflexes?
- Does the person have a reduced level of consciousness?
- Does the person have a tracheostomy?
- Is the person in the supine position during feedings?
- Is the person receiving feedings or medications through a gastric tube?
- Does the person have signs of abdominal distention?
- Are the person's stomach contents more than 150 mL before a scheduled feeding?
- Is there any noise with respiration?
- Is there a productive cough? What is the consistency of the sputum?
- Are the pulse and respiratory rates elevated?

Box 6-6 lists risk factors for aspiration in older adults.

■ Nursing Diagnosis

Risk for aspiration

■ Nursing Goals/Outcomes Identification

The nursing goals for an older individual at risk for aspiration are to (1) remain free from episodes of aspiration and (2) maintain clear, noiseless breath sounds.

■ Nursing Interventions/Implementation

The following nursing interventions should take place in hospitals or extended-care facilities:

1. **Position the person appropriately.** The person should be positioned in a Fowler's or semi-Fowler's position before both oral and gastric tube feedings. This position should be maintained for at least 30 to 45 minutes after each feeding. Elevating the head allows solutions to flow into the stomach and

reduces the chance of regurgitation. If the person must remain flat in bed, a side-lying position is better than a supine position.

2. **Assess for stomach distention.** Stomach distention can be an indication of slow gastric emptying, which can lead to regurgitation and aspiration. Continued complaints of gastric fullness or excessive stomach gas should be monitored carefully and reported. If these problems persist, the amount or type of feeding may need to be changed.

3. **Avoid feeding too rapidly.** Rapid ingestion of food increases the likelihood of regurgitation and aspiration. Oral nourishment should be offered slowly, and adequate time should be allowed for chewing and swallowing.

4. **Avoid liquids and puréed foods.** Semisolid foods are less likely to be aspirated than are liquids or puréed foods. The consistency of liquids can be modified with commercial preparations that are available in most dietary departments.

5. **Monitor respiratory sounds and respiratory rate, and observe the amount and type of sputum produced.** Aspiration of food or fluids may result in coughing, choking, dyspnea, and respiratory distress. Increased amounts of frothy sputum are often noted. If the person has a tracheostomy, feeding solutions should be tinted with blue food coloring. If secretions removed during respiratory suctioning reveal a blue color, aspiration has occurred.

6. **Keep suction equipment available.** Aspiration can result in respiratory distress. Suction equipment should be kept on hand whenever an individual at risk for aspiration is being fed.

7. **Consult with specialists such as speech therapists and dietitians.** A team approach to swallowing disorders and potential aspiration can help reduce the likelihood of problems. Speech therapists often have special training in swallowing disorders and can suggest modifications in feeding practices. Dietitians are specially trained to meet the needs of these individuals and can provide a nutritionally sound diet in a form modified to meet the needs of the person at risk for aspiration.

The following interventions should be taken for persons receiving tube feedings:

8. **Check placement of the nasogastric tube using the approved method.** Nasogastric tubes can become displaced into the lungs, resulting in aspiration. Tube placement should be verified before any solution is instilled. This should be done routinely according to institutional policy.

9. **Measure stomach contents before starting intermittent feeding; then replace stomach contents.** Stomach distention, which is related to decreased gastric emptying time, increases the risk for

---

| Box **6-6** | Risk Factors for Aspiration in Older Adults |

- Neurologic problems, particularly those that affect the cough and/or gag reflexes
- Reduced level of consciousness
- Continuous supine positioning
- Tracheostomy tubes
- Gastric tubes
- Decreased gastric motility; excessive amounts of residual gastric contents or gas

regurgitation and aspiration. If possible, the volume of stomach contents should be measured before intermittent tube feedings. This may not be possible if a small-bore tube is used. If the volume of stomach contents exceeds 50 to 100 mL, the physician should be notified and the feeding withheld. Stomach contents should be replaced through the tube to maintain electrolyte balance.

10. **Maintain clean technique for all feeding tubes, equipment, and formula.** Bacterial contamination of formula increases over time and when breaks in clean technique occur. Be sure to wash your hands before pouring formula or checking placement. Wash the top of the formula can before using. Cleanse ports before and after manipulation. Change feeding bags and irrigation sets according to agency policy—at least every 24 hours. Clean equipment between uses and store properly. Avoid use of food dyes, which have been shown to increase the risk for contamination.

The following interventions should take place in the home:

1. **Explain safety precautions to the individual and the family or caregiver.** Explain the importance of proper positioning, proper rate of feeding, and modifications to food consistency that reduce the likelihood of aspiration.
2. **Encourage enrollment in a home safety course that includes the Heimlich maneuver and cardiopulmonary resuscitation.** Aspiration of solids can sometimes be relieved by the use of the Heimlich maneuver. Respiratory distress related to aspiration may require other emergency interventions until medical assistance arrives. The family should be prepared to provide these lifesaving measures if they plan to provide care in the home.
3. **Use any appropriate interventions that are used in the institutional setting** (Nursing Care Plan 6-1).

⭐ Nursing Care Plan 6-1 | Risk for Aspiration

Mr. Thomas is a 74-year-old man who recently suffered a stroke. His level of consciousness is decreased, he has no gag reflex, and the left side of his face shows some paralysis. His physician has ordered intermittent feedings (every 4 hours) of a commercial nutrient solution through a nasogastric tube.

Nursing Diagnosis
Risk for Aspiration

Defining Characteristics
- Decreased level of consciousness
- Facial paralysis
- Absence of gag reflex

Patient Goals/Outcomes Identification
Mr. Thomas will remain free from episodes of aspiration.

Nursing Interventions/Implementation
1. Assess for signs of stomach distention, cough, or excessive respiratory secretions.
2. Position Mr. Thomas in Fowler's position before feeding.
3. Verify placement of the nasogastric tube using approved methods.
4. Measure the stomach contents. Withhold feeding and notify the physician if the volume of stomach contents is greater than 50 to 100 mL.
5. Return the stomach contents through nasogastric tube.
6. Allow adequate time (approximately 30 minutes) for instillation of 250 mL.
7. Keep the head elevated for 30 to 45 minutes after feeding.
8. Keep suction equipment at the bedside. Check at regular intervals to verify that this equipment is functioning properly.

Evaluation
Physical assessment reveals no signs of stomach distention. The residual stomach contents before feedings range from 25 to 70 ml. No episodes of coughing or silent tearing are noted with feedings. His lungs are clear on auscultation. You will continue the plan of care.

Critical Thinking Questions
The patient's family thinks that the feeding tube is unnecessary and that he should be offered food and fluids by mouth.
1. How would you explain the risks to them?
2. How would you modify the plan of care if continuous feedings were ordered?

Get Ready for the NCLEX® Examination!

Key Points

- Nutritional and fluid problems are common in the aging population.
- Knowledge of a wide range of facts and concepts about nutrition and the nutritional needs of older adults is important. This text addresses the basics only. For greater understanding, texts that specialize in geriatric nutrition should be consulted.
- A wide range of factors increases the risk for malnutrition in the elderly population. These should be taken into account when assessing the nutritional status of older adults.
- Sensory or cognitive changes, weakness, activity intolerance, and loss of interest in food as a result of depression or other emotional disturbances contribute to these problems.
- Signs and symptoms of poor nutrition such as confusion, weight loss, lethargy, and lightheadedness may be mistakenly attributed to an illness or medication reaction rather than to the underlying nutritional problem.
- Indicators of nutritional and metabolic alteration are most commonly observed in the skin, mucous membranes, hair, and nails. Assessment of these structures can tell nurses a great deal about an aging person's nutritional status and fluid balance.
- Good nutrition has been shown to be one of the most significant factors in the prevention of skin breakdown.
- Nurses play an important role in the recognition of nutritional and fluid balance problems, identification of contributing factors, and development of an appropriate plan of care.
- Nurses should recognize the importance of consultation with the dietitian and referral to community agencies that can provide nutritional support.

Additional Learning Resources

SG Go to the Study Guide on pp. 379–397 for additional learning activities to help you master the chapter content.

evolve Go to your Evolve website (http://evolve.elsevier.com/Wold/geriatric) for the following FREE learning resources:
- Animations
- Answer Guidelines for Nursing Care Plan Critical Thinking Questions
- Answers and Rationales for Review Questions for the NCLEX® Examination
- Glossary with pronunciations in English and Spanish
- Video Clips

Review Questions for the NCLEX® Examination

1. An elderly man who resides in a long-term care facility recently began to refuse food and will not open his mouth for solids. He does take liquids by mouth. He repeatedly says, "Leave me alone." He has lost a total of 5 lb over the past month. The best first nursing intervention is to:
   1. Obtain an order to insert a feeding tube from the physician.
   2. Assess to identify changes in physical or emotional status.
   3. Discuss use of high nutrient liquid feedings with the dietitian.
   4. Request assistance with feeding from the family.

2. An elderly woman recently moved to the United States from the Middle East. She does not like to drink cow milk or eat most cheeses. A culturally acceptable food that would best help meet the need for calcium is:
   1. Yogurt
   2. Broccoli
   3. Sardines
   4. Tofu

3. An elderly man who lives alone in an apartment is placed on a sodium-restricted diet because of congestive heart failure. He asks the nurse to help him make good diet choices. The foods he should avoid are: (Select all that apply.)
   1. Canned tomato soup
   2. Deli bologna or ham
   3. Grilled steak
   4. Frozen spaghetti dinner
   5. Pancakes
   6. Boiled eggs

4. An 85-year-old woman was admitted to the hospital. Clinical indicators of inadequate nutrition include which of the following? (Select all that apply.)
   1. Thin, brittle hair
   2. Hgb 10.2; Hct 33
   3. Thin, dry skin
   4. Slow reflexes
   5. Pale conjunctiva

5. An elderly client is taking furosemide (Lasix) to reduce edema. Dietary teaching for this person would best include directions to increase dietary intake of which of the following foods? (Select all that apply.)
   1. Bananas
   2. Apple juice
   3. Tomatoes
   4. Oranges
   5. Grapes
   6. Milk

6. An elderly nursing home resident has poor skin turgor, dry mucous membranes, and very concentrated urine. The best directions for the nurse to give to the nursing assistant include: (Select all that apply.)

1. Make sure the client eats everything served at each meal.
2. Offer small amounts of fluids frequently during the day.

3. Provide good oral hygiene.
4. Identify the beverages that the person prefers.
5. Keep a large container of iced water in the person's room.
6. Give the client hard candy to suck on.

Medications and Older Adults

Objectives

1. Identify factors that increase the risk for medication-related problems.
2. Discuss the reasons each of these factors increases health risks for the aging person.
3. Describe how pharmacokinetics is altered with aging.
4. Discuss the pharmacodynamic changes observed in the aging person.
5. Identify the significance of the Beers criteria.
6. Explain specific precautions that are necessary when administering medication to older adults in an institutional setting.
7. Identify the risks related to aging and pertinent nursing observations for specific drug categories.
8. Discuss how medications fit into the nursing plan of care.
9. Describe specific nursing interventions and modifications in technique that are related to medication administration to older adults.
10. Describe the older person's rights as they relate to medication administration.
11. Identify information that should be provided to older adults regarding medications.
12. Discuss the impact of age-related changes on self-administration of medications.
13. Describe nursing interventions that can reduce problems related to self-administration of medication in the home.

Key Terms

absorption (ăb-SŎRP-shŭn) (p. 132)
distribution (dĭs-trĭ-BŪ-shŭn) (p. 132)
excretion (ĕks-KRĒ-shŭn) (p. 133)
geropharmacology (jĕr-ō-făr-mă-KŎL-ö-jē) (p. 132)

half-life (p. 132)
metabolism (mĕ-TĂB-ō-lĭzm) (p. 133)
pharmacokinetics (făr-mă-kō-kĬ-NĚT-ĭks) (p. 132)
polypharmacy (pŏ-lē-FĂR-mă-sē) (p. 133)

Problems related to medications are common in older adults, and they are costly in terms of both time and money. Medications can alter an aging person's ability to perform normal functions, can result in behavior changes, and can be life threatening. Adverse reactions to medications are common in older adults. Studies have revealed that as many as 17% of hospitalizations of persons older than 66 years of age were related to adverse drug reactions. In addition, one in three older persons is likely to develop iatrogenic (treatment-related) complications secondary to medications taken during a hospital stay. Adverse drug reactions also have been linked to an increased risk for falls and automobile accidents. Studies show that the resulting hospitalizations cost older adults and taxpayers several billion dollars each year.

Estimates indicate that the average person older than 65 years of age takes three or more prescription medications each day. In addition, the average older person also takes three or four nonprescription medications obtained over the counter (OTC). The cost of these medications exceeds $3 billion per year. Studies have shown that 40% of all prescription drugs are written for people age 65 and older. Many elderly prefer to try self treatment with OTC medications before consulting a physician. Studies show that older adults purchase 40% of the OTCs sold and that 90% of this group use OTC drugs at least occasionally.

Considering these numbers, it is no surprise that use, misuse, and abuse of medications present serious threats to the aging population. Medications are potent substances. For every desired effect, many side effects and adverse effects are likely to occur. Although often useful or necessary to maintain health, medications present risks to people of all ages, and older adults are at even greater risk than the younger population (Box 7-1).

RISKS RELATED TO DRUG-TESTING METHODS

In general, the methodology used to test drugs and to establish therapeutic dosages does not take into account the unique characteristics of older adults. Most drug testing is performed on healthy, young adult men. Because older adults normally have had some changes in body function and are more likely to suffer from at least one disease process, they are not physiologically the same as young adults. It seems obvious that an 80-year-old, 94-pound woman with heart disease should not be expected to respond in the same way that a healthy 35-year-old, 200-pound man would.

Box 7-1 **Factors That Increase the Risk for Medication-Related Problems**

- Drug-testing methodology
- Physiologic changes related to aging
- Use of multiple medications
- Cognitive and sensory changes
- Knowledge deficits
- Financial concerns

The drugs and dosages that are appropriate for one may be unsuitable for the other. No medical professional would think of giving an adult dose of medication to a child, yet the same consideration is not always given to the unique situation presented by older adults. Geropharmacology, the study of how older adults respond to medication, is a new but growing area. Until all physicians recognize the uniqueness of older adults and modify treatment accordingly, overmedication is likely to occur.

RISKS RELATED TO THE PHYSIOLOGIC CHANGES OF AGING

People do not experience age-related physiologic changes at the same rate. When considering the responses of older adults to medication, it is more important to consider physiologic age than chronologic age. The more physiologic changes experienced, the greater the risk will be of an altered response to medications. Even the most common physiologic changes of aging can have a significant effect on pharmacokinetics and pharmacodynamics (Table 7-1).

PHARMACOKINETICS

Pharmacokinetics is the study of drug actions within the body, including absorption, distribution, metabolism, and excretion.

Drug Absorption

Most medications are taken orally and are absorbed through the gastrointestinal tract. Gastric acid secretion decreases as we age, resulting in an increased gastric pH.

Table 7-1	**Factors Affecting Drug Response in Older Adults**
EFFECT	**CAUSE**
Decreased drug absorption	Decreased hydrochloric acid; altered gastrointestinal motility
Altered drug distribution	Storing of fat-soluble drugs in fatty tissue; decreased serum albumin for binding of drugs
Altered drug metabolism	Decreased enzyme activity in liver
Decreased drug excretion	Decreased renal blood flow; decreased glomerular filtration rate; decreased number of functional renal tubules

When the concentration of acid is lower than normal, drug absorption is reduced. Decreased acidity also affects the breakdown of capsules and tablet coatings in the stomach, resulting in a variable absorption rate, depending on the way a drug is manufactured.

Decreased gastric motility and a slower emptying rate of the stomach are common with aging. These can increase the amount of time that the medication is in contact with the gastric mucosa and can lead to increased absorption. Decreased peristalsis can also affect the speed at which enteric medication reaches the intestine. It may take longer for a drug to reach its site of absorption; therefore, its onset of action may be delayed. Changes in the ability of the cells in the gastrointestinal tract to absorb and transport the drug can further influence its absorption. If medication is not transferred effectively through the cell membrane, the amount of absorption will be decreased.

Drug Distribution

With aging, there is typically a decrease in total body mass, lean body mass, and total body water and an increase in total body fat. These changes can significantly alter the distribution of medications. Because there is less total body water, water-soluble drugs such as gentamicin, histamine-receptor blockers, and lithium tend to remain in higher concentrations in the bloodstream. This results in increased blood concentration levels of these drugs. An older person who is dehydrated is at even greater risk for reaching excessive blood levels of water-soluble drugs.

As muscle mass decreases and the percentage of adipose tissue increases, fat-soluble drugs such as phenobarbital and the benzodiazepines become trapped in the fatty tissue, resulting in abnormally low blood levels. If the dosage is increased based on these blood levels, an excessive amount of medication may be administered. Because fat-soluble drugs continue to be released slowly from the fat into the bloodstream, older persons may exhibit delayed or hangover effects. The half-life of a single dose of diazepam, which is 36 hours in a young adult, may extend to as much as 100 hours in an older individual.

A decrease in hemoglobin and the plasma protein albumin is common with aging. This results in fewer available sites for protein-bound drugs such as warfarin, phenytoin, theophylline, salicylates, and tolbutamide. The danger of adverse or toxic reactions is high even with smaller doses, because an unbound active drug still circulates in the bloodstream. The risk for toxicity is greater in malnourished older adults. Aging persons who consume high-carbohydrate, low-protein diets are more likely to develop toxicity than are aging persons who consume a well-balanced diet. Because not all of the serum drug assays can distinguish between free and bound medications, these tests may not provide reliable measures of toxicity.

Drug Metabolism

The liver is the primary site of drug **metabolism**. Aging often results in decreased activity of liver cells, decreased metabolic enzymes, and decreased cardiac output, which results in reduced blood flow to the liver. By 65 years of age, the liver has only 55% to 65% of the perfusion of a young adult. This reduction in perfusion decreases the liver's effectiveness in metabolizing drugs. When drugs are not metabolized effectively by the older adult's liver, the risk for toxicity increases. Toxicity is always a concern with medications commonly prescribed for older adults, including digoxin, β-blockers, calcium-channel blockers, and tricyclic antidepressants.

Drug Excretion

Aging kidneys are significantly less effective at removing waste products, including the by-products of medications. As the kidneys become less effective in the **excretion** of drugs, more drug remains in the circulation, leading to elevated drug levels and symptoms of drug toxicity. Circulatory changes that reduce blood flow to the kidneys result in drug accumulation in the bloodstream and increase the risk for toxicity.

Because the changes in kidney function are accompanied by changes in lean body mass, serum creatinine levels often remain constant, masking the decline in function. When the risks for toxicity are assessed, creatinine clearance tests provide a more effective measure of kidney function than does the serum creatinine level.

Medications such as aminoglycosides, digoxin, lithium, procainamide, and cimetidine are likely to reach toxic levels because of poor renal excretion. Nonprescription drugs such as alcohol and nicotine can also affect kidney function and cause changes in drug elimination in older persons.

PHARMACODYNAMICS

Responses to medications are less predictable in the aging person. Pathologic changes in target organs may affect the response to medications. Receptor sites on the target organs may respond more or less sensitively to medications. The receptors may respond normally to some medications but not to others. Receptors often may be more sensitive to medications, placing older adults at increased risk for toxic responses. Brain receptors are particularly sensitive, thus the strong response of most older persons to psychotropic medications. When the receptor sites are less sensitive, the individual may require larger-than-normal doses to achieve therapeutic effects. If receptor sites in the myocardium are affected, older persons may require higher doses of common medications such as propranolol and lidocaine. Administration of these higher doses increases the risk for toxicity.

Polypharmacy

Polypharmacy, the prescription, administration, or use of more medications than are clinically indicated, is a common problem in older adults (Figure 7-1). According to many studies, older adults ingest a far greater number of medications than do younger persons. A recent survey revealed that the average institutionalized older person takes 7.5 medications. Nearly 10% of those living independently take as many as 12 prescription drugs. This number does not include OTC medications that may be taken with or without a physician's recommendation or knowledge. It is estimated that older adults purchase 40% of all nonprescription medications. The more medications taken, the greater the risk for untoward reactions, drug interactions, and drug toxicities. Drug interactions and toxicities in older adults are likely to result in behavioral or cognitive changes, which are often mistaken for dementia.

Many factors contribute to the increased usage of medication among older adults, including an increased likelihood of multiple acute or chronic disease conditions, increased availability of a variety of prescription and OTC medications, changes in patient expectations, and changes in the health care delivery system.

Newer, better, and more potent medications are developed every day. Medical conditions of older adults that were once considered untreatable are now treated routinely using medications. Because older adults tend to have more physical complaints

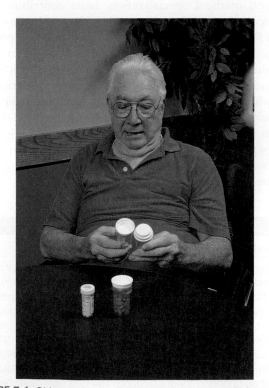

FIGURE 7-1 Older adults' concurrent use of many prescription medications can lead to polypharmacy.

or diseases than do younger individuals, medication usage increases exponentially.

Older adults seek medical intervention for many reasons. Some live with their problems and seek medical attention only when they have serious concerns. By the time such a person seeks medical attention, his or her condition may have seriously deteriorated, requiring the prescription of multiple medications. Other older persons make frequent visits to their physicians, seeking reassurance that nothing is seriously wrong. Rather than spending the time needed to reassure older adults, some physicians issue a prescription as a way to terminate the visit. Unfortunately, this poor medical practice occurs too often and can result in older adults taking unnecessary or marginally necessary medications.

Still other older persons expect their physicians to be able to eliminate all of their problems and ailments with medications. Every television show, magazine article, or recommendation from a friend extolling the benefits of a new medication sends some older adults to their doctors' offices to request or even demand the new medicine. They expect the physician to provide a medication to relieve their ailments, and they often perceive that the physician is not doing anything for them unless some medication is prescribed. Some older adults even go from doctor to doctor until they find one who will give them what they want. Under these pressures, some physicians prescribe medications that they otherwise would not have ordered.

Changes in health care delivery, particularly increased medical specialization, have contributed to medication-related problems. It is increasingly common for an older person to have two or more physicians providing their care. When more than one physician writes prescriptions, the risk for medication reactions and overmedication increases dramatically. If a physician does not know what drugs the patient is already taking, he or she cannot consider those drugs when determining the safety of another prescription. Every physician providing care to an older person must be aware of all medications that person is taking, no matter who prescribed them.

🏥 Clinical Situation

Medication Side Effects

A patient who was using timolol eye drops that were prescribed by an ophthalmologist for glaucoma began to experience joint pain. Not seeing any connection between his eye problems and his aching joints, the patient sought the advice of his rheumatologist. Fortunately, the rheumatologist asked the patient whether he was taking any other medications. When timolol was identified, the rheumatologist recognized the possibility of a drug-induced problem and contacted the ophthalmologist, who then changed the medication. The joint pain disappeared without further medical intervention.

BEERS CRITERIA FOR POTENTIALLY INAPPROPRIATE MEDICATION USE IN OLDER ADULTS

The fact that older adults respond differently than younger adults has been recognized for some time. Until recently, there were no specific guidelines to aid the physician in selection of medications least likely to cause adverse reactions. In 1991, the Beers Criteria, a list of drugs that should usually be avoided by the elderly, was developed. This list was improved and expanded in 1997 and again in 2002. Two separate lists now exist. Part I identifies medications best avoided by the elderly independent of diagnoses or conditions (Table 7-2). Part II uses diagnoses or conditions as the primary consideration (Table 7-3 on pages 138–139). Medicare and Medicaid have developed regulations for skilled nursing facilities that are heavily based on the Beers criteria. Skilled care facilities are required to have protocols that ensure that physician's orders are in compliance. Citations are issued to facilities that fail to comply.

To protect the elderly, physicians and others who have legal authority to prescribe medications should remember six basic guidelines: (1) Start low and go slow, (2) start one drug and stop two, (3) do not use a drug if the adverse effects are worse than the disease, (4) use as few drugs as possible and use nonpharmacologic approaches whenever possible, (5) frequently assess the patient's response, and (6) consider drug holidays.

RISKS RELATED TO COGNITIVE OR SENSORY CHANGES

Cognitive and sensory limitations increase the risks for medication errors in older adults. Cognitive problems come in several forms, including a lack of the literacy skills needed to read the labels and directions, the inability to understand and comply with directions, and the inability to make correct judgments about medications. In severe cases of cognitive impairment, older individuals may not even recognize that they have to take medication. If they do attempt to take medication, serious and potentially harmful errors are often made. Cognitively impaired older adults should not be responsible for medicating themselves but should be supervised by a family member or nurse.

Sensory changes, particularly visual and, to a lesser extent, hearing changes, present problems for older adults. When vision changes render an older person unable to read a medication label or to recognize the different sizes, shapes, or colors of the various medications, serious problems can arise. Many older adults essentially guess about what medications they are taking, often taking the wrong medication at the wrong

Table 7-2   2002 Criteria for Potentially Inappropriate Medication Use in Older Adults: Independent of Diagnoses or Conditions — Beer's Criteria

DRUG	CONCERN	SEVERITY RATING (HIGH OR LOW)
Propoxyphene (Darvon) and combination products (Darvon with ASA, Darvon-N, and Darvocet-N)*	Offers few analgesic advantages over acetaminophen, yet has the adverse effects of other narcotic drugs.	Low
Indomethacin (Indocin and Indocin SR)	Of all available nonsteroidal anti-inflammatory drugs, this drug produces the most CNS adverse effects.	High
Pentazocine (Talwin)	Narcotic analgesic that causes more CNS adverse effects, including confusion and hallucinations, more commonly than other narcotic drugs. Additionally, it is a mixed agonist and antagonist.	High
Trimethobenzamide (Tigan)	One of the least effective antiemetic drugs, yet it can cause extrapyramidal adverse effects.	High
Muscle relaxants and antispasmodics: methocarbamol (Robaxin), carisoprodol (Soma), chlorzoxazone (Paraflex),metaxalone (Skelaxin), cyclobenzaprine (Flexeril), and oxybutynin (Ditropan). Do not consider the extended-release Ditropan XL.	Most muscle relaxants and antispasmodic drugs are poorly tolerated by elderly patients, since these cause anticholinergic adverse effects, sedation, and weakness. Additionally, their effectiveness at doses tolerated by elderly patients is questionable.	High
Flurazepam (Dalmane)	This benzodiazepine hypnotic has an extremely long half-life in elderly patients (often days), producing prolonged sedation and increasing the incidence of falls and fracture. Medium- or short-acting benzodiazepines are preferable.	High
Amitriptyline (Elavil), chlordiazepoxide-amitriptyline (Limbitrol), and perphenazine-amitriptyline (Triavil)	Because of its strong anticholinergic and sedation properties, amitriptyline is rarely the antidepressant of choice for elderly patients.	High
Doxepin (Sinequan)	Because of its strong anticholinergic and sedating properties, doxepin is rarely the antidepressant of choice for elderly patients.	High
Meprobamate (Miltown and Equanil)	This is a highly addictive and sedating anxiolytic. Those using meprobamate for prolonged periods may become addicted and may need to be withdrawn slowly.	High
Doses of short-acting benzodiazepines: doses greater than lorazepam (Ativan), 3 mg; oxazepam (Serax), 60 mg; alprazolam (Xanax), 2 mg; temazepam (Restoril), 15 mg; and triazolam (Halcion), 0.25 mg	Because of increased sensitivity to benzoadiazepines in elderly patients, smaller doses may be effective as well as safer. Total daily doses should rarely exceed the suggested maximums.	High
Long-acting benzodiazepines: chlordiazepoxide (Librium), chlordiazepoxide-amitriptyline (Limbitrol) clidiniumchlordiazepoxide (Librax), diazepam (Valium), quazepam (Doral), halazepam (Paxipam), and chlorazepate (Tranxene)	These drugs have a long half-life in elderly patients (often several days), producing prolonged sedation and increasing the risk of falls and fractures. Short- and intermediate-acting benzodiazepines are preferred if a benzodiazepine is required.	High
Disopyramide (Norpace and Norpace CR)	Of all antiarrhythmic drugs, this is the most potent negative inotrope and therefore may induce heart failure in elderly patients. It is also strongly anticholinergic. Other antiarrhythmic drugs should be used.	High
Digoxin (Lanoxin) (should not exceed >0.125 mg/d except when treating atrial arrhythmias)	Decreased renal clearance may lead to increased risk of toxic effects.	Low
Short-acting dipyridamole (Persantine). Do not consider the long-acting dipyridamole (which has better properties than the short-acting in older adults) except with patients with artificial heart valves	May cause orthostatic hypotension.	Low

Continued

Table 7-2	2002 Criteria for Potentially Inappropriate Medication Use in Older Adults: Independent of Diagnoses or Conditions – Beer's Criteria—cont'd	
DRUG	**CONCERN**	**SEVERITY RATING (HIGH OR LOW)**
Methyldopa (Aldomet) and methyldopa-hydrochlorothiazide (Aldoril)	May cause bradycardia and exacerbate depression in elderly patients.	High
Reserpine at doses >0.25 mg	May induce depression, impotence, sedation, and orthostatic hypotension.	Low
Chlorpropamide (Diabinese)	It has a prolonged half-life in elderly patients and could cause prolonged hypoglycemia. Additionally, it is the only oral hypoglycemic agent that causes SIADH.	High
Gastrointestinal antispasmodic drugs: dicyclomine (Bentyl), hyoscyamine (Levsin and Levsinex), propantheline (Pro-Banthine), belladonna alkaloids (Donnatal and others), and clidinium-chlordiazepoxide (Librax)	GI antispasmodic drugs are highly anticholinergic and have uncertain effectiveness. These drugs should be avoided (especially for long-term use).	High
Anticholinergics and antihistamines: chlorpheniramine (Chlor-Trimeton), diphenhydramine (Benadryl), hydroxyzine (Vistaril and Atarax), cyproheptadine (Periactin), promethazine (Phenergan), tripelennamine, dexchlorpheniramine (Polaramine)	All nonprescription and many prescription antihistamines may have potent anticholinergic properties. Nonanticholinergic antihistamines are preferred in elderly patients when treating allergic reactions.	High
Diphenhydramine (Benadryl)	May cause confusion and sedation. Should not be used as a hypnotic, and when used to treat emergency allergic reactions, it should be used in the smallest possible dose.	High
Ergot mesyloids (Hydergine) and cyclandelate (Cyclospasmol)	Have not been shown to be effective in the doses studied.	Low
Ferrous sulfate >325 mg/d	Doses >325 mg/d do not dramatically increase the amount absorbed but greatly increase the incidence of constipation.	Low
All barbiturates (except phenobarbital) except when used to control seizures	Are highly addictive and cause more adverse effects than most sedative or hypnotic drugs in elderly patients.	High
Meperidine (Demerol)	Not an effective oral analgesic in doses commonly used. May cause confusion and has many disadvantages to other narcotic drugs.	High
Ticlopidine (Ticlid)	Has been shown to be no better than aspirin in preventing clotting and may be considerably more toxic. Safer, more effective alternatives exist.	High
Ketorolac (Toradol)	Immediate and long-term use should be avoided in older persons, since a significant number have asymptomatic GI pathologic conditions.	High
Amphetamines and anorexic agents	These drugs have potential for causing dependence, hypertension, angina, and myocardial infarction.	High
Long-term use of full-dosage, longer half-life, non–COX-selective NSAIDs: naproxen (Naprosyn, Avaprox, and Aleve), oxaprozin (Daypro), and piroxicam (Feldene)	Have the potential to produce GI bleeding, renal failure, high blood pressure, and heart failure.	High
Daily fluoxetine (Prozac)	Long half-life of drug and risk of producing excessive CNS stimulation, sleep disturbances, and increasing agitation. Safer alternatives exist.	High
Long-term use of stimulant laxatives: bisacodyl (Dulcolax), cascara sagrada, and Neoloid except in the presence of opiate analgesic use	May exacerbate bowel dysfunction.	High

Table 7-2 2002 Criteria for Potentially Inappropriate Medication Use in Older Adults: Independent of Diagnoses or Conditions – Beer's Criteria—cont'd

DRUG	CONCERN	SEVERITY RATING (HIGH OR LOW)
Amiodarone (Cordarone)	Associated with QT interval problems and risk of provoking torsades de pointes. Lack of efficacy in older adults.	High
Orphenadrine (Norflex)	Causes more sedation and anticholinergic adverse effects than safer alternatives.	High
Guanethidine (Ismelin)	May cause orthostatic hypotension. Safer alternatives exist.	High
Guanadrel (Hylorel)	May cause orthostatic hypotension.	High
Cyclandelate (Cyclospasmol)	Lack of efficacy.	Low
Isoxsurpine (Vasodilan)	Lack of efficacy.	Low
Nitrofurantoin (Macrodantin)	Potential for renal impairment. Safer alternatives available.	High
Doxazosin (Cardura)	Potential for hypotension, dry mouth, and urinary problems.	Low
Methyltestosterone (Android, Virilon, and Testrad)	Potential for prostatic hypertrophy and cardiac problems.	High
Thioridazine (Mellaril)	Greater potential for CNS and extrapyramidal adverse effects.	High
Mesoridazine (Serentil)	CNS and extrapyramidal adverse effects.	High
Short acting nifedipine (Procardia and Adalat)	Potential for hypotension and constipation.	High
Clonidine (Catapres)	Potential for orthostatic hypotension and CNS adverse effects.	Low
Mineral oil	Potential for aspiration and adverse effects. Safer alternatives available.	High
Cimetidine (Tagamet)	CNS adverse effects including confusion.	Low
Ethacrynic acid (Edecrin)	Potential for hypertension and fluid imbalances. Safer alternatives available.	Low
Desiccated thyroid	Concerns about cardiac effects. Safer alternatives available.	High
Amphetamines (excluding methylphenidate hydrochloride and anorexics)	CNS stimulant adverse effects.	High
Estrogens only (oral)	Evidence of the carcinogenic (breast and endometrial cancer) potential of these agents and lack of cardioprotective effect in older women.	Low

*Proxyphene and its combination products were recalled by the FDA in November, 2010, because of the risk of serious or possibly fatal heart rhythm abnormalities. These drugs should no longer be prescribed or administered.

Abbreviations: CNS, central nervous system; COX, cyclooxygenase; GI, gastrointestinal; NSAIDs, nonsteroidal anti-inflammatory drugs; SIADH, syndrome of inappropriate antidiuretic hormone secretion.

Reprinted with permission: Fick, D.M., Cooper, J.W., Wade, W.E., Waller, J.L., Maclean, J.R., & Beers, M.H. (2003). Updating the Beers Criteria for potentially inappropriate medication use in older adults: Results of a US consensus panel of experts. *Archives of Internal Medicine, 163*(22), 2716–2724. Table 1, p. 2720. Evidence Level VI: Expert Opinion. Copyright © 2003, American Medical Association. All Rights reserved.

time and in the wrong amount because they are unable to read the directions. Liquid medications, particularly injectable medications such as insulin, are commonly overdosed or underdosed because of poor vision. Many of these risks can be reduced by adequately assessing the person's ability to read labels accurately, by proper teaching and by using special labels or magnifying devices that facilitate safe administration.

RISKS RELATED TO INADEQUATE KNOWLEDGE

Inadequate knowledge about medications can result in serious problems for older adults. This lack of knowledge, which can relate to both prescription and nonprescription medications, has many causes and manifests in different ways.

One common sign of lack of knowledge involves sharing medications with friends or relatives.

Table 7-3 2002 Criteria for Potentially Inappropriate Medication Use in Older Adults: Considering Diagnoses or Conditions

DISEASE OR CONDITION	DRUG	CONCERN	SEVERITY RATING (HIGH OR LOW)
Heart failure	Disopyramide (Norpace), and high sodium content drugs (sodium and sodium salts [alginate bicarbonate, biphosphate, citrate, phosphate, salicylate, and sulfate])	Negative inotropic effect. Potential to promote fluid retention and exacerbation of heart failure.	High
Hypertension	Phenylpropanolamine hydrochloride (removed from the market in 2001), pseudoephedrine; diet pills, and amphetamines	May produce elevation of blood pressure secondary to sympathomimetic activity.	High
Gastric or duodenal ulcers	NSAIDs and aspirin (>325 mg) (coxibs excluded)	May exacerbate existing ulcers or produce new/ additional ulcers.	High
Seizures or epilepsy	Clozapine (Clozaril), chlorpromazine (Thorazine), thioridazine (Mellaril), and thiothixene (Navane)	May lower seizure thresholds.	High
Blood clotting disorders or receiving anticoagulant therapy	Aspirin, NSAIDs, dipyridamole (Persantin), ticlopidine (Ticlid), and clopidogrel (Plavix)	May prolong clotting time and elevate INR values or inhibit platelet aggregation, resulting in an increased potential for bleeding.	High
Bladder outflow obstruction	Anticholinergics and antihistamines, gastrointestinal antispasmodics, muscle relaxants, oxybutynin (Ditropan), flavoxate (Urispas), anticholinergics, antidepressants, decongestants, and tolterodine (Detrol)	May decrease urinary flow, leading to urinary retention.	High
Stress incontinence	α-Blockers (Doxazosin, Prazosin, and Terazosin), anticholinergics, tricyclic antidepressants (imipramine hydrochloride, doxepin hydrochloride, and amitriptyline hydrochloride), and long-acting benzodiazepines	May produce polyuria and worsening of incontinence.	High
Arrhythmias	Tricyclic antidepressants (imipramine hydrochloride, doxepin hydrochloride, and amitriptyline hydrochloride)	Concern due to proarrhythmic effects and ability to produce QT interval changes.	High
Insomnia	Decongestants, theophylline (Theodur), methylphenidate (Ritalin), MAOIs, and amphetamines	Concern due to CNS stimulant effects.	High
Parkinson disease	Metoclopramide (Reglan), conventional antipsychotics, and tacrine (Cognex)	Concern due to their antidopaminergic/ cholinergic effects.	High
Cognitive impairment	Barbiturates, anticholinergics, antispasmodics, and muscle relaxants. CNS stimulants: dextroAmphetamine (Adderall), methylphenidate (Ritalin), methamphetamine (Desoxyn), and pemolin	Concern due to CNS-altering effects.	High
Depression	Long-term benzodiazepine use. Sympatholytic agents: methyldopa (Aldomet), reserpine, and guanethidine (Ismelin	May produce or exacerbate depression.	High
Anorexia and malnutrition	CNS stimulants: DextroAmphetamine (Adderall), methylphenidate (Ritalin), methamphetamine (Desoxyn), pemolin, and fluoxetine (Prozac)	Concern due to appetite-suppressing effects.	High

Table 7-3 2002 Criteria for Potentially Inappropriate Medication Use in Older Adults: Considering Diagnoses or Conditions—cont'd

DISEASE OR CONDITION	DRUG	CONCERN	SEVERITY RATING (HIGH OR LOW)
Syncope or falls	Short- to intermediate-acting benzodiazepine and tricyclic antidepressants (imipramine hydrochloride, doxepin hydrochloride, and amitriptyline hydrochloride)	May produce ataxia, impaired psychomotor function, syncope, and additional falls.	High
SIADH/ hyponatremia	SSRIs: fluoxetine (Prozac), citalopram (Celexa), fluvoxamine (Luvox), paroxetine (Paxil), and sertraline (Zoloft)	May exacerbate or cause SIADH.	Low
Seizure disorder	Bupropion (Wellbutrin)	May lower seizure threshold.	High
Obesity	Olanzapine (Zyprexa)	May stimulate appetite and increase weight gain.	Low
COPD	Long-acting benzodiazepines: chlordiazepoxide (Librium), chlordiazepoxide-amitriptyline (Limbitrol), clidiniumchlordiazepoxide (Librax), diazepam (Valium), quazepam (Doral), halazepam (Paxipam), and chlorazepate (Tranxene). β-blockers: propranolol	CNS adverse effects. May induce respiratory depression. May exacerbate or cause respiratory depression.	High
Chronic constipation	Calcium channel blockers, anticholinergics, and tricyclic antidepressant (imipramine hydrochloride, doxepin hydrochloride, and amitriptyline hydrochloride)	May exacerbate constipation.	Low

This practice is common and persists because many older adults are unaware of the dangers. When older adults find a medication that makes them feel better, they may attempt to share the medication with friends who have similar problems. The intention of helping friends is good, but the consequences can be serious and even fatal. All people, particularly older adults, must be aware that it is not safe to take a medication prescribed for someone else. If an older adult believes that a certain medication will help, that person should get the name of the medicine and then contact his or her physician. The physician, not a friend, is best able to determine whether the drug will be safe and beneficial.

Many older adults have misconceptions about OTC preparations. It is estimated that 60% to 70% of older adults use at least one OTC preparation. Many do not think of OTC medications as "real" drugs because no prescription is needed to purchase them. Because they do not consider OTC medications to be real drugs, older adults are not likely to consult with a physician, pharmacist, or nurse regarding their use. Many simply go to the drug store or grocery store and purchase whatever preparation looks like it might help. This uneducated use of OTC drugs can be hazardous to older adults, particularly those who are also taking prescription medications. OTC medications are capable of potentiating or interfering with the effects of prescription medications, possibly resulting in serious harm. OTC drugs can also create or mask symptoms of disease. Use of these drugs can make it difficult for the physician to recognize changes in health status. Older adults must be taught to consult with their physicians or pharmacists before taking any OTC medication.

Alcohol is the most commonly consumed nonprescription drug used by adults. Most older adults do not think of alcohol as a drug, so they do not think about it when taking medications. Alcoholic beverages can cause adverse reactions when taken in conjunction with many prescription and OTC drugs. It is prudent to check with the physician or pharmacist before drinking alcohol. Today most prescription drugs are labeled if there is a risk for interaction with alcohol, but these labels are not always given adequate attention. In addition to OTC medications, herbal or natural remedies are being used with increased frequency, particularly among the baby boom population and ethnic minorities. It is important to consider possible interactions between these substances and more traditional prescription and OTC medications.

Older adults often lack adequate knowledge regarding their prescription medications as well. They are often given one or more prescriptions and simply told to take them according to the directions. The directions provided may be very clear to a knowledgeable health care professional, but they are often misunderstood or misinterpreted by older adults. Even simple misunderstandings can lead to improper self-medication and result in serious consequences. To reduce the risks, older adults often require additional instruction to take their prescriptions safely. Because this is a common problem among older adults, self-administration of medication is addressed in detail later in the chapter.

Clinical Situation

Polypharmacy

Mrs. Smith had been taking a medication for her high blood pressure. This medication was no longer completely effective in controlling the problem, so her physician ordered a newer, more potent antihypertensive. Approximately 25 tablets of the original medication were left in the bottle, which Mrs. Smith left in her medicine chest. After taking the new prescription for a month, Mrs. Smith happened to check her blood pressure with one of the automatic machines located in a drugstore. She found that her blood pressure was just a little bit higher than she thought it should be. Remembering that she had another medicine for blood pressure at home, she decided (without consulting the physician) to take a few of the "less potent" old tablets. Only when she began to feel dizzy and almost fainted did she call the physician.

RISKS RELATED TO FINANCIAL FACTORS

Medications are expensive. A single prescription can easily cost $100 or more a month. If an aging person requires more than one medication, the cumulative cost can be overwhelming. To save money, older adults living on limited incomes may fail to take their medications or they may make changes in the amount or frequency to conserve their supply. Because these changes do not follow the recommended therapeutic schedule, a wide variety of untoward responses can occur. There is hope that this will be less of a problem now that prescription drug coverage is available under Medicare provisions.

Even with insurance coverage, it is probable that a significant percentage of prescriptions written by physicians will not be filled. Some older adults simply say, "I don't like to take pills." Others will get a prescription filled once to see whether it is "worth the price." If the benefits gained from taking the medication are not readily obvious to older adults, they may not get the prescription refilled. Because medications are expensive, many frugal older adults save medications that

were prescribed in the past, even if the drugs are no longer part of their therapy. Older adults are often reluctant to discard costly medications, holding on to them "just in case" they are needed again. This practice can bring serious harm if the medications are kept long enough to become outdated. Outdated medications can undergo chemical changes that make them hazardous. Saving old medications also increases the risk for problems if the older person thinks the drug is appropriate and takes it without checking with the physician.

MEDICATION ADMINISTRATION IN AN INSTITUTIONAL SETTING

It is obvious that medications can present a wide range of problems for older adults. Nurses who work with older adults must consider each of these risks when determining a plan for safe administration. Medication administration is a common part of nursing care of older adults in hospitals, extended-care facilities, and home settings. Approaches and methods may vary according to the setting, but the safety of the older adult remains the primary concern. A great deal of nursing time in hospitals and extended-care facilities is spent on medication-related activities. Because medications play an important role in the health care of most older adults, nurses must take special precautions to ensure that drugs are administered safely.

Safe drug administration begins with a thorough knowledge and understanding of each medication. Any questions regarding medication therapy must be clarified and resolved before a medication is administered. Information regarding medications is contained in many reference books, which should be readily available to nurses. Before administering a medication, nurses should have the following information:

- Therapeutic effects of the medication
- Reasons this individual is receiving the medication
- Normal therapeutic dosage of the medication
- Normal route or routes of administration
- Any special precautions related to administration
- Common side effects or adverse effects of the medication (see Clinical Situation, p. 134)
- Signs of overdose and toxicity

NURSING ASSESSMENT AND MEDICATION

Nurses must be sure to thoroughly assess their older residents before administering any medications. After administration, nurses should monitor older adults continually to determine whether the medication is having the desired effect. This should be done after administering both scheduled and as-needed medications. Residents should also be observed for any untoward effects or significant changes in medical condition or behavior (Box 7-2).

Because normal physiologic changes and the effects of disease place the older person at an increased risk for drug-related problems, nurses should be particularly watchful for any signs of overdose or toxicity. Special age-related risk factors and observations for the more common drug classifications are summarized in Table 7-4.

Box 7-2 CARE Acronym for Medication Assessment

C—Caution/compliance: Assess benefits and risks. Remember, there are many reasons the elderly may not be compliant.
A—Adjust: The dose may change based on age and condition. "Start low, go slow" is the rule for elderly patients.
R—Review regimen regularly: Polypharmacy is common in the elderly. Each new medication increases risk for interactions.
E—Educate: Be sure elderly patients know their drugs, how and when to take them, and when to notify the physician.

Modified from Fordyce M: *Geriatric pearls,* Philadelphia, 1999, FA Davis.

Table 7-4   Common Drug Categories With Precautions Related to Aging

TYPE OF MEDICATION	RISK FACTORS	ASSESS FOR
Cardiac Medication		
Digoxin, propranolol	Dehydration, hypothyroidism, decreased renal excretion, and hypoxia increase the risk for toxicity.	Visual spots, dizziness, headaches, fatigue, drowsiness, mental changes, numbness around lips or of hands, altered pulse rate or regularity, loss of appetite, nausea, vomiting, diarrhea, weight loss
Diuretics		
Bumetanide, furosemide	May result in dehydration. May precipitate hydrochlorothiazide, urinary incontinence, or retention in older chlorothiazide men with prostate hypertrophy. May result in altered electrolyte balance (K+ and Na+), which predisposes patient to digitalis toxicity.	Signs of dehydration, hypotension, weight loss, lethargy, and confusion
Antihypertensives		
Captopril, clonidine, hydralazine hydrochloric acid, methyldopa	High doses may aggravate existing problems in cerebral, coronary, and renal circulation. Hot weather, alcohol, and exercise are likely to increase the risk for hypotension.	Bradycardia, postural hypotension, weakness, headaches, palpitations, nausea, vomiting, diarrhea or constipation, difficulty urinating, and edema
Psychotropics (Including Antianxiety Agents, Antidepressants, and Antipsychotics)		
Flurazepam, triazolam, diazepam, haloperidol Thorazine, thioridazine	Older persons usually require smaller doses to achieve therapeutic response. Tardive dyskinesia is a significant risk with long-term therapy.	Apathy, confusion, drooling, lip smacking, grimacing, difficulty swallowing, decreased mobility, skin reactions, jaundice, impaired sense of balance, alteration in gait, falls, drowsiness, fainting, hypotension, palpitations, constipation, hypothermia, and complaints of feeling cold
Antiinfectives		
Cephalosporins, penicillins, sulfonamides, tetracyclines	Standard dose may result in higher blood levels in older adults. Increased risk for allergic reactions or superimposed yeast infections with aging. Damage to cranial nerve VIII is particularly common in older adults.	Nausea, vomiting, diarrhea, dehydration, signs of oral or vaginal yeast infection, urticaria, and tinnitus
Nonsteroidal Antiinflammatory Agents		
Aspirin, ibuprofen, tolmetin, naproxen	Increased risk for gastrointestinal and central nervous system problems with aging	Signs of gastrointestinal upset including nausea, vomiting, tarry stools, diarrhea or constipation, and occult blood loss; central nervous system side effects including dizziness, confusion, mood swings, depression, and tinnitus
Bronchodilators and Spasmolytics		
Theophylline	Older adults taking allopurinol, propranolol, and cimetidine are at increased risk for toxicity.	Tachycardia, arrhythmias, anorexia, nausea, headaches, or insomnia
Antiulcer Medications		
Cimetidine, ranitidine, aluminum and magnesium hydroxide	May affect the absorption of other medications	Confusion, dry mouth, gynecomastia, impotence, constipation, and diarrhea

⊕ Cultural Considerations

Assessment and Ethnicity

Ethnicity is one factor that should be considered when the nurse assesses a patient's use of and response to medication; however, it should not be used to stereotype any group. Some ethnic variations that have been identified include the following:

- African Americans do not respond as well as whites to propranolol (Inderal) or to the angiotensin-converting enzyme (ACE) inhibitors such as captopril (Capoten). Because of an enzyme deficiency, some African Americans may be more resistant to chemotherapy.
- Codeine and similar drugs are more likely to be effective in individuals of Chinese, Japanese, Thai, and Malaysian descent. Individuals of Asian descent are also more likely to experience alcohol intolerance and may demonstrate excessive responses to antianxiety medications. Use of herbal remedies is common among the Chinese. Common herbs such as ginseng may affect the absorption and elimination of other drugs.
- Hispanics are more likely to experience significant side effects from antidepressants and need to be monitored closely.

Implementation of computerized records as part of the Minimum Data Set 3.0 (see Chapter 8) provides better linkage between nurses and pharmacists. It is hoped that this interdisciplinary approach to medication will promote early recognition of problems or areas of concern regarding the medication regimen.

MEDICATIONS AND THE NURSING CARE PLAN

Medications are only one part of the overall care of the older person and should be included as such. For example, the administration of laxatives should be only a part of a more comprehensive plan to assist bowel elimination, and the administration of analgesics should be only a part of a larger nursing care plan for pain control.

Nursing interventions and precautions related to medications should be addressed in the plan of care. This could include the use of safety devices, call signals, behavior monitoring, or any other specific precaution related to medications. The care plan should indicate when it is necessary to check vital signs, monitor laboratory values, or make any other special observations. All parameters specified by the physician should be readily identified in the care plan—for example, "Hold digoxin if apical pulse is below 60" or "Give 6 units regular insulin at bedtime if the fingerstick blood glucose is over 150."

The care plan should indicate any individual preferences of the older person. Many older adults use a particular order or method to take their medication. This information should be in the care plan so that all staff nurses can be consistent.

NURSING INTERVENTIONS RELATED TO MEDICATION ADMINISTRATION

It is often necessary to modify procedures and techniques of medication administration when working with older adults. Despite modifications, the traditional "rights" of medication administration remain essential to the process.

Right Resident

Proper identification of the resident or patient is an essential part of safe nursing care. This simple task can be a challenge to nurses who work in extended-care facilities. Whenever a large number of residents are up and about, accurate identification becomes more difficult.

The most accurate way to verify identity is to compare the medication record with the identification bracelet (see Figure 7-2). Whenever possible, these bracelets should be used for identification checks. However, not all long-term residents wear identification bracelets, and if they do wear them, the bracelets are often old and blurred. When reliable bracelets are not available, alternative methods must be used.

A resident's pictures are sometimes used as a means of identification. However, pictures that are old or bear little resemblance to the individual are useless. Pictures used for identification must be kept up to date and must be readily available when medications are distributed.

Identification can also be accomplished by asking the resident to state his or her name. Most people respond promptly and appropriately with the correct name. A response to hearing the nurse call a name that

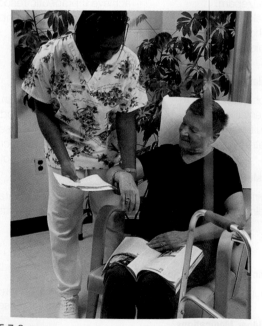

FIGURE 7-2 Before administering any medications, the nurse should check the resident's identification bracelet to be sure the right person receives the right drug.

involves a head shake or a "yes" from a patient is not enough to ensure identification. Many older adults suffering from hearing or cognitive impairment give some sort of response to any name. When an older person is not oriented to a person, bracelets or pictures must be used (Box 7-3).

Attempting to identify a resident by room and bed number is not adequate because cognitively or perceptually impaired individuals often wander into the wrong room or lie down in someone else's bed. Nurses should be careful to avoid the trap of insisting that they "know the residents." Identification must be checked with each medication pass—no matter how long you have been caring for the patient. Serious mistakes can and do occur when nurses take shortcuts with safety procedures. As a method of ensuring accurate identification in accredited agencies, The Joint Commission (TJC) requires the use of two identifiers before the administration of medications.

Right Medication

Before administering a medication, the nurse must ensure that the drug provided by the pharmacy is, in fact, the correct one. This is not as easy as it seems. Because each medication has a generic name and one or more trade names, and, because the appearance of a medication can vary widely depending on the manufacturer, nurses must use a reference source to verify that the right drug is, in fact, available. The physician's orders should be checked carefully, and the pharmacy should be contacted if any questions arise. Many drug names look or sound alike; therefore, it is important to check spellings carefully.

If telephone medication orders are permitted, the nurse taking the order should repeat the entire order to the physician, taking care to clarify the spelling of the drug to avoid the possibility of error.

Right Amount

The goal of drug therapy in older adults is to achieve the maximal therapeutic benefits while giving the smallest amount of medication necessary (Box 7-4). Therefore, the dosage prescribed for an older adult is often lower than what would be prescribed for a younger adult (see Table 7-5). To achieve therapeutic levels without overdosing the older adult, the physician may order lower doses or less frequent administration of a medication. With lower doses, it is imperative for the nurse to verify the strength of the medications (checking decimal points closely). All measurements, particularly for liquids, must be made with great care. Decreased frequency in administration can result in medications that are administered every other day or every third day. Nurses must pay close attention when administering medication to avoid administering it on a day when the drug should be withheld. Any questions regarding the dosage should be clarified with an approved reference, the pharmacist, or the physician before the medication is administered. To prevent errors due to misinterpretation of orders, TJC has published an official "Do Not Use" list of symbols, abbreviations, and mathematical expressions (Table 7-6).

Right Dosage Form

Problems arise when the older person is unable to swallow tablets or cannot swallow at all and relies on a gastric or nasogastric tube for nourishment. For these patients, nurses must consider safe alternatives. If the medication is available in liquid form, the nurse should discuss the possibility of an order change with the physician. Because liquids might be absorbed more rapidly than solids, all changes in medication form require a physician's order. Many times when the drug form is changed, the dosage is also changed. If a liquid form is not available, the tablet or capsule may have to be crushed or broken to facilitate swallowing. Not all medications can be crushed or broken, because these activities can alter the action of the drug (see Box 7-5). If there is any question of whether a medication should be crushed, the pharmacy should be consulted. Lists of common medications that should not be crushed or chewed are available from many sources and should be kept on the nursing unit as quick references.

Box **7-3**	Safety Alert

Identification must be checked (following agency policies) each time a medication is administered. Failure to do this can result in serious errors and harm to older adults.

Box **7-4**	Guiding Rule for Medication Administration in Older Adults

Achieve the maximal therapeutic benefits while giving the smallest necessary amount of medication!

Table **7-5**	Examples of Drug Dosages	
DRUG	**DOSAGE FOR HEALTHY ADULTS**	**DO NOT EXCEED**
Ibuprofen	200–800 mg three to four times/day	1200 mg/day
Indomethacin	25–50 mg three or four times/day	200 mg/day
Naproxen	250–500 mg twice/day	1250 mg/day
Sulindac	150–200 mg twice/day	400 mg/day
Piroxicam	10–20 mg daily	

Data from Skidmore-Roth L: *Mosby's drug reference*, ed 24, St Louis, 2011, Elsevier.

Table 7-6	The Joint Commission's Minimum "Do Not Use" List of Abbreviations and Additional Abbreviations to Avoid*	
DO NOT USE	**POTENTIAL PROBLEM**	**USE INSTEAD**
U (unit)	Mistaken for "0" (zero), "4" (four), or cc	Write "unit"
IU (international unit)	Mistaken for IV (intravenous) or the number 10 (ten)	Write "international unit"
Q.D., QD, q.d., qd (daily)	Mistaken for each other	Write "daily"
Q.O.D., QOD, q.o.d., qod (every other day)	Period after the Q mistaken for "I" and the "O" mistaken for "I"	Write "every other day"
Trailing zero (X.0 mg) [NOTE: Prohibited only for medication-related notations] Lack of leading zero (.X mg)	Decimal point is missed	Never write a zero by itself after a decimal point (X mg), and always use a zero before a decimal point (0.X mg)
MS	Can mean morphine sulfate or magnesium sulfate	Write "morphine sulfate" or "magnesium sulfate"
MSO_4 and $MgSO_4$	Confused for one another.	
> (greater than) < (less than)	Misinterpreted as the number "7" (seven) or the letter "L" Confused for one another	Write "greater than" Write "less than"
Abbreviations for drug names	Misinterpreted due to similar abbreviations for multiple drugs	Write drug names in full
Apothecary units	Unfamiliar to many practitioners Confused with metric units	Use metric units
@	Mistaken for the number "2" (two)	Write "at"
cc	Mistaken for U (units) when poorly written	Write "mL" or "ml" or "milliliters" ("mL" is preferred)
µg	Mistaken for mg (milligrams), resulting in 1000-fold dosing overdose	Write "mcg" or "micrograms"

*Abbreviations on this list should not be used in any form—upper or lower case, with or without periods.
The Joint Commission, 2011. Reprinted with permission.

Right Route

Most medications are prescribed for oral administration. When an oral medication is being administered, the importance of the medication, the preferences of the older person, and his or her capabilities must be considered.

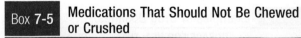

Box 7-5	Medications That Should Not Be Chewed or Crushed

- Enteric-coated tablets (Many appear to have a "candy coating.")
- Capsules (Some may be opened and the contents dissolved; others may not—be sure to check with pharmacy.)
- Time-release tablets or capsules (These often have names with suffixes such as LA [long-acting], SR [sustained-release], ER [extended-release], etc.)
- Sublingual or buccal tablets
- Medications with a bitter taste
- Medications that can irritate oral mucous membranes

Many older adults receive numerous medications. The nurse should give the most important medications first, so if the person refuses to take them all, at least the most essential ones will have been administered. Whenever a person refuses to take his or her medication, it should be noted in the chart, and the nurse in charge should be notified.

Some older adults are capable of and prefer swallowing several tablets at one time to "get it over with." If they experience no difficulty taking their medications this way, there is no reason to try to make them change their habits. Other people prefer to take their medications one tablet at a time. If this is their preference, the nurse should oblige. Still others have trouble swallowing any solid medications.

Tablets, particularly large ones, are likely to cause the greatest problems. Dryness of the mouth related to aging often makes swallowing difficult and results in complaints of pills sticking in the throat. Encouraging older adults to take a drink of water or some other beverage before they try to swallow the tablet may make swallowing easier. Coating the tablet with a spoonful of pudding, ice cream, or applesauce might also help the patient swallow it more easily. Only small amounts of these foods should be used to facilitate swallowing.

? Critical Thinking

When a Patient Refuses Medication

A 78-year-old patient in the hospital for pneumonia has taken his medication without problems in the past. Today he refused all oral medications, including those for his diabetes and hypertension.
- Why do you think he might be refusing his medication?
- How can the nurse determine what is going on in this particular situation?
- What actions should the nurse take?

Crushed medications should not be mixed into a serving of food during mealtime. This practice is unsafe because it often results in a partial missed dose because the entire serving of food may not be consumed and because the nursing assistant assigned to feed the patient is not qualified to administer medications. Again, use of a small amount of applesauce, pudding, or ice cream to facilitate swallowing of a crushed medication is an acceptable practice. Crushing medication and hiding it in food to administer a medication that the patient has refused violate the person's right to choose and is considered unethical. Facility policies should provide directions as to how to proceed when a patient refuses medications as a result of dementia or other cognitive problems.

Administration of medication through a feeding tube is often necessary and must be done correctly. Liquid forms of a medication are preferable and should be requested when available. Large particles of a medication can block the feeding tube and necessitate tube replacement. To prevent blockage, each tablet should be finely crushed and then placed in a plastic medication cup, where it should be thoroughly dissolved in a small amount of warm water. Once they are completely dissolved, medications are administered through the feeding tube. Each medication should be administered separately. The feeding tube should be flushed with a small amount of water before the first medication is given, again after each medication, and once more before the tube is reconnected with the feeding solution. Medications should never be mixed together or with feeding solutions. Medications with an unpleasant taste should be given after all other medications. Offering a sip of ice water before the medication or refrigerating unpleasant-tasting liquid medications can make them more palatable.

Transdermal delivery is becoming an increasingly popular route for drug administration. Transdermal medications are administered using a "patch" consisting of a center that contains the medication surrounded by a skin overlay, which secures the patch to the skin. Transdermal medications are readily accepted by most older adults because they are easy to apply and are effective for extended periods of time. This route is convenient and has a high rate of compliance because it is painless, tasteless, and eliminates the need to consider the timing of application in relation to meals. Transdermal patches cause few gastrointestinal problems and are able to maintain more stable plasma levels, so there are fewer side effects. An additional benefit of the transdermal patch is that drug delivery can be stopped immediately by the removal of the patch.

The major disadvantage of the patch is skin irritation due to either the active ingredient or the adhesive used to secure the patch. Newer techniques have reduced these problems, and the risk can be reduced by rotating the application site and cleaning the skin thoroughly following removal (Box 7-6).

The inhalation route is also used for the administration of medication. Inhalation drugs are typically administered using metered-dose inhalers and nebulizers. The older adult who has arthritis in the hands or lacks coordination may need some assistance using these devices. Effectiveness of drugs administered by inhalation is often affected by the diminished lung capacity and decreased depth and strength of inhalation typically seen with aging.

When a parenteral medication is ordered, other precautions must be taken. Because older adults generally have less muscle mass and subcutaneous tissue than do younger people, injection sites should be selected carefully. Intramuscular injections are best administered using the ventrogluteal site, which is

Box 7-6   Precautions When Using Transdermal Patches

1. Check the dosage strength of the patch.
2. Verify the correct site or sites for administration.
3. Remove any protective liner so that the medication is in contact with the skin.
4. Handle with caution so that the nurse's skin does not come in contact with the medicated portion.
5. Document where each patch is applied. Be sure to rotate sites.
6. Remove all old patches, and clean the skin before applying a new one (pay special attention for clear patches that are difficult to see on the skin).
7. Avoid use of heat over a patch because this causes vasodilation, which increases the rate of absorption.
8. Dispose of old patches by folding sticky edges together and placing in the sharps container. (For environmental reasons, it is not acceptable to use the toilet or wastebasket for disposal.)
9. Teach patient safe application, removal, and disposal of patch. Also teach patients to report use of a patch, as well as any other medications, when seeking medical attention, particularly during emergency care or when magnetic resonance imaging (MRI) is anticipated because many patches contain metal.

easily accessible without excessive repositioning. It is free from any major nerves or blood vessels. This muscle remains large enough for injection even in very slender people. Furthermore, it is well away from areas of possible contamination if the older person is incontinent.

The needle length should be chosen with caution, depending on the injection site. The deltoid muscle is usually a poor site for all but very infrequent administrations of very small volumes. To avoid striking the bone of an emaciated older person, a shorter-length needle (e.g., 1 inch instead of 1.5 inches) may be needed.

Right Time

Some medications are more effective or better tolerated if given under specific conditions. For greatest effect, medications that are ordered before meals should be given when the stomach is empty. Because people produce less gastric acid as they age, a sufficient rate and amount of absorption may depend on having the stomach free of food. Medications that are ordered after meals should be given only after the person has eaten.

Activities of daily living can be affected by medications. Medications should be administered at times when the drugs will interfere as little as possible with normal activities. For example, a diuretic medication should be given early in the day to prevent the older person from having to get up several times at night to urinate.

The timing of eye-drop administration becomes an issue when an aging person requires more than one type of medication in the same eye. Some eye medications are compatible and can be given together, whereas others cannot. The timing and order of administration for eye drops should be clarified with the pharmacy, and the schedule should be clearly stated in the medication administration record.

Right Documentation

Care must be used when documenting medications. Facilities use a variety of different forms and records to document various aspects of care, including medication administration. To ensure that all medications are administered properly, the rules of charting must be followed.

Medications cannot be charted as having been administered until they are actually taken. This means that the nurse must stay in the room and watch the older adult take the medication. It is not safe practice to leave medication at the bedside unless the resident has specific orders that permit self-medication.

Special observations regarding the patient's or resident's response should be included in the daily nursing notes and narrative summaries. The reasons for administration of as-needed medications should be identified each time one is administered, and the effectiveness of these medications should be documented. When a medication is refused or withheld, the reasons should be clearly documented and the physician notified so that the plan of care can be adjusted if necessary.

PATIENT RIGHTS AND MEDICATION

Older adults have the right to know what medication they are receiving and why they are receiving it. Nurses should provide this information when questioned and when a new medication is prescribed.

Older adults also have the right to refuse to take medication. If a person refuses to take medication, nurses cannot use force. A positive attitude and encouragement may help persuade the individual to cooperate. However, when a medication is still refused, the reasons for refusal must be determined and documented, the nurse in charge notified, and any problems communicated to the physician.

The older person must be provided with privacy during injections or any other such procedures. The doors should be closed and the curtains drawn. Failure to do this is a violation of resident rights.

The use of psychotropic drugs as chemical restraints presents a risk to the rights of older adults, and their administration is strictly controlled by the Omnibus Budget Reconciliation Act (OBRA) regulations. Nurses must carefully follow the specific guidelines regarding the administration and monitoring of behavior when an older person is receiving a psychotropic medication. Each abnormal behavior that is an indication for administration of such drugs must be individually identified in the plan of care. During each shift, the nurse must document the number of times these identified behaviors occur. If no symptoms occur at a given dosage of psychotropic medication, the physician will attempt to decrease the dose. This process continues as long as the older person receives these medications.

SELF-MEDICATION AND OLDER ADULTS

IN AN INSTITUTIONAL SETTING

Under OBRA legislation, residents of care facilities should have the option of self-medication if they are capable of doing so safely. A physician's order stating that self-medication is permitted is usually required.

Self-medication by a resident can be time-consuming because the nurse remains responsible for monitoring the resident's compliance and response to the medications. When self-medication is anticipated, the nurse must assess the older adult's ability to understand and comply with the medication regimen. This assessment should include the resident's ability to read labels, follow directions, and measure dosages accurately. After it has been determined that the person can safely assume responsibility for self-medication, the nurse should develop a plan, including (1) delivery of adequate amounts of medication, (2) safe storage of medications that will be kept at the bedside, (3) record-keeping of medications taken, and (4) follow-up assessments of medication effectiveness or side effects.

> ### Coordinated Care
> #### Delegation
> **Medication Administration**
>
> Many long-term care institutions now use specially trained nursing assistants as medication assistants to administer routine oral and some topical medications to stable patients. The responsibility for monitoring the patient's response remains the responsibility of the nurse.

IN THE HOME

Taking medications correctly can be a complex problem for older adults. Because medications are a significant part of the medical plan of care, older adults who live independently must learn to take them properly. The responsibility of assessing medication-taking behaviors and teaching safe self-administration often falls to the home health care nurse (see Home Health Considerations box).

> ### Home Health Considerations
> #### Medications
>
> Nurses who work in home health have a great opportunity to evaluate patients' knowledge of the medications they are taking and their compliance with medication therapy. The number of drugs prescribed and the risk for drug-drug interactions increase when a patient is being seen by more than one physician. Compliance issues are also likely to occur when a patient is taking multiple medications. Here are some steps the nurse can take to increase patient awareness and compliance:
>
> 1. Explain why it is important to do a thorough medical history and review of medications to gain the older adult's cooperation.
> 2. Determine what drugs (prescription, OTC, and herbal) are kept in the house. If possible, go around with the elderly person and identify where medications are stored. Be sure to check places such as medicine cabinets, the kitchen table, counters or cabinets, on top of and inside the refrigerator, at the bedside, and in purses.
> 3. Check whether there are any other "old medications" stored in a shoebox, bag, or anywhere else.
> 4. If possible, gather all of the medications in the house and go through them one at a time. Ask the patient to point out which ones are taken daily, occasionally, and as needed. If more than one elderly person lives in the home, separate the medications and evaluate each separately. Watch for drugs that do not relate to any identified health problems, for any drug duplications due to orders under both generic and trade names, for potential drug-drug interactions, and for inappropriate drug dosages.
> 5. Review each medication to determine whether the patient knows why he or she is taking it, when to take it, and any precautions to use regarding the drug.

6. Discuss what method (if any) the older person uses to verify that the appropriate doses of all medications are taken each day (e.g., Does the person use a daily or weekly pillbox?).
7. After obtaining the patient's consent, discard any expired drugs.

TEACHING OLDER ADULTS ABOUT MEDICATIONS

Older adults and their families or significant others should be given complete information about the prescribed medications and the proper method for taking them. Explanations should be given well in advance of the older adult leaving the office, clinic, or hospital. If possible, nurses should select a time when the older adult's anxiety level is low because the individual will be more likely to remember the important points when calm. If the directions are complex, extra time may be needed to ensure that they are understood completely. Commonly, older persons fail to ask questions because they are afraid of being judged as ignorant or bothersome. This information should be reviewed and repeated if necessary at subsequent visits.

Most medications are taken orally, but increasingly drugs are administered using alternative routes. When medication is taken in any way other than the oral route, the nurse should verify that the older person understands and is able to demonstrate safe self-administration. This includes transdermal patches, suppositories, eye drops or eardrops, and injections. Remember, many things that seem obvious or simple to nurses are complex for others.

In addition to teaching independent older adults about their prescription medications, nurses should teach the importance of consulting with the physician or pharmacist before using alcoholic beverages or taking any OTC medications. Independent older adults should also be reminded never to take medication prescribed for someone else without first consulting the physician.

> ### Patient Teaching
> #### Independent Older Adults and Medications
>
> Older adults who live independently need to know the following:
> - Alcohol and nonsteroidal antiinflammatory drugs (NSAIDs), including ibuprofen, can increase blood pressure and interfere with the action of antihypertensive medications.
> - Excessive use of acetaminophen (Tylenol) can damage the kidneys, and if the patient uses alcohol heavily, it can also damage the liver.
> - Antacids do not protect the stomach from aspirin or NSAIDs.
> - Antacids, calcium supplements, and significant amounts of dairy products should be taken at least 2 hours apart from other medications.
> - The combination of NSAIDs and angiotensin-converting enzyme inhibitors increases the risk for renal failure, especially when the patient is also taking a diuretic.

Each older person who lives independently should have an up-to-date record that identifies his or her major physical problems, physician(s), any allergies, and all current medications. This list must be updated each time a medication is added or discontinued. If the person is not capable of keeping the record up to date, the nurse or family should provide assistance. This record should be taken along each time the individual receives health care services so that all care providers have the necessary information. A written record relieves the older person of the burden of trying to remember too many details, which is particularly difficult when the person is under stress.

Nurses can assist older adults by preparing medication cards or sheets that identify and give the important information about each medication (see Box 7-7). Teaching aids should be kept simple and clear. Writing should be large and legible so that the older person can read it with ease. Family members should be included in the teaching so that they are able to assist the older person if necessary.

SAFETY AND NONCOMPLIANCE (NONADHERENCE) ISSUES

Noncompliance with prescribed medication regimens is common among older adults. Failure to take medication as prescribed results in poorer health, more adverse reactions, more emergency department visits, more hospitalizations, and even more deaths. The financial cost of noncompliance with medication therapy is estimated to be as high as $100 billion a year.

Several factors can increase the risk for noncompliance. Cognitive and sensory limitations increase the risk for medication errors. Keeping track of multiple medications can be confusing to anyone, but it is more likely to present problems for older adults. One or two medications do not seem to cause many problems, but a significant number of older adults become confused and noncompliant when three or more medications are ordered. Special precautions and complicated time schedules compound the problems. To reduce the risk for noncompliance, nurses should encourage older adults to talk to the physician and/or the pharmacist to see whether there is any safe way to reduce the number of medications or simplify the medication schedule. In addition, research has shown that depression, belief patterns, and lack of a social support system contribute to noncompliance.

Techniques that improve safety and compliance include, but are not limited to, the following:

- Associating medication schedules with regular daily events such as meals or bedtime can help older adults remember to take their medications. Additional teaching may be necessary if medications require special timing (e.g., before or after meals). Unless older persons are aware of the reasons and necessity for a schedule, they may not comply and therefore may experience untoward effects.
- Explain the importance of preparing medication in a well-lit area. Poor lighting can further reduce vision in older adults and increase the chance of an error being made.
- Ensure that containers are properly labeled. Visually impaired older adults can continue to self-medicate if measures are taken to compensate for visual problems. Large, preferably upper-case or printed lettering should be used on all labels and teaching materials. All print or writing should be in dark, bold letters. If there is any chance of moisture spilling on the labels, they should be coated in clear plastic or otherwise protected. This prevents blurring of the lettering, which can lead to errors.
- Apply color codes, tape strips, pictures, or textures such as sandpaper to containers to help older adults recognize them. For example, black could indicate medicine that is to be taken with breakfast, red could indicate medications for lunch, and a piece of sandpaper attached to the bottle could indicate bedtime medications. Yellow should be avoided because many older adults have difficulty distinguishing this color. Alternatively, there could be one strip of tape for morning administration, two strips for lunch, three strips for dinner, and four strips for bedtime. The nurse should ensure that the person understands whatever coding system is selected. Medication cups can be marked with dark lines or tape to improve accuracy when measuring liquids, and special magnifiers are available for insulin syringes.
- Modify containers for ease of use. Impaired physical function can interfere with self-medication. Many pill bottles routinely come with safety caps that older adults cannot open. If requested, most pharmacies will provide containers that are easier to open.

Box 7-7	Information to Include on Medication Teaching Sheets

- The name of the medication (trade and/or generic)
- The time or times when the medication should be taken
- Whether the medication should be taken before, with, or after meals
- Any precautions to take when preparing the medication
- How much of the medication to take
- The reason the person is receiving each medication (desired effects)
- The most common side effects
- What action to take if these side effects occur
- What to do if the person forgets to take a dose of the medication
- What to do if the person experiences nausea or vomiting and is unable to take oral medication

- Establish measures to distinguish and separate similar containers. If the older person is receiving eardrops and eye drops, these containers should be stored well away from each other and marked clearly with a large picture of an eye or an ear so that they are distinguishable. This is particularly important because many ear preparations can cause permanent damage to the eye.
- Teach older adults to store medications properly. Medications should be stored away from direct light and moisture, which can cause chemical changes. The tiny pillboxes used by many older adults can be dangerous and should be avoided. Pills left in the boxes may undergo chemical changes. Nitroglycerin can become totally ineffective if stored improperly. Once medications are removed from the prescription bottle, they cannot be readily identified and the older person can easily take the wrong pill. It is safest to leave medications in the pharmacy bottles even though they may be bulky.
- Obtain or devise a system to promote compliance. When older persons are unable to keep their medication schedule straight by using the bottles provided by the pharmacy, other approaches may be necessary. There are several ways nurses can help older adults remember to take their medications. Medication reminder systems help some older adults remember to take medications. These systems typically consist of divided containers that sort the medications by day of the week or by time. They can either be purchased or created using foam egg cartons labeled with the day and time. A simple check of the box reveals whether the medication was taken on time. Some individuals require more medication than fits conveniently into these standard containers or fear that they will drop the egg carton and mix everything up. These individuals may benefit from a system using small zip-closure plastic bags that are labeled (using masking tape) with the appropriate day and time. High-technology solutions such as automated pill dispensing systems with alarms are available, but the cost of most of these devices is significant, and maintenance of the system may be too complex for the average older adult.
- Stress the importance of being alert when taking medications. Sleepiness can interfere with the ability to read labels. If patients are not completely awake, they can easily take the wrong medication. It is not advisable for older adults to keep any medications, particularly those taken to promote sleep, at the bedside. Because sleeping pills dull the ability to perceive things accurately, patients who have trouble getting to sleep may take extra doses of their medication and be seriously harmed.

Older adults can achieve maximal benefits from their medication when nurses pay careful attention to all aspects of medication administration. Careful assessment, good teaching, and well-planned interventions can enable many older adults to function independently.

Get Ready for the NCLEX® Examination!

Key Points

- On average, older adults take three or more medications each day, not including OTC preparations.
- Drug use, misuse, and abuse present serious threats to the well-being of older individuals and increase the risk for hospitalization resulting from adverse drug reactions.
- The chance of adverse reactions is increased by the normal physiologic changes of aging, pathologic changes related to the higher incidence of acute or chronic diseases, and a myriad of other factors.
- The medical community has long recognized that children require special considerations with regard to medication, and we are now aware that the aging population also requires special considerations.
- Geropharmacology, the study of how older adults respond to medications, is an expanding area of study.
- Physicians who prescribe medication, pharmacists who dispense medication, and nurses who administer medication must continue to work together to understand the unique problems and needs of older adults with regard to these potentially dangerous substances.
- Nurses must work diligently to build a knowledge base of the medications administered to their patients or residents, know how to administer each medication safely, know how to assess the aging person's need for and response to each medication, and develop an appropriate plan of care that includes safety concerns and teaching needs.

Additional Learning Resources

SG Go to the Study Guide on pp. 379–397 for additional learning activities to help you master the chapter content.

evolve Go to your Evolve website (http://evolve.elsevier.com/Wold/geriatric) for the following FREE learning resources:
- Animations
- Answer Guidelines for Nursing Care Plan Critical Thinking Questions
- Answers and Rationales for Review Questions for the NCLEX® Examination
- Glossary with pronunciations in English and Spanish
- Video Clips

Review Questions for the NCLEX® Examination

1. Following an appointment with the physician, the nurse is teaching an independent living elderly person about a newly prescribed medication. The factor most likely to interfere with the effectiveness of this process is:

   1. The client wears a hearing aid.
   2. The client has a history of hypothyroidism.
   3. The nurse provided written handouts.
   4. The nurse is in a hurry.

2. An example of a medication that can be crushed is:

   1. A potassium tablet
   2. Enteric coated aspirin
   3. Sublingual nitroglycerine
   4. A calcium tablet

3. The nurse is administering medication through a transdermal patch. Precautions should include: (Select all that apply.)

   1. Remove all old patches before applying a new patch.
   2. Use the same location each time.
   3. Wash and rinse the skin after removing an old patch.
   4. Dispose old patches in the toilet.
   5. Verify the dosage strength of the patch.
   6. Handle the patch so the nurse does not touch the medicated surface.

4. A resident in a long-term care facility has a physician's order for digoxin (Lanoxin) 0.25 mg every morning in tablet form. If the nurse assesses that this resident has been having difficulty swallowing, the nurse should:

   1. Administer the digoxin (Lanoxin) in liquid form.
   2. Crush the digoxin (Lanoxin) for administration.
   3. Withhold the digoxin (Lanoxin) and document.
   4. Discuss the possibility of an order change to liquid form with the physician.

5. Elderly individuals are more likely to experience adverse drug reactions because of:

   1. The number of medications they take daily
   2. Physiologic changes in metabolism and excretion
   3. Higher percentage of body fluid
   4. Cognitive changes
   5. Interactions with foods and OTC preparations
   6. Decreased sense of taste

6. The nurse would instruct the independent living older person to:

   1. Take most medications with milk or antacids to avoid stomach upset
   2. Avoid drinking alcohol if taking acetaminophen (Tylenol)
   3. Keep daily medications in the kitchen cabinet near the sink
   4. Save prescription drugs in case the physician orders them again

Health Assessment of Older Adults

Objectives

1. Identify different levels of assessment.
2. Describe the difference between subjective and objective data.
3. Discuss the importance of thorough assessment.
4. Describe appropriate methods for structuring and conducting an interview.
5. Identify approaches that facilitate a successful physical examination of the older adult.

6. Discuss the modifications used when preparing an older person for a physical examination.
7. Describe the techniques used when performing a physical examination.
8. Explain the adaptations used when assessing vital signs in older adults.
9. Discuss the significance of the Minimum Data Set as a tool for comprehensive assessment of institutionalized older adults.

Key Terms

assessment (ă-SĔS-mĕnt) (p. 151)
auscultation (ăw-skŭl-TĀ-shŭn) (p. 155)
inspection (Ĭn-spĕk'shən) (p. 155)

palpation (păl-PĀ-shŭn) (p. 155)
percussion (pĕr-KŬ-shŭn) (p. 155)
screenings (skrē'nĭng) (p. 157)

Health **assessment** of older adults can be done on several levels, ranging from simple screenings to complex, in-depth evaluations. To perform assessments accurately, nurses and other health care providers who gather information regarding older adults must possess the necessary knowledge and skill to perform the assessments correctly. They must know how to use diagnostic tools and equipment safely. Furthermore, they must be knowledgeable and sensitive to the unique needs and characteristics of older adults.

HEALTH SCREENING

Health **screenings** are done to identify older individuals who are in need of further, more in-depth assessment (Table 8-1). Screening for high blood pressure, hearing problems, foot problems, and problems with activities of daily living are commonly performed at senior citizen centers and health clinics. Screening services are often provided by medical and nursing schools or other health groups committed to helping needy older persons. Many screenings are performed by lay individuals working under the direction of professionals. Special screenings for depression and suicide risk, although less common, are recommended for the older adult population. Some problems are more common among certain ethnic populations. Screening ethnic populations most at risk for problems can promote early identification and treatment of problems (Table 8-2).

Screenings are not designed to provide treatment; rather they are intended to identify older individuals

with significant findings and refer them to the most appropriate health service provider (i.e., physician, social worker, dietitian, or nurse). Early screenings and appropriate referrals help ensure that older individuals who are most in need of care are seen in a timely manner. They also help reduce frustration in older adults and wasteful use of time and resources. Depending on what is being evaluated, health screenings may be conducted in person, by telephone, by telecomputer, or, less commonly, by mail surveys.

HEALTH ASSESSMENTS

In-depth health assessments are time-consuming and must be performed by skilled professionals. Nurses perform health assessments of older adults in the community, in clinics, and in institutional settings. Health assessment includes the collection of all of the important health-related data using a variety of techniques. **Data** are all of the information a nurse gathers about a person. This information is used to formulate nursing diagnoses and to plan patient care; therefore, it is essential that accurate and complete data be collected. Data can be either objective or subjective.

Objective data include information that can be gathered using the senses of vision, hearing, touch, and smell. Objective information is collected by means of direct observation, physical examination, and laboratory or diagnostic tests. Because objective data are concrete by nature, all trained observers should report

Table 8-1	Preventive Medicine: Screening Recommendations for Older Adults
SCREENING TEST	RECOMMENDATION
Blood pressure	Every clinical examination, q 1–2 yr (USPSTF)
Clinical breast examination	Annually if >40 yr (USPSTF)
Mammogram	q 1–2 yr if 50-69 yr q 1–3 yr if 70-85+ yr (AGS, USPSTF)
Pelvic examination/Pap smear	q 2–3 yr; after 3 negative tests, can decrease after age 65–69 yr (AGS, USPSTF)
Cholesterol	q 5 yr No data for >85 yr
Rectal examination	Annually if >40 yr (ACS)
Fecal occult blood	Annually if >50 yr (ACS)
Sigmoidoscopy	q 3-5 yr if >50 yr (ACS)
Prostate examination/ PSA	Annually if >50 yr (ACS) Not recommended (USPSTF)
Tests for hearing impairment, visual acuity, thyroid function, ECG; blood glucose; glaucoma screening	Periodically (USPSTF)
Examination of heart, lungs, nodes, testes, skin, mouth	Annually (ACS)
Mental/functional status, osteoporosis screen, chest radiograph	As needed (USPSTF)

ACS, American Cancer Society; *AGS*, American Geriatrics Society; *USPSTF*, United States Preventive Services Task Force.

Table 8-2	Suggested Preventive Screenings Based on Ethnicity
DEMOGRAPHIC GROUP	PREVENTIVE SCREENINGS
African American	Blood pressure, blood diseases, breast cancer, prostate cancer, weight gain, vision loss, diabetes, cholesterol
Mexican American	Weight gain, diabetes, cervical cancer
Southeast Asian	Depression, diabetes
Filipino American	Blood pressure, diabetes
Pacific Islander	Weight gain, diabetes
American Indians	Weight gain, diabetes, hearing loss
European American	Breast cancer

Modified from GeroNurseOnline.org (geronurseonline.org).

similar findings about a person or that person's behavior at any given point in time. Behaviors such as crying, limping, and clutching the abdomen can be verified by anyone who observes the patient. Rashes, skin lesions, and wound drainage are likewise observable to anyone. Objective data can be made more precise and specific by using meters, monitors, and other measuring devices. A blood pressure reading, a change in weight, the size of a wound, the volume of urine, and laboratory test results are all examples of specific objective data. Whenever possible, objective data should be stated using specific information because accurate and precise data enhance the nurse's ability to determine changes in a person's health status. For example, it is better to actually take a temperature reading than to touch the skin and determine that it feels warm. Both are objective observations, but one is more precise than the other.

Subjective data are information gathered from the older person's point of view. Fear, anxiety, frustration, and pain are examples of subjective information. Subjective data are best described in the individual's own words, such as "I'm so afraid of what is going to happen to me here" or "It hurts so much I could die!"

When performing a health assessment on an older person, the nurse needs to modify his or her usual approaches and techniques to make them more appropriate for older adults.

INTERVIEWING OLDER ADULTS

Interviews such as those conducted during admission to a clinic or institution are likely to be planned and conducted in a formal manner. Other interviews may be spontaneous, informal, and based on an immediate need recognized by the nurse. Before beginning an interview with an older person, the nurse should plan ways to establish and maintain a climate that promotes comfort and develops trust. This includes preparing the physical setting, establishing rapport, and structuring the flow of the interview. During this planning phase, the nurse should take into consideration the unique needs of the older person.

PREPARING THE PHYSICAL SETTING

The environment where the interview will take place should be chosen carefully. Distractions should be minimal; noise from televisions, radios, and public address systems should not be loud enough to distract the older adult or interfere with his or her ability to distinguish words and understand questions. Lighting should be diffuse because bright lights or glare may make it difficult for the interviewee to see clearly. Furniture should be comfortable. Privacy is very important. Conducting the interview in a room where there is little chance of interruption is ideal. If such a place is not available, the patient's room may provide sufficient privacy—the curtains should be drawn and the door closed. The room should be comfortably warm and should be free from drafts that might cause discomfort. Because many older adults experience urinary frequency or urgency, it is advisable either to assist them to the bathroom or to tell them that a bathroom is available nearby should they require it.

ESTABLISHING RAPPORT

It is most appropriate to begin the interview by greeting the older person and introducing yourself. During this first contact, it is best to address the person using his or her formal name (e.g., "Mr. Smith" or "Mrs. Adams"). Appropriate use of names indicates respect and helps build rapport. Use of the individual's first name only without the person's consent is presumptuous and overly familiar. This familiarity may be resented by the older person whether or not it is verbalized. When there is any doubt about the person's preference, it is appropriate for the nurse to ask the person how he or she wishes to be addressed.

The nurse should briefly explain the purpose of the interview so that the individual will know what to expect. An explanation helps reduce anxiety that otherwise might interfere with understanding. The nurse should explain how long he or she expects the interview to last, as well as what will happen after it is completed.

Nurses should focus on and speak directly to the older person being interviewed (Figure 8-1). This notion may seem obvious, but it is often disregarded in practice. Often, a younger family member present during the interview "takes over" the responses for the older person. The conversation then takes place between the nurse and the family member while the older adult remains passive. An assertive older person might speak up and say, "Let me speak for myself," whereas a nonassertive older adult may be left feeling frustrated and unimportant. The nurse should continue to direct the conversation to the older person and, if necessary, tactfully request that the family member allow the older person to respond first before

he or she adds information. Because of necessity, in situations in which the older person is confused, nonresponsive, or does not speak English, the family member will need to be more actively included to translate or provide information.

Cultural Considerations
Assessment and Culture

Americans tend to approach issues directly. This is considered inappropriate in many Hispanic and Asian countries, where more social, tactful, and indirect conversation is thought to be appropriate. It is also culturally appropriate to include family members and to determine who will answer questions and participate in the assessment process.

During the physical examination, the nurse should be careful to maintain the modesty standards set by each culture.
- In some cultures, it may be desirable for a family member to be present during this examination. In most cases, this should be permitted.
- Cultural values may dictate that physical contact with a nurse of the opposite gender is inappropriate. In these cases, the patient or family may request that a nurse of the same gender as the patient perform the examination.

When in doubt, an expert who is knowledgeable about the specific cultural expectations or an authoritative reference text should be consulted.

Rapport is enhanced by first determining the problems or concerns that trouble the patient most and then focusing on those problems. This helps reduce anxiety and increases the older person's perception that the nurse is truly concerned about him or her. Assessment should start with a look at the whole person before focusing on specifics.

STRUCTURING THE INTERVIEW

It is important to plan sufficient time for the interview. Older individuals typically have a long and complex life story to tell. Remember that the speed of recall and verbal responses may be slower with age. The individual may feel pressured or stressed if the pace of the interview is too rapid.

The nurse should try not to accomplish too much during a single interview. The effort involved in communication can be fatiguing to an older individual, particularly one with health problems. It is better to have several brief interactions lasting less than 30 minutes each rather than one long interview that leaves the patient exhausted. Nurses should be sure to stay alert for signs of fatigue (e.g., sagging head or shoulders, sighing, altered facial expression, and irritability), which indicate the need to end the interview.

During the interview, a variety of communication techniques should be used to ensure that the patient accurately understands the information. Nurses should avoid using medical jargon and should use

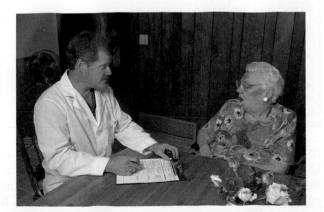

FIGURE 8-1 Conducting an interview.

only words that the older person understands. The nurse should speak slowly and clearly and keep messages simple but should not patronize older adults. The fact that an older person requires extra time does not mean that the person is in any way mentally impaired. Even if the older person has been diagnosed with a mental impairment, he or she deserves respectful and professional responses. Nurses must remain calm and empathetic. When the patient is speaking, the nurse should not interrupt. The nurse must listen to both the verbal and nonverbal messages being sent. Many older individuals tend to ramble in conversation and may need to be brought back on track. If this is necessary, a summary or restatement of the conversation is helpful. It is not appropriate to complete sentences for the older person. The nurse should remain attentive and calm and should allow the patient to complete his or her own sentences. Too often, the nurse's conclusion is considerably different from the patient's.

The nurse should try not to end an interview too abruptly. A statement such as "We're almost done for now" prepares the older person for the end of the interaction. Many lonely persons will try to extend the conversation beyond the time the nurse has available. Setting a time for further interaction by saying, "We'll talk again tomorrow morning" or "I'll set up another appointment so we can talk more" can help maintain rapport. It is essential for the nurse to follow through as promised, or the patient may lose trust and refuse to communicate freely in the future.

OBTAINING THE HEALTH HISTORY

Before starting a physical assessment, the nurse will use interviewing techniques to obtain a health history. This history starts with basic identifying data followed by a history of past health concerns and then a review of current health issues. Some older adults are able to provide information easily, whereas others may be poor historians. Much will depend on the cognitive level of the individual and the complexity of his or her particular medical history. When the older adult is unsure of answers, it is often wise to move on to other topics and attempt to gather the information from a family member at a later time. In addition, the nurse may want to obtain information regarding the person's family and psychosocial status. Information gathered from the history will help the nurse form an overall impression of the older person and can help the nurse focus on those areas most in need of further exploration and assessment (Box 8-1).

PHYSICAL ASSESSMENT OF OLDER ADULTS

Once the history is obtained, the nurse is then ready to proceed to the physical assessment. During this assessment, objective information is obtained to accompany

---

Box 8-1 Health History Data

History should include, but not be limited to, the following information:

IDENTIFYING DATA
- Name
- Date of birth
- Residence
- Ethnicity and cultural preferences
- Language preferences
- Religion
- Marital/significant other status
- Previous and/or current occupation
- Educational background
- Advance directives and any other relevant data

PAST HISTORY
- Perception of general health
- Frequency of medical and dental care, including screenings such as mammography, BP, etc.
- Known or suspected allergies (medicines, food, animals, etc.)
- Immunizations (type and date)
- Exposure to communicable disease such as TB
- Serious childhood illness or injuries (rheumatic fever, fractures, etc.)
- History of serious illnesses (specify illness, date of onset, type of treatment received, resolved vs. ongoing problem)
- Hospitalizations (reason and date)
- Surgeries (type and date)
- Mental health treatment (type and date)
- Review of personal health habits such as diet, fluid intake, exercise practices, sleep patterns, bowel and bladder routines, alcohol, caffeine and tobacco use, etc.

PRESENT MEDICAL HISTORY
- Major current problems or concerns (in person's own words)
- Do the problems relate to an accident or fall?
- Symptoms (location, duration, severity, etc.)
- Date of onset (sudden or gradual onset)
- What makes problem worse or better?
- What was done in response to symptom(s) (home remedies, MD visit, etc.)?
- Medications currently taken (look at bottles if possible)
- Compliance with medication regimen
- Current medical treatments or therapies (oxygen, physical therapy, etc.)

FAMILY AND PSYCHOSOCIAL HISTORY
- Living family members (spouse, children, siblings, etc.) and nature of relationships
- Friends and social activity practices (clubs, church activities, community organizations, etc.)
- Significant deceased family members
- Hobbies and interests
- Pets

---

the subjective information offered by the older person. Objective information further helps the nurse determine the person's abilities and limitations. It may verify the subjective information given by the older person; it may also reveal problems that were previously unrecognized. When assessing older persons, it is important that nurses pay close attention not only to obvious physiologic changes, but also to changes in mood or behavior that may signal a change in condition. Seemingly small pieces of information can be important to the total assessment. Older adults have different physiologic responses than do younger persons. For example, a temperature change of just a few tenths of a degree may indicate the onset of an infection in an older person, rather than rising above the 100° F reading, which is expected in younger people. Other changes can be equally meaningful and may be missed or ignored if nurses are not especially careful (Table 8-3).

Physical assessment should take place in a location that promotes physical comfort of the older person. Often this will be the person's room or a special examination room. Adequate privacy should be maintained by keeping doors and curtains closed. Care should be taken not to chill the older person while examining the body. Blankets and gowns that provide adequate warmth should be used to promptly cover the parts of the body not being assessed. If the examination is being done during physical care (e.g., during the bath), particular attention must be paid to prevent chilling caused by evaporation.

Equipment such as a flashlight, measuring tape, scale, sphygmomanometer, stethoscope, and thermometer should be collected before beginning the assessment to convey a sense of competence and to allow the assessment to progress smoothly.

Table 8-3	Atypical Presentation of Illness
TYPE OF ILLNESS	**PRESENTATION**
Infectious diseases	Absence of fever WBC within normal limits Decreased appetite or fluid intake Behavioral changes Confusion
"Silent" acute abdomen	Mild abdominal discomfort Constipation Vague respiratory symptoms
"Silent" cardiac problems	No complaint of chest pain Vague symptoms of fatigue or nausea Decreased functional status
Pulmonary	May not exhibit paroxysmal edema nocturnal dyspnea or coughing Subtle changes in function, appetite Confusion
Thyroid disease	Hyperthyroidism: fatigue, "slowing down" Hypothyroidism: agitation and confusion
Depression	Vague somatic complaints, including GI symptoms, changes in appetite, constipation, sleep problems

Modified from Ham R, Sloane D, Warshaw G: *Primary care geriatrics: a case-based approach,* St Louis, 2002, Mosby.

Complete physical assessment should be done in an orderly manner so that no important observations are missed. Begin with an overview of the person, including general appearance, hygiene, grooming, alertness, responsiveness, and general mobility; then proceed with more focused assessments. The most common method of physical assessment is a head-to-toe approach in which the entire body is assessed systematically. Other approaches such as body system or functional approaches are also viable. Later chapters provide guidelines for assessing safety needs, nutrition, skin, elimination, activity, sleep, cognitive function, and other areas in more detail.

When performing a physical assessment, nurses use a variety of techniques, including **inspection**, **palpation**, **auscultation**, and **percussion**.

INSPECTION

Inspection is the most commonly used method of physical assessment in which the senses of vision, smell, and hearing are used to collect data. Skill at inspection improves the more often the technique is done. Inspection requires the nurse to be totally active, alert, and aware of everything he or she sees, hears, or smells. Inspection begins the first time we see the older adult. Even during a brief interaction, skilled nurses should be inspecting the individual, looking for anything that may indicate a change in his or her condition.

Inspection can be both general and specific. General inspection is used to detect the need for more specific inspection. For example, if the nurse observes that the older individual is eating poorly, a more specific inspection of the oral cavity may be indicated. If body odor is detected, a more specific inspection of the skin may be indicated. If the nurse hears noisy breathing, a more specific inspection of the lungs may be necessary. If gait is abnormal, a more complete assessment of the joints, muscles, feet, and nervous system is indicated.

Inspection is used when assessing the overall level of function, as well as when looking for specific areas of need within any particular area of function. When inspecting the aging individual, it is important that the nurse pay close attention to details. Adequate light (preferably natural light) should be used when trying to detect subtle changes in skin color. Size and mobility of body parts on one side of the body should be compared with those on the opposite side.

PALPATION

Palpation uses the sense of touch in the fingers and hands to obtain data. Palpation is used for evaluation in many parts of a physical assessment, including pulses, temperature and texture of the skin, texture and condition of the hair, the presence and consistency of tumors or masses under the skin, distention of the urinary bladder, and the presence of pain or tenderness.

When palpating, the nurse should use the fingertips, which are the most sensitive part of the fingers. Warm hands and short fingernails promote comfort and reduce the risk for trauma to fragile older skin. Light touch should be used before deeper touch is attempted. When taking the pulse of an older person, deep palpation may occlude blood vessels. Deep pressure may also increase pain. Painful areas should be palpated last.

AUSCULTATION

Auscultation uses the sense of hearing to detect sounds produced within the body. Heart, lung, and bowel sounds are typically assessed using auscultation. Auscultation involves the use of a stethoscope or other sound amplifier (such as a Doppler) to make the sounds louder and more easily heard. Sounds are described according to their quality, pitch, intensity, and duration. **Quality** describes the sound being heard through subjective terms such as crackling, whistling, or snapping. **Pitch** describes whether the sounds have a low or high tone. **Intensity** refers to the loudness or softness of the tone. **Duration** refers to the length of time a sound is heard. **Frequency** refers to how often a sound is heard. A sound can be continuous or intermittent. When sounds are intermittent, the number of times and the interval between occurrences should be determined.

Auscultation requires a quiet environment and special skills. Nurses who perform auscultation should have special training in the technique and should be knowledgeable regarding the significance of any findings.

PERCUSSION

Percussion is a technique in which the size, position, and density of structures under the skin are assessed by tapping the area and listening to the resonance of the sound. Depending on the amount of vibration (sound) heard, the presence of masses, fluid, or air can be determined. This technique is used least often by nurses. It requires special skill and training.

ASSESSING VITAL SIGNS IN OLDER ADULTS

Assessment of vital signs involves all of the techniques previously discussed. When assessing vital signs, nurses should first complete a general inspection of the older adult to determine whether there are any subjective or objective observations that may affect the procedure or accuracy of the readings. Because activity level, medications, eating, stress, disease processes, and the environment can all affect vital signs, the possible contributions of these factors should be considered.

Baseline vital sign readings should be obtained during the initial contact with the older person. These readings are the basis for comparison with future readings, and they enable nurses to determine whether the person's health status is remaining constant or changing over time.

TEMPERATURE

The general inspection helps nurses select the most appropriate route for temperature assessment. The oral (sublingual) route is used most commonly for temperature assessment. Either an electronic thermometer or a glass thermometer that does not contain mercury can be used to take an oral temperature. Electronic thermometers are preferred because they can give an accurate temperature in less than 1 minute instead of the recommended 3 minutes for a glass thermometer. However, using the oral route is not always possible with older adults. Those who are edentulous (without teeth) or have poor muscle control may be unable to close the mouth tightly enough for an accurate reading to be obtained. Older adults who are unable to follow directions are also poor candidates for oral temperature checks.

Although acceptable, the rectal route should be used with caution. Use of the rectal route can be psychologically traumatic to older adults, particularly if they are alert but unable to cooperate with an oral temperature. The rectal route should not be used in older persons who have undergone rectal surgery or have rectal bleeding. Rectal readings can be affected by the presence of stool in the rectum. Rectal temperature readings reflect changes in core body temperature more slowly than do oral readings.

Use of the axillary route is not common in older adults. This route is time-consuming, and the accuracy of temperature readings may be affected by environmental conditions.

Determination of body temperature using a sensor that measures the temperature of the tympanic membrane has received mixed reviews. This method has advantages and disadvantages. Use of the tympanic sensor takes seconds only, is not invasive, and does not require patient cooperation; however, the readings obtained using this method are not as accurate as originally claimed, particularly when the device is not used precisely as directed. Individual agencies need to determine whether this method of assessment is adequate for their needs.

In general, healthy, active older individuals are able to maintain core body temperature within normal limits. The accepted norm for oral temperature is 98.6° F ± 1° F (or 37° C ± 0.6° C). Studies have shown that older adults, particularly those older than 75 years, have an average core body temperature of 97.2° F (36° C). This decrease may be a result of inactivity, decreased subcutaneous fat, an inadequate diet, or environmental factors. Environmental temperature appears to play a greater role in older adults because their thermoregulatory control systems are not as efficient as in younger individuals.

PULSE

Before the nurse assesses the pulse, the patient should be positioned so that he or she is comfortable and the nurse has access to the desired site. Position should be consistent (e.g., lying, sitting, or standing) each time the pulse is checked; this will provide meaningful readings for comparison.

Pulse can be assessed at various sites on the body, including the temporal, carotid, brachial, radial, femoral, popliteal, posterior tibial, and dorsalis pedis arteries, as well as at the apex of the heart (Figure 8-2). When possible, the pulses on both sides of the body should be assessed and compared.

The radial artery is the site most commonly used for routine pulse assessment. The radial pulse is normally palpable at the lateral aspect of the wrist. This pulse should be palpated gently in older adults because excessive pressure may occlude the blood vessel. The pulse rate should be counted, and the rate, rhythm, and volume should be noted. Consistency of the blood vessel should also be assessed. The normal pulse rate in adults ranges from 60 to 90 beats per minute. Rates outside this range or significant changes from an individual's normal readings indicate the need for further assessment. Older persons, particularly those with a history of cardiovascular problems and those receiving digitalis, require prompt, thorough assessment if there is a significant change in the pulse rate.

The arteries of older adults may feel stiff and knotty because of decreased elasticity. In aging individuals, it is common to observe irregularities in rhythm. These may be related to medical conditions or they may have no identified cause. Detection of an irregular pulse in an aging person whose pulse was previously regular is significant and requires further assessment. A change in pulse volume may indicate the need to assess fluid balance. Weak, thready pulses are often seen in individuals with fluid volume deficits or electrolyte imbalances; full or bounding pulses may indicate excessive fluid

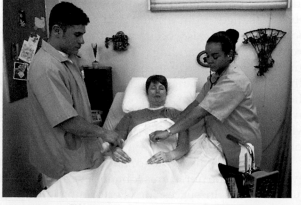

FIGURE 8-2 Assessing vital signs.

volume. Weakness of a radial pulse may make palpation impossible and necessitate use of the apical route.

When assessing the apical pulse, nurses should help their aging patients assume a comfortable position and should drape them to prevent chilling and to provide for modesty. The apical site is located on the left side of the chest. The apical heartbeat is best heard by placing the stethoscope over the fifth intercostal space even with the middle of the clavicle. The apical pulse should be counted for a full minute. Each "lub-dup" sound heard is counted as one heartbeat. The apical pulse should be assessed for regularity and the presence of any unusual sounds.

When assessing the pulse of an older woman with sagging breasts, nurses should lift the tissue gently and place the stethoscope at the lower edge of the breast. Apical pulse may be difficult to assess in obese older adults or in those who have a change in the shape of the chest cavity.

Apical and radial readings, even when taken at the same time by two nurses, may be different. This is referred to as a **pulse deficit.** Inadequate force of the heart or disease of the blood vessels may prevent transmission of blood from the heart to the peripheral vessels. Of the two, the apical pulse rate is considered more reliable.

The peripheral pulses of legs and feet should be palpated and assessed to determine whether they are present and to determine the quality of the pulse. Peripheral pulse rate is not normally counted. Altered peripheral circulation may be an early indicator of decreased cardiac functioning or vascular changes. Pulses on one side of the body should be compared with those on the other side to determine whether changes have affected one or both sides of the body.

Cardiovascular changes with aging, particularly arteriosclerotic changes, often result in a decrease or complete loss of palpable pulses in the lower extremities. The nurse should start with the pedal pulses. If these are not detectable, the nurse should proceed upward toward the trunk and assess the popliteal and then the femoral pulses. If pulses cannot be palpated, it may be necessary to use a sound amplifier called a **Doppler** to evaluate circulation to the extremities.

If peripheral pulses are diminished or absent, the nurse should suspect circulatory impairment and assess the extremity for capillary refill time, temperature, color changes, and the absence of hair, all of which may indicate serious problems.

RESPIRATION

After completing a general assessment of all of the factors that influence respiration, the aging person should be placed in a comfortable position to maximize ease of breathing. The rate, depth, and ease of breathing must be assessed (Figure 8-3). Each combination of inspiration and expiration is counted as one respiration.

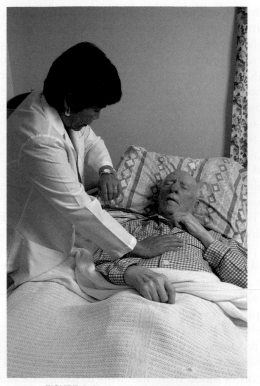

FIGURE 8-3 Measuring respirations.

The normal respiratory rate for older individuals is similar to that of younger adults. A range of 12 to 20 breaths per minute is considered normal. A decrease in the resting respiratory rate is significant in the older person. It may be an indication of impending infection and may appear before an elevation in temperature is observed. Increased respiratory rate is common with anxiety, pain, elevated temperatures, and increased activity.

The depth of respiration tends to decrease with aging. Chest expansion is often decreased because of alterations in the shape of the thoracic cavity, muscle weakness, sedentary lifestyle, or disease processes.

Slightly irregular breathing rhythms are not unusual in the aging population. However, abnormal findings, such as a highly irregular rhythm, dyspnea, or breathlessness with exertion, require further assessment to determine the cause.

BLOOD PRESSURE

Blood pressure readings are an important part of the physical assessment. It is essential that these readings be properly obtained. To obtain the most accurate readings, the patient should be positioned so that the upper arm is at the level of the heart.

Equipment should be chosen carefully if meaningful results are to be obtained. Cuff selection should be based on the patient's upper arm size. It is a common mistake to use a one-size-fits-all blood pressure cuff. Many older persons, particularly those who are frail, have lost a great deal of upper arm mass. A cuff that is too wide for the size of the individual's arm provides falsely low readings. A properly sized cuff is 20% wider than the diameter of the arm at its midpoint. Once the proper cuff has been obtained, it should be applied gently but snugly to the arm. Nurses should pay close attention not to pinch the skin in the cuff, which can easily lead to bruising.

The technique used to obtain the blood pressure measurement should follow the methods approved by the American Heart Association. This includes taking the blood pressure first by palpation, then by auscultation. The practice of pumping the cuff to excessively high pressures can result in inaccurate readings.

Blood pressure readings vary widely among older adults. Some older patients have blood pressure readings in the low-normal range; others have significantly elevated readings. Hypertension is a common problem in the older adult population because of renal and cardiovascular changes of aging. Elevated blood pressure can also be related to emotional upset, pain, exertion, eating, or smoking. This type of elevation disappears when the precipitating event is removed. To obtain accurate readings, nurses should attempt to reduce or minimize these factors before assessing blood pressure. Persistent elevations in blood pressure (i.e., systolic readings 160 mm Hg or higher; diastolic readings 90 mm Hg or higher; or elevations of both systolic and diastolic readings) indicate hypertension. Elevated blood pressure readings should be reported promptly, particularly if they are unusual for an individual.

Many aging individuals take medication for hypertension. Nurses should follow through with careful blood pressure monitoring when these medications are administered, and all precautions related to the specific medication should be followed rigorously.

Aging individuals are susceptible to posture-related changes in blood pressure. Older adults who have an inactive lifestyle and those who take drugs such as vasodilators, antihypertensives, or tricyclic antidepressants are particularly prone to orthostatic, or postural, hypotension. **Orthostatic hypotension** is a sudden drop in blood pressure that occurs when a person changes from a lying to a sitting or standing position. It may also occur when the person moves from sitting to standing. Those experiencing postural hypotension complain of lightheadedness or dizziness when changing positions. In severe cases, the person may even lose consciousness. Orthostatic hypotension is commonly observed in individuals who are on extended bedrest or receiving medication for hypertension.

To determine the existence and severity of postural hypotension, the nurse must obtain several blood pressure readings in succession. Performing this assessment requires a certain amount of skill. The nurse first takes the blood pressure when the patient is at rest in bed. Then the patient sits at the edge of the bed, and the nurse takes the blood pressure again in 1 to 5 minutes. The patient then stands for 1 to 5 minutes, and the nurse takes a third reading. All readings are recorded, along with any subjective information provided by the patient regarding dizziness, loss of balance, or other sensations. A drop of more than 20 mm Hg is always significant and should be reported promptly. A standing systolic blood pressure less than 100 mm Hg should also be reported. If the individual complains of symptoms such as dizziness, safety precautions should be taken (see Box 8-2).

| Box 8-2 | Body Systems Approach to Physical Assessment* |

SKIN

History: Injuries, burns, infections, allergies, anemia, fluid intake levels, when and how skin change occurred, etc.
Techniques: Inspection and palpation
Assess:
- Color (erythema, pallor, cyanosis, jaundice, ecchymosis)
- Pigment changes (hypopigmentation hyperpigmentation)
- Elasticity (turgor)
- Temperature
- Moisture (perspiration, oiliness)
- Texture
- Lesions
  - Primary: Macule, papule, pustule, vesicle, wheal, cyst, tumor
  - Secondary: Scale, scar, fissure, lichen, ulcer
  - Vascular: Senile purpura, hemangioma, spider angioma
  - Itching/tenderness
- Edema
  - Pitting Edema

SCALE	DEGREE	RESPONSE
1+ trace	Barely detectable	Rapid
2+ mild	Less than ¼ in.	10–15 sec
3+ moderate	¼–½ in.	1–2 min
4+ severe	Greater than ½ in.	2–5 min

NAILS

History: Injuries, dietary insufficiency, COPD, etc.
Techniques: Inspection and palpation
Assess:
- Shape
- Color
- Thickness
- Ridges
- Angle of nailbed
- Surrounding tissues (paronychia)

HAIR

History: Cosmetic use, dietary insufficiency, hormone problems, exposure to parasites
Techniques: Inspection and palpation
Assess:
- Color and texture
- Distribution
- Quantity (alopecia, hirsutism)
- Condition of scalp, presence of nits

SKULL, FACE, AND NECK

History: Congestion, drainage, sore throat, difficulty swallowing, dental problems, swelling, exposure to communicable disease, etc.
Techniques: Inspection and palpation
Assess:
- Size, shape, and symmetry (moon face)
- Smile and frown (look for symmetry or drooping)
- Nose (drainage, symmetry)
- Sinuses (check for tenderness or pressure)
- Lips (color, moisture, lesions)
- Mouth, including mucous membranes, teeth, and gums
- Throat and tonsils
- Shape and movement of neck
- Lymph nodes

Continued

Box 8-2 | Body Systems Approach to Physical Assessment—cont'd

EYES

History: Glaucoma, cataracts, refractive problems, dry eyes, tearing, blurring, double vision, etc.
Techniques: Inspection
Assess:
- Placement of globes (bulging or sunken)
- Eyelids (crusting, lashes, ptosis, etc.)
- Conjunctiva (color, drainage, etc.)
- Sclera (color)
- Blinking (15–20 times per min)
- Pupils (PERRLA)
  - Dim room (so pupils dilate)
  - Check size and shape of pupils (should be equal and round)
  - Shine light into one eye (both pupils should constrict)
  - Have patient look at a distance then focus on a finger 4 in. (10 cm) from bridge of nose (both eyes should constrict with accommodation)
  - Eye movements (cardinal fields): Have the patient hold head still; then move a finger (12 in. from face) toward each field, then back to center (may elicit nystagmus)
  - Light reflex: Shine light 12 in. from face (should be symmetrical reflection on cornea)
  - Convergence: Watch as you move finger toward nose
  - Visual acuity: Snellen test (do each eye separately, then together; do first without glasses, then with close reading test—e.g., newspaper)

EARS

History: Difficulty hearing, etc.
Techniques: Inspection
Assess:
- Placement, shape, drainage
- Inspection of external canal (otoscope)
- Hearing acuity (whisper test, audiometry)

RESPIRATORY

History: COPD, difficulty breathing, shortness of breath, lack of energy, cough, hemoptysis, tobacco use, allergies, medications, etc.
Techniques: Inspection, auscultation (palpation and percussion)
Assess:
- Shape of thorax (barrel, sunken)
- Spinal curvatures (kyphosis, lordosis, scoliosis)
- Movement of chest during respiration
- Rate, rhythm, and depth of respiration
- Listen to lung sounds over fields; compare side to side
- Trachea (bronchial sounds)
- Assess above clavicle and scapula to assess apex (bronchovesicular sounds)
- Stay inside scapula when doing midsection; move out when doing bases (vesicular sounds)
- Adventitious lung sounds:
- *Crackles (rales)* — Fine, short, crackling sounds best heard on inspiration, commonly heard in lung bases
- *Wheezes* — Continuous squeaky, musical sounds; best heard on expiration; may be heard all over lung fields
- *Gurgles (rhonchi)* — Continuous low-pitched sounds; coarse with snoring quality; cleared by coughing; heard over trachea and bronchi
- *Friction rub* — Grating sound; similar to the rubbing sound made when sandpaper is used; heard on both inspiration and expiration; heard most often on lower anterior and lateral chest

CARDIOVASCULAR

History: History of heart disease, chest pain, lack of energy, fatigue, high BP, SOB, medications, edema, etc.
Techniques: Inspection, palpation, auscultation
Assess:
- Peripheral pulses (carotid, radial, brachial, pedal, popliteal, femoral) for presence, strength, symmetry
- Apical pulse
- Capillary refill time (normal is less than 3 sec)
- Presence of varicosities
- Signs of thrombophlebitis (tenderness, redness, swelling, positive Homans')

GASTROINTESTINAL

History: GI pain, nausea, vomiting, constipation, flatulence, diarrhea, etc.
Techniques: Inspection, then auscultation before palpation (empty bladder, supine with knees slightly bent)
Assess:
- Shape and contour of abdomen
- Presence of scars
- Bowel sounds in four quads (use diaphragm) every 20 sec

Box 8-2   Body Systems Approach to Physical Assessment—cont'd

MUSCULOSKELETAL

History: Weakness, joint or muscle pain and tenderness, recent injury
Techniques: Inspection and palpation
Assess:
- Size and symmetry of muscles
- Muscle strength bilaterally
- Presence of contractures
- Tremors or spasms
- Swelling or deformity of joints (tenderness or pain)
- Range of motion (smoothness, crepitus)

NEUROLOGIC

History: Any injury or illness affecting CNS or PNS, loss of consciousness, behavioral changes, loss of balance, headaches, or sensory changes
Techniques: Inspection
Assess:
- Orientation
- Speech
- Movement
- Grip strength
- Pupillary responses (presence and rate)
- Balance or gait
- Changes in smell, vision, hearing, sensation, temperature perception
- Reaction to painful stimuli

GENITOURINARY

History: Voiding patterns, frequency, hesitancy, painful voiding, urgency, incontinence, history of STD, discharge or drainage from genitals, open lesions, etc.
Techniques: Inspection, palpation
Assess:
- Bladder fullness/distention
- Amount, odor, color, and consistency of urine

*This approach is useful for focus assessments.

SENSORY ASSESSMENT OF OLDER ADULTS

Simple assessments of vision and hearing ability are based on empiric data (the way the individual responds to visual or auditory clues). Nurses should observe whether the person is able to read or do close work that requires good central vision or whether he or she participates in television viewing or other sight-related activities. If the older person uses eyeglasses, the ability to see with and without them should be assessed.

Talking with older adults can reveal the presence or absence of hearing. Difficulty gaining attention, the frequent need to repeat information, or mistakes in understanding directions are good indicators of hearing problems. If applicable, hearing-aid assessment should take place when the older person is wearing the aid—but only after it has been checked for proper functioning. Special assessment by a vision or audiometric specialist can reveal more precise information regarding vision and hearing.

PSYCHOSOCIAL ASSESSMENT OF OLDER ADULTS

Psychological assessment is performed to determine whether older people are alert and aware of their surroundings or suffer from some level of confusion,

delirium, or dementia. The differences between these conditions are discussed in detail in Chapter 10. Psychological status is best assessed by direct observation and by means of standardized assessment tools. Many assessment tools are available to assist nurses in assessing mental status in older adults. Probably the best known and most highly regarded is the Mini-Mental State Examination (MMSE), a sample of which is provided in Figure 8-4. Performing this

MMSE Sample Items

Orientation to Time
  "What is the date?"

Registration
  "Listen carefully. I am going to say three words. You say them back after I stop. Ready? Here they are...
  APPLE (pause), PENNY (pause), TABLE (pause). Now repeat those words back to me." [Repeat up to 5 times, but score only the first trial.]

Naming
  "What is this?" [Point to a pencil or pen.]

Reading
  "Please read this and do what it says." [Show examinee the words on the stimulus form.]
  CLOSE YOUR EYES

FIGURE 8-4 Mini-Mental State Examination.

assessment requires little time and a pencil and blank sheet of paper only. Scoring of this tool is simple and self-explanatory. Other assessment tools may also be used. Several of these are available in computerized form on the Internet (see Box 8-3).

Assessment of social function is determined by observing the amount, frequency, and type of social interaction in which the older person participates. A variety of levels and degrees of social interaction can be classified as normal as long as the individual is happy or at least content with that level. Chapters 11, 12, and 13 deal more with socialization issues.

Many evidence-based assessment tools are available online from the Hartford Institute of Gerontologic Nursing (www.hartfordign.org/resources/education/tryThis.html.) According to the Hartford Institute, the goal of the *Try This: Best Practices in Care for Older Adults* series of assessment tools is to provide knowledge that is easily accessible, easily understood, and easily implemented and to encourage the use of these best practices by all direct care nurses.

SPECIAL ASSESSMENTS

The Minimum Data Set 3.0

In an attempt to improve the quality of care provided in extended-care facilities, the federal government instituted major reforms through the Omnibus Budget Reconciliation Act (OBRA) of 1987. An important focus of this law was the improvement and standardization of assessment procedures used in these facilities. The first reform produced by the U.S. Department of Health and Human Services was the Resident Assessment Instrument (RAI), introduced in 1990. This tool specified a comprehensive, standardized assessment that was to be completed on admission, with significant change in status, and thereafter on a yearly basis. The first version of the database used to conduct this assessment was a printed document called the **Minimum Data Set (MDS) 1.0.** This tool was designed not only to help assess residents, but also to help caregivers identify problems, develop intervention plans, and monitor outcomes. It was hoped that use of this tool would make the assessment process more consistent and reliable throughout the country. MDS 1.0 did

| Box 8-3 | Examples of Psychological Assessment Tools on the Internet |

- Cornell Scale for Depression in Dementia
- Short Test for Dementia
- Functional Activities Questionnaire
- Clinical Dementia Rating Scale
- Informant Questionnaire on Cognitive Decline in the Elderly (IQCODE)
- Confusion Assessment Method

help improve assessment and care in many cases, but information was often difficult to locate, and interdepartmental monitoring of problems and outcomes was difficult because the assessment was paper-based. The **MDS 2.0** was an upgraded, computerized version of the older document. **MDS 3.0** is a new, state of the art, form designed to improve patient input into the assessment process. (Figure 8-5 shows page one of the form. The full MDS 3.0 can be found on Evolve). It is not merely an update or revision of the previous form. Design improvements in the MDS 3.0 were directed at increased reliability, enhanced accuracy, and expanded usefulness as a tool to improve clinical assessment. This new format went into effect during fall of 2010. All health care agencies that receive federal funding are mandated to use the computerized MDS and must be capable of transmitting the results to state and federal agencies. Data collected from the MDS are used to provide credibility and justify government funding of programs.

The MDS 3.0 is a comprehensive assessment tool that assesses core areas of function. Unusual findings discovered with MDS 3.0 initiate further evaluation using more detailed focus assessments called **Care Area Assessments (CAAs).** These replace the Resident Assessment Protocols (RAPs). RAP triggers are now called **Care Area Triggers (CATs).**

Use of a computer-based system improves the process of assessment and planning. Use of a computer database helps make the process more comprehensive, more complete, and easier for the nursing staff and other departments, once the users become familiar with the program. Computerization of records in this database enhances the flow of information between departments within a facility. For example, the pharmacy can verify that psychotropic and antidepressant medications are administered only when appropriate medical diagnoses exist, and the physicians and nurses can correlate dosage changes with observed behaviors. The dietary department can validate that appropriate diets are ordered based on medical diagnosis and can detect changes in weight that may indicate the need for further intervention. Nurses can identify interventions that will be most beneficial at preventing pressure ulcers, constipation, or other common problems.

The computerized MDS 3.0 enhances the ability to access and correlate data from every long-term care facility in the United States and provides an unprecedented database of information regarding the nursing home population. As the database grows, caregivers will learn more about the population of infirm older adults, their most common medical problems, and the most or least effective treatments and interventions. All data from the MDS 3.0 must be transmitted directly to the Center for Medicare Services (CMS) within 14 days after the facility completes the MDS assessment. States may specify additional reporting requirements.

Resident ______ Identifier ______ Date ______

MINIMUM DATA SET (MDS) - Version 3.0
RESIDENT ASSESSMENT AND CARE SCREENING
Nursing Home Comprehensive (NC) Item Set

CAA's = [ ] PPS = Ⓢ

Section A — Identification Information

A0100. Facility Provider Numbers

A. **National Provider Identifier (NPI):** [ ][ ][ ][ ][ ][ ][ ][ ][ ][ ]

B. **CMS Certification Number (CCN):** [ ][ ][ ][ ][ ][ ][ ][ ][ ][ ][ ][ ]

C. **State Provider Number:** [ ][ ][ ][ ][ ][ ][ ][ ][ ][ ][ ][ ][ ][ ][ ]

A0200. Type of Provider

Enter Code [ ] **Type of provider**
- Ⓢ 1. **Nursing home (SNF/NF)**
- Ⓢ 2. **Swing Bed**

A0310. Type of Assessment CAA

Enter Code [ ][ ] A. **Federal OBRA Reason for Assessment**
- Ⓢ 01. **Admission** assessment (required by **day 14**)
- Ⓢ 02. **Quarterly** review assessment
- Ⓢ 03. **Annual** assessment 1, 8, 11
- Ⓢ 04. **Significant change in status** assessment 1, 8, 11
- Ⓢ 05. **Significant correction** to **prior comprehensive** assessment 1, 8, 11
- Ⓢ 06. **Significant correction** to **prior quarterly** assessment
- Ⓢ 99. **Not OBRA required** assessment

Enter Code [ ][ ] B. **PPS Assessment**

PPS Scheduled Assessments for a Medicare Part A Stay
- Ⓢ 01. **5-day** scheduled assessment
- Ⓢ 02. **14-day** scheduled assessment
- Ⓢ 03. **30-day** scheduled assessment
- Ⓢ 04. **60-day** scheduled assessment
- Ⓢ 05. **90-day** scheduled assessment
- Ⓢ 06. **Readmission/return** assessment

PPS Unscheduled Assessments for a Medicare Part A Stay
- Ⓢ 07. **Unscheduled assessment used for PPS** (OMRA, significant or clinical change, or significant correction assessment)

Not PPS Assessment
- Ⓢ 99. **Not PPS** assessment

Enter Code [ ] C. **PPS Other Medicare Required Assessment – OMRA**
- Ⓢ 0. **No**
- Ⓢ 1. **Start of therapy** assessment
- Ⓢ 2. **End of therapy** assessment
- Ⓢ 3. **Both Start and End of therapy** assessment

Enter Code [ ] D. **Is this a Swing Bed clinical change assessment?** Complete only if A0200 = 2
- 0. **No**
- Ⓢ 1. **Yes**

Enter Code [ ] E. **Is this assessment the first assessment** (OBRA, PPS, or Discharge) **since the most recent admission?**
- 0. **No**
- 1. **Yes**

Enter Code [ ][ ] F. **Entry/discharge reporting**
- 01. **Entry** record
- 10. **Discharge** assessment - **return not anticipated**
- 11. **Discharge** assessment - **return anticipated**
- 12. **Death in facility** record
- 99. **Not entry/discharge** record

Code "-" if information unavailable or unknown

Care Area Assessment Legend

1. Delirium	5. ADL Function/Rehabilitation Potential	9. Behavioral Symptoms	13. Feeding Tubes	17. Psychotropic Drug Use
2. Cognitive Loss/Dementia	6. Urinary Incontinence & Indwelling Catheter	10. Activities	14. Dehydration/Fluid Maintenance	18. Physical Restraints
3. Visual Function	7. Psychosocial Well-Being	11. Falls	15. Dental Care	19. Pain
4. Communication	8. Mood State	12. Nutritional Status	16. Pressure Ulcer	20. Return to Community Referral

Form 1851P 8/10 2010 Briggs Medical Services Company, Des Moines, IA 50306 (800) 247-2343 www.BriggsCorp.com — 1 of 38 — MDS 3.0 Nursing Home Comprehensive (NC) Version 1.00.2 10/01/2010

FIGURE 8-5 Minimum Data Set for nursing home resident assessment and care screening. The full form can be found on Evolve.

The new MDS enables state and federal agencies to evaluate the performance of an individual institution in any number of categories and facilitates a level of comparison between treatment methods that has not previously been available. For example, the frequency, location, and extent of pressure ulcers can be determined and correlated to age, disease, diet, and other factors. It also enables the supervising government agency to compare various long-term care providers with one another.

The ability to assemble these data on a regional or national basis excites the better health care providers, because these correlative data will enable them to identify critical parameters in resident status and develop more effective models for care. Other providers, particularly those who may not meet the expected standards of care, view this oversight capability less favorably.

Because the MDS plays such an important role in determining resident status and planning and evaluating care, it must be completed in a timely manner and updated regularly. Licensed nursing staff must pay close attention to the times specified in the statutes and complete all records in a timely manner.

ASSESSMENT OF CONDITION CHANGE IN THE ELDERLY

Many times, health status changes in the elderly are subtle and not the same as we learned to expect in younger adults. Early recognition and treatment of change in status can prevent serious harm for the elderly. This is true at home, in extended care facilities, and in the hospital setting. A number of evidence-based instruments have been developed to help the nurse perform a systematic and comprehensive assessment.

FULMER SPICES

SPICES is an acronym for six common "marker conditions" that when assessed provide an overview of the person's status. This is a screening tool that can and should be used routinely. Identification of one or more of these problems indicates an increased risk for functional decline and even death. More in-depth assessments are required when a problem is identified. (See appropriate chapters for assessment guidelines.) This assessment is not a total list of significant problems; for example, pain and elimination are not included, but the assessment does address the most common and relevant issues. Additional information and tools designed to help the nurse perform effective assessments of the elderly are available online. Box 8-4 provides a listing of some of the most helpful sites.

S—sleep disorders
P—problems with eating or feeding
I—incontinence
C—confusion
E—evidence of falls
S—skin breakdown

Box 8-4 **Internet Sites for Assessment of Elderly**

There are many helpful geriatric assessment tools available online. These sites contain download or printable forms for use when performing both general and focused geriatric assessments.

Hartford Institute for Geriatric Nursing – http://hartfordign. org/trythis

Interactive textbook on Clinical Symptom Research (cognitive impairment and delirium specific) – http:// symptomresearch.nih.gov/chapter_5/sec5/cebs5pg2. htm

International Society of Geriatric Oncology – http://www.siog.org/index.php? option=com_content&view=article&id=103&Itemid =78http://ge

Merck Manual of Geriatrics – www.merck.com/mkgr/mmg/ home.jsp

National Institute on Aging – www.nia.nih/gov//health

Primary Care Geriatrics – http://www.ttuhsc.edu/som/ fammed/ttmedcast/FunctionalAssessment.pdf

University of Iowa – www.medicine.uiowa.edu/gec/tools/ default.asp

University of Maryland – http://geri-ed.umaryland.edu/ assess_tools.html

University of Missouri – http://web.missouri.edu/~proste/tool/

Stall, Robert S. MD – Educational Web Page - ridoc.net/ assessmenttools.html

---

FANCAPES

When the nurse suspects that an actual emergency or serious problem is present or might be developing, in these situations, deep, focused assessments are more appropriate and necessary. The following mnemonic can be used to organize this assessment:

F—fluid
A—aeration (oxygenation)
N—nutrition
C—cognition, communication
A—activity/abilities
P—pain
E—elimination
S—skin/socialization

Once the status assessment is completed, the nurse must still decide the most appropriate action. A summary of nursing responses is presented in Table 8-4.

Table 8-4 **Should I Call? Presentation and Action to Take**

PRESENTATION/ CONDITION CHANGE	CALL MD OR APRN IMMEDIATELY IF:	CALL 911 IF:
Vital signs	Systolic BP: >200 or <90 Diastolic BP: >115 Resting pulse: >130 or <55 Oral temp: >101 Rectal temp: >102	The vital sign changes are associated with altered and/or severe symptoms of other kinds of distress (e.g., airway obstruction or anaphylaxis)

Table **8-4**   Should I Call? Presentation and Action to Take—cont'd

PRESENTATION/ CONDITION CHANGE	CALL MD OR APRN IMMEDIATELY IF:	CALL 911 IF:
Delirium	Any sudden onset of change in mental status	Change in mental status accompanied by suspected or possible airway obstruction Severe respiratory distress Clinical signs of shock
Edema	Sudden fluid excess noted in associated shortness of breath (SOB), pink frothy sputum, possibly co-occurring with chest pain Abrupt onset of edema in one leg only Loss of sensation in swollen leg Associated tenderness and/or redness in affected leg	Suspicion of a cardiovascular event, such as syncope, tachycardia, or other symptoms of acute coronary syndrome (ACS)
Sleeping difficulties	Only if associated with mental status changes	Not applicable
Bleeding	Uncontrolled bleeding or repeat episode (e.g., prolonged nosebleed) Emesis with frank blood Bloody stools Vaginal bleeding, profuse	Uncontrolled bleeding Bleeding with symptoms of impending shock and/or VS changes Trauma with or without evidence of overt injury
Falls	Obvious deformity of limb or alignment of same Joint or hip pain with reduced range of motion Inability to bear weight Laceration with uncontrolled bleeding	Major trauma event, such as a fall of a significant distance with associated loss of consciousness or VS changes
Chest pain	New-onset or recurrent pain not relieved in 20 min with previously ordered nitroglycerine ×3. Chest pain accompanied by VS changes, dyspnea, diaphoresis, nausea/vomiting.	Complaints of chest pain associated with or followed by LOC changes or obvious arrhythmia with pulse check such as severe bradycardia (<40) or tachycardia (>150)
Medication error	Resident is symptomatic because of the error	Resident is symptomatic *and* there are VS and/or LOC changes
Constipation/ diarrhea/emesis	Severe abdominal pain Rigid abdomen or extreme tenderness on palpation Bowel sounds absent Guarding (tensing of abdominal wall to protect inflamed underlying organs)	Only when associated with other symptoms such as mental status changes or in conjunction with other cardiovascular symptoms that would necessitate transfer
Pain	Associated with a fall/trauma Noticeable and new inability to perform ROM Headache with altered vision and/or LOC	Severe, uncontrolled pain
Dehydration	More than 1 episode of vomiting in 24 hours *and* decreased fluid intake Less than 50% of normal fluid intake over 24 hours	VS abnormalities LOC change Suspected sepsis such as narrowed pulse pressures, tachycardia, fever, mental status changes.
Pressure ulcers/ skin rash	Stage II, III, or IV receiving no treatment and no protocol to cover the condition Signs of wound infection: purulent discharge, erythema, odor Fever	Not applicable
Depression/ suicidal ideation	Expression of suicidal ideation that contains a plan for carrying it out in the assisted living residence (e.g., "I have a lot of medications hidden away to use when I think my time has come.")	Expressed suicidal ideation with a plan and inability to monitor resident in the assisted living residence
Seizures	New onset Status epilepticus	New onset or status epilepticus *associated with*: possible airway compromise, severe respiratory distress, signs of shock
Visual changes	Associated stroke symptoms (e.g., hemiparesis, slurred speech, headache, facial drooping)	Suspected stroke/CVA

Continued

Table 8-4	Should I Call? Presentation and Action to Take—cont'd		
PRESENTATION/ CONDITION CHANGE	**CALL MD OR APRN IMMEDIATELY IF:**		**CALL 911 IF:**
	Complaints of seeing "halos" (a person will look at a light and see a halo or rainbow-colored circle around the light) Any abrupt onset Suspected trauma with severe pain		
Shortness of breath	VS changes or suspected cardiovascular involvement Labored breathing Ashen appearance Cyanosis		Evidence of inadequate oxygenation (cyanosis, increased respiratory rate, paradoxical chest movement, diaphragmatic breathing, use of accessory muscles) despite interventions, such as Egan's Fundamentals of Respiratory Care (2003): Oxygen via nasal cannula: 0.25 to 4 L/min; through simple mask: 5–12 L/min

CVA, cerebrovascular accident; LOC, level of consciousness; VS, vital sign.
From Geriatric Nursing Vol 29; No 1, Jan/Feb 2008. (Adapted with permission from B. Jordan, MS, ARNP, BCPCN, and J Sandberg-Cook, MS, ARNP, BCPCN, Dartmouth-Hitchcok Medical Center, Hanover, NH.)

Get Ready for the NCLEX® Examination!

Key Points

- Although the initial health assessment of an older adult is important, it is only a starting point. It is important to remember that assessment is a continuous and ongoing process.
- As each aging person's condition changes, objective and subjective data will also change.
- OBRA mandates that the total assessment be revised and updated whenever a significant change occurs in a resident's mental or physical condition.
- Because nurses spend the greatest amount of time with older adults, they have the greatest opportunity to assess and recognize significant changes.
- It is the responsibility of nurses to assess continually and to institute changes in care, based on those observations.

Additional Learning Resources

SG   Go to the Study Guide on pp. 379–397 for additional learning activities to help you master the chapter content.

evolve   Go to your Evolve website (http://evolve.elsevier.com/Wold/geriatric) for the following FREE learning resources:
- Animations
- Answer Guidelines for Nursing Care Plan Critical Thinking Questions
- Answers and Rationales for Review Questions for the NCLEX® Examination
- Glossary with pronunciations in English and Spanish
- Video Clips

Review Questions for the NCLEX® Examination

1. The assessment tool that is most commonly used to determine the mental status of the elderly person is the:
   1. Confusion Assessment Method
   2. Mini-Mental State Examination
   3. Short Test for dementia
   4. MDS 3.0

2. The nurse suspects the presence of a urinary tract infection in an elderly person. This is based on an assessment finding of:
   1. Fever
   2. Flank pain
   3. Urinary frequency
   4. Behavioral changes

3. An elderly person who takes antihypertensives or vasodilators has increased risk for developing orthostatic hypotension. For this reason, the nurse needs to frequently assess:
   1. Apical pulse rate
   2. Blood pressure
   3. Body temperature
   4. Respiratory rate

4. When performing an assessment of the gastrointestinal system of an elderly client, the nurse would proceed in what order? Place the parts of a gastrointestinal system assessment in sequence from first to last.
   1. Palpate abdomen.
   2. Observe abdomen for scars.
   3. Obtain a health history.
   4. Inspect the oral cavity.
   5. Auscultate bowel sounds.

5. When performing a physical assessment of an elderly person, the nurse tries to ensure that cultural values are respected by: (Select all that apply.)
   1. Explaining what will take place during the assessment
   2. Describing the nurse's professional credentials before starting the procedure
   3. Draping the patient to maintain modesty
   4. Encouraging a family member to be present if desired by the patient
   5. Having the examination done by a nurse of the same gender
   6. Seeking information from a transcultural nursing textbook

Meeting Safety Needs of Older Adults

Objectives

1. Discuss the types and extent of safety problems experienced by the aging population.
2. Describe internal and external factors that increase safety risks for older adults.
3. Discuss interventions that promote safety for older adults.
4. Discuss factors that place older adults at risk for imbalanced thermoregulation.
5. Describe those older adults who are most at risk for developing problems related to imbalanced thermoregulation.
6. Identify signs and symptoms of thermoregulatory problems.
7. Identify interventions that assist older adults in maintaining normal body temperature.

Key Terms

heatstroke (HĒT-strōk) (p. 174)
hyperthermia (hī-pĕr-THĔR-mē-ă) (p. 174)
hypothermia (hī-pō-THĔR-mē-ă) (p. 173)
thermoregulation (thĕr-mō-RĔG-ū-lā-shŭn) (p. 173)

Safety is a major concern when working with or providing care to older adults. Although older adults compose approximately 11% of the population, they account for approximately 23% of accidental deaths. A report from the National Safety Council reveals that approximately 24,000 people older than 65 years die from accidental injuries each year, and at least 800,000 sustain injuries serious enough to disable them for at least 1 day.

Falls, burns, poisoning, and automobile accidents are the most common safety problems among older adults. Exposure to temperature extremes also places older adults at risk for injury or death. Older adults are more susceptible to accidents and injuries than are younger adults because of internal and external factors. Internal factors include the normal physiologic changes with aging, increased incidence of chronic disease, increased use of medications, and cognitive or emotional changes. External factors include a variety of environmental factors that present hazards to older adults.

INTERNAL RISK FACTORS

Vision and hearing are protective senses. When the acuteness of the senses diminishes with aging, the risk for injury increases. Vision and hearing changes are common with aging. Diminished range of peripheral vision and changes in depth perception are common and can interfere with the ability of older adults to judge the distance and height of stairs and curbs or to determine the position and speed of motor vehicles. Night vision diminishes. In dim light or glare, older adults may be unable to see that a curb, step, or other hazard is present. They may be unable to see or read stationary road signs that provide directions or warnings. Falls or motor vehicle accidents often result from altered vision.

Changes in visual acuity make it more difficult to read labels with small print. This can make it difficult for older adults to read the directions on prescriptions. Many older adults have taken incorrect medications or wrong doses or have even consumed poisonous substances because they could not see adequately to read the labels.

Decreased auditory acuity reduces an older person's ability to detect and respond appropriately to warning calls, whistles, or alarms. For example, older adults may not hear a warning call of impending danger, may not hear a motor vehicle or siren in time to avoid an accident, or may not respond to a fire alarm in time to leave a building safely.

The senses of smell and taste also help protect us from consuming substances that might be harmful to the body. Decreased sensitivity of these senses increases the risk for accidental food or chemical poisoning in the elderly population.

Older adults often experience one or more physiologic changes that increase their risk for falls and other accidental injuries. Any of these changes alone or in combination can reduce the older person's ability to respond quickly enough to prevent an accidental injury. When these problems are combined with chronic diseases or health problems, the risk increases dramatically. Common physiologic changes that affect safety include the following:

- Altered balance
- Decreased mobility

- Decreased flexibility
- Decreased muscle strength
- Slowed reaction time
- Gait changes
- Difficulty lifting the feet
- Altered sense of balance
- Postural changes

Conditions affecting the cardiovascular, nervous, and musculoskeletal systems are most likely to contribute to safety problems. Any cardiovascular condition that results in decreased cardiac output and decreased oxygen supply to the brain can cause older adults to experience vertigo (dizziness) or syncope (fainting). Common disorders with this result include anemia, heart block, and orthostatic hypotension. Studies have shown that approximately 52% of long-term nursing home residents older than 60 years experience four or more episodes of orthostatic hypotension a day.

Older persons with neurologic disorders such as Parkinson's disease or stroke experience weakness and alterations in gait and balance that increase the risk for falls. Neurologic and circulatory changes can also decrease the ability to sense painful stimuli or temperature changes, increasing the risk for tissue injuries, burns, and frostbite. A study has shown that nursing home residents with diabetes are more than twice as likely to suffer from falls as those who do not have diabetes.

Musculoskeletal conditions such as arthritis further reduce joint mobility and flexibility, decreasing the ability of the older person to move and respond to hazards and intensifying the likelihood of accidents or injury. Box 9-1 lists injury risks for older adults.

Medications often contribute to falls, and, because older adults commonly take one or more medications, their risk for untoward effects is increased. Any medication that alters sensation or perception, slows reaction time, or causes orthostatic hypotension is potentially dangerous for older adults. Common types of hazardous medications include sedatives, hypnotics, tranquilizers, diuretics, antihypertensives, and antihistamines. Alcohol, although not a prescription medication, acts as a drug in the body. Alcoholic beverages, particularly in combination with prescription drugs, increase the risk for falls and other injuries. More information regarding safe use of medications is included in Chapter 7.

Box 9-1   Injury Risks for Older Adults

- Impaired physical mobility
- Sensory deficits
- Lack of knowledge of health practices or safety precautions
- Hazardous environment
- History of accidents or injuries

Cognitive changes or emotional disturbance and depression may be overlooked as risk factors for falls or injury. These disturbances reduce the older person's ability to recognize and process information. Distracted or preoccupied older adults are less likely to pay full attention to what is happening or what they are doing. This lack of attention and caution increases the risk for accidents and injury.

FALLS

Falls are the most common safety problems in older adults. Consider the following statistical facts revealed in the literature:

1. One-third to one-half of people older than age 65 are prone to falling.
2. Any fall is the best predictor of future falls. Two-thirds of those who have experienced one fall will fall again within 6 months.
3. The older a person becomes, the more likely he or she is to suffer serious consequences, such as a hip fracture, from a fall.
4. Falls are a leading death caused by injury in people older than age 65 and number one for men over 80 and women over 75.
5. Approximately one-fourth of older adults who experience falls will die within a year and another 50% will never return to their previous level of independence or mobility.
6. The incidence of falls is higher among those residing in long-term care facilities than among those who live independently in the community.
7. The number of hip fractures due to falls is projected to exceed 500,000 per year in 2040.
8. The cost to Medicare and Medicaid will climb dramatically as the elderly population increases. Direct costs related to falls are expected to exceed $32 billion by 2020.

These statistics were dramatic enough that the federal government enacted the *Elder Fall Prevention Act of 2003* to develop a national initiative intended to reduce falls. This act was designed to fund research, promote public education, and provide services proven to reduce or prevent elder falls. In 2009 and 2010, additional legislation designed to reduce the number of falls among older adults was passed. Legislation requiring training on fall prevention for long-term care workers also has been implemented.

Many independent elderly are reluctant to report a fall because of the implication that they are frail and dependent. In addition to causing bodily harm, falls take a psychological toll on the elderly, causing them to lose confidence and decrease mobility. This is unfortunate because early recognition and interventions can reduce the risk for further falls. Studies have shown that supervised exercise focusing on balance, gait, and strength may be of help, as will environmental modifications. Older adults living independently in the community often do not recognize hazards in their home environment because they are too accustomed to their surroundings to view them as potential hazards. The elderly and their family members need to be aware of things they can do to reduce the risk for falls. Some helpful approaches are summarized in Box 9-2.

Fall prevention is everyone's responsibility. Outreach sessions about fall prevention designed to meet the needs of elderly adults, their families, and anyone who has contact with elderly adults could be offered at senior centers, libraries, businesses, and community colleges. Health care settings need to maintain current and complete policies and procedures for fall prevention, new employee training regarding fall prevention, a method for prompt reporting and investigation of all falls, and scheduled multidisciplinary meetings to identify problems and plan interventions.

Coordinated Care
Collaboration

Fall Prevention

Nursing assistants often have good insights into the reasons for a fall. The nurse could ask the CNA for a few suggestions for actions that might help prevent a future fall. These ideas could then be included in the plan of care. Ownership of the idea is likely to improve compliance with the plan. Make sure that the nursing staff and all other departments take fall prevention seriously. Report the presence of any unsafe conditions, no matter how minor they seem. Notify housekeeping, maintenance, or security promptly and then verify that the problem has been corrected. Another strategy is "Catch me doing something right." Too often we are quick to blame someone when a fall occurs. It is a far better practice to praise the staff when you see call lights being answered promptly, spills being mopped up, and proper footwear or assistive devices being used. Some literature even suggests identification of a "Falls Champion"—a staff member who has additional training regarding fall prevention who can then provide training to others, act as a mentor to new staff, and keep a high awareness of the need for fall prevention.

Cultural Considerations
Home Fall Risk Among Chinese Older Adults

A study designed to identify risk factors for falls in the homes of elderly adults residing in China revealed data that are very similar to those found in the United States. In China, falls are identified as the second leading cause of accidental death. As with Americans, many elderly Chinese do not recognize safety hazards because they have lived with them for a long time. Risk areas and hazards in China and the United States are almost identical. Tai chi chuan, an exercise designed to maintain balance, is a common daily practice among the elderly in China. The benefits of this exercise for fall reduction are being researched in the United States.

EXTERNAL RISK FACTORS

Environmental hazards include everything that surrounds older adults. Potential hazards are presented by the people and the variety of objects a person comes into contact with on a daily basis. Even the climate in which a person lives can present an environmental hazard. Environmental hazards are everywhere: in the home, on the street, in public buildings, and in health care settings. Box 9-3 lists tips on preventing injuries in the home. Although injuries can and do occur often in the home, a change in environment, such as hospitalization, travel, or any other move from a familiar environment, increases the likelihood of injury for older adults.

FIRE HAZARDS

Older adults are among the highest risk groups for injury or death due to fire. Hospitals and long-term care facilities are well aware of the danger of fire. Building codes for these institutions require safety doors, fire extinguishers, exit windows, oxygen precautions, and other safety measures. Each institution should have a fire safety plan designed to reduce the risk for fire, a quick notification system to the local fire department, protocols for fire containment, and an evacuation plan. Fortunately, these measures have made institutional

---

Box 9-2 Reducing the Risk for Falls

- *Prepare safe surroundings.* Make sure you have adequate lighting, particularly in stairwells. Keep frequently needed items such as the telephone, tissues, etc., on a table near your chair or bedside. Avoid placing items on the floor, particularly near your favorite chair or bedside. Make sure there are no throw rugs, uneven floors, electric wires, oxygen tubing, or other items that could cause tripping. Mop up spills in the kitchen or bathroom immediately. Do not climb on anything other than an approved step stool to reach high places.
- *Allow adequate time to complete an activity or task.* Haste increases the risk for falls or other injuries. If you feel dizzy or lightheaded, sit for a while before standing.
- *Wear proper-fitting footwear.* Shoes with nonslip soles and low heels are recommended because high-heeled shoes contribute to balance problems. Shoes should have closures

that are easy to manipulate. If shoes have laces, check that they do not come loose and cause tripping. Loose-fitting slippers or shoes can drop off the foot and lead to a fall.
- *Use assistive devices if needed.* A cane or walker provides security by enlarging the base of support. These devices should be kept close at hand to avoid leaning or reaching. The tips should have solid rubber grips to prevent slipping and may need to be modified on icy surfaces to promote gripping.
- *Ask for help when necessary.* This Bible passage provides good advice: "Pride goeth before destruction, and a haughty spirit before a fall." Failure to seek help can lead to serious injury. Older adults should be encouraged to recognize that good judgment is a sign of healthy aging and not a sign of weakness.

Box 9-3	Preventing Injuries in the Home

- *Ensure that all rugs are firmly fixed to the floor.* Tack down loose edges, ensure that rubber skid-proofing is secure, and remove decorative scatter rugs.
- *Maintain electric safety.* Check regularly to ensure that there are no broken or frayed electric cords or plugs. Any defective electric plug or cord should be repaired by an approved repair person. Discard all electric appliances that cannot be repaired. Install ground fault interrupt (GFI) electric sockets near water sources to prevent accidental shocks when appliances are used.
- *Decrease clutter and other hazards.* Throw out unnecessary items such as old newspapers. Keep shoes, wastebaskets, and electric or telephone cords out of traffic areas. Never place or store anything on stairs. Ice should be cleared promptly from sidewalks and outside staircases. Cat litter can be used to provide traction on icy surfaces.
- *Provide adequate lighting.* This is particularly important in stairwells. Switches should be located at both the top and bottom of stairs. Use night-lights in the bedroom, bathroom, and hallways. The kitchen should have adequate lighting in food preparation areas to facilitate label reading and to reduce the risk for injury when sharp objects are used.
- *Provide grip assistance wherever appropriate.* Handrails should be installed in all stairwells to provide support for stair climbing. Grab bars alongside the toilet and in the bathtub and shower also help provide support. Lightweight cooking utensils with large handles and enlarged stove knobs make cooking easier and safer for older adults.
- *Place frequently used items at shoulder height or lower where they can be reached easily.* Keeping frequently used items available decreases the need to use climbing devices. Use only approved devices such as step stools when reaching for items that cannot be reached easily. Ladders are not recommended for use by older adults, but if they are used, ensure that they are fully open and locked. Excessive reaching should be avoided, and another person should stand by to steady the ladder, reducing the risk for tipping.
- *Take measures to prevent burns.* Avoid smoking or the use of open flames whenever possible. Do not wear loose, long sleeves when cooking on a gas stove. Check that the hot water tank setting does not exceed 120° F. Use a mixer valve to prevent sudden bursts of hot water. Have a plan for leaving the residence in case of fire.

fires an uncommon occurrence. Fires in the community are another story. Studies show that over 1200 Americans over age 65 die each year as a result of fires. Residential fires injure an average of 3000 older adults each year. Most of the injuries are a result of cooking accidents, whereas the majority of the deaths are smoking-related. Many of these deaths could be prevented by instituting these basic fire safety precautions in the home:

- Make sure smoke detectors are installed. Check that the batteries are working and replace them twice a year. Do not disable the device if cooking fumes or steam causes it to sound. Instead, move the device or try a different type of detector.
- Use caution with cigarettes or open flames. Do not leave them unattended or on an unstable surface where they could fall onto flammable floors or furniture. Empty all smoking materials into a metal container so no smoldering materials can combust. NEVER smoke in bed.
- Make sure there are no open flames from cigarettes, matches, candles, etc., if oxygen is in use. Oxygen does not burn, but it supports the combustion of other flammable items.
- Check extension cords for fraying or loose plugs. Do not pull cords out by tugging on the wire. Be careful not to overload an outlet. Avoid using extension cords; get an electrical block with a circuit breaker instead.
- Be sure to turn off the stove or oven if you are leaving the area. Keep baking soda and a pot lid available to smother a fire if it occurs. *Do not* use water, particularly if grease is involved.

- Never cook while wearing long, loose sleeves that could catch fire, causing serious burns.
- If you live in a rental unit, report any fire safety hazards such as blocked exits, cluttered hallways, or other problems to the owner or management promptly. If these problems are not resolved, notify the fire department.
- Have an escape plan. Plan more than one escape route if possible. Practice how you would get out, particularly if you use a wheelchair or other mobility aids. Keep a flashlight, eyeglasses, and a whistle (to warn others or to help them find you) at the bedside. If the fire is in your residence, get out to safety before calling the fire department. Close the door behind you to prevent the spread of the fire. DO NOT try to fight the fire yourself.
- DO NOT use elevators when there is a fire.

HOME SECURITY

People, particularly strangers, present a risk to the elderly. Older adults are more vulnerable than younger persons to attack and injury from those who prey on weaker or more defenseless people, such as the infirm or elderly. Older adults need to be aware of the risks presented by strangers and learn to institute measures to reduce the likelihood of injury (Box 9-4).

VEHICULAR ACCIDENTS

Probably the most dangerous hazards, because of their size and speed, are motor vehicles. Motor vehicle accidents are more likely to occur with aging, whether the older person is a pedestrian or a driver.

Box **9-4** **Home Security Guidelines**

- *Think and plan ahead to reduce risks to personal safety.* Unfortunately, we live in a society that is less safe than the one in which older adults grew up. Precautions that may not have been necessary in the past should now be part of each person's daily planning.
- *Identify ways an intruder could enter the home.* Defective locks on windows or doors should be replaced. Locks should be secured and checked each time the person enters and leaves. Lost or stolen keys may necessitate lock changes.
- *Maintain regular contact with friends and family.* Daily phone calls or some sort of signaling system should be used to indicate that everything is all right.
- *Use the telephone safely.* Keep a phone at the bedside and near the favorite sitting area. This eliminates the need to hurry to another room. If possible, obtain a phone with large numbers, which enables accurate dialing in a stressful situation. An autodial function with emergency numbers is also helpful. An answering machine is useful in screening unwanted or late-night calls. Women living alone should never broadcast this fact to strangers. Using a male voice on the answering machine is a wise precaution.
- *Answer the door safely.* Ensure that doors are secure with a peephole at eye level for viewing visitors before opening the door. Make sure that outside lighting is available and working so that nighttime visitors can be observed. Ask for proper identification before opening the door for a stranger. Do not open the door if there is any doubt about who is there; authentic sales agents or service employees will wait and not be offended by having their identification checked with their company.
- *Bank safely.* Withdraw cash in small-denomination bills. Do not carry or display large amounts of cash. Secure money immediately in a wallet, money belt, or handbag. It is wise not to put large sums of money in a shoulder or strap handbag that can be pulled away easily. It is better to keep wallets in an internal pocket or body pouch. Keep large amounts of cash and valuables in a bank or other financial institution. Vary the day and time that banking is done. When using an automated teller machine, avoid nighttime visits and whenever possible, have another person along for safety.
- *Prepare for emergencies.* Have emergency numbers posted in large, clear lettering near each telephone. If entry door locks have dead bolts, they should be left unlocked with the key in place while the older person is inside. This reduces the risk of the older person being trapped in the building in case of fire and enables emergency care providers to enter the housing unit if services are needed.

Studies reveal facts that demonstrate the magnitude of the problem. Crossing roads is a significant problem for elderly pedestrians. One study revealed that only 1% of independent persons older than 72 years were able to cross a street before the traffic signal changed. Although the incidence of pedestrian accidents is low, the risk for serious injury is great. Some communities with high numbers of elderly have adopted modifications that make street crossing safer. These include pedestrian-controlled timers, safety islands, and restrictions on vehicle turns at intersections. Active lobbying by seniors in other communities could help initiate some of these safety innovations.

Older adults are often unwilling to stop driving in spite of the serious risks to themselves and others. Independence is the main reason voiced by elderly adults for continued driving. A driver's license is a ticket to freedom. From adolescence on, Americans' preferred method of transportation is the car. In some parts of the country, driving seems to be more a necessity than a luxury. Rural and suburban areas may not have viable alternatives other than reliance on another person to provide transportation. Currently, there are few legal measures in place to determine when an older adult's driving privileges should be terminated, but many proposals are being discussed in states all across the country. This is a difficult issue, often pitting younger family members against aging parents. Not infrequently, health care providers are caught in the middle of the dilemma.

Driving by the elderly is a major concern in communities in which large numbers of senior citizens reside. In 2003, 7541 people age 65 and older died in motor vehicle crashes, and it is estimated that approximately 200,000 were treated for motor vehicle accidents. While these numbers include both passengers and drivers, the issue of older drivers is increasingly in the news and the issue will only get larger as the Baby Boom generation ages. Drivers over age 65 have the highest crash rate per mile driven. By 2020 more than 40 million drivers will be over age 65. The number of drivers over age 70 is expected to triple in the next 10 years. Although it has not been shown that older drivers pose a greater risk for injury or death to others, they themselves are more likely to die from injuries sustained in a motor vehicle accident than are younger drivers. The fatality rate for drivers over age 85 is nine times higher than for drivers 25 to 69 years of age, based on a mile-for-mile basis.

Several factors contribute to these statistics. Age-related vision changes result in altered depth perception, changes in night vision, and diminished ability to recover from glare. Hearing changes can interfere with the ability to recognize sirens or other auditory warnings. Decreased muscle strength, reduced flexibility, and slower reflexes reduce the ability to respond to hazards while controlling a motor vehicle. Other medical conditions or medications may also have effects on driving ability. One of the growing risk factors is related to changes in cognitive functioning, particularly due to Alzheimer's disease. Estimates indicate that between 30% and 45% of people with early Alzheimer's disease continue to drive. Only six states (California, Delaware, Nevada, New Jersey, Oregon, and Pennsylvania) require the physician to report mental impairment.

The National Motorists Association takes the position that changes in understanding, judgment, and memory pose a greater threat on the roads than do physical changes. Yet advocates for Alzheimer's victims often recommend limiting rather than terminating driving privileges.

> Baby Boomers are a large segment of the automobile market. As this group ages, automakers are adapting their vehicles to be more friendly to older adults while still marketing a stylish image to entice Baby Boomers to buy their cars. Modifications include larger numbers on the instrument panel, easier-to-grip handles, adjustable pedal height, back-up sensors, higher and wider bucket seats, and many other features. Senior citizens are encouraged to ask auto dealers about which "senior-friendly" features or options are available.

Although people are usually aware of the need to modify activity levels as they age, older adults may not be equally aware of the need to make adjustments in driving. Initiating safe driving modifications can enable older adults to enjoy the freedom of movement provided by automobiles while protecting themselves and others (Box 9-5). Sometimes these adjustments are not enough, and the difficult decision to stop driving must be made. Warning signs that indicate a person should stop driving include, but are not limited to, the following:

- Nervousness or lack of comfort behind the wheel
- Difficulty staying in one lane
- More "near misses"
- More dents or scrapes on the car (or hitting or scraping the garage, mailbox, etc.)
- Other drivers "honking" at you more often
- Friends or family not wanting to ride with you
- Confusing the brake and gas pedals
- Difficulty turning to look over your shoulder when backing up
- Medical conditions or medications that affect your ability to maneuver the car
- Being easily distracted or having difficulty concentrating while driving
- Getting lost more often
- Receiving more warnings or traffic tickets

When older adults stop driving, they need alternative means of getting around. Family and friends are often more than willing to provide transportation. Volunteers from churches or civic agencies may also provide rides for senior citizens. Some communities provide low-cost bus or taxi services. The local Agency on Aging can provide information regarding services that are available in a particular area. Often elderly clients complain that alternative transportation is too costly. This can be countered by statistics that estimate the yearly cost of owning and operating a car at about $6000 per year. That amount will pay for quite a bit of alternative transportation.

THERMAL HAZARDS

Another external factor that presents risks to older adults is extremes in environmental climate. Older persons in extreme conditions (temperatures below 60° F or above 90° F) are at increased risk for developing problems related to thermoregulation (Box 9-6). It is estimated that 10% of all persons older than age 65 have some thermoregulating defect that puts them at risk. Older persons who are sick, frail, inactive, or taking medications such as sedatives, tranquilizers, antidepressants, and cardiovascular drugs that prevent the body from regulating temperature normally are at serious risk when exposed to even minor climate changes.

Box 9-5 Safe Driving Practices for Older Adults

DO
- Plan ahead to know where you are going
- Add extra time so that you do not feel rushed
- Limit your driving to places close to home and easy to get to
- Avoid distractions such as talking, playing the radio, or using a cell phone
- Wear your seat belt at all times
- Wear appropriate eyeglasses and hearing aids
- Pace trips to allow for frequent rest breaks
- Use extra caution when approaching intersections
- Drive at a safe distance behind other cars

AVOID DRIVING
- If taking medications that affect driving skills
- During rush hour
- At night, when lighting is limited, or during inclement weather
- On busy streets and in congested traffic areas
- On limited-access roads with high speed limits and complex intersections such as freeways

---

Box 9-6 Thermoregulation Risks for Older Adults

- Exposure to excessively cold or hot environments
- Limited financial resources to pay for heat or clothing that is suitable for environmental temperature
- Neurologic, endocrine, or cardiovascular disease
- Hypometabolic or hypermetabolic disorders (diabetes, cancer, hypothyroidism, hyperthyroidism, malnutrition, obesity)
- Infection or other febrile illness
- Dehydration or electrolyte imbalances
- Inactivity or excessive activity
- Temperature-altering medications (alcohol, antidepressants, barbiturates, reserpine, benzodiazepines, phenothiazines, anticholinergics)

Even active, healthy older persons are at increased risk when exposed to extremely hot or cold temperatures.

Hypothermia and Hyperthermia

As the cost of heat increases, older adults may try to save money by lowering their thermostat setting. This can be dangerous because a drop in environmental temperature below 65° F can result in hypothermia for elderly persons in their eighties and nineties. Likewise, air-conditioning costs are considerable, and many elderly adults may be reluctant to use it even when available. The National Institute on Aging offers free "Age Pages" that provide information on how to avoid hypothermia and hyperthermia. This information can be obtained online (www.nia.nih.gov) or by phone (800-222-2225). The National Energy Assistance Referral (NEAR) Program can help seniors pay their heating bills. NEAR phone operators (800-674-6327) will give callers the number to reach their state Low-Income Home Energy Assistance Program (LIHEAP) office, as well as referrals to local agencies that offer assistance with paying energy bills.

Thermoregulation, the ability to maintain body temperature in a safe range, is controlled by the hypothalamus. The normal core body temperature is maintained between 97° F and 99° F. Body temperature can be affected by a wide range of internal and external factors. Internal factors include muscle activity, peripheral circulation, amount of subcutaneous fat, metabolic rate, amount and type of foods and fluids ingested, medications, and disease processes. External factors include humidity, environmental temperature, air movement, and amount and type of clothing or covering.

Heat is produced by metabolic processes and by muscular activity such as shivering and conserved by vasoconstriction. Heat is lost through vasodilation and perspiration. Anything that changes the balance of heat lost and heat retained can cause problems.

Hypothermia is defined as a core body temperature of 95° F or lower. Older adults are highly susceptible to hypothermia for several reasons. Normal changes that occur with aging affect the body's ability to regulate temperature. Changes in the skin reduce the older person's ability to perceive dangerously hot or cold environments. Decreased muscle tissue, decreased muscle activity, diminished peripheral circulation, reduced subcutaneous fat, and decreased metabolic rate affect the amount of heat produced and retained by the body. As a person ages, metabolism slows, activity decreases, and shivering diminishes. When the older person is exposed to low environmental temperatures, body temperature drops further. These changes further decrease activity and heat production and allow the body temperature to decrease even further. If this cycle is not stopped, the person may die. The National Institute on Aging estimates that more than 2.5 million older adults are at risk for hypothermia, and the Centers for Disease Control and Prevention reports that approximately 700 deaths per year were attributed to exposure to excessive cold.

Disease processes such as hypothyroidism, hypoglycemia, and malnutrition can also cause a decrease in heat production. Medications that decrease environmental awareness, such as barbiturates, tranquilizers, and antidepressants, can increase the risk for hypothermia. Alcohol ingestion is highly dangerous because it decreases environmental awareness and, at the same time, increases vasodilation with resulting heat loss.

While decreased body temperature is the major symptom of hypothermia, an older person may manifest other signs or symptoms (Box 9-7). One of the first signs of hypothermia in older adults is growing mental confusion that can progress from simple memory loss or changes in logical thinking to total disorientation. Pulse and respiratory rate slow with hypothermia and may be difficult to detect in severe cases. The skin becomes cool or cold to the touch, and pallor or cyanosis is often present (particularly on the extremities). The face may appear swollen or puffy. Muscles appear to be stiff, and fine tremors may occur. Changes in coordination, including poor balance or gait changes, are common. Behavior changes such as lethargy or apathy may occur, but irritability, hostility, and aggression are also possible responses. Shivering, an indication that the body is having difficulty maintaining adequate body temperature, may or may not be evident in older adults, because this response often diminishes or disappears with aging. Because many of the signs and symptoms of hypothermia are similar to those of other disorders in older adults, they can easily be missed or mistaken for something else. The National Institutes of Health suggests an assessment of the "umbles"—mumbles, stumbles, fumbles, and grumbles—to look for possible indications of hypothermia.

With proper precautions, hypothermia is preventable. Approaches to prevention are identified in the nursing interventions section later in the chapter.

Box 9-7 Signs of Hypothermia

- Mental confusion
- Decreased pulse and respiratory rate
- Decreased body temperature
- Cool/cold skin
- Pallor or cyanosis
- Swollen or puffy face
- Muscle stiffness
- Fine tremors
- Altered coordination
- Changes in gait and balance
- Lethargy, apathy, irritability, hostility, or aggression

When hypothermia is suspected, immediate intervention is necessary to prevent serious complications or death. If the elderly person is unconscious, call 911; special care will be required to prevent cardiovascular complications and to rewarm the person. This should be done even when the person appears to be dead because a pulse may not be palpable as a result of severe vasoconstriction. If the person is conscious, get him or her out of the cold and into a warmer environment. Remove cold and/or wet clothing and wrap the person with blankets or other insulating coverings. Warm blankets may be used, but avoid heating pads, electric blankets, or immersion in a hot bath because these may cause cardiovascular problems and cause damage to fragile skin. Warm, not hot, beverages are appropriate and beneficial if the person is able to drink.

Hyperthermia, a higher than normal body temperature, occurs when the body is unable to get rid of excess heat. Deaths directly or indirectly caused by hypothermia average about 700 per year in the United States. Men die from hyperthermia about twice as often as women. Of these deaths, 40% occur in adults over age 65. Hyperthermia can be caused by excessively high environmental temperatures, an inability to dissipate heat, or increased heat production due to exercise, infection, or hyperthyroidism.

Many parts of the country experience extremely high temperature during summer months. When this heat is combined with high humidity, the normal cooling mechanisms of the body are ineffective. Even under moderate conditions, it takes longer for older adults to begin sweating, and, because of diminished thirst and decreased body water, they produce less perspiration. These factors render older adults more likely to develop heat exhaustion and heatstroke.

Hyperthermia can place a significant strain on the heart and blood vessels of older adults. Cardiovascular problems and heat are a deadly combination. Endocrine problems such as diabetes and psychiatric disorders also increase the risk for hyperthermia. Medications commonly used by the elderly can compromise the body's normal adaptation to heat. Diuretic medications prevent the body from storing fluids and can diminish superficial vasodilation. Anticholinergic medication used to treat Parkinson's disease (e.g., benztropine and trihexyphenidyl) can interfere with perspiration as does a wide range of psychotropic medications. Consumption of alcohol should be avoided because it can decrease awareness of symptoms and contribute to fluid loss.

Symptoms of hyperthermia are progressive. Mild, early signs of heat stress include feeling hot, listless, or uncomfortable. Cramps in the legs, arms, and abdomen are early indicators of elevated body temperature. Indications of a serious heat-related problem may include hot, dry skin without perspiration; tachycardia; chest pain; breathing problems; throbbing headache; dizziness; profound weakness; mental or perceptual changes; vomiting; abdominal cramps; nausea; and diarrhea.

Heat exhaustion occurs gradually and is caused by water or sodium depletion. Both active and inactive older adults can develop heat exhaustion if they do not consume adequate fluids and electrolytes when exposed to hot environments. If heat exhaustion is not recognized and treated, it can progress to a more severe condition called *heatstroke*.

Heatstroke, a condition in which the body temperature can climb as high as 104° F, is a life-threatening emergency. Heatstroke is a very real concern for active older persons, particularly those living in hot climates. Strategies that can prevent or reduce the incidence of hyperthermia are listed under Nursing Interventions in each of the Nursing Process sections that follow.

SUMMARY

Psychological trauma caused by falls, assaults, motor vehicle accidents, fires, thermal events, or other injuries can be more serious than the physical trauma itself. Fear of injury often confines older adults to their homes and can cause them to lose confidence in their ability to perform even simple actions. They may restrict their activity, thereby contributing to further loss of strength, decreased mobility, social isolation, and increased dependence. If too much function is lost, institutionalization may be necessary.

❖ NURSING PROCESS FOR RISK FOR INJURY

■ Assessment/Data Collection

- Does the person have a history of falls or other injuries?
- If yes, how often has the person fallen? When and where did the fall occur? What types of injuries are most common?
- How often does the person suffer injuries?
- What is the person's level of vision? Hearing? Temperature perception?
- Does the person have any impairment in gait or balance?
- Does the person use any assistive devices such as a cane, walker, etc?
- What kind of footwear does the person wear most often?
- Does the person suffer from any cognitive impairment?
- Is the person forgetful?
- Does the person smoke? Light candles in the home? Use a gas stove?
- Does the home have a smoke detector? Is it working?
- Does the person live alone?
- What medications does the person take?
- Does the person suffer from dizziness or fainting?
- What are the person's hemoglobin and hematocrit levels?

- Is the person able to follow directions?
- Does the person drive? Does he or she wear a seat belt when riding in a car?
- If living at home, where does the person store medications?
- Where does the person store chemicals and cleaning supplies?
- Are there any safety hazards in the home environment? Scatter rugs? Electric wires? Others?

■ Nursing Diagnoses

Risk for falls, risk for injury, risk for trauma, risk for poisoning

■ Nursing Goals/Outcomes Identification

The nursing goals for an older person at risk for injury, trauma, or poisoning are to experience a decrease in the frequency and severity of injuries and to identify unsafe conditions and behaviors.

■ Nursing Interventions/Implementation

The following nursing interventions for those at risk for injury, trauma, or poisoning should take place in hospitals or extended-care facilities:

1. **Evaluate the person for the risk for falls.** Older individuals who experience dizziness or fainting with position changes are at increased risk for falls. These symptoms are often caused by a sudden drop in blood pressure (orthostatic hypotension). These individuals should be instructed to move slowly and to remain seated until the dizziness passes. Episodes of orthostatic hypotension are more likely to occur early in the morning, particularly before

breakfast, and may be aggravated by dehydration or medications. Episodes of dizziness may have other causes and should be reported to the physician so that the cause can be determined. Evaluate laboratory values for the presence of anemia, which can increase the risk for falls. Be sure to notify the physician of any abnormal values so that appropriate interventions can be initiated. All new admissions should be assessed for problems with balance and gait so that appropriate safety strategies can be initiated.

Older individuals should be encouraged to move at a comfortable pace and not to hurry. Hurrying increases the risk for falling. They should be encouraged to wear comfortable footwear that helps with support and balance. Assistive devices that improve stability by providing a wider base of support (e.g., canes and walkers) may be needed (Figure 9-1).

Check high-risk individuals frequently. The call signal should be readily available whether the person is in bed or in a chair. Lounges and bathrooms should be equipped with call signals. Calls from older adults should be answered promptly. If older adults have to wait too long for assistance, they may attempt to stand or walk even if they know it is unsafe.

Provide adequate assistance based on the patient's abilities and limitations. Use lifts and other transfer devices when appropriate. Care should be taken to prevent injury to both the patient and the caregiver.

2. **Modify the environment to reduce risks.** To prevent falls resulting from visual changes, stairwells should be well illuminated both day and night. The edges of stairs, shower lips, and any other

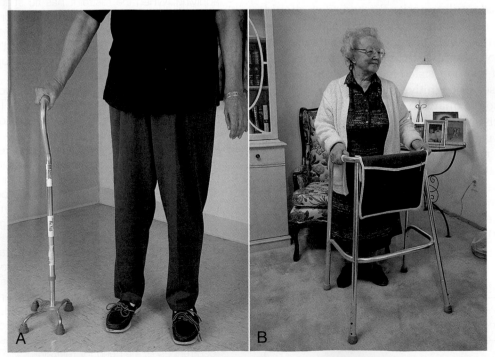

FIGURE 9-1 Assistive devices promote support and safety. **A,** Quad cane. **B,** Walker.

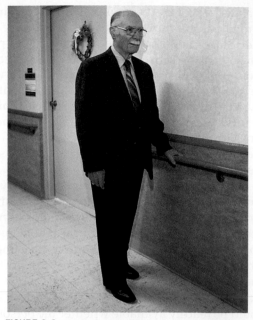

FIGURE 9-2 Handrails provide support when walking.

elevations should be marked using a dark or contrasting color stripe to help the aging individual recognize the edge. Hallways should have strong grip rails to provide support during ambulation (see Figure 9-2). All clutter such as newspapers, wastebaskets, shoes, and other clutter should be removed from the floor. Provide non-skid footwear. Be sure to lock all devices with wheels such as beds and wheelchairs. Use low beds or keep beds in low position unless the caregiver is at the bedside. If the caregiver has to leave the person, even briefly, the bed should be lowered. Whenever the bed is elevated, the side rail opposite the caregiver should be up to reduce the chance of falls. Electronic sensors or alarm systems designed to signal when an at-risk person attempts to stand up from a chair or get out of bed unassisted may be helpful, particularly in cases of cognitive impairment where the elderly person is unaware of the risk for falling.

Medication carts should be locked and properly stored when not in use. Medications should never be left at the bedside unless this is permitted by the physician. Medications intended for one individual can easily be taken by a confused person who wanders into the room. Cleaning carts and supplies should also be locked in a cabinet or closet when not in use (Box 9-8).

Box 9-8   Safety Alert

All poisonous agents, including cleaning solutions, must be stored in locked cabinets or closets where they are out of the reach of residents. Cleaning carts should be kept within sight of staff.

Restraints must be used with caution—and only when there is a documented reason for them and only after the person or his or her guardian agrees to their use (see following Coordinated Care box). This includes use of foot pedals, vest and waist restraints, and even chair tables and safety belts. Omnibus Budget Reconciliation Act (OBRA) regulations are very specific about when and what types of restraints are permitted. Most facilities require a physician's order to use restraints.

Coordinated Care

Collaboration

Use of Restraints

All staff, including nursing assistants, should be thoroughly trained regarding the use of each type of restraining device. Close attention should be paid to when, what, how, and why restraints are used.

- **When:** Restraints should be used only when other less restrictive methods have been tried first and found to be ineffective. Restraints should never be used as a form of punishment. Physician's orders are necessary for both physical and chemical restraints. Informed consent should be obtained from the patient or legal guardian before restraints are used.

- **What:** The least restrictive device that allows the highest level of function but still provides protection should be used. For example, a waist bar or lap board in a wheel chair is likely to be preferable to a full-vest restraint.

- **How:** Read all manufacturers' directions and agency policies before applying a restraint. Use the correct-size device. Make sure to identify the front and back of the device before applying. When the restraint has tie straps, care must be used to attach them to a part of the bed or chair that moves with the patient so that they do not become overly constricting. Use only quick-release hitch knots that are affixed in locations where the nurse, but not the patient, can easily reach them. When restraints are in use, the patient must be checked frequently. Restraints should be released at least every 2 hours, and tissues beneath the restraint must be inspected for signs of altered circulation or other tissue damage.

- **Why:** Inappropriate use of restraints increases the risk for harm to the patient. The potential for lawsuits charging abuse or neglect increases when restraints are in use. To reduce the risk for legal liability, the nurse should document carefully. Documentation must include the following: (1) a baseline assessment of physical condition, including vital signs, infections, pain, fluid and nutritional status, elimination status, medications, vision, hearing, mental status, and typical behavior patterns; (2) information describing specific behaviors that necessitated the need for restraints, including persons or events that may have triggered the behavior; (3) data identifying the type and time the devices were used; (4) the patient's response to restraint; and (5) interventions identified as part of the plan of care designed to prevent recurrences of the need for restraint.

Restraints

Identify as many alternatives to using restraints as you can.

- Why do you think that these alternative actions will decrease the need for restraints?
- How many of these actions have you seen used in care settings?
- Have you tried any yourself? How effective was the alternative intervention?

Complementary and Alternative Therapies

Music Therapy

Research has found that older patients who listen to music they enjoy exhibit significantly more positive behaviors while out of restraint than do older patients who are not exposed to music. No single type of music is right for everyone. Family members may be helpful in identifying favorite music, or the staff may try different types of music and observe the patient's response. Some may prefer classical; others like big band; still others love gospel music. Considering the demographics, the music of the Baby Boomers (e.g., Elvis, James Taylor, the Beatles) may soon be what is played.

The following interventions should take place in the home:

1. **Assess the environment for hazards and modify it to reduce the likelihood of injury.** The home environment can be dangerous for older adults. To reduce the likelihood of poisoning, all cleaning supplies should be stored well away from food or medications. If the older person has impaired judgment, it may be necessary to keep all poisonous substances in a locked cabinet or closet. All medications should be labeled clearly in large letters so that individuals can distinguish their names and directions. Check refrigerator for spoiled or outdated food.

Individuals with circulatory changes should be taught the importance of checking the temperature of bath water with a thermometer. They should not add hot water when sitting in a tub or adjust the temperature of the water while in the shower. Use only nonskid shower mats. Any spills should be mopped up promptly to reduce the risk of slipping.

Aging individuals should be discouraged from climbing because falls from higher places are more likely to cause serious injury. In general, chairs, footstools, and other pieces of furniture are unsafe. If the person needs to reach a high area, a good step stool with a broad base of support should be used. Select furniture that is steady and easy to get out of without assistance.

Stairs should be kept free of clutter. Handrails in stairwells should be sturdy and in good repair. Install grip rails in showers, tubs, and around toilets, making sure they are tightly attached to the structure (studs) of the wall not just the plaster.

Make sure there is adequate lighting without glare, particularly in stairwells and bathrooms. Keep a flashlight at the bedside for emergencies or when a light cannot be easily reached. A floor should be checked for hazards such as clutter, scatter rugs, or loose carpet edges that, when rolled up, may trip a person. All hazardous items should be removed or repaired to reduce the risk for falls.

Make sure smoke detectors are installed and that they are working correctly. Change batteries twice a year in the spring and fall when clocks are changed for daylight savings time.

Encourage use of a medical alert, "panic button," emergency call device that is worn as a necklace or bracelet. This can be activated to summon help if a fall occurs. In addition, the person should be assessed for a depressed mood. Studies have shown that the incidence of falls is three times higher among depressed individuals living at home.

2. **Recruit the assistance of a family member or friend to check on the older person at regular intervals.** Regular visits to the home permit a quick check of the most obvious hazards. Any unsafe conditions can be corrected before an injury occurs. The nurse should review the most common concerns with the visitors so that they are more alert and aware. Although frequent checks will not always prevent injury, they can reduce the chance of an injured older person lying helpless for extended periods. Some older persons invest in special call signal devices that can be worn on their bodies. These call signals can be activated in case of emergency to summon help. They should be purchased only after the reputation of the company who sells and services the device has been carefully checked with an agency such as the Better Business Bureau. Many of these so-called safety systems are worthless and provide a false sense of security to older adults.

3. **Use any appropriate interventions that are used in the institutional setting.**

❖ NURSING PROCESS FOR HYPOTHERMIA/HYPERTHERMIA

■ Assessment/Data Collection

- What is the person's body temperature?
- How does it change throughout the day?
- Is the person inactive or excessively active?
- Does the person show any signs of infection, including behavioral changes?
- Does the person complain of feeling hot or cold?
- Does the person have any disease conditions that increase the risk for ineffective thermoregulation?
- Does the person suffer from electrolyte imbalance?
- Does the person consume alcohol or other temperature-altering medications?

- Does the person suffer from dementia, depression, or other conditions that decrease awareness?
- Does the individual have adequate financial resources to pay for housing that has adequate heat and ventilation?
- Does the individual have clothing suitable for the environmental conditions?

See Box 9-6 for a list of thermoregulation risks for older adults.

▪ Nursing Diagnoses

Hypothermia, hyperthermia, risk for imbalanced body temperature, ineffective thermoregulation

▪ Nursing Goals/Outcomes Identification

The nursing goals for an older person with hypothermia, hyperthermia, imbalanced body temperature, or ineffective thermoregulation are to maintain core body temperature within the normal range and to state the appropriate modifications in dress, activity, and environment needed to maintain body temperature within the normal limits.

▪ Nursing Interventions/Implementation

The following nursing interventions should take place in hospitals or extended-care facilities:

1. **Monitor the environmental temperature, humidity, and air movement.** Room temperature should be maintained at a comfortable level between 70° F and 75° F. Relative humidity between 40% and 60% is comfortable for most people. Ventilation should provide an exchange of air without drafts that may cause chilling. Limit the time an elderly person is exposed to extreme temperatures, either hot or cold.
2. **Monitor body temperature at regular intervals.** The temperature of any person at risk for hyperthermia or hypothermia should be monitored regularly. In many cases, a thermometer that registers temperatures below 95° F is needed for accurate measurement. Electronic thermometers or thermal ear sensors provide accurate temperatures when used correctly.
3. **Provide clothing and bed covers that are suitable for the environment.** Extra clothing and blankets may be necessary for inactive persons. Knit undergarments, layered clothing, bed socks, nightcaps, and flannel sheets or blankets are particularly effective at retaining body heat. Make sure to use adequate covers or an adequately warmed room when bathing a frail elderly person. In the summer, clothing should be lightweight, loose, and nonconstricting to allow adequate movement of air over the body.
4. **Promote adequate fluid and food intake.** In cold weather a diet rich in protein and additional snacks can help maintain subcutaneous fat needed for insulation and promote adequate muscle mass needed to sustain heat production.

In hot weather, older adults should have fresh fluids at the bedside at all times. Pitchers of a cool sugar-free beverage should be available in day rooms, activity centers, and lounges. Because older adults may have a diminished sense of thirst, frequent reminders to drink may be necessary.

5. **Monitor activity level in accordance with environmental temperature.** Increased physical activity helps older adults keep warm in cool weather. Excessive activity should be avoided during hot weather, particularly during daytime hours when heat is greatest.

The following interventions should take place in the home:

1. **Verify that the residence has adequate heat in cold weather and adequate ventilation in hot weather.** Many older adults, particularly those who live alone and those with limited financial resources, live in marginal or substandard housing. There is often inadequate heat to provide warmth in winter or inadequate ventilation to keep cool in the summer. If the home is poorly heated, the person should be encouraged to stay active and dress warmly. If the house is too hot or is poorly ventilated, the person could be encouraged to reduce activity and dress in cool clothing. If air-conditioned public buildings such as shopping plazas, libraries, or senior citizen centers are accessible, older adults should be encouraged to spend the hottest times of day in such facilities.
2. **Identify community resources that can help older adults maintain a safe environment.** Many public utility companies have special programs designed to ensure that older adults have adequate heat in winter. Some also provide fans or air conditioners in the summer. Often these are available to older adults at reduced prices. Special payment plans that spread the cost of heating or air conditioning over the year are also available in most areas of the country. Such plans can enable older adults to budget their limited resources while maintaining a safe thermal environment.
3. **Teach good health habits.**
4. **Use any appropriate interventions that are used in the institutional setting.**

To Prevent Hyperthermia

(1) Decrease physical activity during the daytime. (2) Do heavy chores such as laundry early in the morning or in the evening. (3) Perform outdoor activities after sunset. (4) Dress in light-colored, loose-fitting cotton clothing. (5) Keep out of direct sunlight—use hats, umbrellas, awnings, or other types of sunscreens to reduce sun exposure. (6) In excessive heat, take cool baths or showers several times a day, or apply cool,

wet towels or ice packs to the axillae and groin. (7) Drink a minimum of 8 to 10 glasses of water or cool beverages each day regardless of thirst. When there are medical restrictions on fluid intake, the physician should be consulted regarding the recommended amount of intake. (8) Avoid drinking hot beverages and alcohol. (9) Eat several small meals instead of a few large ones.

To Prevent Hypothermia

(1) Keep the heat within the safe temperature range of 70° F to 75° F. (2) Stay active. (3) Wear several layers of clothing rather than one heavy layer. Wool, knits, and flannel are particularly warm. (4) Drink 8 to 10 glasses of fluid daily, including warm beverages. (5) Avoid consuming alcohol. (6) Eat several small, warm meals throughout the day.

Get Ready for the NCLEX® Examination!

Key Points

- The normal physiologic changes of aging, increased incidence of chronic illness, increased use of medications, and sensory or cognitive changes place the aging population at increased risk for injury.
- Risk for injury increases dramatically when older adults are exposed to multiple environmental hazards.
- The most common injuries experienced by older adults include falls, burns, poisoning, and automobile accidents.
- Nurses can play an important role by helping older adults recognize their risk factors, by planning coping strategies to promote safety, and by modifying their environment to minimize the likelihood of injury.

Additional Learning Resources

SG Go to the Study Guide on pp. 379–397 for additional learning activities to help you master the chapter content.

evolve Go to your Evolve website (http://evolve.elsevier.com/Wold/geriatric) for the following FREE learning resources:
- Animations
- Answer Guidelines for Nursing Care Plan Critical Thinking Questions
- Answers and Rationales for Review Questions for the NCLEX® Examination
- Glossary with pronunciations in English and Spanish
- Video Clips

Review Questions for the NCLEX® Examination

1. A factor that contributes to the development of hypothermia in older adults is decreased:
   1. Activity level
   2. Sensory perception of cold

   3. Percentage of body fat
   4. Nutritional and fluid intake

2. Which manifestation(s) indicate(s) serious heat-related problems? (Select all that apply.)
   1. Cramps in the legs
   2. Vomiting
   3. Heavy perspiration
   4. Profound weakness
   5. Mental changes
   6. Throbbing headache

3. The nurse should instruct the nursing assistant who is caring for a client who is receiving antihypertensive medication to:
   1. Have at least two people assist with ambulation
   2. Allow them to stand up slowly from sitting or lying position
   3. Take the blood pressure if they complain of diplopia
   4. Provide additional salt with their meals

4. The nurse is aware that the best predictor of an elderly person falling is:
   1. A history of previous falls
   2. Use of multiple medications
   3. Sensory deficits
   4. Alterations in balance

5. List three nursing interventions the nurse could implement that would reduce the risk for falls.

Cognition and Perception

Objectives

1. Describe normal sensory and cognitive functions.
2. Describe how sensory perception and cognition change with aging.
3. Discuss the effects of disease processes on perception and cognition.
4. Describe methods of assessing changes in perception and cognition.
5. Identify older adults who are most at risk for experiencing perceptual or cognitive problems.
6. Identify selected nursing diagnoses related to cognitive and perceptual problems.
7. Describe nursing interventions that are appropriate for older individuals experiencing problems related to perception or cognition.
8. Discuss pain assessment and management as they relate to older individuals.

Key Terms

aphasia (ă-FĀ-zē-ă) (p. 181)
catastrophic reactions (p. 188)
cognition (KŎG-nĭ-tĭn) (p. 180)
confusion (kən-fȳ'uzhən) (p. 185)
delirium (dĕ-LĬR-ē-ŭm) (p. 187)
dementia (dĕ-MĔN-shē-ă) (p. 187)
dysarthria (dĭs-ĂR-thrē-ă) (p. 193)
dysphasia (dĭs-FĀ-jē-ă) (p. 193)
hemianopsia (hĕm-ē-ŭn-ŌP-sē-ă) (p. 184)

intelligence (ĭn-tĕl'ə-jəns) (p. 180)
memory (mĕm'ə-rē) (p. 180)
otosclerosis (ō-tō-sklĕ-RŌ-sĭs) (p. 181)
perception (pər-sĕp'shən) (p. 180)
presbycusis (prĕz-bē-KŪ-sĭs) (p. 181)
presbyopia (prĕz-bē-Ō-pē-ă) (p. 181)
stimuli (STĬM-ū-lī) (p. 181)
sundowning (SŬN-doun-ĭng) (p. 188)

The cognitive-perceptual health pattern deals with the ways people gain information from the environment and the way they interpret and use this information. Perception includes the collection, interpretation, and recognition of stimuli, including pain. Cognition includes intelligence, memory, language, and decision making. Cognition and perception are intimately connected to the functioning of the central nervous system and the special senses of vision, hearing, touch, smell, and taste.

NORMAL COGNITIVE-PERCEPTUAL FUNCTIONING

The environment excites or stimulates the senses. The senses, in turn, pass these stimuli into the cerebral cortex, where recognition (perception) and interpretation (cognition) occur. Specific regions of the cerebral cortex are responsible for detecting and processing the stimuli acquired by the various senses. Malfunction of the sensory organs or of the interpretation centers in the brain results in disturbed perception and cognition.

If the senses do not function appropriately, stimuli do not enter the brain and there is not enough information for accurate interpretation. Individuals with sensory deficits in one area may attempt to compensate for these deficits by gathering more information from those senses that function normally. People with hearing deficits often lip-read or otherwise rely on visual cues. People with visual deficits rely more heavily on the senses of hearing and touch. People with multiple sensory deficits have great difficulty collecting information and often experience serious cognitive and perceptual problems. Adult hearing impairment has been associated with social isolation and depression. People with sensory deficits have a normal ability to think and learn, but for them, the process is more difficult. The story of Helen Keller's life illustrates the difficulties experienced by a sensorially deprived person.

As discussed in Chapter 3, numerous sensory changes occur with aging. Common visual changes

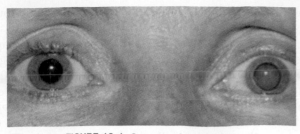

FIGURE 10-1 Cataract of the left eye.

include farsightedness, caused by a loss of elasticity of the lens and resulting decrease in the power of accommodation (**presbyopia**); decreased ability to respond to changes in light, resulting in night blindness; and cataracts (Figure 10-1), which cloud the lens and result in blurred vision and sensitivity to glare. Common auditory changes include loss of hearing acuity, particularly of higher-pitched sounds (**presbycusis**); loss of hearing resulting from decreased sound transmission (**otosclerosis**); and ringing in the ears (tinnitus), which can be caused by Ménière's disease, age-related changes, or medications. Older adults are increasingly susceptible to misperception and therefore misinterpretation when one or more of these changes are present.

Cognition, or thought, takes place in the cerebral cortex of the brain. Cognitive development starts at the time of birth and perhaps even earlier. When the human brain is repeatedly exposed to stimuli, connections develop between nerve fibers of the cerebral cortex. Each time stimuli are introduced to the brain, they are associated (at an unconscious level) with the pool of facts, memories, and experiences that are stored there. Once these connections are firmly established, information is said to be learned. Once learning has taken place, information or skills can be retrieved as needed. Memory enables people to retain and recall previously experienced sensations, ideas, concepts, impressions, and all information that has been previously learned. The human mind is extraordinary in its ability to learn and process extensive amounts of information. It is able to retrieve information on demand, correlate random pieces of information, make judgments, solve problems, and create ideas.

COGNITION AND INTELLIGENCE

We all have different levels of cognitive ability. People often speak of intelligence quotients (IQs) when they try to describe cognitive ability. However, IQ can be deceptive because there are different types of intelligence, and standardized testing procedures do not measure all types of intelligence.

Fluid intelligence is the ability to perform tasks or make judgments based on unfamiliar stimuli. This is sometimes referred to as the ability to "think on your feet." **Crystallized intelligence** (often called *wisdom*) is the ability to perform tasks and make judgments based on the knowledge and experience acquired throughout a lifetime. Because young people have less knowledge

and experience, they must rely more on fluid intelligence. With advanced age comes an abundance of skills and knowledge that has been acquired over time, and crystallized intelligence is used more often.

Intelligence is often measured by means of tests. Although intelligence tests are commonly used, they have distinct limitations. Most written tests measure verbal and mathematic ability. Thus, a person who has had little formal education can have a high level of cognition and yet score poorly on standardized intelligence tests. Cognition is not the same as education. Cognition is the ability to think and reason. Many people have good cognitive skills but poor education.

Intelligence tests are normally timed. Because all individuals do not process information at the same speed, two individuals with a similar pool of knowledge and skills may be judged very differently, simply because they respond at different speeds. Those with a rapid rate of information processing are typically judged more intelligent than those who take longer to process information, even if the end result is the same. This is probably reflective of our culture, which values speed.

COGNITION AND LANGUAGE

Language is a product of cognitive function. In both spoken and written forms, language allows humans to communicate ideas and thoughts. Language develops early in life. By age 2, the average child has a vocabulary of several hundred words. Very specific areas of the brain are dedicated to language, and they change significantly as language skills improve.

Sensory and cognitive problems can result in poor language development or loss of language skills. Damage to the language centers of the brain can result in **aphasia**, a condition in which people are unable to understand or express themselves through language.

Aging persons commonly experience sensory changes that interfere with the collection of information. Visual and hearing changes, changes in taste and smell, and changes in touch and sensation all interfere with the ability to collect accurate information from the environment (Figure 10-2).

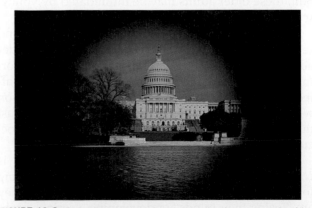

FIGURE 10-2 One type of vision disturbance that is common in older adults: restricted peripheral visual field.

Box 10-1	Possible Indicators of Hearing Loss

- Difficulty understanding women or children
- Trouble following a conversation if more than one person is talking
- Difficulty hearing over the phone
- Difficulty hearing because of background noise
- Complaints that other people are mumbling
- Increased volume of radio or television, particularly if those with normal hearing complain about the loud volume
- Straining to hear conversation at a normal volume

Many older people who are considered confused actually suffer from disturbed sensory perceptions. An older person who does not hear well (Box 10-1) or see well may walk into traffic or make mistakes about directions; these mistakes are not made because the individual is confused, but rather because he or she does not have enough sensory information to make an appropriate decision. Multiple competing stimuli can also cause problems if older adults are unable to focus on the important stimuli and disregard nonessential stimuli.

Intelligence does not automatically decrease with aging; the ability to learn does not either. Some people seem less intelligent as they age because of their tendency to be slower and more cautious in their responses. Rather than be embarrassed, older adults often take more time to be certain of the answer before they respond. This hesitancy or uncertainty may be mistaken for a lack of intelligence, which it is not.

Lack of formal schooling may make older adults appear less intelligent. They may lack polish in their speech and have a more limited vocabulary than do better-educated people. Many older adults who grew up in difficult times ended their formal educations at a young age because they had to work to help support the family. When today's older adults entered the workforce, advanced education was not needed to earn a decent living. Many continued to read and learn and often exceeded what school would have provided. Still, these older adults may be intimidated by young, well-educated caregivers.

The speed at which information is processed and recalled changes with age. It is common for older adults to take longer to recall a specific piece of information. Short-term memory is more likely to be affected than is long-term memory. An older person who cannot remember what he or she had for breakfast may be able to describe in great detail an event that occurred 50 years ago.

Some degree of forgetfulness or memory loss is common with aging. This problem can be disturbing to the alert aging person. Many begin to fear that they are "losing their minds" or developing a serious problem. Careful assessment is needed to distinguish mild memory loss from an early indication of a more serious cognitive disorder.

There is no known reason why memory loss happens, but studies have shown that by 75 years of age, even an alert older person may lose as much as 30% of memory. The more memories a person has developed throughout life, the more he or she will retain, so well-educated older adults tend to retain a higher level of function than do less well-educated older adults. Even without formal education, many older persons are able to compensate for memory gaps by relying more on the large pool of experience gathered over a lifetime.

> Healthy older people are able to learn new information, no matter what their age. Although the ability to acquire new information appears to decrease with age, it may be more a matter of a lack of desire to learn than an inability to acquire and retain the information. If a healthy older person wants to learn something, he or she is usually capable of doing so. Once information is learned, the alert older person can recall it as well as a younger person can.

❖ NURSING PROCESS FOR DISTURBED SENSORY PERCEPTION

An older person can experience disturbances in one or more of the senses. The extent of these disturbances can range from very small changes to total loss of sensory function. The more serious the disturbance, the greater the risks are. Different nursing approaches are necessary for different types of sensory disturbances.

■ Assessment/Data Collection

Has the person mentioned any changes in the taste or smell of food?

- Can the person detect whether something is cold or warm?
- Can the person feel whether something is smooth or rough?
- Does the person have known vision problems (e.g., glaucoma, macular degeneration, cataracts, refractive errors)?
- Does the person see small details or shadows?
- Does the person frequently walk into or trip over objects?
- Can the person read? If not, why not? If yes, can he or she read newsprint or only large-print headlines?
- How close to the television does the person sit?
- Does the person wear eyeglasses? If yes, are they single-lens, bifocal, or trifocal?
- When was the person's vision last checked?
- Does the person respond when people speak to him or her at normal volumes?
- Can the person hear a whisper from someone behind or to the side of him or her who cannot be seen?
- Does the person turn the volume of the television or radio to a very loud level?

- Does the person turn his or her head to hear?
- Does the person wear a hearing aid?
- Does the person respond appropriately or inappropriately to questions?
- Can the person follow directions?

Box 10-2 lists risk factors for problems related to cognition and perception in older adults.

■ Nursing Diagnosis

Disturbed sensory perception: visual, auditory, kinesthetic, gustatory, tactile, olfactory

■ Nursing Goals/Outcomes Identification

The nursing goals for older individuals with disturbed sensory perception are to (1) demonstrate improved ability to detect changes in the environment, (2) interact appropriately with the environment, and (3) demonstrate the ability to compensate for deficits by using prosthetic devices and alternative senses.

■ Nursing Interventions/Implementation

The following nursing interventions should take place in hospitals or extended-care facilities:

1. **Ensure that all caregivers are aware of the person's sensory problems.** The Kardex should identify any vision or hearing problems and should be displayed in a prominent place on the patient's records. Nursing assistants and ancillary personnel should be made aware of sensory problems and appropriate methods of communication before attempting to provide care for an older individual with sensory deficits.

2. **Make appropriate sensory contact before beginning care.** If the aging person is hard of hearing, the nurse should avoid startling him or her. Approaches should be made so that the older individual can see the nurse, or the individual should be touched gently on the hand before more personal

contact is made. If the person is visually impaired, the nurse should speak up and introduce himself or herself when entering the room. This lets the person know who is there, even if he or she cannot see a face clearly.

3. **Determine the best methods for communicating with older adults.** Nurses must be patient and relaxed when working with older adults (Figure 10-3). When working with sensorially altered older persons, it is best to keep messages as simple as possible, use easily understood words, and speak clearly. It may be necessary to reword a statement if the first attempt is not understood. When explaining care or treatments, nurses must be careful to avoid information overload. When writing messages, they should ensure that the writing is clear and large enough to be seen easily.

When dealing with older adults who are hearing-impaired, it is helpful to speak in a low tone of voice because hearing losses are usually in the higher frequencies of sound. Because many hearing-impaired people compensate by lip-reading, it is best to stand in good light while facing the person and to speak slowly but not unnaturally so. Nurses must not chew gum or eat while conversing. If one of the older person's ears is better than the other, talking into the good ear may help. Background noise from television or radio should be kept to a minimum because it may distract older adults or interfere with verbal communication.

Facial expressions, gestures, and other visual cues that are appropriate to the message should be used. These cues can help the person understand what the nurse is talking about. For example, if the nurse's intended message is "Please come with me," the nurse can hold out his or her hand and begin to walk. If it is time to groom someone's hair, the nurse can show the person the brush and comb to help make the message clear.

Box 10-2	Risk Factors Related to Cognition and Perception in Older Adults

- Vision problems (total blindness, presbyopia, macular degeneration, cataracts, hemianopsia, detached retina, diabetes, glaucoma, and significant refractive errors)
- Hearing problems (presbycusis, otosclerosis, and conductive sensorineural deafness)
- Dementia (including Alzheimer's disease)
- Disturbed cerebral circulation (stroke, aneurysm, and head injury)
- Drugs that affect the sensorium (alcohol, narcotic analgesics, tranquilizers, sedatives, and hypnotics)
- Disturbed neurologic function resulting in decreased levels of consciousness
- Disturbed metabolic states (hypoglycemia and metabolic alkalosis)
- Environments with either inadequate or excessive sensory stimulation

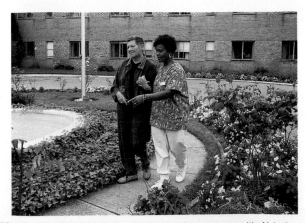

FIGURE 10-3 Nurses can use touch to calm a person with Alzheimer's disease.

Persons with hearing impairments are not likely to understand messages spoken through the call signal speakers that are used in most care settings. In most facilities, even people with good hearing have problems with these devices. Caregivers should respond promptly and in person to calls from the sensorially impaired. More information regarding communication with older adults is provided in Chapter 5.

4. **Modify the environment to reduce risks.** Lighting is important for older adults. Because it takes the eye longer to adjust to bright light as we age, stairs and other hazardous areas should be designed to prevent glare. When an older person has a condition in which a portion of the visual field is lost (hemianopsia), the furniture should be arranged to maximize the person's ability to see (Figure 10-4). Personal belongings should be placed toward the good side, and the person should be taught to turn his or her head and "sweep" the environment to pick up more visual cues.

5. **Verify that prostheses such as eyeglasses and hearing aids are functional.** Obtaining the proper corrective lenses is not a one-time requirement. As the eyes continue to change, a prescription that was once adequate may lose its effectiveness. Simply because a person wears eyeglasses does not mean that he or she can see clearly, particularly if the person has had the eyeglasses for some time. Eye examinations should be performed regularly and prescriptions changed whenever required. Many aging individuals suffer from multiple refractive errors and require bifocals or trifocals to achieve adequate focus. Bifocals and trifocals can present problems because the wearers must move their heads to shift the line of vision to the proper section, depending on what they wish to view. Some people find this so disturbing that they choose not to wear the correct prescription. Problems such as these should be reported to the physician so that an acceptable solution can be found.

Eyeglasses must be cleaned regularly. Fingerprints and other debris can distort vision and make the glasses useless. To be of benefit, eyeglasses must also fit the person properly. Many glasses are too loose and slide down the nose; others are too snug and create uncomfortable pressure areas on the nose or ears. Often, older adults wear glasses with broken frames that are taped together. If the glasses do not help vision or they are uncomfortable, older adults are likely to avoid wearing them. Nurses should arrange a consultation with an eye specialist to get such problems corrected.

Hearing aids are worn by many older persons. These devices do not duplicate normal hearing and are not beneficial for everyone. Hearing aids can be built into eyeglasses or inserted into the ear canal. Some of the older units hang over the external ear; newer models are almost invisible when worn (Figure 10-5).

Many persons have difficulty adjusting to hearing aids and complain that they are bothersome. When first fitted with a hearing aid, the person may be able to tolerate it only for a few minutes a day. As the person adjusts to the device, the amount of time it is worn should be gradually increased. Older persons who are adjusting to wearing a hearing aid often report that it makes them nervous or jumpy to hear so many sounds. They should be reassured that this is normal and that the jumpiness will go away as they become used to wearing the hearing aid. Many people who wear hearing aids report that the sounds they hear are "tinny" or "noisy" and that they hear feedback whistles or hums. These noises are usually caused by incorrect insertion or improper adjustment of the controls on the device.

Hearing aids require a certain amount of care and maintenance. Because they are fragile, care should be taken not to drop them. Most are made of plastic and should be kept away from very hot or very cold places. Before being inserted into the ear, hearing aids should be checked for cracks or rough edges that could injure the ear. The ear mold should be

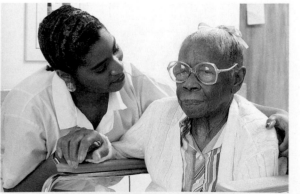

FIGURE 10-4 Nurses should approach patients who have a left-sided hemiparesis from the right side. This older woman may not be able to see people to her left.

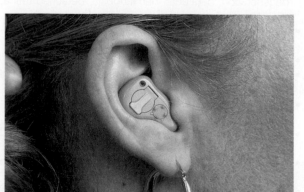

FIGURE 10-5 A hearing aid in the ear canal is barely visible.

cleaned regularly. Special attention should be paid to the removal of cerumen, which may plug the canal and reduce the effectiveness of the device. Batteries should be checked and changed regularly because the hearing aid will not work properly without a good power source. To prolong the life of the batteries, the hearing aid should be shut off when it is not in use. Batteries should be checked for corrosion and contacts should be cleaned, particularly if the device becomes wet. Storing unused batteries in the refrigerator can prolong their life. Old batteries should be discarded after a change so that they are not mistakenly saved and reused. This mistake can lead to confusion and frustration.

Caregivers who are not familiar with hearing aids should receive special training in how to place them in the ear canal properly. Hearing aids are useless unless they are worn properly. Nurses should always verify that a hearing aid has been applied to the correct ear. If the person wears two aids, they should be marked so that the correct device is placed in the correct ear. If the device still does not function properly, nurses may need to consult with an audiologist or speech therapist. If the older person is reluctant to wear the hearing aid, the nurse should do a thorough assessment to determine why he or she is refusing. A thorough reevaluation of hearing may be necessary. The following interventions should take place in the home:

1. **Modify the home environment to compensate for sensory changes.** Modifications in the home will help older adults cope with sensory changes. Increasing the amount of light is the least expensive and most beneficial change. Lights should be positioned so that glare is avoided. Incandescent bulbs are better than fluorescent bulbs because they do not have a distracting flicker. Burned-out bulbs should be replaced promptly. It is even better if light bulbs are replaced when they begin to dim rather than waiting until they burn out.

Use of contrasting colors helps older adults determine edges and borders. Contrasting strips should be applied to areas where there is a change in elevation, such as shower entrances and steps. Contrasting door frames, dishes, pillows, personal care items, and toilet seats will help older adults distinguish these items more easily.

2. **Assist sensorially impaired persons in developing techniques or acquiring devices that will help compensate for losses.**
Hearing-Impaired Persons. Nurses should explain ways that hearing-impaired persons can improve communications. These include (1) telling others that they are hard of hearing, (2) focusing on the speaker and paying attention to what is being said, (3) facing the speaker or asking the speaker to face them, (4) asking the speaker to speak slowly and clearly but not to shout, and (5) asking the speaker to repeat when information is not clear.

Many special devices are available for hearing-impaired persons. Local telephone companies can provide special equipment such as amplifiers or video display terminals that enable older adults to maintain contact with others. Doorbells and mats that flash a light when someone is at the door are available. Alarm clocks that vibrate rather than ring can be purchased from specialty or department stores. Hearing-impaired individuals with adequate vision should be made aware of closed-caption television broadcasts, which provide typed narration of news and many entertainment programs.

Visually Impaired Persons. Telephone dials can be modified with overlay rings that have large numbers to assist in dialing. Most newer telephones can be programmed with commonly used numbers so that the person needs to push only one button to dial. Handheld or floor standing magnifying devices help with reading or close work. Large-print books and magazines are available in most public libraries. Written materials can also be enlarged on photocopy machines to make reading easier. Books on audiotape are also available in stores and many libraries. Talking clocks that fit in a pocket are available.

❖ NURSING PROCESS FOR DISTURBED THOUGHT PROCESSES

Anything that damages or interferes with the normal functioning of the cerebral cortex can result in cognitive (i.e., thinking and judgment) problems. All changes in cognitive function must be given immediate attention. Prompt assessment of the type and severity of the disorder, along with identification of the cause or causes, enables the caregiver to plan the most appropriate interventions for each individual. Cognitive function can be affected by sensory changes, physiologic factors, or emotional disorders. Cognitive problems can range from mild and reversible forms of disorientation to severe and irreversible forms of dementia. Depression, hypothyroidism, and vitamin deficiencies are common treatable causes of pseudodementia (Box 10-3).

Sensory changes can result in behaviors that mimic cognitive problems but actually are not. The two should not be confused. Sensory misperception should be ruled out before further cognitive assessment is performed.

The term **confusion** is used to describe a wide range of behaviors. Both lay people and professionals use this term far too frequently—often incorrectly and inappropriately.

Confusion is defined as a mental state characterized by disorientation regarding time, place, or person that leads to bewilderment, perplexity, lack of orderly thought, and the inability to choose or act decisively and to perform activities of daily living. Confusion is categorized in different ways by different authorities, but one common system identifies three major forms: acute confusion, idiopathic confusion, and dementia.

Clinical Situation

Cognition and Perception

Imagine that you are an aging person hospitalized for chest pain. You have trouble seeing (particularly because you cannot reach your glasses in the drawer) and are hard of hearing (you are wearing your hearing aid, but the batteries do not work). The medication you took has made you a little light-headed, and your bladder seems to fill every 30 minutes. You send a call signal to go to the bathroom, but no one comes and you are getting desperate. You try to get up, but the rails are in your way and you fall to the floor. Before anyone comes to help, you can wait no longer and void on the floor. By the time someone gets there, you are frightened and angry. You yell and slap at the person. The next thing you know you are restrained in bed, and a tube has been put in your bladder. If you could read the nurse's note, you would see this statement: "Confused, agitated, and combative. Restrained for protection. Catheter inserted for incontinence."

Box 10-3	Dementia: Types and Causes

ACUTE REVERSIBLE DEMENTIA
Hypoxia caused by:
- Hypotension
- Anemias
- Ventilatory problems
- Heart failure

Environmental changes
Fluid and electrolyte imbalance
Metabolic disturbances:
- Acidosis
- Hypoglycemia
- Hyperglycemia
- Elevated blood urea nitrogen

Drug toxicity
Malnutrition
Transient ischemic attacks
Decreased sensory input
Sensory overload
Hypothyroidism
Brain tumor
Infection
Subarachnoid hemorrhage
Subdural hematoma

CHRONIC IRREVERSIBLE DEMENTIA
Alzheimer's disease
Anoxia
Untreated acute dementia
Pick's disease
Creutzfeldt-Jakob disease
Alcoholism
Untreated abnormal blood pressure
Hydrocephalus
Heavy metal toxicity
Multiple cerebral infarction

From Wolanin MO: *Geriatr Nurs* 4:227, 1983.

Acute confusion, often called **delirium**, is characterized by disturbances in cognition, attention, memory, and perception. This type of confusion is usually caused by a physiologic process that affects the autonomic nervous system. Conditions that can cause delirium include uncontrolled pain, infection, metabolic disturbances, vitamin deficiencies, uremia, hypoxia, hypercalcemia, endocrine imbalance, myocardial infarction, constipation, drug toxicity, and drug withdrawal.

A mnemonic tool used to focus an assessment is found in Table 10-1 (DELIRIUM).

Acute delirium has a sudden onset of hours or days. It is characterized by rapid mood swings, disorganized sleep cycles, changes in psychomotor activity (hypoactivity, hyperactivity, or both), tremors or spasmodic activity, rapid speech patterns, loss of attention, and a wide range of cognitive changes (Tables 10-2 and 10-3). Older individuals with underlying emotional instability can exhibit a full-blown psychotic episode with delusions and auditory or visual hallucinations. The severity of symptoms may vary throughout the day, and symptoms are often worse at night. Because the cause of dementia is usually physiologic, acute confusion does not respond well to behavioral approaches

---

Table 10-1	Mnemonic Assessment for DELIRIUM	
COMPONENT	**CONSIDERATIONS**	
Drug use	Any recent change in medications, increase or decrease in dosage, change from specific brand to a generic. Pay special attention to sedative-hypnotics (including alcohol), antidepressants, opioids, antipsychotics, anticholinergics, anticonvulsants, antiparkinsons, and H₂ blockers	
Electrolyte imbalance	Abnormal levels of calcium, sodium, or magnesium often related to malnutrition or dehydration	
Lack of drugs	Missed medication doses	
Infection	Check for UTI, signs of inflammation, respiratory congestion, etc.	
Reduced sensory input	Visual or hearing impairment, failure to use glasses or hearing aids, social isolation	
Intracranial problems	Recent head injury (fall or vehicular accident), history of stroke, meningitis, history of seizure	
Urinary retention and/or fecal impaction	Recent anesthesia, history of benign prostatic hyperplasia, recent catheter removal	
Myocardial problems	Increased anginal symptoms, abnormal electrocardiogram (EKG), recent post cardiac surgery status	

Table **10-2**	Differences between Delirium and Dementia

DELIRIUM	DEMENTIA
Rapid onset measured in hours or days	Usually a slow, insidious onset of symptoms over months or years
Reduced level of consciousness	Initially no change in level of consciousness
Variable course over 24 hours	Stable over 24 hours
Increased or decreased psychomotor activity Disturbed sleep–wake patterns Disorientation and perceptual disturbances possible visual and auditory hallucinations Memory impairment Decreased attention span with disorganized thinking	Impaired memory with loss of abstract thinking, judgment, language skills (aphasia), motor skills (apraxia), and ability to recognize familiar people or objects (agnosia)
Generally reversible if underlying problem is identified and treated; may recur with acute illness	Generally not reversible

Table **10-3**	Nursing Interventions for Delirium and Dementia

DELIRIUM	DEMENTIA
Designed to treat underlying pathologic condition and maintain physiologic integrity	Designed to maintain or maximize level of function
Includes administration of fluids, nutrition, oxygen, antianxiety medications, and so on	
Designed to control environmental stressors, to protect safety, and to promote comfort	Includes environment modification, activity-based therapies, and communication strategies

such as reorientation. Once the cause is identified and treated, the symptoms generally disappear. Failure to identify and correct underlying physiologic problems can result in serious physical harm or even death.

Idiopathic confusion does not have an identifiable physiologic basis. It is most likely to occur when there is a stressful disturbance in lifestyle or life patterns such as what occurs with the death of a loved one, depression, or relocation to a hospital or new living quarters. The onset of symptoms is likely to correlate to specific occurrences or situations, although this is not always the case. Idiopathic confusion tends to affect memory and the ability to concentrate. Affected older adults are often depressed. Common symptoms of

idiopathic confusion include appetite changes, loss of interest in activities, changes in sleep patterns, agitation, feelings of worthlessness or guilt, fatigue, or other physiologic complaints. The ability to perform routine activities of daily living is not usually affected, but the willingness to perform these activities may be. Individuals experiencing this form of confusion usually respond well to reorientation interventions and approaches that reduce stress levels. Symptoms may be reversible but may not disappear completely.

Dementia is a slow, insidious process that results in progressive loss of cognitive function. Dementia is caused by damage to the cerebral cortex that is most commonly a result of disease conditions (e.g., Alzheimer's disease; Box 10-4), multiple infarcts of the cerebrum secondary to stroke, or other pathologic conditions of the brain. Drug intoxication, Huntington's

Box **10-4**	Facts About Alzheimer's Disease

- Alzheimer's disease is not a normal part of aging. It is a progressive, degenerative, irreversible form of dementia.
- The disease was first identified in 1906 by Alois Alzheimer, a German neurologist.
- Most cases of Alzheimer's disease occur in people older than 65 years of age, but it can occur as early as 30 years of age.
- The incidence of the disease doubles approximately every 5 years from ages 65 to 85.
- Alzheimer's disease affects both men and women of all religions, races, and socioeconomic backgrounds.
- The cause of the disease remains unknown, but genetic, chemical, viral, and environmental factors are suspected. Family history and the presence of the apolipoprotein E gene appear to indicate an increased risk for development of the disease.
- Alzheimer's disease causes gradual changes such as plaques and tangles in the nerve cells of the brain that can be detected on autopsy.
- Neurologic changes result in a loss of the ability to process information normally.
- The first signs of Alzheimer's disease are subtle changes in behavior. The disease affects each individual differently; the type and severity of symptoms, as well as the order of their appearance, differ from person to person.
- People suffering from Alzheimer's disease lose the ability to think, remember, understand, and make decisions. Consequently, they are often unable to perform even the most basic activities of daily living. The ability to control basic body functions such as elimination is also lost.
- People with Alzheimer's disease suffer personality changes. They lose the ability to control moods and emotions, leading to unpredictable and often inappropriate behavior. Unusual behaviors include wandering, pacing, hiding things, swearing, disturbed sleep patterns, and repetitive actions.
- There is no known cure for Alzheimer's disease. A variety of medications is being tested for use with this disease, with varying degrees of success.

disease, Creutzfeldt-Jakob disease, Pick's disease, cerebral hypoxia, hyperthyroidism, subdural hematoma, and brain tumors are less common causes. Dementia is characterized by changes in memory, judgment, language, mathematic calculation, abstract reasoning, and problem-solving ability; impulsive behavior; stupor; confusion; and disorientation. Changes related to dementia are progressive and believed to be irreversible. In the early stages, many cases of dementia are mistakenly considered a part of normal aging, which can result in delayed diagnosis and treatment. The stages of dementia are listed in Box 10-5. Many older adults who suffer from the early stages of dementia are able to recognize that something is wrong, but they do not know what it is. They may be rather creative in the types of excuses used to explain their problems. However, in the later stages, impaired cognitive function is dramatic and obvious, even to a casual observer.

Common behaviors seen with advanced dementia include wandering, excessively emotional reactions (**catastrophic reactions**), combative behaviors, suspiciousness, and hallucinations or delusions. These agitated behaviors, which are often worse late in the day, are referred to as the **sundown syndrome** or **sundowning**. Affected persons often do not recognize even their closest family members and friends. These abnormal behaviors are frightening to the family and anyone who cares about the affected individual.

People suffering from dementia are at increased risk for injury and personal neglect. They are unable to recognize or understand hazards in the environment. Self-care deficits in eating, bathing, grooming, and toileting are common.

In the early stages of dementia, the family may be able to provide adequate care at home. With advanced stages, full-time supervision and total physical care are often required. Dementia is likely to result in institutional placement.

Dementia affects up to 10% of adults older than age 65 who live in the community. The incidence of dementia in those 85 years or older is estimated as high as 50%. Approximately half of institutionalized older adults suffer from some form of dementia.

? Critical Thinking

Dementia

What amount of personal connection have you had with a person who has Alzheimer's disease or another form of dementia? If possible, identify one specific individual whom you can recall well.
- In what context did you interact with this person (home, hospital, extended care)?
- How much continuous time did you spend with this person?
- What behaviors did you observe?
- How did you respond to these behaviors?
- Did you find interacting with this person to be stressful? In what way?

    Now imagine being a spouse or child caring for this individual in a home setting.
- How do you think this person's experiences differ from yours?
- What types of stressors do you think the person experiences?
- What could you suggest to help this person cope?
- What support services are available in your community?

■ Assessment/Data Collection

- Does the person mention any changes in memory?
- Does the person's family or significant others notice memory changes?
- Does the person have difficulty remembering recent or remote events?
- Can the person grasp new ideas, or does he or she have difficulty with this?
- Can the person make appropriate, informed decisions?
- Does the person find it difficult to learn new things?
- What helps the person learn new things?
- What is the person's dominant language?
- Does the person speak other languages?
- What is the person's language/vocabulary level?
- What is the person's education level?
- How long is the person's attention span?
- Are there significant behavior changes, including hyperactivity (agitation, excitability, distractibility) or hypoactivity (lethargy, apathy, somnolence)?
- Is the person restless, uncooperative, belligerent, angry, withdrawn, or threatening?
- Has the person experienced any delusions or hallucinations?
- Are there particular times of day when behavior is most noticeably different?
- Does the person have a history of stroke or other brain disease?

Box 10-5 Stages of Dementia

STAGE 1
- Forgetfulness
- Decreased judgment
- Loss of spontaneous emotional response
- Decreased ambition
- Decreased mental abilities, including verbal and mathematic skills

STAGE 2
- Increased level of forgetfulness
- Significantly impaired judgment
- Irritable behavior
- Agitation
- Confusion as to person, place, and time
- Episodes of incontinence

STAGE 3
- Inability to communicate
- Loss of contact with environment
- Total physical dependency
- Total incontinence

- Have there been any recent changes in medication or dosage?
- Are there any signs of infection (urinary tract infection, pneumonia)?
- What is the level of hydration?
- Is the person constipated?
- What is the person's oxygen saturation?
- What are the results of the Folstein Mini-Mental State Examination (MMSE)? (See Chapter 8 for more details about this tool.)

See Box 10-2 for a list of risk factors for problems related to cognition and perception in older adults.

■ Nursing Diagnosis

Disturbed thought processes

■ Nursing Goals/Outcomes Identification

The nursing goals for older individuals with altered thought processes are to (1) remain free from injury, (2) assist in activities of daily living to the highest level possible, and (3) seek assistance when needed.

■ Nursing Interventions/Implementation

The following nursing interventions should take place in hospitals or extended-care facilities:

1. **Assess behavior on admission and at regular intervals.** Correct identification of the type of cognitive loss is important so that appropriate medical and nursing interventions can be planned and implemented. When a sudden change in behavior is observed in a person who has had normal cognition, a physiologic problem is usually suspected, diagnosed, and treated. However, for persons who already have a history of cognitive changes, it is more difficult to identify these changes. Progression from mild confusion to dementia is common but can be missed unless caregivers pay close attention to subtle changes in behavior.
2. **Provide assistive sensory devices.** Confusion is worse when there is inadequate or inaccurate sensory input. Nurses must ensure that older individuals wear eyeglasses, hearing aids, dentures, and other adaptive devices designed to maximize sensory perception when necessary.
3. **Orient the person to person, place, and time, and provide any other important situational information.** The person should be called by the name he or she responds to best. Most often, this is the first name, such as Mary, Jim, or Alice. Nurses can refer to calendars or clocks to orient to time of day, week, and month. Calendars can be used to show the aging individual when important events such as birthdays, holidays, and special activities will occur. The nurse should remind the person where he or she is and describe daily events and procedures before they happen. If the person becomes combative, the nurse must not argue with him or her. Instead, the nurse should focus on the feelings that the person exhibits by using reflective statements such as, "I know that this isn't what you want to do right now, but it's dinnertime and the food is here."
4. **Provide a structured environment that ensures safety yet enables the person to keep active as long as possible.** Nurses should ensure that the environment is free from hazards that could lead to falls. Individuals who get up frequently might benefit from wearing shoes even when in bed so that they have better balance and footing when they get up.

Some people suffering from dementia become less active; others demonstrate pacing or other repetitive movements. To maintain strength and joint mobility, inactive persons should be encouraged to perform some physical activity that they like each day. Specific activities should be identified and time should be structured into the care plan. Activity, occupational, and physical therapists can help develop a plan to meet individual needs (Box 10-6).

Individuals who pace should be allowed to do so without restraint. Pacers should be encouraged to take rest periods during the day so that they do not exhaust themselves.

Wanderers may need to be housed on a care unit with controlled exits that set off alarms when anyone passes through the door. Wandering can also be monitored by use of an electronic bracelet that sounds an alarm when the wearer tries to leave the unit or building. In home or hospital settings where these controls are not practical, bed or chair alarms (weight sensitive pads that set off alarms when the person is off the pad) can be used to let nurses know that the person has gotten out of his or her bed or chair. Adequate lighting is important

---

Box 10-6   General Approaches for Dealing With Confused Older Adults

- Provide a calm, safe, and structured environment with a controlled number of stimuli.
- Use a calm, gentle, one-on-one approach.
- Speak normally and informally as though the person is not confused.
- Allow plenty of time; avoid hurrying.
- Determine the confused person's reality; avoid confrontation or forced reorientation to objective fact.
- Encourage reminiscence using family pictures, common activities, or objects.
- Provide familiar clothing and personal items from home.
- Redirect attention or use some other form of distraction to reduce anxiety resulting from disturbing thoughts.
- Provide safe, repetitive activities within individual capabilities (e.g., winding yarn and folding towels).
- Provide continuity of care with a limited group of caregivers.
- Develop and maintain daily routines for care and activities.
- Avoid sudden changes in routine, room, or caregivers.

to reduce the likelihood of falls and to reduce fear induced by misperception of shadows.

Light Therapy

Studies have shown that bright light therapy may improve the length of sleep and decrease some of the agitated behaviors commonly associated with sundown syndrome.

5. **Provide continuity.** Too many new faces or changes are frightening and disturbing to confused older adults. Whenever possible, care should be provided by a consistent group of caregivers who are able to develop a trusting relationship. The aging person should have access to familiar personal belongings such as pictures or a blanket or purse. These can provide comfort and help the person keep some contact with reality.

6. **Administer psychotherapeutic medications as ordered.** A few medications are available to aid in the treatment of cognitive disorders such as Alzheimer's disease. These medications do not cure or reverse existing cognitive loss but are often beneficial in slowing the progression of loss. The most commonly prescribed medications include tacrine (Cognex), donepezil HCl (Aricept), rivastigmine (Exelon), and memantine (Namenda).

7. **Avoid use of physical and chemical restraints.** Keeping confused persons restrained in beds or chairs tends to increase their level of confusion. The use of physical and chemical restraints can be harmful and can actually make the behavior worse. Restraints are a form of imprisonment, and their use without a valid medical reason can be grounds for legal action. Restraints were traditionally used to protect people from falls or other injury. Too often, however, they were used so that nursing staff did not have to take time to adequately meet the older person's needs. Rather than protecting older adults, restraints can cause harm and lead to physical deterioration. It may be more appropriate to keep the bed in low position or position a mattress on the floor next to the bed to reduce the risk for injury if the person does fall.

Current Omnibus Budget Reconciliation Act (OBRA) legislation recognizes the problems involved with restraint and currently restricts the use of chemical restraints to specific situations. It is not appropriate to treat nonaggressive behavior with psychotropic medication. Nonaggressive individuals are more likely to respond to alternative therapies such as music, dance, exercise, art, or other forms of activity therapy (see Complementary and Alternative Therapies box). Verbal agitation is not typically responsive to medication. Under current guidelines, only constant yelling or screaming are a valid justification for antipsychotic medication. When psychotropic medications are used, they should be administered at the lowest dose and for the shortest possible time.

Music Therapy

Music therapy has been shown to be beneficial in working with cognitively impaired older adults, including those suffering from dementia. It is hypothesized that musical stimuli activate the creative right side of the brain, which, in turn, facilitates the entry of information to the logical left side of the brain, thus enhancing cognitive function. Following are some behavioral responses to music:
- Improved mood
- Decreased depression
- Muscle relaxation
- Diminished fear and apprehension
- Improved physical movement during therapy

8. **Structure participation in activities of daily living.** If affected persons are able to perform any of their own physical care, they should be encouraged to do so, particularly in the early stages of dementia. This helps them maintain physical strength, and it promotes self-esteem for those who are aware that they are losing functional ability. Routines should be kept simple. The care plan should be individualized for each person and followed consistently by all caregivers. Simple step-by-step directions should be provided. Choices should be kept to a minimum because they tend to increase anxiety and agitation (Figure 10-6). Clothing should be kept simple and should be modified to make dressing and undressing easy, thereby reducing frustration. Hair should be styled so that care is quick and easy. Shorter styles make shampooing and grooming easier and less time-consuming. Mealtimes should be kept as pleasant as possible. Finger foods are more easily managed than are foods that require the use of silverware. Soup or beverages can be served in cups with handles that are easier to control. To

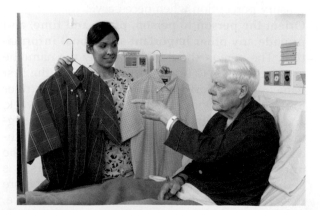

FIGURE 10-6 The nurse offers simple clothing choices to the patient.

prevent burns, careful attention should be paid to the temperature of hot beverages or soups. Trays should be prepared before serving to minimize delay and frustration. Meat should be cut into easily digested pieces because the person may forget to chew before swallowing. Reminders to swallow are necessary in some cases. Toileting schedules can help reduce episodes of incontinence. Many confused older adults become increasingly agitated when they need to eliminate, even if they do not recognize the sensation.

9. **Structure the environment to minimize disruption; avoid sudden changes of room or environment.** Frequent change of staff, large numbers of strange people, excessive noise, and excessive amounts of activity can be overly stimulating to those who suffer from dementia; therefore, they should be kept to a minimum. Sudden changes of room or even rearrangement of the furniture and belongings can cause increased confusion, apprehension, and agitation. Whenever possible, room changes should be avoided. If it is necessary, the new room should be as similar to the old one as possible. Personal effects should not be moved unless necessary for safety.

10. **Develop a plan to deal with "acting out" behaviors.** Excessive stimulation and stress are likely to trigger catastrophic reactions or delusional behavior. Making decisions and responding to questions are stressful to those suffering from dementia and should be avoided. Certain actions on the part of nurses will help the person regain control. Distractions such as a walk or a cup of tea can be used to divert the person's attention. If this does not work, it may be necessary to take the person to his or her room or a quiet place free from the stimuli that caused the upset. Simple touch and reassurance, even sitting quietly with the person, may be enough to reestablish control.

> It is essential that nurses remain calm when confused individuals act out. It is not easy for nurses to deal with repeated irritating or hostile behaviors, but they must remember that anger, arguments, and explanations only confuse the person and make the situation worse. Even if nurses do not say anything negative to the person, body language may communicate a lack of acceptance. Frustration can be perceived by older persons, despite their confusion. If nurses are unable to control their personal behavior, it may be necessary to leave the situation and seek support from other staff members to regain self-control.

11. **Use effective communication skills.** Use of effective communication techniques can promote positive interactions with confused older adults. Smiles, eye contact, and gentle touch should be used. Nurses should express genuine interest and warmth and listen to the confused person, even if the words do not make sense. The person must be allowed adequate time to express himself or herself. When giving information, the nurse should keep the messages short and simple, using words that are familiar to the person, and speak in a calm, natural tone of voice.

12. **Consult with family and the multidisciplinary team.** The family may be able to provide valuable information regarding the older person's likes, dislikes, routines, and fears. When they have been providing care in the home, families may also be able to provide suggestions for approaches that have worked in the past. Care of confused older adults requires cooperation and coordination between various departments so that continuity can be maintained. Regular "staffings" that include all relevant departments and disciplines provide an opportunity to review the person's current status and revise the plan of care.

The following interventions should take place in the home:

1. **Help the family accept the diagnosis.** The diagnosis of dementia is difficult for loved ones to accept. They must be allowed opportunities to verbalize concerns and express their feelings of anger, frustration, or helplessness.

2. **Help the family adjust to the demands of providing care for a cognitively impaired older person.** Persons with severely altered thought processes cannot be left alone. It is difficult to devise a plan that enables families to supervise impaired older adults while also allowing them to continue with their own lives. Nurses can do several things to help families cope with this situation. Nurses can explain and demonstrate the types of behaviors, actions, and communication techniques that are likely to be effective. They can help families make modifications in the home environment that will provide optimal safety yet maintain some semblance of a normal home. Nurses can also recommend books and pamphlets that provide families with more detailed and specific information. Several good books on the care of patients with Alzheimer's disease are available in bookstores. The Alzheimer's Association has many good reference books and pamphlets, including a handbook titled *Home Care of the Alzheimer Patient*.

3. **Provide emotional support and help the family identify coping strategies.** Coping with the day-to-day responsibilities of caring for a cognitively impaired older person is highly stressful. Regular visits to assess how the family is coping, as well as time spent listening to concerns, help family members deal with their fears and anxieties.

4. **Identify community resources.** Support groups for the families of Alzheimer's disease or other dementia sufferers are available in many communities.

Nurses should keep abreast of support groups that are available in each community so that they can supply this information to concerned family members. Nurses should encourage family members to participate in these groups. Respite care programs are also available in many communities. These programs provide supervised care for a few hours—and even for days at a time—so that the family members can spend time doing the things they need or want to do without worrying about care responsibilities.

5. **Help families make arrangements for institutional placement, if necessary.** If the demands of caring for the impaired person become physically or psychologically excessive for the spouse or family, nursing home placement may be necessary. The family often needs assistance in making contact with these facilities or with a social worker who can help them with the planning. In addition to helping with the planning, nurses should provide emotional support to the family. The decision to move a loved one to a long-term care facility is exceedingly stressful, and the family is likely to experience feelings of helplessness or guilt.

6. **Encourage families to plan for end-of-life decisions.** The family needs to discuss issues such as a guardianship or health care decision maker. They should be encouraged to seek advice from the primary caregiver and a lawyer before severe mental deterioration occurs.

7. **Use any appropriate interventions that are used in the institutional setting.** (See Nursing Care Plan 10-1.)

★ Nursing Care Plan 10-1   Disturbed Thought Processes

Mr. Quick has a history of organic brain syndrome. He is not oriented to person, place, or time. He often cannot remember whether he has eaten or what he should be doing at any given time. His behaviors are sometimes socially inappropriate; for example, he wanders into rooms and takes the belongings of other residents. He has a very short attention span and is unable to follow most directions. He likes to wander the halls and often laughs to himself. He sometimes sits in the dayroom if the radio is playing and taps his foot to the music.

Nursing Diagnosis
Disturbed thought processes

Defining Characteristics
* Lack of orientation to person, place, and time
* Impaired ability to follow directions
* Short attention span
* Inappropriate social behaviors
* Inappropriate affect
* Repetitive behaviors

Patient Goals/Outcomes Identification
Mr. Quick will sustain no harm.

Nursing Interventions/Implementation
1. Address Mr. Quick by name.
2. Make eye contact before attempting to communicate.
3. Use pictures and familiar objects to orient him to his own room. Place a recognizable picture or other device at the door.
4. Provide a simple calendar or clock to help orient him to time.
5. Use simple language and short sentences.
6. Use concrete objects or other visual cues to explain things.
7. Allow adequate time for social interaction and communication.
8. Encourage participation in music therapy sessions.
9. Assess for changes in mental processes.
10. Notify the physician of significant changes in mental status.

Evaluation
Mr. Quick is still not oriented to person, place, or time. He continues to wander the halls on the unit when not distracted. He will sit still to fold and unfold towels or other repetitive tasks. He sings and claps along during music therapy sessions. You will continue the plan of care.

Critical Thinking Questions
1. What other activities can you identify that would be appropriate for Mr. Quick?
2. What safety precautions are needed if he continues to wander in the halls?

❖ NURSING PROCESS FOR IMPAIRED VERBAL COMMUNICATION

The ability to communicate by using words or language is a uniquely human skill. It is so much a part of our daily lives that we do not even consider the possibility of losing it. Yet many people are forced to live without the ability to speak or communicate through words. Individuals who experience cognitive or sensory changes commonly lose the ability to use words to communicate effectively.

Speech is the term used to refer to spoken language. Speech requires coordinated functioning of the brain, cranial nerves, pharynx, larynx, and lungs. The normal physiologic changes of aging affect the quality of speech. Normal speech in older adults tends to be slower, softer, less fluent, less rhythmic, and breathier than in younger individuals, and it often has a tremulous quality. Patients who suffer from neurologic damage affecting muscle control may experience more than usual difficulty with speech articulation, a condition called dysarthria. Speech is only a part of language.

Language is a broad term that includes all modes of spoken or symbolic communication. Language allows us to send and receive messages from other humans. We use language to convey our ideas and to make our wishes known to others. Without the ability to communicate, we are isolated from the world around us. Persons who lose the ability to use language or to speak are likely to experience problems. Older people with impaired verbal communication skills often become depressed, agitated, and frustrated, and they feel excluded from normal social interactions.

Language is a complex and not completely understood function of the brain. Both hemispheres of the cerebral cortex contribute to the process of encoding and decoding language, but two regions of the brain play key roles in language and speech: **Broca's area,** which is located in the posterior frontal lobe, and **Wernicke's area,** which is located in the posterior temporal lobe. If either of these areas is damaged by trauma or oxygen deprivation for prolonged periods of time from occlusion or hemorrhage, serious language problems can occur. The most common language problem seen in older adults is called **aphasia** (or dysphasia).

Dysphasia should not be confused with dysphagia, which is difficulty swallowing. Stroke or head trauma can cause both problems. Speech pathologists are an excellent resource for information about speech problems and swallowing disorders.

Aphasia has been classified in several different ways. The most common classification includes **receptive aphasia,** in which the person has difficulty understanding language; **expressive aphasia,** in which the person is unable to express himself or herself using language; and **global aphasia,** in which the person loses the ability both to understand language and to express himself or herself using language. Each of these categories has several subclassifications.

Receptive aphasia is not the same as deafness. Communication problems in deaf people are caused by mechanical or neurologic defects that do not allow sounds to enter the nervous system. Persons suffering from receptive aphasia hear sounds normally but are unable to give these sounds meaning. In some cases, this loss is complete; in others, only specific language reception is lost. Some persons cannot understand spoken words but can understand written words. Others can repeat the spoken words but cannot give any meaning to them. Still others can understand single words but not sentences or word combinations.

Like receptive aphasia, expressive aphasia comes in more than one form. Broca's aphasia is a common form in which the person is able to understand verbal and written language but is unable to speak words fluently. The area of the brain that coordinates the muscles of speech is damaged. This form of aphasia is particularly frustrating because the person knows what he or she wants to say but cannot get the words out. In **Wernicke's aphasia,** the person is able to speak, but the words produced may be nonsensical or have little connection with reality (Table 10-4).

The term *global aphasia* is used when receptive and expressive language skills are lost. Persons suffering from global aphasia are profoundly affected. If any communication ability remains, it is in the form of a single sound that may be repeated with a variety of pitches, rhythms, and emphasis.

When an older person loses the ability to talk with others, he or she finds it difficult, if not impossible, to maintain normal roles and relationships. Even those who fully retain their intellectual function and understanding are viewed differently if they cannot speak clearly. Once the ability to communicate has been damaged, these older persons find that they are no longer treated as capable, competent adults, but are instead treated as though they were deaf or mentally impaired. Friends, family, and even health care professionals are

Table **10-4** Comparison of Common Types of Aphasia	
BROCA'S APHASIA	**WERNICKE'S APHASIA**
Lesion in frontal lobe	Lesion in temporal lobe
Expressive or motor	Receptive or sensory
Speech is slow, labored, hesitant, nonfluent, poorly articulated	Speech is rapid, fluent, normal in tone, clearly articulated, and long and rambling
Short sentences with little grammatic structure	May follow stereotyped patterns
Nonsense or jargon speech indicates noncomprehension	

increasingly likely to avoid people with impaired communication skills. This avoidance is rarely deliberate; it occurs out of frustration or ignorance. Avoidance by others increases the likelihood of frustration, depression, social isolation, and loss of self-worth in older adults.

▪ Assessment/Data Collection

- Does the person have any sensory limitations? (See the assessment of disturbed sensory perception on pages 182–183.)
- Has the person experienced any injury or surgery that altered the normal speech mechanisms?
- Does the person have a history of cerebrovascular injury or disease?

▪ Nursing Diagnosis

Impaired verbal communication

▪ Nursing Goals/Outcomes Identification

The nursing goals for older individuals with impaired verbal communication are to (1) communicate needs with a minimal amount of frustration, (2) demonstrate an increased ability to communicate needs and feelings, and (3) express satisfaction with or acceptance of alternative methods of communication.

▪ Nursing Interventions/Implementation

The following interventions should take place in hospitals, in extended-care facilities, and at home:

1. **Assess the older person's communication problems and abilities.** Communication problems and abilities differ from person to person. It is important that nurses understand the specific problems and capabilities of each person so that the plan of care can be individualized to best meet the individual's needs.
2. **Identify specific approaches that are effective for each person.** Many techniques can facilitate communication. Nurses should try a variety of these to determine which are most effective. When working with a person who has impaired verbal communication, the nurse can use the following approaches: (1) Face the person when speaking, and establish eye contact; (2) speak slowly and clearly and in a low tone of voice; (3) speak in a normal tone of voice, and avoid shouting; (4) allow adequate time for communication (do not hurry the communication); (5) pace communication to avoid fatigue; (6) keep messages simple with one- or two-word phrases; and (7) use touch therapeutically.
3. **Document in the care plan the selected techniques that facilitate communication.** The specific approaches or techniques that are effective should be clearly documented in the plan of care so that all caregivers can use them consistently. This will reduce the frustration of both the affected person and the staff.
4. **Explain effective communication techniques to family members and friends.** Communication techniques should be explained to visitors, including family, friends, and clergy. This promotes positive interactions and enables both the affected person and his or her visitors to have a good experience. The more positive the interaction, the greater the likelihood of regular visits and interaction with the affected individual. This enables the person to maintain a somewhat more normal pattern of social interaction. It is wise to avoid large groups of visitors, which might interfere with the person's concentration and result in confusion, frustration, and fatigue.
5. **Teach verbally impaired older adults methods for their specific communicating needs.** If the person is unable to communicate verbally, nurses should provide flash cards, pads, pencils, picture boards, or magic slates. If unable to use these, the person should be encouraged to use gestures. Open-ended statements such as "Show me what you would do with (the item in question)" may help the individual describe his or her needs.
6. **Consult with a speech therapist/pathologist to determine the most effective communication strategies.** Speech therapists are specially trained to identify and treat communication disorders. Whenever possible, speech therapists should be consulted as soon as a communication problem is suspected. The recommendations should be incorporated into the plan of care and supported by all caregivers (Nursing Care Plan 10-2).

❖ NURSING PROCESS FOR PAIN

The origin of some stimuli, such as pain, is within the body. Either physiologic damage or psychological distress can result in the sensation we call *pain*. Pain is a subjective perception. It is what the person tells you it is. Everyone experiences pain in a unique way. Because no two people mean exactly the same thing when they say they have pain, nurses must attempt to detect and determine the severity of another person's pain through careful assessment.

Nurses can neither see pain nor measure pain with a meter, but they can detect its presence by careful listening and observation. Much information regarding the severity, quality, and location of pain can be gained from listening to how the person describes his or her pain; observing the individual's level of activity; and watching body language for subtle cues such as grimacing, guarding of a body part, or drawing away when a body part is touched. Various visual pain scales (Figure 10-7) can help determine the severity of pain.

Response to pain differs from person to person. Culture, sex, spiritual beliefs, and age all play a role in what a person considers painful and how he or she responds to it. Some people believe that pain and suffering are punishments or ways to atone for

⭐ **Nursing Care Plan 10-2** | **Impaired Verbal Communication**

Mr. White, age 68, suffers from Alzheimer's disease. He is able to understand simple commands and follow them. His speech is brief, hesitant, and garbled. It takes a long time for him to say anything. He often shakes his head and pauses when trying to think of words. He often repeats the phrase "Help me, help me." At times he becomes very frustrated when he cannot make his wishes known to his family or the staff. He spends much of his time alone in his room and has been observed crying after a particularly frustrating visit with his family.

Nursing Diagnosis
Impaired verbal communication

Defining Characteristics
• Garbled speech
• Inability to express ideas and feelings
• Inability to find words
• Inability to complete sentences

Patient Goals/Outcomes Identification
Mr. White will maintain the optimal level of interaction with family and staff.

Nursing Interventions/Implementation
1. Ask *yes/no* questions whenever possible.
2. Observe nonverbal communication.
3. Use touch to communicate empathy.
4. Speak slowly using short, simple sentences.
5. Repeat, rephrase, and restate messages.
6. Decrease environmental distractions.
7. Establish eye contact before starting communication.
8. Provide visual cues whenever possible.
9. Use pictures of familiar items.
10. Allow ample time for responses.
11. Explain basic communication techniques to family.
12. Consult with speech therapist regarding other communication techniques that may benefit Mr. White.

Evaluation
Mr. White follows some simple one- or two-word directions once his attention is obtained. He points to common objects on a picture board and occasionally leads caregivers to an object when told to "Show me." He continues to have episodes of crying and pleas of "Help me." His family states that he "seems less upset" when they sit with him in a quiet area or when they look at a family picture album. You will continue the plan of care.

Critical Thinking Questions
1. What other approaches could the nurse use to decrease Mr. White's frustration?
2. What intervention might help the family deal with Mr. White's diminishing communication ability?

wrongs they have done in their lives. Others believe that pain is a test of their faith.

Some cultures teach that a person should be stoic or uncomplaining or that pain should be hidden and tolerated with a minimal amount of intervention. Other cultures teach that it is acceptable to express pain by crying, moaning, and yelling. These individuals expect relief from the pain as quickly as possible. Nurses coming from one cultural perspective may be totally puzzled when confronted by patients from another. Nurses who think that a person who is quiet cannot be in pain often fail to look for pain in quiet patients. Nurses who are silent sufferers often become upset with the dramatic behavior of more demonstrative people.

Older adults are at increased risk for pain because of the higher incidence of disease conditions with aging. Some older adults have a decreased ability to sense pain, whereas others are highly sensitive to painful stimuli. There is no proof that pain decreases with aging. Pain influences the way older adults feel about themselves and how they interact with others. Chronic or unrelieved pain can lead to behavior changes. Older persons who demonstrate anger, depression, or isolation from others should be evaluated for pain.

Many older adults deny pain because they fear they will be avoided or lose their independence. They live with pain because they think that it is a normal part of growing old. It is not. Pain is an

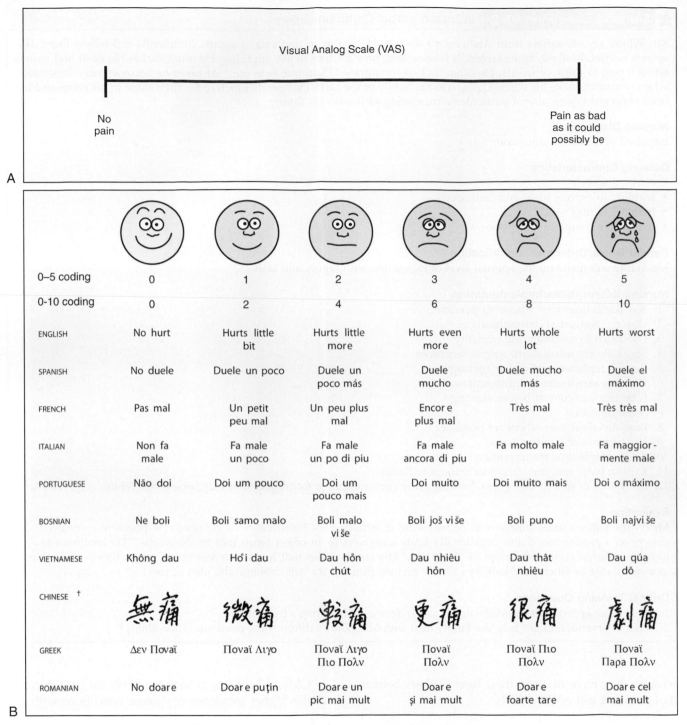

FIGURE 10-7 A, Visual analog scale. **B,** Wong FACES Pain Rating Scale.

indicator that something is wrong in the body. It does not have to be tolerated simply because the sufferer is old.

Determining the presence of pain in confused older persons is difficult. If pain is not recognized and assessed, serious harm may result. Failure to recognize pain can cause delays in the treatment of serious medical conditions and delays in response to a change in condition.

Confused older adults have difficulty interpreting painful stimuli, identifying the location, and communicating the nature of their distress to caregivers. They do not always respond to pain in the typical ways that nurses expect. Changes in body language, vital signs, and level of confusion are possible indicators of pain. The presence of pain is likely to result in agitation; increased pulse, respiratory rate, and blood pressure; and an increased level of confusion.

■ **Assessment/Data Collection**

- Does the person complain of pain?
- Is the pain constant or intermittent?
- Where is the pain?
- Is the pain generalized or localized?
- How does the person describe the pain (e.g., burning, stabbing, radiating, and gnawing)?
- How long has the person had the pain?
- Does the pain interfere with activities of daily living?
- Does the pain interfere with sleep?
- What helps the person control the pain?
- Does the person take any medication for the pain?
- What medication does the person take, and how often?

■ **Nursing Diagnoses**

- Pain
- Chronic pain

■ **Nursing Goals/Outcomes Identification**

The nursing goals for acute or chronic pain are to (1) report an improved comfort level or decrease in pain, (2) verbalize the ability to cope with pain, and (3) demonstrate techniques that provide relief from pain.

■ **Nursing Interventions/Implementation**

The following nursing interventions should take place in hospitals or extended-care facilities:

1. **Thoroughly assess the nature and severity of the pain.** Not all pain is the same. It is easy to miss significant changes in an older person's condition, particularly someone who suffers from chronic pain. A thorough assessment should be done to determine whether current pain is similar to previous pain or is different in degree, location, or severity. The mnemonic PQRST provides an organized plan so that all relevant areas are considered (Table 10-5). An alternative pain assessment tool uses the mnemonic COLDSPA which stands for character of the pain, onset, location, duration, severity, pattern and associated symptoms.

   If the person is cognitively impaired or noncommunicative, it is particularly important to watch nonverbal cues. Often, a close family member who knows the person's normal responses can help nurses interpret the person's behavior.

2. **Provide comfort measures.** Often, simple comfort measures (e.g., repositioning, giving a backrub, and toileting) can reduce pain. Fear and anxiety

Table 10-5 **PQRST Method for Pain Assessment**

COMPONENT	ASSESSMENT QUESTIONS	EXAMPLES
Provocation or Palliation	What activities or circumstances precede or cause the pain?	Pain occurs only when stomach is empty. Pain occurs after exercise.
	Did the pain occur suddenly or gradually?	Pain builds from mild to severe.
	What makes the pain better or worse?	Pain decreases with rest.
Quality	What does the pain feel like? (Try to elicit patient's own words.)	Dull, aching, sharp, burning crushing, stabbing, tearing, cramping, throbbing, grinding.
Region, Radiation, or Referral	Where is the pain located? Can the patient touch the specific area?	Pain localized in temporal region of skull.
	Does the pain remain localized to a small area or does it involve a larger area of the body?	Entire abdomen hurts.
	Is pain present in one or more areas of the body?	Pain in pelvic area and region of the scapula.
	Does the pain begin in one area and then move to another area? If so, where does the pain move to?	Pain starts in chest and radiates down left arm.
Severity	How severe is the pain on a scale of 1 to 10?	Pain reported at level 7.
	Which illustration best represents pain? (Use a picture board ranging from a happy face to a face with a frown and tears.)	
Timing	When did the pain start?	Pain first noted at 7 a.m.
	How long does the pain last?	Pain has been present for 6 hours.
	Is the pain continuous or intermittent?	Pain "comes and goes."
	Does the pain occur only at certain times of the day?	Pain noticed only during evening.
Additional questions	Has the patient experienced any pain like this in the past?	History of intermittent headaches.
	Is the current pain similar or different than previous episodes?	Current headache much more severe than ever experienced previously.
	Did the patient take any medication for pain?	
	Has the medication been effective at relieving pain? How effective? How long was it effective?	Acetaminophen reduces, but does not eliminate, the discomfort for 2 to 3 hours.

can increase pain. Listening to older adults and providing emotional support often help reduce pain.

3. **Avoid actions that increase pain.** Simple actions such as jarring the bed or moving an individual too rapidly can increase pain. Because movement may increase pain, care should be used when moving, transferring, or otherwise touching persons in pain. Often a simple touch, an explanation of what to expect, or acknowledgment of the pain shows that the nurse is sensitive to the feelings of the older person.

4. **Anticipate situations likely to cause pain.** Because confused persons are unable to report pain accurately, nurses need to anticipate activities or procedures that are likely to cause pain and institute measures to prevent or reduce it.

5. **Teach nonpharmacologic approaches to pain control.** Many nonpharmacologic approaches are available for pain control. Biofeedback, meditation, hypnosis, and imagery are all useful in pain control. These techniques often are not attempted with older adults because caregivers think that they will not accept or understand the techniques. Many older adults are not only capable of learning these techniques, but they are pleased to have some control in the relief of pain.

6. **Administer medications as ordered.** Studies have shown that nurses tend to underestimate rather than overestimate pain in others. This leads to more suffering than is needed. Nurses are often afraid that administering medication will lead to addiction or dependence. In fact, timely administration of medication before pain becomes severe actually decreases the total amount of medication used. The types and dosages of medications used to control pain in older adults are highly individualized and may differ from those used with younger adults.

The following interventions should take place in the home:

1. **Help older adults and their families develop a plan to cope with pain.** Pain, particularly the chronic pain endured by many older persons, can be physically and psychologically exhausting for the affected person and his or her loved ones. Nurses should help those living at home to develop a plan built on the interventions that are most effective for them. Older adults and their families should be shown how to incorporate these pain-relief measures into daily activities so that pain is kept to a minimum and the person is able to lead as normal a lifestyle as possible.

2. **Use any appropriate interventions that are used in the institutional setting.**

Get Ready for the NCLEX® Examination!

Key Points

- Perceptual changes are among the most common problems experienced by older adults.
- Disturbed vision and hearing present multiple concerns related to safety and lifestyle.
- Pain, although not a routine problem of aging, can interfere with the older person's ability to lead a fulfilling life.
- Nurses must be alert to cognitive and perceptual changes and identify ways to support as normal a lifestyle as possible.
- Providing care for older individuals who are experiencing severe cognitive changes, particularly those with dementia, challenges the skills and capabilities of nurses, families, and all health care providers.
- Ongoing assessment of perceptual and cognitive functioning is necessary to detect subtle but potentially dangerous changes.
- Prompt recognition of problems and careful selection of appropriate interventions will allow the aging person to maintain the highest level of function possible.

Additional Learning Resources

SG   Go to the Study Guide on pp. 379–397 for additional learning activities to help you master the chapter content.

⊝volve Go to your Evolve website (http://evolve.elsevier.com/Wold/geriatric) for the following FREE learning resources:
- Animations
- Answer Guidelines for Nursing Care Plan Critical Thinking Questions
- Answers and Rationales for Review Questions for the NCLEX® Examination
- Glossary with pronunciations in English and Spanish
- Video Clips

Review Questions for the NCLEX® Examination

1. Hearing aids are worn by many older people. Which statement regarding hearing aids is false?

    1. Batteries should be stored in the refrigerator.
    2. Ear molds should be cleaned regularly.
    3. Most people easily adjust to hearing aid use.
    4. Hearing aids are fragile.

2. The nurse should use care when assessing pain level in the elderly because: (Select all that apply.)

   1. Chronic pain is more common with aging.
   2. Older people are able to tolerate more pain than younger persons.
   3. Older people have decreased sensory perception of pain.
   4. Cognitive changes may alter the ability to report and describe pain.
   5. Elderly people may deny pain for various reasons.
   6. Behavioral changes may be indicators of pain.

3. The condition which is least likely to be reversible is:

   1. Dementia
   2. Delirium
   3. Confusion
   4. Depression

4. The nurse explains to a family member that the most appropriate environment for a person suffering from dementia is one that has:

   1. Lots of color and textures
   2. Subdued lighting and soft music
   3. Bright lights and a TV for stimulation
   4. Common and familiar objects

5. When an elderly person with dementia resists efforts to reposition or ambulate, the nurse should suspect the person is:

   1. Having a medication reaction
   2. Being stubborn
   3. Becoming more confused
   4. Experiencing pain

11

Self-Perception and Self-Concept

Objectives

1. Discuss the concepts of self-perception and self-concept.
2. Describe how self-perception and self-concept change with aging.
3. Discuss the effects of disease processes on self-perception and self-concept.
4. Identify signs of later-life depression.
5. Identify suicide risk in older adults.
6. Describe methods of assessing changes in self-perception and self-concept.
7. Identify older adults who are most at risk for experiencing problems related to self-perception and self-concept.
8. Identify selected nursing diagnoses related to self-perception or self-concept problems.
9. Describe nursing interventions that are appropriate for older adults experiencing problems related to self-perception and self-concept.

Key Terms

anxiety (p. 201)
body image (p. 204)
depression (p. 201)
fear (p. 201)
feedback (p. 200)

helplessness (p. 201)
hopelessness (p. 201)
powerlessness (p. 201)
self-esteem (p. 200)

NORMAL SELF-PERCEPTION AND SELF-CONCEPT

The attitudes and perceptions people have about themselves, their abilities, and their self-worth make up what is often called *self-identity*. People form their self-identities from their values, life experiences, and interactions with others. People with good self-worth and high self-esteem share certain characteristics. They have strong personal values and believe that they have the ability to control their lives. They have had positive life experiences and have received positive feedback from others. People with poor self-worth and low self-esteem tend to have weak personal values and think that they have little control over their lives. They have had primarily negative life experiences and have received negative feedback from others.

We form our self-identities by comparing ourselves and our experiences with some ideal. This can be an internal ideal drawn from our personal values or an external ideal drawn from the society around us. Many people experience problems with self-worth because they always measure themselves against external standards. Contemporary standards are communicated repeatedly by advertising and the media. People who are young, thin, rich, successful, and attractive are idealized. Anyone who does not meet these superficial and artificial standards is somehow judged inferior and thus is viewed negatively by our society. Few people are able to meet all of the idealized criteria. This results in a large number of people (of all ages) in contemporary society who suffer from negative self-esteem.

In trying to meet external standards, people are likely to lose themselves and their internal values. The more we look to the external forces, the less likely we are to have high self-esteem. The more we look internally for our self-worth, the more satisfied we will be in the long run. Shakespeare summed it up nicely in *Hamlet:* "This above all: to thine own self be true/And it must follow, as the night the day, thou canst not then be false to any man." (I, iii, 75).

It is easy to say that people should draw on internal ideals to maintain self-esteem, but this is difficult in light of external pressures and feedback. In today's society, people usually have more negative experiences than positive ones. Therefore, problems relating to self-perception and self-esteem are common in people of all ages. Problems relating to self-esteem are particularly common among the poor, the infirm, and older adults. Studies have shown that women tend to have lower self-esteem until they reach their eighties or nineties. Not surprisingly, it was also found that health and wealth have positive effects on self-esteem.

Actions That Caregivers Can Use to Promote Self-Esteem

- Help older adults find interests, activities or hobbies, even learn a new skill.
- Encourage volunteering, social interaction, and participation in social gatherings.
- Seek guidance or mentoring from older adults and listen to their advice. Avoid "talking down" to older adults.
- Keep older adults informed, and encourage them to maintain control of their health.

Feedback from others affects our perception of ourselves. People who have caring friends and families tend to have higher levels of self-identity and self-esteem. Strong families and friends provide support for one another. They help one another keep things in perspective by providing positive feedback and buffering one another from an often negative world. A good family and good friends play an important part in building and maintaining our self-esteem. Persons who lack supportive family and friends are likely to have a poor perception of self and low self-esteem. Those who come from dysfunctional families or who are separated from loved ones run a high risk for poor self-perception and low self-esteem. These people are more likely to suffer from negative feedback because they lack the necessary support to provide balance.

A real or perceived ability to make choices plays an important role in self-perception and self-esteem. People who feel capable of controlling what happens perceive things far differently from those who perceive no control over their lives. Our sense of self-control starts with our bodies. Adults are used to having control of their bodies and bodily functions. Control of the movement of body parts and of elimination are so basic we do not even think of them—at least not until we lose control of them for some reason. Consider how you would feel if tomorrow you woke up and could not move or could not control your bladder or bowels. Would your sense of self-worth and self-esteem change? Adults are also used to having control and making choices regarding their activities. Choices regarding activities of daily living (e.g., hygiene practices, amount and type of clothing, amount and type of food, and amount and type of exercise and sleep) are determined by and are reflections of an adult's self-perception and level of self-esteem. Loss of control results in **depression, powerlessness, helplessness, hopelessness, fear,** and **anxiety.** Loss of control destroys self-esteem (see Health Promotion box).

Health Promotion

Six Ways the Elderly Can Improve Self-Esteem by Taking Control

1. **Take control of your attitude.** Attitude is an important part of aging. Health is not the best measure of successful aging—attitude is. A positive attitude is the starting point to taking control of other areas of life. Have a "can do" frame of mind. Seek out small changes at first—ones that you can make easily. A success will increase positive attitude and enhance your motivation to keep trying.

2. **Take control of your health.** See your physician and dentist regularly. Follow a regular exercise plan. Eat balanced meals. Get enough sleep.

3. **Take control of your appearance.** Stand up straight and hold your head high. Take time to dress up, have your hair styled, wear make-up, get a manicure, shave, buy some new clothes (or use some of the items that have been given as gifts and are hiding in your closet or drawers).

3. **Take control of your time.** Be as active as you can. Establish a schedule that gets you up and moving. Plan to get out for visits, shopping, or activities—or just a walk several times a week. Better still, at least once a day.

4. **Take control of your social life and relationships.** Call friends and family; do not wait for them to call you. Go to church or a social gathering, join a book club, or do anything you enjoy where you may meet new people and form new friendships.

5. **Take interest in both old and new activities.** Recognize any physical limitations but do not use them as an excuse for inactivity. Take up old hobbies or find new ones. Find out what classes are offered at the senior center, library, or community college. Find a part-time job, or volunteer.

Problems related to self-perception and self-esteem are not as obvious as are physical problems. By their very nature, self-perception and self-concept are subjective. Many people find it difficult to talk about their feelings, often finding themselves unable or unwilling to put their feelings into words. More often, our perceptions of self-worth and self-esteem are exhibited to others through behavior. Significant behaviors include the amount of attention paid to personal hygiene and grooming, the type and frequency of emotions exhibited, body posture, the amount and type of eye contact, and voice and speech patterns. People with very high self-esteem appear to be very much in control of themselves and their lives. They are usually well groomed, maintain an erect body posture, make eye contact with others, speak clearly in a normal tone of voice, and exhibit emotions appropriate to a given situation.

People with very low self-esteem often appear disinterested and out of control. They often appear unkempt or disheveled. They may slump or slouch, and there seems to be little purpose to their movement.

Eye contact is infrequent. The amount of communication with others is reduced, is negative in nature, and is often mumbled or abrupt. Emotions can vary from expressions of sadness to full-blown anger.

Most people's self-esteem and behavior fall between these two extremes. As long as behavior falls within the accepted range of normal, people tend to disregard or overlook what is going on inside other people. Only when behaviors move outside of the normal range do we seriously attempt to understand what is happening inside the person to cause those behaviors.

SELF-PERCEPTION/SELF-CONCEPT AND AGING

Erikson has identified the major task of late life as maintenance of ego integrity (the sense of self-worth) versus despair. Attitudes toward aging, the level of self-esteem throughout life, the extent of physical change caused by aging and illness, the presence or absence of emotional support systems, and the ability to maintain a degree of control—all of these have an impact on whether aging adults will be successful in accomplishing this task.

Aging individuals develop their own perceptions of aging. It is difficult to see oneself getting old. Many older adults express dismay with the realization and can even identify a particular moment when they perceived themselves as old. One older woman recently attended her fiftieth high school reunion. She reported having a good time but wondered what she was doing with all of these "old people." A subtle but real change in her self-perception occurred after that incident. Before then, she did not feel old; afterward, she was more aware of her age. Successful aging is not so much a matter of years lived or health status, but rather a matter of perception and attitude. Successful aging has sometimes been described as "mind over matter." If you don't mind, it doesn't matter.

Poor self-concept, depression, and other negative feelings can be seen in the older population, although they are not as common as once believed. Studies have shown that the percentage of older adults experiencing problems appears to be no higher than among other age groups. Older adults who have had a poor self-concept throughout their lives are not likely to gain self-esteem with aging. Older adults who had a healthy level of self-esteem during their younger days may experience some problems during aging, but these are most often a result of societal attitudes.

Ageism is still prevalent in our youth-oriented society, which far too often portrays older adults as physically and mentally inept, nonproductive, and dependent. Considering these negative images of aging, it is easy to understand why many people do all within their power to avoid the physical signs of aging. It is difficult for some younger people to understand how radically the changes of age or illness can destroy self-image and self-esteem in older adults. Many younger persons feel that measures such as hair transplants or cosmetic surgery look absurd. They mock older adults, further lowering the aging person's self-worth. It will be interesting to see what these insensitive people do as they age. One can only wonder what societal attitudes toward aging will be and how they will change as Baby Boomers move into old age.

Older people who accept the negative societal perceptions are likely to suffer more than do those older adults who refuse to accept these stereotypes. Unfortunately, those who start with the poorest self-concept are the ones who are most likely to accept the negatives and are particularly vulnerable to loss of self-worth. Physical, social, and economic changes that occur with aging result in changes in the way older adults perceive themselves and their bodies. The greater the amount of change, the more likely the person is to experience problems related to self-concept. Small changes in appearance or function (e.g., wrinkles or aches and pains) nibble at the edges of self-worth. Serious illnesses (particularly those that result in obvious disfigurement or major loss of function, such as strokes) take a large toll on the aging person's perception of self.

Frequent and significant losses (including decreasing physical health; decreasing mental quickness; loss of significant others; loss of pride in appearance, roles, or possessions; and loss of independence) threaten the perception of control that is important to most adults. These losses can result in a variety of problems, which often increase in severity if left unchecked.

Institutional placement further damages self-worth by stripping older adults of many of the personal belongings that make up the visible part of their identity. Facilities that are able to accommodate more than a small amount of clothing and a few mementos of a lifetime are rare. A lifetime of 80 years is often reduced to a small closet and bedside stand.

Although losses of physical and functional abilities are damaging to self-worth, loss of the emotional support of loved ones is even more devastating. Death is an increasingly common visitor to older adults. This does not make it less frightening; rather it is a reminder of one's own mortality. The friends and loved ones who made life worthwhile slip away, one by one. The positive messages that a person is worthwhile, lovable, and loved become less frequent, and the reasons for living disappear. Losses resulting from death or separation from friends and family can leave older adults without those sources of positive feedback that nourish self-worth.

We cannot prevent loss resulting from death, but loss resulting from separation is another matter. Older adults who are separated from their families and significant others are at increased risk for experiencing diminished self worth. Breakdown of the extended family and increased geographic mobility may result in isolation of older adults, though some studies have shown that this is not as great a problem as often cited. Although a large percentage of the elderly do not reside with family members, they often live alone by choice. A majority of older adults report that they continue to have regular and frequent contact with grown children either in person or by phone.

Separation from family is often associated with placement in an institutional setting. In spite of the fact that institutional placement is usually the last choice after all other alternatives have failed, older adults often feel rejected and isolated when nursing home placement is necessary. It is a natural response for older adults to feel they have been "put away" because they have little value or worth. These individuals often feel unimportant, unloved, and unwanted. Even if this is completely untrue, the perception greatly decreases their sense of self-worth. If family and friends visit often and show positive concern, self-esteem can be maintained. Unfortunately, this is not always the case. It is in institutional settings—where nobody really knows or cares about the inner person—that many older adults lose their remaining sense of self-esteem and self-worth.

DEPRESSION AND AGING

Depression is more common in the aging population than often suspected or recognized. Studies indicate the magnitude of the problem. It is estimated that among people over age 65, depression is a problem for as many as 1% to 9% of community-dwelling elderly, 10% to 26% or more of long-term care residents, and 11% to 46% of hospitalized older adults. Research estimates that only 1 in 6 elderly who suffer from depression is recognized and treated. Depression is more difficult to recognize because typical indicators may be similar to those seen with a variety of medical disorders. For example, weight changes, changes in sleep patterns, decreased energy, and changes in psychomotor activity are signs of depression but also signs of numerous medical problems. Sudden behavioral or personality changes are not a normal part of aging. Depression may be related to a wide range of factors, including loss of independence or loved ones or increased medical problem such as hypothyroidism, anemia, and diabetes. Use of medications to treat disease such as antihypertensives, antiarrhythmics, anticholesterolemics, cardiac glycosides, analgesics, and hormones such as corticosteroids and progesterone are all associated with increased incidence of depression. Careful assessment is necessary to recognize

problems with depression before they result in other, even more serious problems. Some changes that warrant further investigation include the following:
- Stopping normal routines
- Neglected self-care
- Unwillingness to talk
- Agitation and irritability
- Suspiciousness or unjustified fears
- Mood swings
- Isolation and withdrawal
- Increased use of alcohol or mood-altering drugs
- Unexplained injuries
- Verbalization of worthlessness
- Verbalization of suicidal thoughts

SUICIDE AND AGING

The elderly make up about 12% of the total U.S. population, but they account for 17% of the suicides. Older adults at risk for suicide because of depression often present themselves to health care professionals with a variety of physical complaints. Many times, an elderly person has been seen by a health professional shortly before committing suicide (often the previous day), but the real significance of the complaints was missed. More elderly women experience depression but depressed older men and older adults with a history of affective disorders are most at risk for committing suicide. Severe emotional or physical pain, a recent loss, or stressful event such as diagnosis of a terminal disease are present in a large percentage of those who attempt to take their own lives.

Older adults have a higher rate of successful suicides than do other age groups. They tend to use more violent methods to end their lives. Firearms, overdose, and suffocation are common methods used. Seniors are less likely to communicate their intentions, although statements regarding helplessness or hopelessness, sudden interest in firearms, sudden revision of a will, or verbalization about suicide should never be ignored. Family members and health care professionals can help by being aware of warning signs and risk factors. Prompt referral to a mental health professional is wise if problems are suspected.

■ Nursing Process for Disturbed Self-Perception and Self-Concept

When an older adult has a poor self-concept, fears and anxieties increase. As control over one's life decreases, self-esteem plummets even lower, and older adults fall victim to feelings of hopelessness and powerlessness, which lead to depression. Depression leads to isolation from others, further decreasing the sense of self-worth.

■ Assessment
- Does the person verbalize fears or concerns?
- Are these fears of a known or an unknown source?

- Does the person verbalize loss of control over his or her life?
- Has the person recently experienced significant losses?
- Has the person recently moved or been separated from significant others?
- What is the person's general appearance and posture?
- Does the person make or avoid eye contact?
- Does the person verbalize concerns regarding changes in his or her appearance?
- Does the person make negative comments regarding himself or herself?
- Does the person avoid looking in the mirror or at altered body parts?
- Does the person question his or her worth?
- Does the person verbalize feelings of failure?
- Does the person verbalize hopelessness or despair?
- Does the person spend most of the time alone, or does he or she interact with others?
- Does the person accept directions from caregivers passively, or does the person express the desire to make his or her own decisions?
- Does the person exhibit aggression, anger, or demanding behaviors?
- Are there any signs of autonomic nervous system stimulation (e.g., increased pulse or respiratory rate, elevated blood pressure, diaphoresis)?
- Does the person manifest any behaviors typical of emotional upset (e.g., pacing, hand wringing, crying, repetitive motions, tics, aggressiveness)?
- Are there changes in vocal quality (e.g., quivering)?
- Does the person complain of headaches?
- Does the person have difficulty focusing on activities, remembering things, or making decisions?
- Has the person experienced changes in eating or sleeping patterns?
- Has the person started to give away treasured possessions?
- Does the person use alcohol or other mood-altering drugs? Which drugs? How much? How often?
- Does the person verbalize the desire to end his or her life?

Box 11-1 provides a list of risk factors for altered self-perception and self-concept in older adults.

Box 11-1	Risk Factors Related to Self-Perception and Self-Concept in Older Adults

- Conditions that result in change of body appearance (burns, obesity, skin lesions, chemotherapy, disfiguring endocrine disorders such as acromegaly or Cushing's disease, surgical removal of body parts)
- Inability to control bodily functions
- Significant losses (of significant others, possessions, social roles, financial status)
- Recent relocation (particularly if involuntary)
- Chronic pain

❖ NURSING PROCESS FOR DISTURBED BODY IMAGE

People experiencing body image disturbance are likely to refuse to look at or touch the affected body parts. In severe disturbances, the individual may deny that the change has occurred and act as though nothing has happened. Many persons who suffer with this problem are unwilling to discuss their concerns with others for fear that they will be rejected or made to feel different. If they are willing to verbalize their concerns, they may speak of themselves in a disembodied way, as though the deformity or change is not really happening to them. They may speak of themselves negatively or with a great deal of disgust that they are no longer who they once were. They may become preoccupied with their body function and excessively concerned about every minor change. They may need reassurance that nothing else will happen to them. Many persons with altered body image refuse to participate in their own care and resist any plans for rehabilitation. They are likely to verbalize feelings of worthlessness and powerlessness.

■ Assessment/Data Collection

See the assessment for disturbed self-perception and self-concept starting on page 203.

■ Nursing Diagnosis

Disturbed body image

■ Nursing Goals/Outcomes Identification

The nursing goals for older adults with disturbed body image are to (1) verbalize concerns regarding changes in body appearance or function, (2) identify their personal strengths, (3) acknowledge and look at the actual changes in body appearance, (4) verbalize willingness to modify lifestyle to accommodate physical changes, and (5) demonstrate readiness to participate in therapy and use necessary assistive devices.

■ Nursing Interventions/Implementation

The following interventions should take place in hospitals, in extended-care facilities, and at home:

1. **Assess the older individual's perceptions of self, including strengths and support systems.** Even with serious impairment, older adults can have strengths that will help them cope with change. Nurses need to identify the unique strengths of each person so that these can be drawn on when planning care.
2. **Establish a trusting relationship.** To help older adults work through and accept physical changes or deformities, nurses must demonstrate acceptance both verbally and nonverbally. Actively listening to concerns and planning care to include opportunities for the patient to verbalize his or her feelings can help build trust.

3. **Provide care in a nonjudgmental manner.** Because nurses are the people most likely to actually see any deformity, it is particularly important that they show no sign of revulsion or disgust when providing care. Nurses must take particular care not to show even subtle body language or facial expressions that could be perceived by older adults as a sign of nonacceptance.

4. **Encourage the person to look at and touch affected body areas.** Nurses are so used to seeing physical deformities (e.g., stomas and amputations) that they may not be aware of just how frightening these are to the affected person. Many people need time and encouragement to even look at the affected body part. Some depersonalize the change and refer to "it" as though the deformity was something apart from themselves. Looking at and touching the deformity will help the person accept reality. Until he or she is able to do this, the individual will not be ready for teaching or self-care.

5. **Focus on abilities, not disabilities.** To become motivated, a person must feel that he or she is capable of doing the activity. Most older adults—even those with severe deformities—are capable of doing something. Focusing on what can be done instead of on what cannot be done promotes feelings of self-worth.

6. **Assist in selecting clothing and/or dressing older adults in a manner that deemphasizes body changes.** Clothing that draws attention away from obvious deformities helps maintain body image. Sweaters, lap robes, and properly fitted clothing can be used to make deformities less obvious.

7. **Ensure that the person is carefully groomed.** Soiled clothing should be changed promptly. The face and hands should always be kept clean and free from food or other debris. Little things such as neatly combed or styled hair, a shave, or the application of a tasteful amount of makeup can make the person feel better about his or her appearance. How a person looks makes a difference in how that person feels. Remember, though, that an older person should never be made to look "cute." Older adults should always be groomed appropriately for their age.

8. **Coordinate rehabilitative care with other departments.** Physical therapy, occupational therapy, speech therapy, pharmacy, and other departments may be involved in the care of individuals who have experienced significant changes in body function. Nurses spend the most time with these individuals and are most aware of the total effect of various therapies. Nurses should coordinate these activities in the care plan to ensure that all groups are working toward the same goals. It is also important for nurses to monitor their patients' responses to the therapy and their ability to tolerate the effort required in therapy.

❖ NURSING PROCESS FOR RISK FOR SITUATIONAL LOW SELF-ESTEEM

Older adults are at risk for losing self-esteem for many reasons. Those who have low self-esteem are likely to display certain characteristic behaviors. Body language of persons with low self-esteem is similar to that of depressed individuals. They are often observed with their head slumped on the chest or shoulder; the facial expression is one of sadness; and they usually avoid eye contact. These individuals are likely to speak of themselves in negative terms. Statements such as "Don't waste your time on me" or "I can't do anything right" are indicative of low self-esteem. The speech of individuals with low self-esteem is full of statements of sadness, loss, depression, anxiety, and anger. They can see little that is positive about their lives and tend to focus on negative experiences. People with low self-esteem pay little attention to hygiene or grooming. They tend to be very passive, letting caregivers control all facets of their lives. They may demonstrate extreme dependence on others, even if they are capable of doing things for themselves. They are unlikely to initiate activities, and if they do, they are likely to leave activities unfinished. They are resistant to positive feedback and may argue or become angry with anyone attempting to give it. Older adults with low self-esteem are likely to avoid social contact; if forced to be in contact with others, they tend to avoid interaction and stay at the edges of the group or activity.

■ Assessment/Data Collection

See the assessment for disturbed self-perception and self-concept on pages 203-204.

■ Nursing Diagnosis

Risk for situational low self-esteem

■ Nursing Goals/Outcomes Identification

The nursing goals for older adults with self-esteem disturbances are to (1) identify personal strengths, (2) express feelings and concerns, and (3) practice behaviors that promote self-confidence.

■ Nursing Interventions/Implementation

The following nursing interventions should take place in hospitals, in extended-care facilities, and at home:

1. **Explore feelings and concerns.** To plan effective interventions that will improve feelings of self-worth, nurses must be aware of the unique concerns and feelings of each older individual.

2. **Demonstrate acceptance of older adults as people with value and self-worth by responding to concerns, encouraging them to make choices, following through with their requests, and including them in care planning.** Taking time to actually listen and respond to the needs communicated by

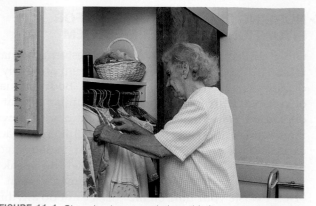

FIGURE 11-1 Choosing her own clothes, this long-term resident is actively participating in her own care and is able to retain her sense of self-worth.

older adults is the best way of demonstrating acceptance. Too often, the nurses "listen" and then do something completely different from what the older person requested. This is a subtle way of indicating that the person does not matter. If nurses are unable to comply with the aging person's requests, an explanation should be given so that the individual understands the reasons.

3. **Encourage participation in self-care activities.** Participation in self-care activities allows older adults to retain a sense of self-worth. Even small acts such as washing their own faces or eating a piece of toast can help make older adults feel some control over their own lives (Figure 11-1).

4. **Provide opportunities for reminiscence. Reminiscence,** sometimes called *life review,* is a phenomenon that is especially important to older adults. Nurses tend to focus on the present. Because there is so much to do, we do not take time to listen to old stories. We are so busy making sure that older adults are oriented to the present that we tend to forget about their past. Some nurses think that talking about all of the "old stuff" is downright boring. Nurses even make the mistake of thinking that participating in these often sentimental and nostalgic conversations is inappropriate, unnecessary, and not a part of nursing care at all. These errors can result in nurses missing important information regarding the mental health and self-esteem of the aging person.

All people, particularly older adults, need to feel that their existence has made a difference. As death approaches, older adults need to feel that their lives have had purpose and meaning. Absence of self-worth leads to despair and hopelessness. Erikson stressed the importance of seeing value in the life stories of older adults.

People of all ages reminisce (i.e., think back to earlier times in their lives). This process helps people work through previous problems and recognize previous successes. It helps resolve conflicts and enables older adults to cope with the present and future and to go on with life and living. Life review is not just looking back at the good old times; rather it is a process of determining that one's life has had value and merit. It is a way to meet the challenges of the present, and it is a way to prepare for death.

Older adults who have completed a life review—either on their own or with assistance—seem to have a certain serenity. They accept that, although not perfect, their lives have been worthwhile. Some find areas of discontent that they are still able to correct: They can still find lost friends, finish incomplete personal business, and make amends. Life review is a healthy process. It is a normal and necessary way that all individuals, particularly older adults, can maintain mental health.

Reminiscing can be done individually or in groups. Older adults who reminisce alone (as many do) are often highly critical of themselves, feeling that they did not make the right choices and do the right things. By reminiscing with others, the true value and merit of life often become clearer. Group sharing tends to be less intense than one-on-one communication. In addition, the memories of one person often trigger similar recollections among other group members. Different perspectives on situations can help older adults see themselves and their responses in a different light.

When working with a group of older adults, nurses should ensure that the group is not too large, or some individuals will not have an opportunity to participate. Five to eight people can effectively participate in a group at one time. It is essential that nurses remain open and actively listen to all participants. Reminiscence therapy may even be beneficial to individuals suffering from Alzheimer's disease by stimulating remnants of long-term memory.

Various devices can be used to stimulate reminiscences. Items such as picture albums and old movies, magazines, newspapers, or songs can be used to start the conversation. Activities such as writing poems, assembling picture albums, making collages, or writing an autobiography may be helpful. Open statements such as "Tell me about when you started your family or tell me about your job" can be helpful as well.

5. **Encourage the family to participate in reminiscence by providing pictures or items that bring back memories of happy times** (Figure 11-2). Families should be encouraged to take the opportunity to share in the memories of their older members. Many families find boxes of old pictures among the older person's belongings. Sometimes the people and events are familiar; other times they include many unknown and unfamiliar individuals. A review of these pictures often helps trigger memories in older adults and enables them to show a side of themselves that their adult children and grandchildren never knew anything about. Pictures of

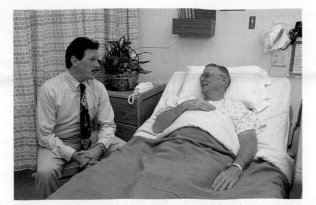

FIGURE 11-2 Reminiscing with the patient about his family history promotes self-esteem in older adults.

a smiling young couple kissing, dancing, taking their children to the park, or taking part in any number of other activities can help the older person remember better times. It can also help the family realize that, like themselves, their parents really were young once—facing the same dreams and challenges. This knowledge can help them grow closer and more aware of the continuity of family and can provide an opening for older people and their families to share feelings that they might otherwise feel uncomfortable addressing (Figure 11-3).

6. **Encourage families to communicate positive feelings to the older person.** Too often, especially at funerals, grief-stricken family members are heard to say, "I wish I had told my mother (or father) how much she (or he) meant to me." The best

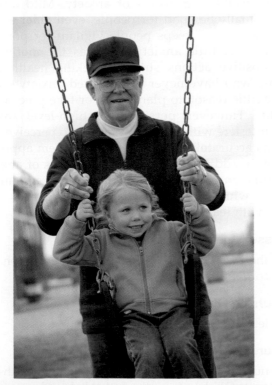

FIGURE 11-3 Bringing young and old together is an important part of the self-esteem of older adults.

way to prevent these regrets is to say and do these things when the older person is still alive. It means a lot to all of us to hear that we are appreciated and loved. It means even more to older adults, who may be questioning whether their lives have had any meaning. Young family members are often hesitant to say positive things face to face because they assume that the older person knows how they feel or because they just feel awkward saying them. It is interesting to observe how many people have no trouble saying something negative but seem unable to put something positive into words. It is no wonder that so many people, particularly older adults, have an altered sense of self-worth.

The greeting card industry has capitalized on this fact by mass-producing cards to help people convey feelings they cannot verbalize. Many older adults treasure greeting cards they receive from family because this is the closest they get to true communication of feelings from family members. Sometimes families need to be reminded and encouraged to meet the need for positive support. Anything nurses can do to help families recognize the importance of positive communication will help older adults (Box 11-2).

■ Nursing Process for Fear

Fear is a feeling of dread or apprehension regarding an identified source. Fear is not unique to older adults, but as functional abilities decrease, fears may become

---

Box 11-2 | Computers to Enhance Communication

Computer use among older adults lags behind that of younger generations, but it has been shown to have many benefits when introduced and encouraged. The following are some benefits that have been identified by research:

• Enhanced self-esteem
• Increased sense of productivity
• Decreased depression
• Improved social interaction
• Improved mental stimulation

The most common types of computer activities studied included word and board-type games, computer art activities, and e-mail communications.

To mediate some age-related changes in vision, hearing, and mobility, computer manufacturers are constantly improving their technology, including features such as touch screens and voice-activated commands.

I can attest to at least one senior citizen's positive experiences on the computer. Seeing the pride and confidence that my father-in-law (91 years "young") in Wisconsin demonstrated said it all when he was sending digital photos of a new great-grandchild to grandchildren in Hawaii, Alabama, Virginia, and California. He says he still prefers "snail mail" that he can hold onto and read at his leisure; on the other hand, if e-mail is the way his grandchildren around the world want to communicate, he is all in favor of it because he hears from them more often.

more obvious. The most common fears identified in older adults include fears of change and disruption in their lives or routines, crime and victimization, loss of loved ones, disease, injury, pain and suffering, loss of independence, financial destitution, and loneliness. It is interesting to note that death was not the most feared item; in fact, many older people express less fear of death than do younger persons. They may state that they fear the unknown, but not death itself. Many even view death as a release from fears and an opportunity to rejoin loved ones.

Fear is closely related to anxiety. Individuals with known fears usually also experience anxiety, although anxiety can occur without a known fear. People respond to fear in different ways. Some might verbalize feelings of helplessness, others might withdraw from contact with other people, and still others might respond aggressively. Aggressive responses to fear are often misinterpreted by caregivers as anger. Fear can also result in physiologic symptoms resulting from stimulation of the sympathetic nervous system. Such symptoms include dilated pupils, dry mouth, trembling, elevated blood pressure, increased pulse and respiratory rate, palpitations, diaphoresis, diarrhea, and urinary frequency. Physiologic stimulation caused by high-level anxiety can be dangerous to aging individuals who are already compromised by endocrine, respiratory, cardiovascular, or neurologic disease.

■ Assessment/Data Collection

See the assessment for disturbed self-perception and self-concept on pages 203-204.

■ Nursing Diagnosis

Fear

■ Nursing Goals/Outcomes Identification

The nursing goals for fearful individuals are to (1) identify specific fears, (2) identify coping strategies that were helpful in the past and use these when fears arise, and (3) use strategies that help control fear.

■ Nursing Interventions/Implementation

The following interventions should take place in hospitals, in extended-care facilities, and at home:

1. **Provide opportunities for older adults to express their fears.** Fear is debilitating. It stops people from being able to take positive actions. Identifying fears is the first step in dealing with them. If older adults demonstrate signs of fear during care, nurses should stop the activity and give the individual the opportunity to express his or her fears. These fears should then be taken into account when planning a strategy to reduce or eliminate them. Nurses should be careful not to minimize or deny the person's fears. Avoid using clichés such as "Don't

worry, we know what we're doing," because such statements convey the idea that the person's feelings are not valid.

2. **Remove or reduce the most common sources of fear.** Each of us fears different things. Fear of falling and fear of loud noises are common from the time of birth. Falling is a very real fear to older adults who require assistance in transfers, particularly transfers that involve hydraulic devices. This fear can be reduced by ensuring that there is adequate help and by providing ongoing reassurance during the transfer.

3. **Provide explanations for all care procedures.** Fear of the unknown is common at all ages. Many activities and treatments that are familiar to nurses are extremely strange and frightening to older adults, who may fear that the procedure will cause bodily harm or pain. Nurses should be careful to explain why the procedure must be done, what will happen, and what the person can do to help. Explanations do not always remove the fear, but they usually do reduce it.

❖ NURSING PROCESS FOR ANXIETY

Anxiety is an unsettled or uneasy feeling caused by a vague or unidentified threat. Anxiety can be mild, moderate, or severe; in extreme cases, it can reach the level of panic. Anxiety can be acute or chronic. Anxiety is more prevalent among older adults than among any other age group, with studies revealing that as many as 10% of older adults report chronic, often debilitating, forms of anxiety. Mild anxiety can actually be good for people, even older adults. A little anxiety keeps people vigilant for potential hazards. A little anxiety provides the motivation for positive actions such as seeking health care. Those who have never experienced anxiety would have little reason to plan ahead or take precautions in life. However, persistent or high-level anxiety can interfere with a person's ability to perceive situations accurately and to respond to them appropriately. In addition to behavioral changes of anxiety, stimulation of the sympathetic nervous system can result, with physiologic changes identical to those seen with fear.

■ Assessment/Data Collection

See the assessment of disturbed self-perception and self-concept on page 203.

■ Nursing Diagnosis

Anxiety

■ Nursing Goals/Outcomes Identification

The nursing goals for older adults diagnosed with anxiety are to (1) identify methods that help reduce anxiety and (2) experience fewer episodes of anxiety.

■ **Nursing Interventions/Implementation**

The following nursing interventions should take place in hospitals, in extended-care facilities, and at home:

1. **Encourage older adults to verbalize their thoughts and feelings.** Once thoughts and feelings are put into words, individuals are often more able to recognize the causes of their anxiety. Once the causes are recognized, strategies can be designed to help the person cope with anxiety. Other people (e.g., nurses) can often see patterns in the verbalized thoughts and feelings of anxious people. This perspective is more objective and often helps the person with anxiety gain a better understanding of himself or herself. Allowing the older person to verbalize anger and irritation or to cry may enable the person to calm down.

2. **Provide a quiet environment and reduce excessive stimulation.** Excessive noise or activity usually increases anxiety. A quiet room with minimal contact and stimulation may help calm older adults. Reassurance with gentle touch and empathetic communication may also help. Stimulating beverages such as coffee should be avoided.

3. **Provide distraction or diversion.** Moderate anxiety may decrease if the individual becomes involved in another activity that he or she finds pleasant. Quiet activities such as listening to music, watching television, or working on a craft are soothing to many older adults (Figure 11-4).

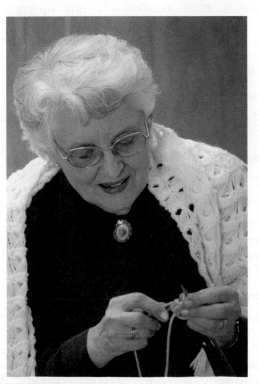

FIGURE 11-4 Crafts such as knitting may help lessen anxiety and maintain activeness in older adults.

❖ NURSING PROCESS FOR HOPELESSNESS

Hopelessness is a subjective state in which people feel unable to solve problems or establish goals. They feel that they have no alternatives or choices, even when they actually can control what occurs. Hopeless persons express feelings of complete apathy in response to problems. They are often heard making statements such as "What's the use in trying; nothing will go right anyway" or "Nothing ever goes right for me." Because hopeless persons cannot see any possible solutions, they tend to be passive and uninterested. They find it difficult, if not impossible, to solve problems or make decisions. The body language of hopeless individuals is that of despondency. In most cases, these persons display few emotions (although some respond with anger). Self-destructive behaviors are common among hopeless older adults. Failure to eat, to take prescribed medication, or to follow up with medical care are often signs of hopelessness. In extreme cases, hopeless individuals may become suicidal. The suicide rate in older adults is higher than that in any other age group, and the numbers appear to be rising. Any older person who demonstrates severe signs of hopelessness should be watched closely. Hopeless older adults who abuse alcohol or other depressant medications are at higher-than-average risk for suicide.

■ **Assessment/Data Collection**

See the assessment of disturbed self-perception and self-concept on pages 203-204.

■ **Nursing Diagnosis**

Hopelessness

■ **Nursing Goals/Outcomes Identification**

The nursing goal for older adults diagnosed with hopelessness is to identify activities or interventions that promote hopefulness.

■ **Nursing Interventions/Implementation**

The following interventions should take place in hospitals, in extended-care facilities, and at home:

1. **Visit older adults frequently and spend time exploring the factors that contribute to feelings of hopelessness.** It is necessary to spend time with older adults to develop enough trust for them to share their concerns. Regular visits that are not related to direct physical care show that nurses are concerned with the person. It is important to get the person to verbalize his or her feelings. Unless nurses know the specific concerns, it is impossible to design approaches that will help a particular aging individual. Hopelessness is often related to other problems, particularly spiritual distress, grief, and depression.

2. **Assess the potential for self-destructive behaviors or suicide.** Frequent verbalization in older adults of the wish to harm themselves or to commit suicide must be taken seriously. Depressed older adults and those who have recently experienced significant loss are at highest risk for suicidal thought. Older adults who live alone are more likely to try to take their own lives. Some commit suicide passively by refusing to eat, refusing medical care, or failing to comply with medical treatments such as taking medications. Other older adults choose a very active form of suicide such as drug overdose, shooting, or hanging. Frail older adults are more likely to attempt passive forms; the stronger person is more likely to choose an actively destructive method (Boxes 11-3 and 11-4).

Box 11-3	Suicide and Older Adults

- At least 6000 people 65 years of age or older commit suicide each year.
- White men are the most likely group to commit suicide.
- Medical illness is a major contributing factor to suicide.
- Social isolation, serious depression, and a history of self-destructive behaviors increase the risk for suicide.
- Life events such as loss of a loved one, uncontrollable pain, and major life changes such as retirement increase the risk for suicide.

Box 11-4	Interventions Related to Suicide

ASSESS FOR SIGNS OF DEPRESSION
- Changes in appetite or sleep patterns
- Unexplained fatigue
- Apathy or loss of interest in life
- Trouble concentrating or indecisiveness
- Social withdrawal from family and/or friends
- Loss of interest in normal activities or hobbies
- Loss of interest in personal appearance
- Crying for no apparent reason

ASSESS FOR OTHER BEHAVIOR CHANGES
- Giving away treasured possessions
- Talking about death or suicide
- Taking unusual or unnecessary risks
- Increased consumption of alcohol or drugs
- Failure to follow through with prescribed medication or diet
- Purchase of a weapon

DEMONSTRATE INTEREST AND BECOME INVOLVED WITH THE PERSON
- Take clues of suicide seriously; do not ignore them.
- Ask the person whether he or she is considering suicide.
- Avoid judgmental statements.
- Offer hope and help the person seek alternatives.
- Promote a safe environment by removing easy suicide methods.
- Seek help from persons or agencies that specialize in suicide prevention.

❖ NURSING PROCESS FOR POWERLESSNESS

Powerlessness occurs when older adults feel they have lost control of what happens to them. Such feelings may result from the loss of control of physical functions or body parts or from loss of a body part. Powerlessness is common with hospitalization or placement in an extended-care facility. Nurses often contribute to feelings of powerlessness by taking over or taking charge of older adults. Doing too much for a person is perhaps more damaging than doing too little. By their very competence, caregivers can intimidate older adults and destroy any initiative for them to even attempt self-care. Individual dignity and control are too often sacrificed to efficiency. This is particularly true of older adults who require more time to accomplish tasks. It is easier for the staff to do something for older adults than to wait for them to do it.

Life in an institutional setting tends to be regimented and restrictive. In an attempt to meet the needs of many people, it is easy to lose track of the uniqueness of the individuals. The needs of the institution often take priority over the desires of the individual. If the importance of older adults is not recognized by caregivers, the institution will completely control the lives of each individual.

Persons who are acquiescent and relinquish control of their lives to others without question are often viewed as the "good" or adjusted residents. Those who protest and demand their own way are viewed as the "bad" or maladjusted residents (see Figure 11-5). These are mistaken notions. Persons who give up control are more at risk for low self-esteem, hopelessness, powerlessness, and social isolation than are those who manipulate, argue, or complain to maintain some control over their lives.

■ Assessment/Data Collection

See the assessment of disturbed self-perception and self-concept on pages 203-204.

■ Nursing Diagnosis

Powerlessness

■ Nursing Goals/Outcomes Identification

The nursing goals for older adults diagnosed with powerlessness are to (1) identify actions in which they can exert control and (2) make decisions and have input in the plan of care.

■ Nursing Interventions/Implementation

The following interventions should take place in hospitals, in extended-care facilities, and at home:
1. **Allow older adults to make choices whenever possible.** Even in institutional settings, choices should be made by older adults as often as possible. Menus can be planned to include options such as sandwiches for people who do not like the menu items. A variety

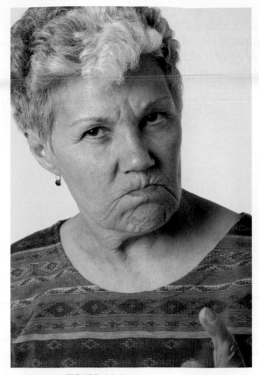

FIGURE 11-5 Assertiveness.

of suitable clothing can be displayed before dressing so that individuals can select the articles they desire. Enough activities should be available so that the person can find one that interests him or her.

2. **Encourage older adults to do as much as possible for themselves.** When people perform their own care, they feel more in control. Such control of simple things can help maintain a sense of being able to influence what happens.

3. **Adapt the environment to encourage independent activity.** Nurses should evaluate the environment, taking into consideration the strengths and limitations of older adults. Many older adults lose their sense of power because things in the environment are outside of their control. When older adults must always ask for things or call on nurses for help, the nurses control the situation. Modifying the environment so that all necessary or desired items (e.g., walkers) are close at hand gives control back to older adults. Elevated toilets can reduce the need to call for assistance. Providing snacks and beverages in a readily accessible place such as a lounge provides control.

4. **Explain the reasons for any changes in the plan of care.** At times, the plan of care may need to be changed. When this is necessary, older adults should be informed as soon as the change is known. The reasons for the change should be explained so that the person understands that the change occurred because of certain circumstances and not simply because the nurses are assuming control of the patient's right to make choices.

5. **Avoid being overprotective or directive.** Nurses and other caregivers often do not allow older adults to use their abilities. In the name of concern and caring, caregivers do too much for older adults. This can lead to one of two possible outcomes: either the older person becomes angry and tells the caregiver to leave him or her alone, or the older person gives up and lets the caregiver do everything. In the first case, the person may not get help when he or she really needs it. In the latter, the person is likely to experience a rapid loss of ability. The best approach is a balanced one in which caregivers support and encourage older adults to perform as much for themselves as is safely possible. Unless the situation is harmful, nurses may have to learn to accept less than perfection and avoid redoing what the person has done for himself or herself. Redoing what has already been done can strip away the older person's dignity and make him or her feel impotent and childlike. Therefore, help should be provided only when it is needed and only to the extent it is needed.

6. **Respect older adults' right to refuse.** The ultimate power held by patients is the right to refuse care. Older adults who are in control of their mental faculties retain this right, and nurses cannot force them to do anything against their wishes. When a person refuses food, care, or medication, nurses should first determine the reasons for the refusal. Once the reasons are known, nurses should develop a plan to reduce or remove the objections. Unless the reasons for refusal are known, any approaches are likely to be unsuccessful. A good explanation of the importance of the treatment or medication often can overcome objections and relieve conflict. In other cases, minor modifications such as changing the method or timing of medications will work. For some individuals, consultation with the dietitian, physician, or other specialist is needed to solve the problem. If alert older persons continue to refuse care despite attempts to gain acceptance, nurses should accept the refusal. This does not mean that further attempts to gain compliance cannot or should not be made in the future. When a person refuses some or all parts of his or her care, nurses should document all of the facts of the situation, as well as all interventions that were tried.

If older adults are unable to make judgments because of impaired cognitive function, a different situation exists. In these cases, the families or guardians should be actively involved in planning care. These individuals may be able to suggest ways to get the person to cooperate. Persons who hold legal guardianship can speak for patients in determining what should be done. Nurses should also discuss these concerns and problems with the physician. Changes in the medical plan can often eliminate problems. (See Nursing Care Plan 11-1.)

⭐ Nursing Care Plan 11-1   Powerlessness

Mrs. Green, age 90, was living independently until recently, when she suffered a fall that resulted in a broken hip. Her family is unable to provide the ongoing care she requires because they, too, are getting old and they live in a different state. Mrs. Green is a new resident of Golden Grove Nursing Home. She is very passive and allows the staff to do everything for her, despite that she is capable of doing many things for herself. She does not express any feelings or preferences about her care, meals, or anything else. When asked about her perceptions, she says, "It doesn't matter. You'll do whatever you want anyway." She prefers to remain in her room.

Nursing Diagnosis
Powerlessness

Defining Characteristics
• Passive behavior
• Apathetic responses
• Verbalization of lack of control
• Nonparticipation in care

Patient Goals/Outcomes Identification
Mrs. Green will participate in decision making regarding her care and identify actions within her control.

Nursing Interventions/Implementation
1. Visit daily for 10 to 15 minutes to allow Mrs. Green to verbalize her feelings and concerns.
2. Respect Mrs. Green's right to private space. Allow her to choose what belongings she wants and where she wants them.
3. Actively include her in care planning, present her with options, and then follow through with her choices.
4. Explain the reasons for any changes that must be made.
5. Keep the call signal handy and respond promptly when called.
6. Meet her requests promptly.
7. Encourage participation in personal care.
8. Assist her in identifying areas in which she can retain control.

Evaluation
The nursing assistant reports that Mrs. Green is demonstrating more assertive behaviors, such as insisting on choosing her own clothing and stating preferences about meals. She has been heard saying, "I will do that later when I am ready." You will continue the plan of care.

Critical Thinking Questions
As her hip has healed, Mrs. Green's behavior has changed, and she is now described by the staff as being demanding and critical of the staff.
1. What do you think has caused the change in behavior?
2. How could you assess and validate your conclusions?

Get Ready for the NCLEX® Examination!

Key Points
• Both age-related and disease-related changes affect older adults' self-images; societal values and life experiences also play a role.
• Self-concept is closely related to the older person's values, beliefs, roles, and relationships.
• When older adults suffer losses in any important area of life, self-concept is threatened.
• If older adults are able to maintain a sense of self-worth and personal value, few problems occur.

• If older adults believe that they are of little value, serious problems, including fear, anxiety, hopelessness, and powerlessness, will result.
• Disturbances in self-concept and self-esteem can significantly affect the older adult's response to care.
• Nurses should pay close attention to what older adults have to say about themselves.
• Measures should be taken to provide emotional support, enhance personal control, and promote self-esteem in older adults.

Additional Learning Resources

SG Go to the Study Guide on pp. 379–397 for additional learning activities to help you master the chapter content.

evolve Go to your Evolve website (http://evolve.elsevier.com/Wold/geriatric) for the following FREE learning resources:
- Animations
- Answer Guidelines for Nursing Care Plan Critical Thinking Questions
- Answers and Rationales for Review Questions for the NCLEX® Examination
- Glossary with pronunciations in English and Spanish
- Video Clips

Review Questions for the NCLEX® Examination

1. Depression in the elderly is:
   1. Uncommon and rarely in need of treatment
   2. Most common among the elderly who live independently
   3. Easily recognized and treated with psychotherapy
   4. Often mistaken for a medical problem

2. The nurse should assess for changes in behavior that are likely to indicate depression such as: (Select all that apply.)
   1. Increased alcohol consumption
   2. Changes in daily routines
   3. Agitation and irritability
   4. Isolation and withdrawal
   5. More frequent calls to family
   6. Complaints of palpitations, trembling, and dry mouth

3. Ways the nurse can promote self-esteem in an elderly client is by:
   1. Using affectionate names like "dear" or "honey"
   2. Selecting clothing that the nurse thinks looks good
   3. Developing a detailed plan of care, stressing grooming
   4. Following through promptly on client requests

4. A verbal clue that an elderly person is experiencing low self-esteem would be:
   1. "I need help now."
   2. "I can't do anything right anymore."
   3. "I wish I were young again."
   4. "I can't do things like I used to."

5. When assessing an elderly client's risk for suicide, the nurse recognizes that:
   1. Suicide is uncommon in the elderly population.
   2. Medical status has poor correlation to suicide attempts.
   3. White females are most likely to commit suicide.
   4. Risk for suicide increases at times of major life changes.

6. Reminiscence is most appropriately used to: (Select all that apply.)
   1. Enhance long-term memory
   2. Promote a sense of self-worth
   3. Stimulate short-term memory
   4. Promote a sense of community
   5. Increase awareness of current events
   6. Provide an opportunity for social interaction

Roles and Relationships

Objectives

1. Describe normal roles and relationships.
2. Describe how patterns of roles and relationships change with aging.
3. Discuss the effects of disease processes on the ability to maintain roles and relationships.
4. Describe methods of assessing changes in roles and relationships.
5. Identify older adults who are most at risk for experiencing problems related to changes in roles and relationships.
6. Identify selected nursing diagnoses related to role or relationship problems.
7. Describe nursing interventions that are appropriate for older individuals experiencing problems related to changing roles and relationships.

Key Terms

dysfunctional (p. 218)
grief (p. 217)
heterogeneous (p. 215)
homogeneous (p. 215)

relationships (p. 214)
role (p. 214)
social isolation (p. 219)

NORMAL ROLES AND RELATIONSHIPS

A role is a socially accepted behavior pattern. People tend to establish their identities and to describe themselves based on the roles they play in life. Man, woman, husband, wife, adult, senior citizen, parent, child, son, daughter, student, teacher, doctor, nurse, worker, and housewife are some common roles. People play many roles over a lifetime and often must attempt to play several roles simultaneously.

Roles are identified, defined, and given value by the society in which a person lives. Each member of society learns the status of various roles and learns to expect certain behaviors, symbols, and relationships that are acceptable for each role. These behaviors, symbols, and relationship patterns can differ widely, depending on the values and norms of the society in which the individual lives. The value assigned by society indicates the status of each role. Those in high-status roles generally possess more privileges and receive more rewards. For example, modern society gives bosses higher status than employees; teachers higher status than students; employed persons higher status than unemployed persons; and younger, more productive members of society higher status than older, retired members.

Relationships are connections formed by the dynamic interaction of individuals who play interrelated roles.

Cultural Considerations

Asian and Pacific Islanders

- Asian and Pacific Islanders include more than 20 distinct ethnic groups.
- Many of these groups are influenced by the teachings of Confucius, which dictate the importance of the family over the individual.
- In keeping with this, children are expected to exhibit "filial piety," which includes honoring and caring for aging parents in the home.
- Belief in this concept may cause a great deal of conflict and guilt for younger family members who have become Americanized in their lifestyles.

Most people develop a wide range of relationships within their families, at work, and during day-to-day social activities. The way individuals occupying each role interact with each other describes their relationships. Relationships can be short or long-term, personal or impersonal, intimate or superficial. Relationships change over time and are affected by the role changes of the people involved.

Each culture and subculture sets standards for designated roles and relationships. People in various roles or relationships are expected to behave in accord with accepted standards, which include things such as the amount and type of clothing or jewelry that are appropriate. Standards specify the type of housing, the means of transportation, and even the type and amount of food consumed. Standards specify how individuals in the culture relate to each other in social and work situations. For example, the role perception for a middle-class American businessman is that he is expected to wear a suit and tie with minimal jewelry, live in an apartment or house in the suburbs, drive a conventional car, eat healthful meals, show up for work on time, and show respect to the boss. If this businessman showed up late for work in jeans and a sweatshirt, wearing an earring and riding a motorcycle, and then later eating a hamburger and telling the boss not to "bug" him, most people would be shocked. Yet this same behavior is not considered atypical for a college student—even one who is studying to be a businessman.

A simple, or homogeneous, society is one in which all members share a common historical and cultural experience. There is little confusion or conflict in a homogeneous social system because the symbols, behaviors, and relationships are perceived in the same way by all members of the society. Everyone knows the accepted roles and how people in each role are expected to relate to each other. Therefore, there is little question and few problems with regard to role or relationship expectations.

A more complex, or heterogeneous, society is one in which the members of many diverse subcultures with different historical and cultural experiences must interact. These subcultures may have their origin in race, religion, ethnic heritage, or age. Because subcultures do not share the same experiences, their symbols, behaviors, roles, and relationships are not perceived in the same way by all members of the larger society. Roles and role expectations are not always clear, and this lack of shared perceptions often leads to misunderstandings, confusion, and conflict.

The American culture is very heterogeneous and is becoming even more so. Problems are likely to occur when people with different role and relationship perceptions are required to interact with each other. The greater the differences in role perceptions, role symbols, and role relationships, the greater the likelihood that cross-cultural misunderstandings will occur. This explains the confusion or stress many people experience when they interact with individuals of different ages or from different cultural backgrounds. It also explains why a person who was raised in a specific culture is more comfortable with similar individuals and finds it difficult to establish close relationships with people from different cultural backgrounds. Furthermore, it explains why people of different ages may have difficulty understanding each other. The diversity of the population contributes to the prevalence of role and relationship problems in contemporary American society.

However, this is not the only role or relationship issue people face. In addition to the interpersonal conflict or confusion seen in modern society, individuals can also experience internal role conflict and confusion. Problems occur when the demands of multiple roles and relationships must be met at the same time, particularly when the expectations of one role conflict with those of another. For example, a woman today is often expected to be wife, mother, and employee. She may be expected to keep up the home, prepare meals, supervise the children, be active in school or community programs, be a social and sexual companion to her spouse, and be a productive worker—capable of doing everything, while working with everyone, and always arriving on time with a smile on her face. Unless today's woman is superwoman, she is bound to fall short of someone's expectations.

Most people occupy multiple roles and develop a variety of relationships throughout their lives. People think of themselves and establish their identities in terms of their roles and relationships. If you ask people to describe themselves, you typically receive a list of roles or relationships (e.g., mother, engineer and supervisor) rather than a list of personal characteristics.

Because people form their self-image based on their roles and relationships, they are likely to have difficulty accepting changes in either. Our identity and sense of self are threatened when roles are lost and the relationships associated with those roles change. The longer the role was held and the more intense the relationships, the greater the grief will be. When a person's role changes, the symbols and indicators of role and status also change. Loss of symbols or status is often as painful as the loss of the role. People may grieve a change of role or loss of relationship as much as they grieve the loss of a loved one.

ROLES, RELATIONSHIPS, AND AGING

The longer a person occupies a particular role, the more familiar and, consequently, more comfortable the person becomes with it. The more comfortable people are in their roles and relationships, the harder it is to adjust to changes.

Older adults must adjust to many predictable role and relationship changes associated with aging, including retirement, altered relationships with adult children, changes in housing, loss of valued possessions, loss of friends resulting from relocation or death, loss of a spouse to death, loss of health, and loss of independence. All of these changes and losses are potentially traumatic to older adults.

Some older adults resent the fact that society forces them to retire. Age 65 was once the typical retirement age, but that is no longer the case. This change has occurred partially because of financial reasons, but also because many older people do not want to retire.

Many of these people feel that they would lose too much of their identity if they retired. They say, "I don't know what I would do if I couldn't work." Older persons who do retire may adjust well or poorly, depending on the adequacy of their other roles to keep them satisfied. In general, the more roles and relationships a person develops at younger ages, the better his or her ability to adjust will be when some of those roles and relationships are lost.

When an occupational role no longer exists, the individual often grieves its loss. Many people look forward to retirement, but once retired find that they miss both the status that role gave them and the interaction with other people. They often resent the fact that they are no longer viewed as productive, contributing members of society. They are no longer lawyers, plumbers, nurses, or teachers; they are just retired people.

The Baby Boomer generation may revise this view of roles and retirement. Perhaps the fact that many have changed jobs and even careers several times during their working years has given them a different perspective on what they can do with the rest of their lives. Either from desire or necessity, 83% of this cohort plan to keep working after retirement. Some need to continue to work because of loss of pensions or retirement investments due to downturn in the economy. Others want to work and "try something new" or "stay active and engaged." Many expect to never fully retire and plan to work as long as their health permits. A significant number of those who are not interested in employment plan to volunteer, travel or seek other outlets for their energy.

Early Baby Boomers seem to be having less difficulty adjusting to retirement than those who preceded them. Many report being highly satisfied with their lives and are in many cases developing new roles and forming new relationships. A common comment heard from this group is, "I don't know how I ever had time to work full-time. I've got too many things to do." This is more likely to be the case for those who have entered retirement in good health and with substantial economic resources. Only time will tell if this pattern continues.

To maintain a connection with those who are still employed, many retired older adults continue to think of themselves as a part of their occupation. A nurse remains a nurse for life, a plumber remains a plumber, and so on. Even if they have not worked in the occupation for years, most older persons continue to identify with their previous occupational roles. This may be particularly obvious in older adult professionals (e.g., physicians, lawyers, professors and ministers) who never stop using their titles. Many expect to retain the same status level and respect as was paid to them when they were actively employed and are highly insulted if this respect is not forthcoming.

There are some roles from which a person cannot officially "retire." Homemaker is one such role. Older persons who have spent the largest part of their lives managing a home—doing the cooking, cleaning, sewing, and other duties required of a homemaker—may feel lost when they are forced by circumstances of ill health or finances to give up the home. Many older adult homemakers (primarily women) have few other roles and feel a great sense of loss when institutionalized. Those who took the time to develop hobbies or social interests and relationships outside of the home tend to adapt better than do those who had no interests other than their homes.

Older adults do not give up the role of parent just because their children are adults. The role of parent is usually identified as being self-sufficient and in control. Role conflict and altered family relationships are likely to occur when older adults attempt to continue to direct their children's behavior long after the children are adults or when the parents lose the ability to function independently and are forced to become dependent on their children. Successful adjustment to changes in the parenting role is difficult and requires a great deal of patience, tact, and accommodation on the part of all family members. Families who have a history of altered parenting or poorly developed family relationships are likely to have serious problems, often leading to abuse or isolation of the older person from his or her family.

In addition to being the parent of adult children, many older adults are grandparents. The role of grandparent is often described as being much more pleasant than that of being a parent. As one grandmother said, "I can have all of the fun and enjoyment of children without the responsibility." Another grandmother replied, "Yes, it's nice when they come to visit, but it's also nice when you can send them home."

Grandparenting allows older adults to share their wisdom and experiences with a new, young generation. Because grandparents are often under less daily stress and are not the primary disciplinarians of the children, they are usually more relaxed and have more time to spend on nonessential activities such as conversation and play (Figure 12-1). It is common for retired grandparents with time on their hands to entertain children with stories or teach them skills, hobbies, or games that the grandparents learned as children. When positive interactions take place between grandparents and grandchildren, a close bond is often formed that benefits both parties (Figure 12-2). Mobility and the resulting separation of family members often make it difficult for this relationship to develop. Both parties are usually worse off for not knowing the other.

Many older persons have occupied the role of spouse for 30, 40, or 50 or more years. With the death of a partner, these persons are deprived of a significant role and relationship. Marriage is one of the most personal and intimate relationships. A successful long-term marriage requires a great deal of effort; the loss

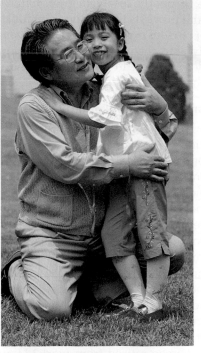

FIGURE 12-1 Grandparenting.

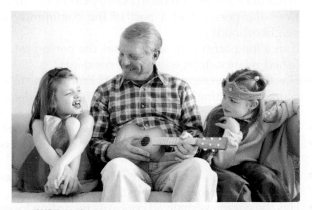

FIGURE 12-2 An older man plays with his grandchildren.

of this intensely personal relationship triggers a high level of emotional distress. Many widowed older adults experience severe grief and social isolation as a result of the loss. They describe themselves as feeling as though a part of them is missing, of feeling half-alive. Many widows and widowers find their grief so overwhelming that they cannot even continue to perform normal activities of daily living.

The loss of friends due to relocation or death also results in changed social roles and relationships. Many activities require more than one person to be fun. Many older adults have formed friendships or social groups over the years. As more and more of the members move away or die, the older person is likely to become increasingly socially isolated. Older persons who outlive their families and friends often feel that their lives are without purpose.

Many older adults change housing arrangements out of choice or necessity. The house may be too big, too expensive, or too difficult to maintain. This is particularly true when the health of one or both occupants fails or when a widow is unable to keep up the home after loss of the spouse. Moving to smaller accommodations commonly necessitates the sale or distribution of personal possessions accumulated over a lifetime. This loss of possessions makes the process of moving even more traumatic for older adults. In some ways, they are "giving away" their lives.

Loss of health and independence are probably the most traumatic losses because they involve changes in the very essence of who people are. When older adults lose health and independence, they lose control over their own destiny. They are at the mercy of others (either family or strangers) for care and sustenance.

As previously discussed, societies establish and define the boundaries of various roles. Individuals are judged by how well they understand and comply with their assigned roles. "Old person" is a role that has many connotations and expected behaviors. In contemporary American society, an ageist definition of the role of older adults would include adjectives such as helpless, infirm, cranky, and useless. Some older adults accept this stereotype and act the part. However, more and more older adults are continuing in productive roles and maintaining successful relationships well into their eighties and nineties. Indeed, it is expected that the Baby Boom generation will try to reinvent aging and break the old stereotypes. Just as they have challenged societal norms from early youth, Baby Boomers are likely to redefine the meaning and intent of life's later years. Old age has been called the "roleless role," a time in which many of the things that gave meaning to life are gone. However, the role is not the person—and the person is more than the sum of the roles played. If Baby Boomers are able to find ways to maintain a sense of purpose and growth into old age, they will have accomplished a remarkable feat.

❖ NURSING PROCESS FOR DYSFUNCTIONAL GRIEVING

Grief is a strong emotion. It is a combination of sorrow, loss, and confusion that comes when someone or something of value is lost. This reaction can come in response to the loss of a person, role, relationship, health, or independence.

Grief affects thoughts, emotions, and behavior and creates a wide range of physical sensations. The normal grief response follows a somewhat predictable pattern, although the exact amount of time any given individual needs to work through a loss differs (Table 12-1).

Grief is normal after the loss of a significant role or relationship (Box 12-1). Grieving leads to dysfunction when the person has an exaggerated or prolonged period of grief. Continued sadness, anger, or denial is

Table 12-1	Phases of Grieving
Shock and Numbness (First 2 Weeks)	
Feelings: Disbelief, denial, anger, guilt	*Behaviors*: Crying, searching, sighing, loss of appetite, sleep disturbance, limited concentration, muscle weakness, inability to make decisions, emotional outbursts
Searching and Yearning (2 Weeks to 4 Months)	
Feelings: Despair, apathy, depression, anger, guilt, hopelessness, self-doubt	*Behaviors*: Restlessness, poor memory, impatience, lack of concentration, crying, social isolation, loss of energy
Disorientation (4 to 7 Months)	
Feelings: Depression, guilt, disorganization	*Behaviors*: Resistance to seeking help or reaching out to others, trying to live as if nothing happened, restlessness, irritability
Reorganization (Up to 18 to 24 Months)	
Feelings: Sense of release, decreased sense of obsession with loss, renewed hope and optimism	*Behaviors*: Renewed energy, reorganization of eating and sleeping habits, improved judgment, renewed interest in activities and goals for the future

Data from Davidson G: *Processing sudden loss*, 1999, Available at www.beyondindigo.com/articles/article.php/artID/56.

Box 12-1 Normal Loss/Grief Reactions

PHYSICAL
- Persistent fatigue
- Tightness in chest
- Muscle weakness
- Shortness of breath
- Susceptibility to minor illnesses
- Hypersensitivity to noise
- Dry mouth
- Headaches
- Grinding teeth
- Tension
- Nausea
- Hyperacidity
- Dizziness

EMOTIONAL
- Anger
- Anxiety
- Ambivalence
- Depression
- Fear
- Irritability
- Loneliness
- Numbness
- Panic
- Sadness
- Guilt
- Shock
- Helplessness
- Apathy

COGNITIVE
- Confusion
- Forgetfulness
- Disorientation
- Disbelief
- Preoccupation
- Decreased attention
- Inability to concentrate

BEHAVIORAL
- Absent-mindedness
- Crying
- Decreased motivation
- Restlessness
- Social isolation
- Inconsistency
- Irritability
- Diminished productivity
- Sleep disturbances
- Appetite disturbances

indicative of poorly resolved grief. Often, grief is so severe that it prevents the person from functioning normal. Older persons experiencing **dysfunctional** grief may completely shut themselves off from normal support systems, lose interest in all activities, and even fail to perform the basic activities of daily living.

■ Assessment/Data Collection

- What is the person's marital status (i.e., single, married, widowed, divorced)?
- If the person has lost a spouse or significant other, how long ago did this occur?
- Does the person live alone or with others?
- If the person lives with others, who are they, and how are they related? What is the family structure?
- How does the person describe relationships within the family?
- What family interactions have you or others observed?
- Does the person belong to any social groups?
- Does the person have close relationships with friends?
- Is the individual employed? What are the relationships at work?
- Has the person retired from work? How long ago? What are his or her feelings regarding retirement? What does the person do to occupy his or her time?
- Does the person feel a part of the community or neighborhood?
- If in a long-term care setting, has the person established relationships with other residents?
- Has the person recently relocated? From home to an acute-care setting? From home to an extended-care facility? From one unit or room to another?
- Does the person spend a great deal of time alone?
- Does the person speak excessively with others or remain silent?
- Does the person exhibit signs of withdrawal, anger, depression, sorrow, fear, or shock?
- Has the person verbalized concerns regarding losses of persons, jobs, or abilities?
- Has the person's sleep or eating patterns changed?
- Has the person's ability to concentrate changed?

Box 12-2 provides a list of risk factors for problems related to changes in roles and relationships in older adults.

■ Nursing Diagnosis

Dysfunctional grieving

Box 12-2 Risk Factors Related to Changes in Roles and Relationships in Older Adults

- Recent loss of a spouse, child, close friend, significant other, or cherished pet
- Recent loss of lifelong or valuable roles
- Recent major adjustment in his or her living situation
- Inability to perform familiar roles owing to loss of functional abilities

■ Nursing Goals/Outcomes Identification

The nursing goals for older individuals with dysfunctional grieving are to (1) verbalize their grief, (2) use available support systems, and (3) participate in activities of daily living.

■ Nursing Interventions/Implementation

The following nursing interventions should take place in hospitals, in extended-care facilities, and at home:

1. **Establish a trusting relationship to encourage verbalization of feelings regarding the change or loss.** Before sharing their true feelings, older adults must develop trust in their nurses. Trust comes only when they believe that the nurses truly care about them as unique human beings and that the nurses will be understanding and sensitive to their feelings. It takes time and effort to develop trust.

    Trust cannot be forced. It may take days, weeks, or even months for a grieving person to share his or her deepest feelings. Although trust cannot be forced, nurses can take actions to promote its development. These actions are summarized in Box 12-3.

2. **Assess the source and acknowledge the reality of the grief.** Grief is very much like pain. It is a complex and personal emotion. Because most people find it difficult to deal with grief, they avoid grieving persons and avoid discussing anything that approaches the source of the grief. These behaviors leave the problem unresolved. To help with grief, it is essential that the grieving person identify and confront the loss. Nurses can help by spending time with grieving individuals and by allowing them the opportunity to verbalize their grief. Once older adults are able to verbalize and acknowledge their grief, nurses can use problem-solving methods to help them develop coping strategies.

3. **Encourage older adults to participate in activities of daily living.** Grieving individuals are often totally preoccupied with their loss. Although this preoccupation is understandable, it is incompatible with normal living. The more a grieving person is able to maintain contact with day-to-day activities, the sooner he or she will be able to go on with life. Nurses can help by providing structure to the day.

Box 12-3	Actions That Promote Trust

- Spend time with the person.
- Actively listen to what the person says.
- Address the person by name.
- Smile.
- Use a warm, friendly voice.
- Make appropriate eye contact.
- Respond honestly to questions.
- Provide consistency of care.
- Respect confidentiality.
- Follow through on commitments.

A plan of care that allows for preferences while setting limits helps provide this structure. A daily schedule that is well planned and predictable often enables grieving older adults to regain some control and to cope with the changes. Encouragement and positive feedback for participation in daily activities help motivate positive behaviors.

4. **Identify sources of support.** Although nurses can provide some support to grieving older persons, many others can also help. Family, friends, spiritual advisers, counselors, therapists, and support groups are all valuable sources.

    Many pamphlets, books, and other materials are available to help people who are experiencing grief. Many can be found in libraries, physician's offices, or other locations where older adults congregate.

❖ NURSING PROCESS FOR SOCIAL ISOLATION AND IMPAIRED SOCIAL INTERACTION

Social isolation, the sense of being alone, is a common problem among older adults. Those experiencing social isolation are likely to be uncommunicative and withdrawn and to have few visitors or other social interactions. Social isolation is a result of many factors and can be unintentional or intentional. The more people are separated from family and friends, the greater the likelihood of social isolation will be.

Most social isolation is unintentional. Separation resulting from death is a common and unavoidable part of aging. Many older people simply outlive their families and friends. These people are likely to become isolated unless they establish new social outlets. Separation resulting from relocation is also common. Today, it is unusual for family members to remain in a single community. Young family members move to find job opportunities; older adult family members move to retirement communities.

Decreased physical mobility and limited finances can result in social isolation. Physical changes can restrict an older person's ability to move about and make social contacts. Financial limitations can lead to separation from others because of the lack of adequate money to buy appropriate clothing or transportation to social activities.

Intentional isolation is less common and is most likely to occur when older adults fear not being accepted by others. Those who suffer from grief may be too upset or absorbed in their own problems to interact with others. Older persons experiencing changes in body image from procedures such as amputation or colostomy are also likely to isolate themselves from others. Older persons who have cognitive or perceptual problems may isolate themselves because they do not understand what is going on around them.

■ Assessment/Data Collection

See the assessment for dysfunctional grieving on page 218.

■ **Nursing Diagnosis**

Impaired social interaction

■ **Nursing Goals/Outcomes Identification**

The nursing goals for older individuals with impaired social interaction are to (1) demonstrate increased participation in social activities and (2) identify actions or resources that will help reduce social isolation.

■ **Nursing Interventions/Implementation**

The following nursing interventions should take place in hospitals, in extended-care facilities, and at home:

1. **Assess the reason or reasons for the social isolation.** Because many factors can lead to social isolation, nurses should identify those that affect each individual. Interventions should be directed at specific problems.

2. **Promote social contact and interaction.** Telephone calls and mail can be used to maintain contact with family and friends. Telephones should be readily available and located so that older adults can have privacy yet comfort when using them (see Figure 12-3). Telephones can be equipped with amplifiers for those who are hard of hearing. Mail should be delivered promptly. Visually impaired older adults should be offered help in reading mail.

   Social rooms and lounges should be available for older adults to use for visits. If the individual is confined to bed, privacy to conduct visits in the room should be given.

   Information about all activities in a facility should be well communicated to older adult residents. Nurses should offer encouragement to those who are reluctant to participate in activities.

   Careful planning is needed to prevent social isolation in older individuals with restricted physical mobility. Nursing care should be scheduled so that there is adequate time for social interaction. The care plan should provide for any assistance required to enable participation in social activities.

3. **Spend one-on-one time with the isolated person.** Those who cannot or will not participate in social interaction need extra attention from the nursing staff. One-on-one interaction, even for brief intervals during the day, helps these persons maintain some social contact. Over time, nurses can attempt to motivate these individuals to try other forms of social contact.

4. **Initiate referrals.** Often, the social worker, chaplain, or activities department can help socially isolated older persons identify acceptable social activities.

❖ **NURSING PROCESS FOR INTERRUPTED FAMILY PROCESSES**

Normal changes in family processes were discussed in Chapter 1. When older persons or their families verbalize concern or confusion related to a change in roles or relationships, family dynamics should be assessed. Alterations in family processes can occur at any age but are most common when an aging family member becomes dependent.

■ **Assessment/Data Collection**

See the assessment for dysfunctional grieving on page 218.

■ **Nursing Diagnosis**

Interrupted family processes

■ **Nursing Goals/Outcomes Identification**

The nursing goals for older individuals with altered family processes are to (1) express their feelings regarding changes in roles and relationships and (2) work with family members to develop strategies for coping with changing roles and relationships.

■ **Nursing Interventions/Implementation**

The following nursing interventions should take place in hospitals, in extended-care facilities, and at home:

1. **Assess interactions between older adults and their families.** Nurses should spend time sitting in when family members visit their aging relatives. Nurses should be alert for signs of destructive emotions such as anger or frustration. If these are evident, a rest time or coffee break should be suggested to reduce the tension and allow the family members a chance to calm down. When they have been separated, nurses can try to explore their feelings individually and suggest coping strategies.

2. **Encourage all family members to verbalize their feelings.** It is best to explore the feelings of family members independently. Many people, both old and young, are afraid to express their real feelings in the presence of other involved parties. Nurses should spend time with older adults and each

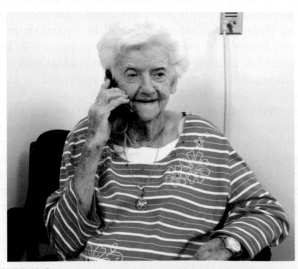

FIGURE 12-3 A resident maintaining social contact by using the telephone.

individual family member in private settings. During this time, it is important to convey to all concerned family members that all feelings, including those of anger and frustration, are acceptable and will be held in confidence. Expressing the negative emotions that are triggered by the stress of coping with changing roles and relationships is not easy for most people and will take time. Once feelings are identified, positive coping strategies can be developed.

3. **Assist family members in identifying personal and family strengths.** Each person and each family has weaknesses and strengths. The key to maintaining or repairing family dynamics is identification of the strengths. Love, concern, and shared spiritual values can be used as a basis for positive relationships.

4. **Encourage family members to visit regularly.** When an aging family member is hospitalized or resides in an institutional setting, the family may feel useless or unnecessary. Some family members feel that their presence is not desired by the nursing staff. Nurses should recognize that family members are able to relate to older adults in unique and special ways. Rather than make the family uncomfortable, the nursing staff should do everything possible to make them feel welcome and at ease. Greeting family members by name helps forge bonds of mutual caring. Responding promptly to requests and showing small considerations (e.g., offering the family members a cup of coffee) can go a long way in making them feel valued.

5. **Encourage the family members to assist in elder care.** Family members are often able and willing to help the nursing staff care for aging loved ones.

Assisting with care provides the family with the opportunity to show their concern for the aging person. Assisting with care should not be expected or demanded, but it should be encouraged if the family appears willing. The amount of involvement will differ from family to family. Some family members may desire to perform a great deal of the care, even bathing and feeding. Others are more comfortable helping with less technical things such as hair grooming or shaving. Nurses can help families by providing all necessary equipment, by teaching families safe and effective ways to perform tasks, and by providing positive comments for a job well done.

6. **Assist families in identifying factors that are interfering with normal interactions.** Normal physiologic changes, illness, disability, side effects of medication, decreased finances, and other events can affect the behavior of older adults and interfere with normal family interactions. Nurses should do a thorough assessment to determine the factors at play in any given situation. Once the causative factors are identified, nurses can work with older adults and their families to develop a plan that eliminates or reduces the problems and thereby facilitates more-normal interactions.

7. **Explore community resources.** If the family dynamics are severely altered, nurses may be unable to meet the family's needs. Special assistance in the form of support groups, geriatric social workers, or geropsychiatric clinics are available in many communities. Nurses should be aware of the resources available in a specific community and make information about these resources available to all family members. (See Nursing Care Plan 12-1.)

✱ Nursing Care Plan 12-1 | Social Isolation

Mrs. Hixton is an alert, generally healthy 77-year-old widow who lives alone in the home she and her husband shared until his death from cancer last year. Her daughter lives several hundred miles away and calls occasionally. The home hospice nurse who visited regularly during her husband's illness stops by as part of her routine follow-up and finds that Mrs. Hixton spends most of her time in the house with the shades drawn and goes out only to buy groceries and other necessary items. She drives to church weekly but does not speak to other church members. She speaks hesitantly to the nurse and makes little eye contact during the conversation. With tears in her eyes, she states that "Nobody cares about me anymore; they all have somebody, but I have nobody."

Nursing Diagnosis
Social isolation

Defining Characteristics
- Feelings of rejection and being alone
- Absence of supportive family or friends
- Withdrawal from contact with others
- Sad, dull affect
- Lack of eye contact
- Preoccupation with own thoughts

Continued

★ Nursing Care Plan 12-1 Social Isolation—cont'd

Patient Goals/Outcomes Identification

Mrs. Hixton will demonstrate increased participation in social activities and identify actions or resources that will help reduce social isolation.

Nursing Interventions

1. Allow Mrs. Hixton time to verbalize feelings of sadness or depression relating to the loss of her spouse.
2. Encourage her to develop a list of family members and friends with whom she previously socialized.
3. Encourage her to make contact with her daughter by phone on a weekly basis.
4. Identify social activities that were previously of interest to her.
5. Encourage participation in a grief counseling group.
6. Consult with minister regarding visitations.

Evaluation

Mrs. Hixton hesitantly expressed willingness to attend one session of grief counseling. During this session she sat quietly and listened to others explain what they were going through. At the next home visit she told the nurse, "I think I'll go to another session. There was another woman there who's having the same problems I am. She offered to have coffee with me." You will continue the plan of care.

Critical Thinking Questions

1. What could the nurse do to help Mrs. Hixton prepare for her next grief counseling session?
2. What could the nurse do if Mrs. Hixton had a negative experience at the group counseling session?
3. What are possible interventions the nurse could use if Mrs. Hixton refused to attend further sessions?

Get Ready for the NCLEX® Examination!

Key Points

- People play many roles and have many integral relationships over a lifetime.
- When aging results in loss of these roles and changes in relationships, grief is a normal response.
- If the grief response is severe, the older person may lose all interest in life.
- Grieving people are often unwilling to participate even in normal daily care or activities.
- To break through grief, nurses must attempt to build a trusting relationship in which the older person can work through the loss and grief. It is hoped that this will enable the person to find new meaning in life and to build new relationships.
- Older adults may become isolated from social interaction.
- Social isolation may result from ineffective methods of coping with grief or from impaired family dynamics.
- Roles and relationships are maintained through communication with others.
- If the ability to communicate with others is impaired (as is the case with many of the common disorders of aging such as stroke or dementia), the ability to maintain relationships is affected.
- Older persons with impaired communication are likely to feel isolated from family and friends and from normal social interactions.
- Nurses who work with older adults should understand the effects of changes in roles and relationships.

- An understanding of the significance of these losses enables nurses to assess the behavior of older adults more effectively and to plan interventions that will be of benefit.

Additional Learning Resources

SG Go to the Study Guide on pp. 379–397 for additional learning activities to help you master the chapter content.

evolve Go to your Evolve website (http://evolve.elsevier.com/Wold/geriatric) for the following FREE learning resources:
- Animations
- Answer Guidelines for Nursing Care Plan Critical Thinking Questions
- Answers and Rationales for Review Questions for the NCLEX® Examination
- Glossary with pronunciations in English and Spanish
- Video Clips

Review Questions for the NCLEX® Examination

1. An elderly woman was widowed about a year ago. Normal expected behavior at this stage of grieving includes:

   1. Loss of appetite, sleep changes, and difficulty making decisions
   2. Improved energy, interest in new activities and goals
   3. Restlessness, poor memory and irritability
   4. Crying, social isolation, lack of concentration

2. An elderly person exhibits passive behavior, apathy, and unwillingness to participate in daily care or activities. He verbalizes a lack of control over his life. The most appropriate nursing diagnosis is:

    1. Anxiety
    2. Fear
    3. Altered self-esteem
    4. Powerlessness

3. The characteristics that place an elderly person at increased risk for social isolation include: (Select all that apply.)

    1. Sensory changes
    2. Decreased physical mobility
    3. Advanced age
    4. Limited financial resources
    5. Incontinence
    6. Physical deformity
    7. Belongs to an ethnic minority group

4. The most appropriate intervention to use for an elderly client who always stays in his or her room is to:

    1. Tell the elder, "It's time to go out and see people."

2. Use a wheelchair to transport the elder to the activity room.
3. Spend one-on-one time discussing the elder's concerns.
4. Call the family and request that they visit more often.

5. The person who is most likely to experience relationship issues is one who:

    1. Has a large pool of family and friends
    2. Has few interests
    3. Likes solitary activities and states, "I like to be left alone"
    4. Has multiple chronic medical disorders

6. The nurse in charge wants to help the unlicensed personnel respond most appropriately to grieving residents in a long-term care facility. To develop an effective training plan, the nurse would:

    1. Look at current magazine articles for ideas
    2. Ask the staff what would best help them
    3. Ask the residents what they think the staff needs to know
    4. Consult the DON for ideas

Coping and Stress

Objectives

1. Explain the concepts of stress and coping.
2. Identify the physical, emotional, and behavioral signs of stress.
3. Describe methods for reducing stress.
4. Discuss changes in stress and coping that occur with aging.
5. Identify older adults who are most at risk for experiencing stress-related problems.
6. Discuss methods of coping with stress and depression.
7. Identify selected nursing diagnoses related to stress-related problems.
8. Describe nursing interventions that are appropriate for older individuals who are experiencing problems related to stress and coping.

Key Terms

coping (p. 227)
distress (p. 224)
imaging (ĬM-Ĭ-jĬng) (p. 228)
mantra (MĂN-trǎ) (p. 230)

meditation (p. 228)
relaxation (p. 228)
self-hypnosis (p. 228)

NORMAL STRESS AND COPING

Stress is a normal part of life. No one lives without it. Stress occurs when a person is faced with a real or perceived threat or experiences a significant or life-altering change. Stressors include *external physical threats* such as extreme heat or cold, noise, or physical trauma; *internal* or *psychological threats* such as thoughts and feelings; and *external social threats* such as job pressures or changeable social relationships. Stress often results from a combination of these factors. The more stressors a person faces, the greater the level of stress will be. Stress occurs whether the threat or change is positive or negative.

Each of us faces a steady stream of life events with which we must cope. Some are temporary or minor events, such as taking a test or giving a speech, which may cause mild distress for a short period. Major life events such as the death of a spouse, serious injury, birth of a child, or marriage are likely to cause significant stress that lasts for a longer period. People experiencing high levels of stress feel exhausted, anxious, and vulnerable.

Different experiences are stressful to different people. Individual perceptions play an important role in determining what constitutes a stressor. For example, muscle pain is a stressor to most people but not to an athlete who views it as a measure of training. Public speaking is highly stressful to most people, but not to a politician who does it every day.

Various rating scales have been developed to quantify the amount of stress caused by common social and psychological occurrences in the lives of older people (Table 13-1). In these rating scales, various events are based on the proportional amount of **distress** involved. These scales are useful general guides when one attempts to measure the amount of stress caused by a particular event. Stress is cumulative, and a combination of several smaller stressors can have the same effects as a major stressor. The more stressors a person faces at a time, the greater the likelihood will be of physical, cognitive, and behavioral changes.

When confronted with stressful events, the body undergoes predictable physiologic responses that prepare it to withstand the threat and to maintain homeostasis. The general adaptation syndrome, described by Dr. Hans Selye, describes the collective responses of the body to stress. According to this theory, stress activates both the sympathetic and parasympathetic components of the autonomic nervous system, initiating a series of physiologic responses.

The general alarm reaction, often called the *fight-or-flight response*, occurs first. In this stage, the body undergoes a predictable range of responses or physiologic changes that are designed to overcome the threat. If these physiologic responses are effective, the body enters a stage of resistance during which it returns to normal functioning. If the responses are not effective, the body depletes its energy reserves and enters the stage of exhaustion. In the most severe cases, this exhaustion can result in death.

PHYSICAL SIGNS OF STRESS

Physical signs of stress are similar in both the young and older adults. These are summarized in Table 13-2.

Table **13-1**	Stokes/Gordon Stress Scale: Selected Items	
RANK	**EVENT OR SITUATION**	**WEIGHT**
1	Death of a son or daughter (unexpected)	100
2	Decreasing eyesight	99
2	Death of a grandchild	99
3	Death of spouse (unexpected)	97
4	Loss of ability to get around	96
4	Death of a son or daughter (expected, anticipated)	96
5	Fear of your home being invaded or robbed	93
5	Constant or recurring pain or discomfort	93
6	Illness or injury of close relative	92
7	Death of spouse (expected, anticipated)	90
7	Moving in with children or other family	90
7	Moving to an institution	90
8	Minor or major car accident	89
8	Needing to rely on cane, wheelchair, walker, or hearing aid	89
8	Change in ability to perform personal care	89
10	Loneliness or aloneness	87
11	Having an unexpected debt	86
11	Your own hospitalization (unplanned)	86
12	Decreasing hearing	85
13	Fear of abuse from others	84
13	Being judged legally incompetent	84
13	Not feeling needed or having a purpose in life	84
14	Decreasing mental abilities	84
15	Giving up long-cherished possessions	82
15	Wishing parts of your life had been different	82
16	Using your savings for living expenses	80
17	Change in behavior of a family member	79
18	Taking a relative or friend into your home to live	78
19	Concern about elimination	77
19	Illness in public places	77
20	Feeling of remaining time being short	76
20	Giving up or losing driver's license	76
20	Change in sleeping habits	76
21	Difficulty using public transportation	75
23	Uncertainty about the future	73
25	Fear of your own or your spouse's driving	71
27	Concern for completing required forms	69
27	Death of a loved pet	69
29	Reaching a milestone year	67
32	Outstanding personal achievement	64
33	Retirement	63
35	Change in your sexual activity	59

Modified from Stokes SA, Gordon SE: *User's manual*, SGSS, Pleasantville, NY, 1988, Pace University.

COGNITIVE SIGNS OF STRESS

In addition to physiologic changes, stress affects the way we think, feel, and act. Although some stress is normal and necessary, high stress levels can be physically and mentally exhausting.

Mild stress results in an increased state of alertness. Individuals experiencing mild stress are able to pay attention to details, to learn, and to solve problems. With increased stress levels, these abilities decrease rapidly.

Persons experiencing severe stress are likely to miss obvious details and might forget even the most basic information. Problem-solving ability is severely affected. Under stress, people are likely to develop tunnel vision, in which they become narrowly focused on one aspect of a problem and ignore other important facts. These individuals are likely to act irrationally or impulsively and make poor choices. Some become incapable of making any decisions at all. Some research even indicates that stress can cause physiologic changes in the brain that have an adverse effect on memory.

Emotional Signs

People experiencing high levels of stress are likely to complain of fatigue, tension, and anxiety. They often report a sense of foreboding or a feeling that something is wrong. They may appear distracted, irritable, short-tempered, or even angry. People living with high-level stress often verbalize feelings of poor self-worth or low self-esteem. They may appear to be so wrapped up in their own problems that they have little capability for or interest in interacting with others. When stress becomes severe, people may experience signs of clinical depression or even verbalize suicidal thoughts.

Depression, which is a major problem among older adults, is not easily identified or diagnosed. Depression is often missed because it occurs in conjunction with the numerous physical and social changes that occur with aging. Depression is more than the down moods that everyone experiences. Depression is a whole-body syndrome that causes physiologic, emotional, and cognitive changes in older adults. The notion of mental illness is unsettling to many older people, who feel that seeking help for mental problems is a sign of a weakness that they should be able to overcome alone. Older persons are more likely to seek attention for physical symptoms than they are for feeling depressed. Symptoms such as chronic pain, appetite loss, sleeplessness, loss of interest, and even dementia-like behavior are often attributed to other problems, and the underlying depression is missed. This is unfortunate, because 60% to 80% of the identified cases of depression can be treated using psychotherapy, medication, or a combination of both.

Depression, while common, is not a normal part of aging. In fact, studies have shown that most older people are satisfied with their lives. It appears that

Table 13-2	Physical Signs of Stress
BODY SYSTEM	**CHANGES SEEN WITH STRESS**
Cardiovascular	Sensation of racing or pounding heart. Elevated pulse rate. Increased BP. Cold, clammy hands and feet. Increased blood glucose level to provide energy for muscles.
Respiratory	Increased respiratory rate and depth. Possible hyperventilation with a tingling sensation in the extremities, faintness, dizziness, and even convulsions if the acid-base balance is seriously altered.
Musculoskeletal	Increased blood glucose level to provide energy for muscles. Increased muscle tension in the back, neck, and head. Complaint of tension headaches, teeth grinding, and backaches.
Gastrointestinal	Decreased peristalsis and decreased production of digestive enzymes. Loss of appetite, nausea, abdominal distention, vomiting, and heartburn. May contribute to development of gastric or duodenal ulcers. Decreased peristalsis resulting in excess intestinal gas and constipation, but diarrhea is also quite common.
Urinary	Decreased urine production but increased urinary frequency.

working through the stressors of a lifetime has enabled many older people to develop a high level of self-knowledge and strong coping skills. Depression appears to be most common when older adults are under physiologic stress. Depression is also likely to occur when older adults perceive that they have lost control of a situation, that they lack the support of significant others, or that their normal coping mechanisms have been overwhelmed by the number or severity of stressors (Boxes 13-1 and 13-2).

Behavioral Signs

People attempt to cope with stress in different ways. Some avoid all interactions or tasks that might increase their stress level, whereas others take on additional duties in an attempt to block out the source of their distress. In either case, performance is likely to suffer. People under stress tend to be disorganized, make more errors, and leave tasks incomplete. They may appear and even sound muddled.

Box 13-1	Symptoms of Depression as Listed in *DSM-IV-TR*

- Changes in appetite and weight
- Disturbed sleep
- Motor agitation or retardation
- Fatigue and loss of energy
- Depressed or irritable mood
- Loss of interest or pleasure in usual activities
- Feelings of worthlessness, self-reproach, or excessive guilt
- Suicidal thinking or attempts
- Difficulty with thinking or concentration

From *Diagnostic and statistical manual of mental disorders*, ed 4, Text revision (DSM-IV-TR). Washington DC, 2000, American Psychiatric Association.

Box 13-2	Goals of Treatment for Depression

- Decreased symptoms of depression
- Reduced risk for relapse and recurrence
- Improved quality of life
- Improved medical health status

The thoughts, statements, and actions of stressed people often jump around in a scattered or disconnected manner. They may pace, hum, or perform other ritualistic actions such as finger drumming, key jangling, or toe tapping. Temper tantrums, shouting, and other aggressive behaviors can occur without warning.

Self-medicating is one response to dealing with depression and other situational problems. It is certainly not a recommended method, but one that is all too common among all age groups, including the elderly. The substances most commonly abused include tobacco, alcohol, and prescription drugs. Some elderly also abuse illicit street drugs, and this number is expected to climb as Baby Boomers get older. Most older adults are aware that tobacco has harmful effects and continue to use the substance in spite of warnings. Although it is physically damaging, tobacco does not have the same effects on the mind and behavior as do alcohol and drugs.

While some people have abused substances from early in life onward, as many as one-third of addictions occur later in life. Drugs such as anxiolytics, tranquilizers, analgesics, and other mood-altering drugs are among the most common prescriptions given to elderly adults. Many times an older person receives prescriptions from several physicians, thus increasing the availability and potential for abuse. As discussed in Chapter 7, many older adults do not adhere to the directions given on a prescription. They alter doses and frequency to suit themselves, increasing their risk for tolerance and dependence. Because the use of alcohol is legal, socially acceptable, and readily available, it is most often an abused substance.

Alcohol tolerance changes as a result of altered physiology. Decreased lean muscle mass, changes in liver enzyme function, and increased nervous system sensitivity to alcohol decrease the safe level of intake for the elderly. Older adults who have abused alcohol for many years consume larger amounts and more often than those who start abusing alcohol later in life. Long-time abusers are more likely to have classic symptoms of alcoholism, experience disturbed family or social relationships, and experience withdrawal when alcohol consumption is stopped suddenly. Late-life abusers are more likely to drink in response to stressful events. They suffer fewer physical symptoms, are less likely to experience withdrawal, and are more likely to have intact relationships. Both groups are likely to drink alone, at home, and in response to stressful or negative emotional perceptions.

Most physicians and nurses overlook alcohol problems in the elderly. Signs of alcohol and drug abuse are sometimes missed because they mimic changes seen with aging such as bone density changes, urinary incontinence, altered sleep patterns, unsteadiness, hypertension, stomach complaints, falls, and so on. Substance abuse should be evaluated even though they seem unlikely. Although more men have substance abuse problems, elderly widows who live alone are also a high-risk group.

Mental health resources and support groups are available in many communities to help with substance abuse. Many are tailored to meet the specific needs of the elderly.

STRESS AND ILLNESS

Stress and illness are closely linked. Research has shown that both mental and physical illness results in stress and that stress increases the risk for both mental and physical illness. A physically ill person is less able to cope with additional physical or psychological stressors, which take energy away from the already depleted reserves and decrease the ability to cope. Stress can interfere with the ability to learn, function, and follow through with the plan of care. Decreasing the number of stressors or the level of stress can prevent illness or improve a person's ability to cope with existing illnesses.

Stress has been shown to have negative effects on many body systems. Because stress activates the sympathetic nervous system (fight-or-flight response), the older person under high levels of stress is at increased risk for angina, heart rhythm abnormalities, and even heart attack. Stress is associated with hypertension and may increase the risk for stroke. The immune system is affected, increasing susceptibility to infections and potentially impairing an older person's response to immunizations such as the pneumonia vaccine. Gastrointestinal problems such as ulcer, GERD, and irritable bowel disease are more likely to occur or worsen when an older person is under stress. Stress can exacerbate sleep problems and often triggers painful headaches or muscle spasms.

People differ in their abilities to cope with stress. Those who do not learn to cope effectively with normal day-to-day stressors cannot function normally when the stress level is high and thus are at risk for becoming physically or mentally ill. Those who do learn good coping strategies can maintain their ability to function despite high-level stress. Many different coping or defense mechanisms are used as part of day-to-day living

Box 13-3	Common Coping or Defense Mechanisms

- *Repression*—The removal of anxiety-producing thoughts or experiences from conscious awareness
- *Denial*—Refusing to acknowledge some painful aspect of external reality that is obvious to others
- *Rationalization*—Creating an acceptable reason for unacceptable thoughts or actions
- *Intellectualization*—Making generalizations to avoid disturbing thoughts or feelings
- *Displacement*—Transferring emotions about one situation or person onto another
- *Suppression*—Avoiding thinking about distressing situations
- *Projection*—Attributing one's own feeling to another
- *Sublimation*—Channeling negative energy into socially acceptable behaviors
- *Substitution*—Keeping so busy with activities that there is no time to think about stressors

(Box 13-3). People who are able to cope effectively usually rely on several of these mechanisms. Coping mechanisms are neither good nor bad; they become dysfunctional only when used excessively or inappropriately as a way of avoiding dealing with the stressors.

STRESS AND LIFE EVENTS

While stress can cause physical illness, physical illness also increases stress. An elderly person suffering from numerous chronic and acute conditions is under greater stress than one who is healthier. Stress can increase as a result of loss—the loss of friends, family members, and particularly, a spouse can be highly stressful. Other life events, such as a change in residence or financial worries, can also contribute to stress.

STRESS-REDUCTION AND COPING STRATEGIES

There are two basic categories of coping style: problem-focused strategies and emotion-focused strategies. Problem-focused coping strategies attempt to change or eliminate the stressful event or threat. Emotion-focused strategies attempt to change the person's response to the stressful event or threat. The type of strategy used depends on the personal significance of the event and the perceived ability to alter the outcomes.

One effective way of reducing stress is to avoid or escape the stressor(s). When an event has little personal significance or when there is little likelihood of having an impact on the outcome of an event, avoidance may be the best choice. When people know that certain events are likely to increase their stress level, the best alternative may be to avoid these situations whenever possible. It is often simpler and wiser to avoid stress than to endure it. When facing a major stressor, it is wise to eliminate as many smaller stressors as possible so that energy is available to cope with the major problem.

When stressors cannot be avoided, when their personal significance is high, or when the person believes he or she can affect the outcome, other methods can be used. Confrontational, cognitive, and problem-solving methods are effective means of dealing with these types of stressful situations.

To use a problem-solving method, a person must first identify and examine his or her stressors. Once the stressors are identified, their importance to the individual can be determined. Only then can alternative actions to reduce the stress be explored. For example, the individual can continue to face the stressor (e.g., an annoying coworker) and live with the consequences (**confrontational**), change jobs (**escape**), decrease contact with the stressor (**avoidance**), or consciously work to change one's attitude toward the annoying person (**emotional distancing**). The choice made is based on a deliberate decision. The mere fact that the person retains control and makes a choice helps reduce the stress level.

Many people need to be taught how to use the problem-solving method for coping with stress in their lives. Learning to use this process with small or minor stressors can help people learn to cope with major stressors. Some find that physical activity helps them cope with stress. Exercise may reduce excessive levels of stress-related hormones and may allow the body to regain homeostasis. The particular physical activity chosen should be one that the stressed individual enjoys and participates in willingly. Physical activity should be carried out in moderation, not to a level of exhaustion where it becomes another form of stress.

Relaxation techniques can be used to help people cope with stress. The most common forms of relaxation techniques include progressive relaxation, **meditation**, **imaging**, biofeedback, and **self-hypnosis**. In addition to these techniques, the support of friends and family

Complementary and Alternative Therapies

Stress Reduction

- *Concentration meditation*—A variety of activities focusing on breathing, body sensation, or mantras may divert the mind from worries and concerns that increase stress.
- *Movement meditation*—Activities such as yoga, tai chi, Qigong, walking, or dancing use motion and focused attention to reduce both mental and physical stress.
- *Prayer and reflection*—Prayers and reflection on sacred verses or poems, either alone or in a group, can be calming and reduce stress.
- *Massage*—Focused manipulation of muscles reduces tension, decreases pain, and promotes a bond of caring, all of which reduce stress.
- *Reiki*—This Japanese technique for stress reduction and relaxation also promotes healing. It is administered by "laying on hands" to increase an unseen "life force energy" that causes us to be alive. When this energy is low, we are more likely to feel stress; when it is high, we are more capable of being happy and healthy.

Complementary and Alternative Therapies

Geriatric Massage

- Geriatric massage is a modification of standard massage designed to meet the needs of older adults.
- Benefits of massage include improved circulation, relief of pain and increased range of motion, decreased anxiety or depression, improved sleep, and enhanced sense of well-being. These services can be provided by certified therapists available in many communities.
- Massage treatments are not covered by Medicare or Medicaid, but they may be covered by private insurance programs.
- A typical session lasts no more than 30 minutes to decrease the risk for fatigue.
- Gentle motions designed to stimulate circulation and relax muscles are used over most of the body. Passive movement and gentle stretching with occasional stronger movements are used on larger joints in the shoulders, legs, and hips to improve joint mobility and flexibility.
- Smaller joints in the hands and feet are gently massaged to relieve pain and improve mobility.
- Massage is not a replacement for physical therapy or exercise.
- Not all older adults are candidates for full body massage. Use of this technique should be discussed with the physician before initiation.

benefits most people. Talking through problems and stresses can facilitate problem solving. If the level of stress is too severe for routine stress-reduction techniques, professional help from counselors, ministers, or mental health professionals may be necessary.

Stress is as much a fact of life for older adults as it is for the younger population. However, the amount and types of stressors do seem to change with aging (see Table 13-1). Many negative life events have been identified as stress producers in older adults; however, there are fewer positive life events that produce stress as we age. Many of the stressors of older adults involve losses. Loss of a spouse or child, home, vision, or driver's license can result in the loss of a purpose in life and may place a severe strain on the coping abilities of older adults. Too many or too frequent stressors can overwhelm older adults, particularly those already under physiologic stress because of physical illness.

The ability to cope with stress differs widely among older adults. In general, those who have learned good coping strategies and have used them throughout a lifetime will continue to do so into old age. Those who did not learn at a younger age how to cope with stress will continue to experience problems.

Because of the unchanging nature of so many of the stressors seen with aging, older adults are more likely to emotionally distance themselves from situations they cannot change. They are increasingly likely to seek support in spiritual or philosophic beliefs that help them cope with these uncontrollable situations.

❖ NURSING PROCESS FOR INEFFECTIVE COPING

Ineffective coping occurs when a person is unable to solve problems or adapt to the stressors in his or her life. Individuals experiencing ineffective coping often verbalize feelings of anxiety, anger, or depression and can often be heard using phrases such as "I just can't cope anymore." In addition, they may complain of changes in physical function that occur as a result of stress. Loss of appetite, nausea, "sour stomach," altered bowel or bladder elimination patterns, and sleep disturbances are common complaints. Older persons who are having problems coping often appear to be agitated. This agitation can interfere with the ability to make even simple decisions, solve problems, and participate in self-care activities. In severe cases, the person may appear angry and hostile or may withdraw from contact with others. If these individuals live independently, they may abuse tobacco, alcohol, or drugs in an attempt to cope with their stress (Box 13-4 and Figure 13-1).

■ Assessment/Data Collection

- Does the person verbalize feelings of tension, stress, frustration, or depression?
- Does the person complain of changes in eating habits?
- Does the person complain of changes in bladder or bowel elimination patterns?
- Is the person experiencing changes in sleep patterns?
- Does the person have difficulty making decisions or solving problems?
- Does the person appear agitated, aggressive, angry, or hostile?
- Is the person depressed or withdrawn?
- Does the person smoke or consume alcohol excessively?
- Has the person experienced an increased frequency of illness or accidents?

Box 13-4   Alcohol-Related Problems in Older Adults

- The incidence of alcohol-related problems in community-dwelling older adults ranges from 1% to 6%. In those hospitalized for medical problems, the incidence increases to 7% to 22%. In those hospitalized in mental health or psychiatric units, the incidence increases even more, from 28% to 44%.
- Alcohol-related problems often go undetected in older adults because symptoms are often mistaken for dementia or medical problems. For example, gastrointestinal problems are more likely to be correlated to antiinflammatory medications than to alcohol consumption.
- Alcohol use in the aging population contributes to liver disease, dementia, peripheral neuropathy, insomnia, poor nutrition, incontinence, depression, inadequate self-care, and medication reactions. Use of alcohol increases the risk for falls, hip fractures, and other accidents.
- Older men are more likely to use alcohol to cope with financial problems, whereas older women are more likely to use alcohol to cope with death or loss of relationships.

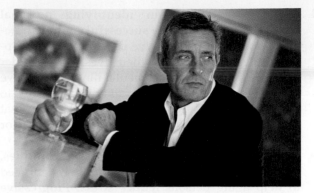

FIGURE 13-1 Loneliness and hopelessness can be manifestations of alcohol abuse.

See Box 13-5 for a list of risk factors for problems related to coping or stress in older adults.

■ Nursing Diagnosis

Ineffective coping

■ Nursing Goals/Outcomes Identification

The nursing goals for older individuals with ineffective coping are to (1) communicate feelings of stress, (2) identify personal strengths and effective methods of coping, and (3) participate in decision making.

■ Nursing Interventions/Implementation

The following nursing interventions should take place in hospitals or extended-care facilities:

1. **Maintain continuity of care to develop a stable, trusting relationship.** Before older persons will verbalize their concerns, they must develop trust in their caregiver(s). This trust is best gained by keeping the number of caregivers to a minimum. A plan of care should be developed with the individual. To reduce stress, this plan should be followed with minimal changes.
2. **Encourage older adults to verbalize their feelings.** Verbalization provides older adults with an opportunity to express their concerns and solve problems. Merely putting feelings into words often reduces the stress that comes from holding back anxious thoughts. Nurses should be careful to remain nonjudgmental and should allow older adults to express a full range of feelings, including fear, anger, hostility, and grief.
3. **Ensure that older adults receive adequate nutrition, rest, and pain relief.** Persons who are hungry, fatigued, or in pain are likely to have difficulty coping with other stressors. Nurses should plan care to minimize these basic physical stressors.

Box 13-5   Risk Factors Related to Problems with Coping or Stress Tolerance in Older Adults

- Recent social, physical, emotional, or financial losses
- Physical illness
- Major life changes

4. **Assist older adults in identifying personal strengths and previously successful coping strategies.** Most older people have used a variety of coping strategies throughout their lives. Unless older adults suffer from chronic mental illness, they have probably managed to cope rather successfully to have reached old age. The coping behaviors that were used throughout life can act as a basis for coping with current situations.

5. **Explain a variety of stress-reduction techniques.** A variety of stress-reduction techniques can be used to help aging persons reduce stress. **Progressive relaxation** is a simple technique that can be used by older adults. To learn to relax, the person is first taught to identify the difference between muscle tension and relaxation. Once he or she can identify the different sensations, the person is taught to alternately tighten and relax muscles, starting at the feet and working upward through the body. This is done until the entire body is relaxed. With practice, this technique can be done quickly, effectively, and at will.

Self-hypnosis takes relaxation a step further and allows individuals to actually place themselves in a trancelike state. This technique is more complex and more difficult to learn than are other relaxation techniques. Commercial audiotapes are available to teach self-hypnosis.

Imaging is a relaxation technique in which individuals are taught to think of a calm, peaceful setting. This can be whatever setting the individual finds most relaxing. The person should visualize this setting and try to picture it in detail, taking pleasure from each aspect of the environment. Then the person imagines *being* in this environment, relaxing and enjoying the experience.

Meditation is a somewhat more difficult—but highly beneficial—relaxation technique. Time and effort are required to learn to meditate effectively. Individuals must learn to shut out external stimuli and focus on calming their thoughts. To gain this internal focus, most meditators use a mantra, which is a word or sound that is repeated over and over again. To facilitate meditation, the individual should be provided with a quiet place where distractions can be minimized and should be assisted into a position that promotes comfort and relaxation.

6. **Encourage older adults to participate in activities (Figure 13-2).** Physical and diversional activities can reduce stress by focusing excess nervous energy in productive ways, but persons experiencing stress may be reluctant to participate. These individuals should be encouraged but never forced to attend these activities, because forcing only increases stress.

7. **Consult with mental health specialists, ministers, or counselors.** Many techniques are available to help older adults cope with stress. If the problem is severe or if nurses are unable to help older adults cope with stress, it is wise to consult with a specialist.

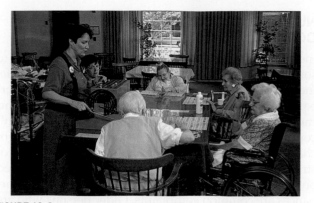

FIGURE 13-2 Regularly scheduled socializing activities serve to combat isolation among older adults.

The following interventions should take place in the home:

1. **Encourage the family to provide emotional support to older adults.** It is often difficult for older adults (or anyone else) to cope with stress alone. Families should be encouraged to spend time with older adults, listening, and providing emotional support. If the family dynamics are disturbed and the family is a source of stress, it may be necessary to reduce family contact and help the older person identify other sources of emotional support such as friends, ministers, or others.

2. **Identify community resources that can provide support to older adults and their families.** Many older persons and their families have difficulty coping on their own. Most communities have mental health clinics or senior citizen help lines to assist in times of stress.

3. **Use any appropriate interventions that are used in the institutional setting.**

❖ NURSING PROCESS FOR RELOCATION STRESS SYNDROME

Relocation stress syndrome describes the physiologic or psychological stress that occurs when a person is transferred from one environment to another. Relocation stress is a common problem with aging and can occur with many types of relocation, including the following:

- From a private home to the home of a family member
- From home to an apartment or other shared living arrangement
- From one area of the city to another
- From home to a hospital
- From home to a long-term care facility
- From home to a hospital and then to a long-term care facility
- From one unit in the hospital or long-term care facility to another unit in the same facility
- From one room to another in a hospital or long-term care facility

Older persons who are required to change residence are likely to experience losses, fears, and concerns that increase stress. Loss of independence, loss of personal possessions, loss of friends and neighbors, fear of the unknown, and concern about the future all increase stress. Stress is greatest when many losses or changes have occurred, when these changes occur in rapid succession, when the changes are unexpected, and when the individual has had little or no say in the decision-making process.

Older persons experiencing relocation stress syndrome exhibit emotional, behavioral, and physical signs of stress. Most newly relocated older persons experience feelings of powerlessness, helplessness, and insecurity. They often verbalize an unwillingness to relocate or dissatisfaction with the new living arrangements. They are likely to express feelings of grief, anger, apprehension, anxiety, loneliness, depression, and confusion. To cope with these feelings, older adults may demonstrate a variety of behaviors.

Some attempt to maintain control of the situation by demanding attention and verbalizing many needs. They may be more dependent on caregivers than their physical condition justifies. Others attempt to cope with the stress by becoming hostile or angry. They often deny the necessity of the change and refuse necessary assistance or care. Still others cope by withdrawing and isolating themselves from contact with staff, other residents, and even family. These behaviors are usually a result of lack of trust or feelings of powerlessness in the new setting.

In addition to behavioral changes, recently relocated older adults are likely to experience physical signs of stress. Changes in eating habits, weight loss, gastrointestinal changes, changes in elimination patterns, and changes in sleep patterns are commonly seen in newly relocated older persons.

■ Assessment/Data Collection

See the assessment for ineffective coping on page 229.

■ Nursing Diagnosis

Relocation stress syndrome

■ Nursing Goals/Outcomes Identification

The nursing goals for older individuals with relocation stress syndrome are to (1) recognize the reasons for the move or change, (2) identify ways to maintain control and decision-making powers in the new environment, (3) verbalize concerns about new living arrangements, and (4) identify methods for coping with change.

■ Nursing Interventions/Implementation

The following nursing interventions should take place in hospitals or extended-care facilities:

1. **Encourage verbalization of feelings, fears, and concerns about the move or change.** When a person holds in all fears and concerns, his or her stress level remains high. Allowing older adults to discuss their concerns openly and freely initiates the problem solving process. Anger is common when older adults disagree with the move. This anger should be accepted as a normal and even healthy response.

2. **Discuss the reasons for the move or change.** Nurses and families should be open and honest about the reasons for a move or change. Any questions the individual has should be answered as completely and honestly as possible. Attempting to shield older adults from the often harsh reality is likely to result in anger and loss of trust.

3. **Include older adults in care planning.** Whenever possible, active participation of older adults in care planning should be encouraged. This allows older adults to maintain some degree of control over decisions that affect their lives. Whenever possible, choices should be offered and the individual's preferences should be respected.

4. **Encourage a positive attitude about the move or change.** Nurses should help older adults identify the benefits that will come with the change and should avoid making personal or negative comments about the move.

5. **Maintain continuity of care to enhance feelings of trust.** When an aging person is newly relocated, the number of persons providing care should be kept to a minimum and care should be given in a consistent manner. The individual's preferences should be respected and his or her needs met promptly. This helps build a sense of trust and decreases the stress that results from rapid or unpredictable changes.

6. **Encourage the use of familiar objects and belongings.** Older adults should be encouraged to bring as many prized personal possessions as space allows. Personal belongings enhance the sense of belonging. Seeing and using familiar items makes a new environment seem more familiar and reduces stress. Personal possessions should be positioned or displayed so that the person can easily reach or see them. Because most people feel that their personal belongings are extensions of themselves, these belongings should always be treated with care and respect by caregivers.

Relocation to a new environment can be confusing and even disorienting to older adults. Selected equipment such as calendars, clocks, night-lights, and personal belongings will help older adults make a smoother adjustment to a new environment.

The following interventions should take place in the home:

1. **Allow older adults to participate in decision making and planning for the change.** It is important to include older adults in decisions that will have a

significant impact on their lives. When a major change (e.g., a change in residence) is necessary, the older person, his or her family, and possibly, a social worker should make decisions together. The person should know the reasons for the change and the available options. When choices are available, the preferences of the individual should be respected. Enabling older adults to retain control of these choices reduces the sense of powerlessness and thus stress.

2. **Anticipate fears and concerns, and allow adequate time to implement the change, when possible.** Nurses should help older adults and their families anticipate and plan for the change. In cases in which a change in environment occurs because of a medical emergency, planning is not possible. In many cases, however, there is adequate time to prepare older adults for a change. This time should be used to allow the individual to accept the fact that a change of environment is necessary. In addition, the individual can sort through personal belongings and distribute or discard them as desired. Scheduled visits to the new environment before the actual move allow the person to become more familiar with the physical structure and people.

3. **Use any appropriate interventions that are used in the institutional setting.** (See Nursing Care Plan 13-1).

⭐ Nursing Care Plan 13-1   Relocation Stress Syndrome

Mrs. Mack, an 81-year-old woman, recently moved into Brookline Care Center. You observe that she looks sad. She spends most of her time alone, sitting in her room looking out the window. She repeatedly asks, "Why did they have to do this to me? I was happy where I was. I just wanted to stay there until I died." Mrs. Mack makes many demands of the staff and asks many questions. She complains that she has difficulty sleeping in strange surroundings with other people so close by.

Mrs. Mack's chart reveals that she has a variety of health problems, including heart trouble and a history of high blood pressure. Until recently, she lived independently in her own apartment and required minimal help with getting to doctors' appointments and grocery shopping. Recently she had become more forgetful, and her daughters were increasingly concerned about her safety and well-being living alone. Both daughters agreed that a care center would be most appropriate, and they found one near one of their homes that was reasonable in cost and that had a vacancy. They made arrangements for the move and notified the landlord before discussing the plans with Mrs. Mack. The daughters moved a few of her personal belongings with her, but many were sold or given to family members.

Nursing Diagnosis
Relocation stress syndrome

Defining Characteristics
- Sad affect
- Apprehension
- Verbalization of concern about move
- Increased dependency
- Increased demands and verbalization of needs
- Change in sleeping patterns

Patient Goals/Outcomes Identification
Mrs. Mack will verbalize an understanding of the reasons for her move, identify concerns about her new environment, and identify ways to cope with the change.

Nursing Interventions/Implementation
1. Encourage Mrs. Mack to verbalize her feelings about the move.
2. Allow expressions of anger or frustration about the family's actions.
3. Encourage Mrs. Mack to discuss her feelings with her family.
4. Explain the reasons that necessitated the move.
5. Involve Mrs. Mack in decision making and care planning.
6. Maintain stable care assignments to build trust.
7. Encourage a positive attitude about change.
8. Offer opportunities to participate in social activities.
9. Encourage her family to bring in more valued personal belongings.
10. Consult a social worker or minister as appropriate to facilitate positive family interactions.

Evaluation
Mrs. Mack's family has brought additional family pictures, some favorite pillows, and a lap robe that had been stored in a closet. They also purchased a small color television with a special earphone for listening in bed. Mrs. Mack states, "I still don't like it here, but I know that my family thinks it is best for me. They are trying to make it better I guess." You will continue the plan of care.

Critical Thinking Questions
1. What behaviors would indicate that Mrs. Mack is adjusting to the change in living accommodations?
2. What additional nursing interventions can you identify that might help Mrs. Mack and her family reduce their stress?

Get Ready for the NCLEX® Examination!

Key Points

- Stress is a fact of life.
- Although the stressors may change throughout life, stress affects people of all ages. The major stressors of aging relate to losses.
- Loss of ability, loss of loved ones, loss of home, and many other losses are stressful to older adults, affecting physical and emotional status.
- Stress can result in behavioral changes. Excessive levels of stress are harmful.
- Each individual uses a variety of coping mechanisms to deal with stress.
- The effectiveness or ineffectiveness of these coping strategies is of concern to nurses.
- Interventions that reduce stress and support positive coping mechanisms can be beneficial.

Additional Learning Resources

SG Go to the Study Guide on pp. 379–397 for additional learning activities to help you master the chapter content.

evolve Go to your Evolve website (http://evolve.elsevier.com/Wold/geriatric) for the following FREE learning resources:
- Animations
- Answer Guidelines for Nursing Care Plan Critical Thinking Questions
- Answers and Rationales for Review Questions for the NCLEX® Examination
- Glossary with pronunciations in English and Spanish
- Video Clips

Review Questions for the NCLEX® Examination

1. When assessing an elderly person, the nurse suspects an increased level of stress when observing the following physiologic data: (Select all that apply.)
   1. Increased urine production with retention
   2. Hyperventilation
   3. Warm hands and feet with sweating
   4. Headache
   5. Rapid pulse
   6. Elevated blood pressure
   7. Loss of appetite and nausea

2. The drug most commonly abused by older adults is:
   1. Cocaine
   2. Marijuana
   3. Heroin
   4. Alcohol

3. Which findings in the patient's history lead the nurse to suspect alcohol abuse? (Select all that apply.)
   1. Poor nutrition
   2. Liver disease
   3. Financial problems
   4. Strong family relationships
   5. Peripheral neuropathy
   6. Poor self-care
   7. Repeated falls or accidents
   8. Heart disease

4. An elderly client tells the nurse that he feels "stressed" and asks what the nurse would recommend. The best response would be:
   1. "See your doctor for an antianxiety medication."
   2. "Get more sleep and try a glass of wine with dinner."
   3. "Are you aware of the tai chi class at the recreation center?"
   4. "Just let go of whatever is bothering you."

5. An elderly person experiencing depression is most likely to have difficulty:
   1. Recalling past events
   2. Orienting to person and place
   3. Identifying recent changes in environment
   4. Concentrating on an activity

6. An elderly person tells the nurse that visiting the doctor is very stressful for her. It is most appropriate for the nurse to:
   1. Suggest that she postpone the visit and go when she is more relaxed
   2. Tell the person that she needs to work on changing her attitude
   3. Help her develop strategies for dealing with her concerns
   4. Stress that it is important and she needs to go and get it over with

Values and Beliefs

Objectives

1. Discuss the impact of personal values and beliefs on everyday life.
2. Identify values and beliefs commonly found in today's older adult population.
3. Discuss how beliefs and values affect the health practices of older adults.
4. Explain the relationship of values and beliefs to health practices.
5. Compare the spiritual practices of major religions as they relate to death.
6. Discuss how culture and ethnicity affect health beliefs and practices.
7. Describe methods of assessing beliefs and values.
8. Identify older adults who are most at risk for experiencing problems related to values and beliefs.
9. Identify selected nursing diagnoses related to values or beliefs.
10. Describe nursing interventions appropriate for older individuals who are experiencing problems related to values or beliefs.

Key Terms

deity (p. 238)
orthodox (p. 238)
religious (p. 234)

ritual (p. 238)
spiritual (p. 237)

Most older persons have established a pattern of values, goals, and beliefs that guide their decisions and choices. These values and beliefs have their origins in the individual's religion, philosophy, family, culture, and society.

Values and beliefs are essential to the human spirit. They are the intangibles that set humans apart from other animals. Values and beliefs affect all aspects of our lives and play an important role in promoting health and coping with illness. Values and beliefs influence how we live and how we die.

Values influence the decisions we make throughout life. They are the "rights and wrongs," the "thou shalts," and "thou shalt nots" that we use to steer our way through the myriad choices made during a lifetime. The choices of spouse, living arrangements, dress, eating patterns, and patterns of health maintenance are all influenced by our personal value system.

The personal value system is developed early in childhood. Many experts believe that most of our values are well established by the time we reach 10 years of age. The idea that the values that guide our lives for 80 or 90 years are established so early is significant, and the implications for parents, schools, and society are tremendous.

Values are based on the beliefs that are stressed by the family, culture, church, school, and media while a person is growing up. The beliefs that were reinforced while we were young will most likely have the greatest influence on our personal value system.

Because people develop their values based on a unique combination of time, place, and experiences, no two have the exact same beliefs and values. People of similar ages, cultural backgrounds, and experiences are likely to share similar beliefs and values. People of different ages, cultural backgrounds, and experiences are likely to hold different beliefs and values.

For example, people who formed their values during the Great Depression see the world quite differently than do those born during World War II or during the baby boom of the 1950s. People reared with strict moral or religious values are likely to have beliefs different from people raised without moral or religious training. People raised in traditional nuclear families are likely to have values different from people raised in other family structures. Those raised before the advent of television are likely to have values different from those raised with television. People growing up when war is viewed as a patriotic duty have values different from those reared during a time when any war is viewed as immoral.

People see the world through their own value and belief structure and use this as a filter by which they judge other people and events. Most of us have difficulty understanding people whose values are different from our own. It is human nature for each person to think that his or her personal beliefs and values are somehow superior to those of others. People with belief and value patterns similar to one's own are likely

Cultural Considerations

Jewish Spirituality

- Different levels of observance exist. Highly Orthodox groups strictly follow ancient Talmudic law. Reformed and Conservative groups accept many beliefs and practices but are less strict in other observances.
- Special dietary practices (Kosher) are very complex and may require guidance from a Rabbi or other authority. Hygiene rituals, including circumcision and special bathing rituals, are part of tradition.
- The Sabbath starts at sundown on Friday and lasts until sundown on Saturday. No work is to be done on the Sabbath.
- Ritual garb includes the tallit, or prayer shawl, which is the most authentic Jewish garment. It is a rectangular-shaped piece of fabric with special fringes called *tzitzit* on each of the four corners. Also important is the yarmulke, or kippah, which is a head covering worn to remind the faithful of God's presence and that there is something higher and greater than man.
- Many special holy days and holidays such as Hanukkah, Yom Kippur, and Passover are recognized throughout the year.
- Prayer is a part of daily life; it provides time for looking inward and is a means of examining one's relationship to God. Ritual prayer is connected to awakening, meals, and bedtime. Groups of 10 men, a *minyan*, is desirable for prayer. A book of prayer called a *siddur* may be used to guide prayer.
- Burial typically takes place within 24 hours of death. From the time of death until the burial, a guardian (*shomer*) stays with the deceased, reciting words from the Book of Psalms. Embalming and cremation are not permitted. The body is dressed in plain white shrouds, regardless of position. The casket must be made completely of wood so that the body should not decompose sooner than the coffin. Seven days of mourning (*shivah*) begin immediately following burial.

Cultural Considerations

Muslim/Islamic Spirituality

- Islam includes a wide variety of groups that vary in their level of orthodoxy.
- The emphasis of Islamic teachings is summed up in the holy book, the Koran (*Qur'an*).
- The Five Pillars of Islamic faith include (1) to proclaim the Shahadah (confession of the faith); (2) to perform the mandatory five daily prayers on time; (3) to fast during the month of Ramadan, the ninth in the lunar calendar, from dawn to sunset; (4) to pay Zakat religious tithes to the poor, and (5) to make a pilgrimage in Mecca, at least once in a lifetime.
- There are no priests or ministers. Religious scholars or teachers called *Imams* are regarded as authorities on theological questions.
- Pork and its derivatives are prohibited. Alcoholic beverages and drug abuse are forbidden.
- Modesty for women, particularly in dress, is highly important. Many Muslim patients request that care be provided by women only.
- At death the body is washed and then wrapped in a cotton sheet. A simple prayer is said for the soul of the deceased person. Autopsy is allowed if necessary and/or required by law. Cremation is not allowed; the body should return to the earth in natural form.

Cultural Considerations

Latinos and Spirituality

- Many Latinos perceive cultural insensitivity and language barriers as contributors to poor quality nursing and medical care.
- Latino culture closely connects faith in the caregivers with the ability to recover and heal effectively. They often verbalize that nurses need to address the person's total life concerns and stressors, not just their physical complaints.
- In times of illness, it is common for older adult Latinos to seek out *remedios* (folk remedies), *curanderos* (traditional Mexican healers), prayers, and over-the-counter medications before they seek attention from organized medical facilities.

Cultural Considerations

African Americans and Spirituality

- Spirituality and religious practices are very important in many families of African descent.
- Belief that illness is caused by failures of faith or by the devil is common, and prayer is an important tool to deal with illness.
- Many different religions are practiced by the African-American community, and the nurse needs to be careful not to stereotype but to determine the specific beliefs and practices of each individual.
- Some African Americans may seek to attend religious services several days a week or may desire frequent visits from their minister. Others, particularly Muslims, may observe dietary restrictions, including fasting and abstaining from pork products.
- Jehovah's Witnesses typically refuse blood products on religious grounds.

Cultural Considerations

American Indians and Spirituality

- American Indians, who make up approximately 1% of the U.S. population, are culturally diverse, represented by 517 tribes and more than 150 languages.
- More than half of American Indians live in the Southwest, but tribal groups can be found in most states.
- Some common beliefs that relate to life and death include a belief: (1) in a Creator or Great Spirit; (2) that all things in the world, living or not, have spirits; (3) that those educated in sacred traditions are to pass them from one generation to the next; and (4) that interdependence with family and tribe is of high value.
- For many American Indians, health and spirituality are inseparable. They may verbalize a need to be alone to practice cultural rituals or to seek guidance from the elders to maintain harmony of mind, spirit, and body.
- Elders are to be respected for their age and wisdom.

Euro-Americans and Spirituality

The influence of Christianity began during the height of the Roman Empire and has continued for over 2000 years. One group, Roman Catholics, have long claimed to be the only Christian church. Their position has caused a great deal of controversy. Conflict between Catholic beliefs and those of the Jews, Muslims, and other religions resulted in everything from heated arguments to bloody wars. Dissatisfied groups "reformed" and split off from the Catholic mainstream. Religious unrest affected Europe throughout history. Families have divided and countries have been formed or destroyed based on religious beliefs. Many immigrants left European countries and immigrated with the hope of finding both economic and religious freedom. People who came to America were not only seeking religious freedom, they were also seeking a place where they could practice their own form of religion free of interference from the state or rival denominations. While Christian churches remain separate and distinct, contemporary interaction between denominations has improved somewhat since the 1960s when the Catholic pope started "ecumenical" outreach to improve understanding between Christian groups. The secular nature of modern society also has diminished some real or perceived animosity between churches.

Christian denominations include Catholics, Episcopalians, Anglicans, Lutherans, Methodists, Presbyterians, Congregationalists, Baptists, Mormons, Fundamentalists, and "nondenominational" Christians. There are many subgroups of each denomination. Specifics regarding each groups beliefs and practices should be sought from the client's minister or clergy.

1) While each Christian church has unique perspectives, some things that most Christians believe include:
   a) God is the creator of everything seen and unseen
   b) Christ is the son of God and is one with God in the trinity.
   c) Christ suffered, was crucified, died and was buried, rose from the dead, and ascended into heaven.
   d) Christ will return to judge the living and the dead. Those who repent will have their sins forgiven and can be saved.
2) Most Christian churches have a specified and hierarchical organizational structure.
3) Clergy are typically educated in the tenets of the specific faith and then "ordained" as a minister of the faith.
4) Most have an organized set of rituals or sacraments to address life events such as marriage, holidays, death, etc.

Cultural Competence

Nurses working in home health care need to have a great deal of awareness and sensitivity to cultural values and beliefs so that they are able to work within a variety of cultural contexts. The nurse who is perceptive of cultural beliefs, values, norms, practices, communication style, and behaviors is more likely to be effective in providing care that is accepted and appreciated by culturally diverse patients. The perception that the nurse is showing respect for a patient's diversity can often make the difference between successful health interventions and avoidance of the health care establishment. The following are some websites that contain information regarding cultural competence:

• http://www.culturediversity.org/
• http://www.xculture.org/training/overview/cultural/assessment.html
• http://medicine.ucsf.edu/resources/guidelines/culture.html

to be viewed positively, and interactions are likely to be of a friendly nature. People with beliefs and values that are different from one's own are likely to be viewed negatively, and interactions may be difficult or even antagonistic.

Misunderstanding and conflict often occur when people with two different or contradictory sets of values interact. Statements such as "He just doesn't understand me" or "I just don't understand her" usually indicate a conflict in beliefs or values. Consider the number of times you have heard parents say this about their children and vice versa. Consider the number of times a member of one ethnic or religious group says it about another. Consider the times nurses say this about a patient of a different age, race, or background.

Understanding the values and beliefs of others is not easy, yet the willingness to try to understand or empathize is an important part of nursing care. To be effective, nurses must be willing to really listen to each person for whom they care and avoid judging others by their own values. It is difficult to withhold judgments based on personal values and to approach others with understanding. Nonjudgmental interaction requires a high level of patience and excellent communication skills.

Values and beliefs are not easily changed. This is true for ourselves and others. The most effective way to change beliefs and values is through education, which can be gained through reading, academic study, and interaction with individuals of diverse backgrounds. Patient teaching and positive interactions can help people change their beliefs. Increasing their personal knowledge about the beliefs and values of the more-common cultural, religious, and social groups can help nurses change beliefs. Open-mindedness and understanding of the wide range of beliefs and values existing in an increasingly diverse world enable nurses to work effectively with a variety of people.

COMMON VALUES AND BELIEFS OF OLDER ADULTS

Although the older adult population is no more homogenized than are younger age groups, aging individuals are likely to share some beliefs and values. People 60 years of age or older developed their value systems in a world that was very different from the world today. Many of the beliefs and values that are important to older adults have no significance to younger persons. This is difficult for older adults to understand, and it is difficult for younger family members or caregivers to appreciate. The value and belief patterns of older adults are likely to challenge the understanding of predominantly younger nurses. Nurses must be careful to determine what beliefs and values are at work before making judgments or planning interventions. Unless the underlying belief or value is correctly identified, nurses are likely to choose ineffective interventions that lead to frustration or anger for all involved.

ECONOMIC VALUES

Many of today's older adults were strongly affected by the depression of the 1930s. They were taught the value of a dollar and to "waste not, want not." Financial independence is important to these individuals, and they may experience intense feelings of shame if forced to accept charity. They may save or hoard items, even items that present health hazards because they value saving rather than wasting. Many older people are dismayed when nurses or family members throw away food or medical supplies and may attempt to retrieve these items, particularly when they are left alone. They may store an excessive number of personal belongings and clutter up their homes until these belongings become a safety hazard. Older adults may refuse to see a doctor or wait until they are seriously ill because they are concerned about the costs. They may refuse to buy medication, take less than the prescribed amount of medication, or fail to discard old prescriptions because of cost concerns. Baby Boomers grew up in a more affluent world and are more likely to value material possession and spend rather than save. This is likely to result in increased fear of retirement and more elders remaining in the workforce. Research shows significant financial discrepancies between Baby Boomers, depending on race and gender.

INTRAPERSONAL VALUES

Many older adults were raised valuing respect and obedience to elders. They often cannot understand why their families do not automatically accept what they say and follow their directions. As discussed in Chapter 12, interactions within the family can present many challenges. The more divergent the values of the various family members, the more likely there are to be misunderstandings and conflict. Nurses are often called on to act as mediators when conflicts arise or to provide support to an older person who feels rejected or misunderstood by his or her children.

CULTURAL VALUES

Cultural values and beliefs unite families, neighborhoods, and communities. Shared cultural values define an authority structure, establish norms for language and communication, and establish a basis for decision making and lifestyle choices. The U.S. society has sometimes been called a "melting pot," implying that we have blended together and become the same type of people, sharing the same cultural values. Sociologists have suggested that we are in fact more of a "fruit salad" made up of many different and unique peoples mixed together with some blending of values and beliefs. Over a period of 300 years, millions of new immigrants from around the world have come and formed a country with a unique culture of its own. Our country was established by immigrants who were trying to escape persecution and find opportunities that were not available in their homelands. We have a culture that is still influenced by a troubled history of slavery and warfare with its native citizens. An ongoing influx of newcomers from diverse cultures presents constant challenges to our society. A heterogeneity of cultures creates a vibrant and dynamic society, but it also creates many opportunities for prejudice and misunderstanding.

Although most people express a dislike for any form of prejudice or segregation, these problems still exist in this country. In spite of affirmative action, many members of minority groups are still not fully assimilated into the dominant culture. This is partially a result of discrimination by the dominant culture but is also effected by the desire of minority groups to maintain their own uniqueness and cultural practices.

New immigrants experience a period of "culture shock" when entering a new cultural environment where their historic values and practices differ from the dominant culture. Response to this experience varies widely. Some are willing to modify or suppress their historic cultural values, accept those of the dominant society, and assimilate into the mainstream fairly quickly. Others try to hold fast to their cultural uniqueness and resist assimilation into the larger society. They may isolate themselves into an enclave for mutual support and actively resist assimilation. Still others try to find a middle ground, neither isolating nor fully assimilating. Members of the same family may experience different reactions from others, leading to intrafamily culture conflict.

Many older adults have lived in this country for years but still identify more with their ethnic group or country of origin than with the dominant society. At times of stress, individuals are more likely to revert to beliefs and values established during childhood. Nurses need to work at developing an understanding of diverse cultural values and beliefs to provide appropriate care. Numerous textbooks and articles are available to help the nurse identify general cultural perspectives and practices. These are helpful; however, it is usually better to have a direct, honest conversation with the individuals, their families, and significant others to identify their unique cultural beliefs and perspectives.

SPIRITUAL OR RELIGIOUS VALUES

Most people believe in and value something beyond the here and now. Spirituality is based in a recognition that there is a relationship between the person and a transcendent supreme being, a life force, an ultimate reality, or an undefined something that is greater than ourselves. **Spiritual** beliefs can motivate us to take actions or to avoid certain actions. These beliefs give meaning to life and to all of the positive and negative experiences that occur during a lifetime. They can inspire positive emotions such as awe, love, hope, and trust or negative emotions such as hatred, anger, fear, and despair. Individuals usually build their value system and set their priorities based on their spiritual beliefs. Spirituality can exist without a formal or organizational structure or may be practiced as part of an identifiable spiritual community.

Many of today's oldest adults were raised in an organized religion that played an important role in the formulation of their values and beliefs. Regular attendance at places of worship, although highly valued by many older adults, is less common today than it was even a few years ago. This may, in part, result from transportation problems or safety concerns that make regular attendance difficult. Many older persons experience severe distress when they are no longer able to worship regularly because of illness, hospitalization, or relocation to an institutional setting.

Changes in the structure of organized religions and the current trend toward cooperation among religious groups trouble many older persons who were taught the value of their own beliefs and are suspicious of religions other than their own. The interdenominational or nondenominational services that are provided in many institutional settings are often rejected by older adults as heresy. Older adults may have developed closeness to a specific spiritual adviser and may be uncomfortable if this person is unavailable. Spiritual counseling often explores intimate secrets and fears. Older persons may be unwilling to interact with a stranger, even if this person is a qualified minister. Increased participation of women in the ministry upsets some older people who believe that only men were intended to be spiritual advisers. No matter how qualified, a woman chaplain may be rejected by an older person who holds these views.

Many older adults persist in older religious practices, which have changed over time. For example, many older adult Catholics will not eat meat on Fridays, although Catholic law now allows meat to be eaten on Fridays throughout most of the year. Older adult Jews may continue to value orthodox dietary and hygiene practices, although many younger Jews have accepted less rigid standards. If the person has persisted in these practices over a lifetime, change is highly unlikely. In these cases, nurses and the health care system must be flexible enough to enable these persons to maintain their beliefs and still maintain adequate hygiene and nutrition.

Baby Boomers were likely raised with some organized religious beliefs but are likely to have changed to less traditional spiritual practices more in keeping with a secular world. As a person ages and death nears, the need to make peace with his or her deity often becomes significant. Spiritual beliefs can be a source of strength, and even people who did not seem to place a high value on religion when they were younger often see a need to seek spiritual guidance when they get older (Figure 14-1). People who questioned the existence of a deity may change their minds when faced

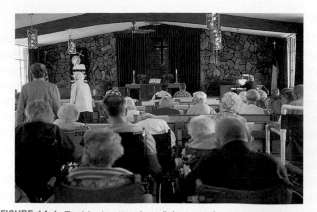

FIGURE 14-1 Residents attend a religious service at a nursing center.

with the reality of their own deaths. Some never express these needs but will accept spiritual counsel if it is offered. Some continue to reject religious counsel, which is also their right.

Decisions regarding the end of life, including the use of high-technology interventions, living wills, euthanasia, or physician-assisted suicide, are usually based on religious beliefs and value systems. Many older adults wish to have a spiritual advisor available for guidance when serious, often life-or-death, decisions are made. Decisions that are made based on religious beliefs must be respected by health care providers, even when their own beliefs and values are different. Survival may be less important to an older person than the violation of long-held beliefs. Coherent older people have the right to make informed choices and have them respected.

Religious rituals are important in many faiths. Prayers, chanting, posturing, cleansing, anointing, and other ritual behaviors are part of the practices of many religions and are used as affirmations of faith. Objects such as icons, menorahs, rosaries, amulets, medals, and holy water are visual symbols of belief that provide comfort and reassurance. A number of books—including the Bible, Koran, Torah, Vedas, and Book of Mormon—are important to the practices of their respective religions (Figure 14-2). Many older

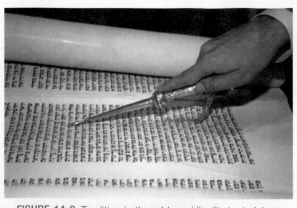

FIGURE 14-2 Tradition in thought—spirituality in Judaism.

Complementary and Alternative Therapies

Prayer

Prayer, which has been practiced by many religious traditions for thousands of years, is a means of communicating with a deity or higher power and is considered by some as a way to escape or transcend tribulations on earth. Prayer can be ritualized and structured or free and informal. Many times prayers are accompanied by rituals or symbols such as candles, incense, beads, etc. Prayer can be incorporated into the plan of care as a complementary therapy designed to promote the patient's spiritual needs.

adults find great comfort in these texts, often memorizing large segments. Older adults who may be unable to read because of the changes associated with aging or illness find comfort in the mere presence of these valued tenets of their faith. Often, the family or spiritual support person will provide these symbols and texts if the older person or nurse requests them. Some religious-sponsored institutions provide them routinely. Individuals with strong religious values and practices often prefer to be hospitalized or live in institutional settings operated by their preferred religious denomination, if these are available in the community.

Many older adults reach the end of life at peace with themselves. It is common for an older adult to say, "I'm ready to go. I've led a good life, not perfect, but I'm ready to meet my maker." Some are not anxious to see life end, but they accept the inevitability. Others, however, have not reached this level of comfort and appear to be in distress as the end of life nears. This may be due to guilt, uncompleted business, poor relationships, or other factors. Spiritual distress is characterized by a lack of hope or an inability to see a purpose or meaning in one's life. People experiencing spiritual

? Critical Thinking

Spiritual Assessment for Nurses

- Do you consider yourself to be spiritual or religious? Why or why not?
- What do you value most?
- What gives meaning to your life?
- Do you belong to an organized church?
- Do you actively participate in church services or functions? How often?
- Are there any specific rituals you need to observe?
- Are there any dietary restrictions in your religion?
- Do you need any objects/articles to support your spiritual practices?
- Do you believe that religion makes a difference in a person's life and death?
- Are there any special things others should know regarding death and dying in your religion?
- In what ways do you think your spiritual beliefs affect your perception and response to the spiritual needs of patients?

Box 14-1   SPIRIT Mnemonic for Spiritual Assessment

S: Spiritual belief system (religious affiliation)
P: Personal spirituality (personal belief system)
I: Integration into a spiritual community (sources of support)
R: Ritualized practices (daily practices, restrictions, and their significance)
I: Implications for medical care (spiritual aspects incorporated into care)
T: Terminal event (end of life)

From Maugans TA, as presented in Larson K: *Geriatric Nursing* 24:6, Nov/Dec 2003.

distress are often fearful or angry. To be open to the spiritual needs of others and work effectively with patients experiencing spiritual distress, the nurse should explore his or her own spiritual feelings and beliefs (see Critical Thinking box and Box 14-1).

❖ NURSING PROCESS FOR SPIRITUAL DISTRESS

■ Assessment/Data Collection

- What is the person's cultural background?
- Does the person have any specific cultural or religious beliefs related to health?
- Is religion or belief in a deity a significant factor in the person's life?
- Does the person attend religious services regularly?
- What is the person's religious denomination, sect, church, etc.?
- Does the person have a preferred spiritual counselor? Does he or she see this person regularly?
- Is the person interested in talking to a priest, minister, rabbi, or other spiritual advisor?
- What religious books or symbols are meaningful to the person?
- Has aging or illness had an impact on the person's beliefs, values, or spiritual practices?

Box 14-2 provides a list of risk factors for alterations in values and beliefs in older adults.

Nursing Diagnosis

Spiritual distress

Nursing Goals/Outcomes Identification

The nursing goals for older individuals suffering from spiritual distress are to (1) identify and verbalize sources of value conflicts, (2) specify the spiritual

Box 14-2   Risk Factors Related to Problems With Values and Beliefs in Older Adults

- Major life stressors such as severe illness or impending death
- A recent significant loss or change in role
- Values and/or beliefs different from those of caregivers or the dominant cultural values
- Removal from a familiar spiritual support system

assistance desired, (3) discuss values and beliefs regarding spiritual practices, and (4) express feelings of spiritual comfort.

Nursing Interventions/Implementation

The following nursing interventions should take place in hospitals or extended-care facilities:

1. **Determine whether there are special spiritual practices and/or restrictions.** Nurses should identify the unique spiritual needs of older adults. Depending on the religion, denomination, or sect within a larger group, specific religious beliefs and practices can vary widely. Many articles and texts identify the major beliefs and practices of the major denominations, but nurses should clarify each individual's interpretation of and compliance with these beliefs and practices. This is particularly important if the religion requires or prohibits certain diets or health behaviors. Every effort should be made to allow older adults to continue practices and rituals as long as they do not interfere with health maintenance. If there is a conflict between spiritual values or practices and health needs, it is wise to consult with an authority of the specific church to identify acceptable strategies or compromises. Failure to consider the older person's spiritual beliefs can result in anger, despondency, and noncompliance with the plan of care.

2. **Identify significant persons who provide spiritual support.** Most religions recognize certain persons as spiritual leaders or guides. These leaders help others learn and practice the beliefs of the specific faith. Priests, rabbis, ministers, deacons, and religious sisters are commonly recognized as spiritual counselors or chaplains in institutional settings. These individuals are the recognized authorities who are trained to provide counsel to their own members and often to members of different faiths. Many older persons have a special closeness to a specific spiritual counselor whom they trust and will appreciate a call or visit from their regular spiritual advisor or minister, particularly when hospitalized or in danger of death. Nurses can contact these individuals or can request that the family initiate contact. This task should not be put off as nonessential, because many people gain as much sustenance from spiritual counsel as they do from medical treatment. In addition to providing counsel to the elderly patient, the spiritual counselor can help the family meet their spiritual needs during stressful situations. A trained chaplain or spiritual counselor can also act as a liaison among the patient, family, and clinical staff by interpreting spiritual practices and concerns.

3. **Determine whether there is any way nurses can aid older adults in meeting their spiritual needs.** Nurses should do an assessment to determine whether any assistance is required to enable older adults to meet their spiritual needs. Nurses are often asked to assist older adults in spiritual practices by contacting spiritual advisers, providing spiritual articles, or facilitating religious rituals.

4. **Provide opportunities for the person to express his or her spiritual needs and concerns.** Listen, in a nonjudgmental manner, to whatever the elderly person wishes to verbalize. When problems or concerns exist, it often helps to verbalize them to someone else. In most of these cases, the speaker does not want to have a mutual conversation, but rather to unburden themselves or to get their fears out in the open so that they can begin to deal with them. The nurse should help the person explore issues rather than try to stop the thoughts or provide reassuring platitudes in an attempt to make the person feel better. Life review or reminiscence may be helpful in aiding the person through these doubts and concerns.

5. **Determine spiritual objects that have meaning to the person; obtain these if possible.** Objects that are symbolic of faith should be placed where they can be seen or touched by older adults; they should not be hidden or put away in a drawer. All religious items should be shown due respect by caregivers. Even if the caregiver is of a different faith, it is important to recognize and respect the symbols of another person's religion.

6. **Provide opportunities for spiritual guidance with due respect for privacy.** Because spiritual practices often include the sharing of private thoughts and fears, older adults should be given opportunities to be alone to pray or meditate if desired. A chapel or quiet room free from distractions is desirable. If the person wishes to meet with a spiritual adviser or to perform religious rituals, he or she should have the opportunity to do so. This may require planning so that no interruptions (e.g., cares or treatments) interfere with the religious activity.

7. **Encourage contact with a spiritual counselor in times of crisis.** In times of spiritual crisis, such as the loss of a loved one or imminent death, privacy is particularly important. Severe grief can result in questioning of spiritual values. Contact with a spiritual counselor can help older adults work through feelings of anger, resentment, or ambivalence toward their spirituality. The spiritual counselor can provide support to dying persons and can assist the families in their time of grief. Special care should be taken to arrange for spiritual rituals related to death such as confession, communion, or anointing. Before preparing the body after death, nurses should be aware of the acceptable practices within specific religions.

The following interventions should take place in the home:

1. **Make arrangements that allow older adults to maintain religious practices.** Arrange for transportation to the place of worship (Figure 14-3). Many religious organizations can find rides for members who are not able to walk or drive. Sometimes, even this is not possible because of severe health problems or immobility, in which case most spiritual advisers are willing to visit in the home or facility if they are notified that a member desires their services.

2. **Use any appropriate interventions that are used in the institutional setting.** (Nursing Care Plan 14-1.)

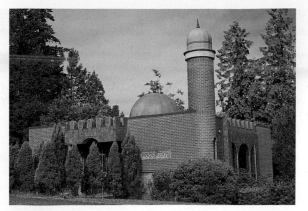

FIGURE 14-3 The main place of worship for Muslims, the mosque.

★ Nursing Care Plan 14-1 | Spiritual Distress

Mr. Quinn, age 78, has attended a Christian church regularly and has expressed a strong belief in a "merciful God." A week ago, he learned from his doctor that he has terminal cancer and has approximately 3 months to live. After talking to the doctor, he went to the chapel and cried. Since then he has spent a great deal of time in his room reading the Bible. He often verbalizes statements questioning the value of prayer and states that "God hasn't shown me any mercy, but I probably have to suffer for all I've done wrong in my life."

Nursing Diagnosis
Spiritual distress

Defining Characteristics
- Withdrawal
- Verbalization of hopelessness and abandonment by God
- Verbalization of feelings of guilt

Patient Goals/Outcomes Identification
Mr. Quinn will recognize that illness places stress on a belief system and will express feelings of spiritual comfort.

Nursing Interventions/Implementation
1. Listen to Mr. Quinn's concerns and feelings in a nonjudgmental manner.
2. Request a visit from the hospital chaplain (if desired, contact a personal minister).
3. Provide privacy for spiritual counseling and sacraments.
4. Keep the Bible and a prayer book readily available.
5. Assist Mr. Quinn to the chapel as requested.

Evaluation
Mr. Quinn visits the chapel daily and has a weekly visit with his minister. After each visit he appears more calm, stating that "I still don't know why this is happening to me, but I'll just have to put my trust in God." You will continue the plan of care.

Critical Thinking Questions
1. What type of verbal or nonverbal responses from the nurse would best demonstrate nonjudgmental acceptance of Mr. Quinn's feelings?
2. What could the nurse do if Mr. Quinn states, "I don't believe in a merciful God anymore" and refuses visits from a chaplain or other spiritual counselor?

Get Ready for the NCLEX® Examination!

Key Points

- Everyone's values and beliefs are unique. They are a product of the individual's culture, education, religion, and society.
- These values and beliefs form the basis of the older person's choices, perceptions, and behaviors.
- The values and beliefs held by older adults may significantly differ from those held by younger individuals.
- If not identified, these differences can result in misunderstandings, confusion, and conflict between older adults and their families or younger health care providers.
- Nurses can reduce problems related to differences in values and beliefs by openly communicating with older adults and by gaining more in-depth information regarding social, spiritual, and cultural diversity.

Additional Learning Resources

SG Go to the Study Guide on pp. 379–397 for additional learning activities to help you master the chapter content.

evolve Go to your Evolve website (http://evolve.elsevier.com/Wold/geriatric) for the following FREE learning resources:

- Animations
- Answer Guidelines for Nursing Care Plan Critical Thinking Questions
- Answers and Rationales for Review Questions for the NCLEX® Examination
- Glossary with pronunciations in English and Spanish
- Video Clips

Review Questions for the NCLEX® Examination

1. To provide culturally sensitive care, the nurse needs to know that the Jewish Sabbath:
   1. Starts at sundown of Friday and ends at sundown on Saturday
   2. Starts at midnight Friday and ends at midnight Saturday
   3. Starts at sundown Saturday and ends at sundown Sunday
   4. Starts at midnight Saturday and ends at midnight Sunday

2. The nurse observes an elderly patient who saves unopened crackers, jelly, and juice packages from the meal tray. This behavior most likely indicates:
   1. That the person would like an additional snack
   2. That the person is frugal and does not want to waste good, usable items
   3. That the person has problems with hoarding that needs to be evaluated
   4. A habit that means nothing in particular

3. An elderly Latino patient wants his family to bring folk remedies to the long-term care facility. The nurse's best response would be to:
   1. Tell them that these are harmful and to be avoided
   2. Remind them that only the physician can order treatments
   3. Encourage them to bring whatever is requested
   4. Identify the benefits and risks of these remedies

4. Identify two of the five Islamic Pillars of Faith
   1. _____
   2. _____

5. During an assessment, a newly admitted patient who is an aging Baby Boomer tells the nurse that he never goes to church and is not sure he believes in a god. The best response would be to:
   1. Further explore his spiritual beliefs
   2. Document that he is an atheist or agnostic
   3. Ask whether he would like to talk to a chaplain
   4. Avoid further discussion of the topic

End-of-Life Care

Objectives

1. Discuss personal and societal attitudes related to death and end-of-life planning.
2. Identify factors that are likely to influence end-of-life decision making.
3. Explore caregiver attitudes toward end-of-life care.
4. Discuss the importance of effective communication at the end of life.
5. Identify cultural and spiritual considerations related to end-of-life care.
6. Describe nursing assessments and interventions appropriate to end-of-life care.
7. Discuss the role of the nurse when interacting with the bereaved.

Key Terms

anorexia (ăn-ŏ-RĔK-sē-ă) (p. 253)
cachexia (kă-KĔK-sē-ă) (p. 253)
Cheyne-Stokes (chān stōks) (p. 253)
ethical dilemmas (p. 245)

hospice (HŎS-pĭs) (p. 246)
morgue (mŏrg) (p. 255)
palliative (PĂL-ē-ă-tĭv) (p. 247)

During the seventeenth century, the poet John Donne wrote, "No man is an island . . . any man's death diminishes me, because I am involved in mankind; and therefore never send to know for whom the bell tolls; it tolls for thee." A death was acknowledged by a solemn ringing of church bells, much the way bells are rung at many funerals today. At that time, death, although not welcome, was accepted as part of the life cycle. Infants, children, and young adults routinely died of infection, accident, and acute illness. Death was a familiar experience to all members of society. Because most people died at home receiving care and comfort from family members, people of all ages, even young children, were exposed to the realities of death.

Our end-of-life experiences are very different today. Medical science and technology have enabled us to cure or treat conditions that once would have been fatal and have extended life expectancy to unprecedented levels. Now, death is more commonly an experience of older adults, with almost 80% of all deaths occurring in the older-than-65 population. Death among older adults usually is not typically caused by an acute illness or accident but is far more likely to be a result of a progression of chronic and debilitating conditions (Box 15-1). Sudden, unexpected death is uncommon in the elderly, as is a steady, slow progression to death. More common is a repetitive cycle of significant health crises (often requiring hospitalization) followed by periods of remarkable improvement—somewhat like the old Timex watch advertisement: "They take a licking but keep on ticking." However, this sequence does take a toll. Bit by bit, the recuperative powers of elderly adults are diminished. Ultimately, their reserves become depleted until they are unable to muster enough energy to recover and they die.

DEATH IN WESTERN CULTURES

A person might think that contemporary American society would have developed a logical, efficient plan to help people as they near the end of life. Instead, many older people and their families are faced with fragmented, disorganized, and often, inadequate guidance. They are forced to attempt to make sense of the ever-changing rules and regulations set up by private or governmental bureaucracies. This increases stress and frustration for the dying person and his or her family members, and effective end-of-life care is too often delayed to be of maximal benefit. Although we have not yet solved all of these problems, many organizations, agencies, educators, and health care providers are working toward that goal. Many groups, including the Institute of Medicine, the American Association of Colleges of Nursing, the Robert Wood Johnson Foundation, and the Open Society Institute's Project on Death in America, have publications and websites to detail the work that is taking place.

ATTITUDES TOWARD DEATH AND END-OF-LIFE PLANNING

The combination of extended life expectancy and technology has changed the average person's experiences and perceptions regarding death. The process of dying

<table>
<tr><td>**Box 15-1**</td><td>**Causes of Death in Adults Ages 65 and Older**</td></tr>
</table>

- Diseases of the heart
- Malignant neoplasms
- Cardiovascular diseases
- Chronic obstructive pulmonary disease
- Pneumonia and influenza
- Diabetes mellitus
- Alzheimer's disease
- Nephritis, nephrotic syndrome, nephrosis
- Accidents
- Septicemia

has been separated from most people's personal experience. Many people reach middle or even late adulthood having little or no direct experience with death. They may know someone who has died and they may have attended a memorial or a funeral service, but few have actually been present with a loved one at the time of death. Attention to end-of-life care has increased in recent years. This interest is being driven, in large part, by the members of the baby boom generation who are dealing with end-of-life concerns related to their parents. Soon these Baby Boomers will make up a large part of the senior citizen population who will need to prepare themselves for the end of life.

In the past, it was easier to make end-of-life decisions. In fact, often there was no need to make a decision. Physicians could unequivocally state, "We have done everything possible." Today, there is always a chance that some new drug, some new procedure, or some new technologic breakthrough might save ourselves or our loved ones from death. The variety of treatment options available to people of all ages makes end-of-life decision making more difficult. Personal values, cultural and spiritual beliefs, and life experiences all affect the choices made.

Some older adults and their families continue to look to technology to prolong their lives and desire to receive every possible treatment available. Other older people would prefer a comfortable death in the presence of loved ones to a traumatic death with heroic lifesaving measures being used. Many older people say that they do not fear death as much as they fear how they will die.

Many people are uncomfortable talking about death. Family members, nurses, and other caregivers must overcome this discomfort so that they can provide good care for older people nearing the end of their lives. Discussions regarding the end of life usually are not as traumatic for the older adult population as they are for younger people. By the time people reach their seventies and beyond, most have experienced the death of loved ones. Parents, spouses, siblings, friends, and even children or grandchildren have died from myriad causes and under widely differing circumstances. Experience with these deaths generally helps aging adults determine what they do or do not want done as the reality of death approaches. Most alert older adults are quite candid in expressing their wishes if approached in a sensitive but a matter-of-fact way.

Ideally, discussions regarding end-of-life care and death planning will occur before a health crisis arises. Too often, important decisions regarding end-of-life care are avoided or delayed, as though denying thoughts about death will keep it from becoming a reality. This is unfortunate because it often shifts the burden to family members who are trying to come to grips with the approaching death of a loved one.

Several situations may help open the door to discussion about a person's preferences regarding end-of-life decisions. Family members may find it appropriate to discuss a parent's preferences after watching a television show or discussing a news article that deals with dying. Other opportunities for discussion of an older person's wishes may occur during gatherings where the family reminisces about other family members who have died or after the death of a friend or family member. Nurses who work in clinics or ambulatory care settings may use comments such as "Even though I'm OK now, I know I won't last forever" as a way to open the door to a discussion of end-of-life planning. Admission to an acute care setting for treatment of a serious or life-threatening illness can present a good opportunity to the nurse to initiate a discussion regarding end-of-life wishes. Once the initial danger has passed and the patient's status has stabilized, there is usually a high level of consciousness regarding death. People who have resisted making plans can no longer avoid the necessity. The nurse may provide the materials needed to initiate advance directives or may refer the patient and family to a social worker or appropriate community resources.

ADVANCE DIRECTIVES

Specific end-of-life decisions can be expressed in advance directive documents such as a living will or durable power of attorney for health care, which are discussed in Chapter 1. These documents specify the type and amount of intervention desired by an individual. Once initiated, they remain in effect until changed. Copies of advance directives should be given to the physician, hospital of choice, extended-care facility, power of attorney for health care, and anyone else deemed appropriate. This can prevent last-minute confusion and possible violation of a person's wishes. If the patient has selected not to have resuscitation attempted, this desire should be posted in the home, noted on the chart, and, ideally, identified on a bracelet or necklace so that the person's wishes are respected in case of an emergency.

There is no single right plan for the end of life. The best plan is usually one that the individual believes offers the greatest rewards or highest quality of life. In general, patients who are positive about their choices and their physician's abilities obtain the best results. However, to make a wise decision, information is needed. Some factors the person may wish to discuss with the physician before making any decisions about a treatment plan include (1) the amount of time a treatment will add to life; (2) the quality of life with this treatment; (3) the amount of pain, disability, or risk involved with the treatment; (4) the amount of time involved in the treatment; (5) the cost of treatment and whether it is covered by insurance; (6) the need for and availability of caregivers; and (7) the availability, benefits, and risks of other treatment options. If a person is not satisfied with the information received from a specific physician, the person has the right to request further consultation with other physicians.

No one knows for sure what he or she will choose when faced with a terminal diagnosis. Guidance and support from physicians, clergy, nurses, social workers, and family can help a dying person make these significant decisions, but each person must ultimately make his or her own choices. It is important to remember that decisions can change as situations change. A competent person retains the right to change his or her mind about treatment at any time.

CAREGIVER ATTITUDES TOWARD END-OF-LIFE CARE

Even health care providers who must routinely face critically ill or dying patients may have difficulty accepting death. Many physicians and nurses have become so focused on preventing illness or curing disease that they are more likely to view death as a personal or professional failure rather than the inevitable end to the human experience. Caregivers, including physicians, nurses, social workers, family members, and any others playing a role in end-of-life care, need to learn to recognize their own attitudes, feelings, values, and expectations about death. They need to explore the professional literature that discusses legal, ethical, financial, and health care delivery issues related to end-of-life care. They need to learn to collaborate with each other to assess and treat the whole person as he or she nears the end of life, including physical, psychological, social, cultural, and spiritual needs. Caregivers need to be able to communicate effectively and respond to the patient, as well as address the needs of the family and significant others as they face grief, loss, and bereavement at the end of life. They need to overcome any feelings of frustration or ineffectiveness as they recognize that a time will come for each person when the focus of care needs to change. Caregivers need to learn when and how to shift from the aggressive medical interventions designed to cure or extend life to more palliative and holistic interventions designed to enable the dying person and his or her significant others to experience a "good" death characterized by comfort, peace, dignity, and caring.

VALUES CLARIFICATION RELATED TO DEATH AND END-OF-LIFE CARE

Beliefs, attitudes, and values regarding the experience of death and end-of-life care vary widely. People's responses are influenced by their age, gender, culture, religious background, and life experiences. Just as patients and their families must explore their values when making end-of-life decisions, so must those who provide care. Physicians, nurses, social workers, and others would benefit from spending some time identifying their personal values related to the end of life. This process will help them identify those values that are likely to influence their decision-making processes and behavior when caring for dying patients.

Ethical dilemmas relating to end-of-life care are more likely to occur when the value systems of the patient and of the caregiver differ significantly. Understanding the value systems of others can help the nurse provide quality end-of-life care, even when the nurse does not share the same values.

? Critical Thinking

Values Clarification Exercise Related to the End of Life

Complete the following statements and reflect on your answers. What do they tell you about your perceptions and values regarding end-of-life issues?

1. Death is . . .
2. Death means . . .
3. After death . . .
4. Decisions about my end-of-life care should be made by . . .
5. Talking about dying makes me feel . . .
6. When I am nearing the end of life, I want my family to . . .
7. When I am nearing the end of life, I want my caregivers to . . .
8. As death nears, I am afraid of . . .
9. I am in pain as I near the end of life . . .
10. I am dying and I do not want . . .
11. Because I am old, death . . .
12. After I die, I want people to . . .

? Critical Thinking

Personal Beliefs and Attitudes about Death

• What are your personal experiences with death?
• Have you lost a close friend, family member, or patient to death?
• How did you feel when you heard that the person had died?
• If you have had more than one experience, did you respond differently to the deaths? Why do you think you responded differently?
• Have you ever been with a person at the time of death?
• What thoughts crossed your mind as the person died?
• Were other people present?
• What was said or done?
• What spiritual or cultural rituals were performed at the time of death or burial?

? Critical Thinking

Ethical Dilemmas

The chapter has identified the most commonly identified wishes of individuals nearing the end of life.
• What should happen if one or more of these wishes conflicts with those of the caregivers?
• What if a spouse values the companionship of the dying person and wants all possible life-extending actions to be provided in conflict with the patient's advance directives?
• What if a physician or family member determines that a patient cannot cope with hearing a terminal diagnosis?
• What if the nurse thinks that the amount of pain medication ordered is excessive?
• What should be done if death seems imminent during the middle of the night when no family is present?

Box 15-2   Summary of Patients' Wishes Related to End of Life

Most dying patients desire to:
• Be able to issue advance directives to ensure their wishes are respected
• Be afforded dignity, respect, and privacy
• Know when death is coming and what to expect
• Have access to information and options related to care
• Retain control of decision making regarding care
• Have control over symptom and pain relief
• Have access to emotional, cultural, and spiritual support
• Retain control regarding who may be present at the end of life
• Know options (e.g., hospital, home care and hospice) and have a choice regarding where and how death will occur
• Have time to say goodbye to significant others
• Leave life when ready to go without unnecessary or pointless interventions

WHAT IS A "GOOD" DEATH?

Many groups in the United States and abroad have conducted research to identify the specific end-of-life outcomes that are most valued and desired by those nearing the end of life and by their families. Themes throughout all of the studies indicate that given their choice, most people wish to be treated with respect and dignity and to die quietly and peacefully with loved ones nearby. Box 15-2 identifies the common threads identified by these studies.

WHERE PEOPLE DIE

Although 90% of people surveyed in a Gallup poll indicated that they desired to die at home, less than one fourth of deaths actually occur there. Trends in some states do appear to show that the number of deaths occurring at home is increasing. Exact numbers vary significantly from state to state, but most deaths still take place in institutional settings. Approximately half of deaths occur in hospitals, and another one fourth occur in extended-care facilities. These numbers are only approximations because it is common for the dying person to be transferred from one setting to another when death is imminent.

A growing trend in end-of-life care is hospice care. Much of this growth has occurred since 1983, when Medicare Hospice Benefit began funding this type of care. A hospice was traditionally a place of rest for a traveler. Hospice care now reaches approximately 17% of those nearing the end of life. The majority of hospice care is provided at home or in extended-care facilities; only 20% takes place in a hospital setting. The focus of hospice care is palliative, providing comfort and meeting the needs of patients and their families (Figure 15-1). Hospice care usually is available for the last 6 months of life and can be extended if the patient survives beyond this time. Extensions are fairly uncommon, and, because of delays in starting hospice care, the median length of care is less than 30 days. This shortened intervention permits few people to achieve maximal potential benefits.

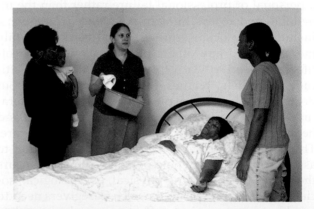

FIGURE 15-1 Hospice is a philosophical concept of providing palliative or supportive care to dying people.

PALLIATIVE CARE

According to the World Health Organization, **palliative** care focuses on reducing or relieving the symptoms of a disease without attempting to provide a cure; it neither hastens nor postpones death. Palliative care affirms life while accepting death as its normal conclusion. Interventions are designed to optimize the patient's ability to live as active and complete a life as possible until death comes. Competent adults, regardless of age, who are suffering from life-threatening diseases such as cancer or advanced chronic conditions such as emphysema or end-stage renal disease can, and often do, make the decision that they no longer desire aggressive treatment such as chemotherapy, assisted ventilation, or dialysis. This does not mean that these patients forego all medical intervention; for example, a wound would still be treated and a fracture would still be placed in a cast. Individuals who choose palliative care typically choose to decline other procedures such as cardiopulmonary resuscitation (CPR), artificial ventilation, and artificial feeding, which may prolong the dying process. Medical treatment and nursing care focus on actions that enable the dying person to have the highest quality of life for whatever time remains in his or her life.

COLLABORATIVE ASSESSMENT AND INTERVENTIONS FOR END-OF-LIFE CARE

Good end-of-life care requires the commitment and collaboration of all caregivers. No matter who is designated as the primary caregiver, all parties, including the family, physicians, nurses, social workers, clergy, psychologists, dietitians, pharmacists, therapists, and volunteers must work together effectively for the good of the dying person. Everyone needs to work together cooperatively and creatively and with a positive attitude to solve any problems that might arise. Problem solving requires mutual respect and prompt, effective communication among all team members. Team members also need to recognize the physical and emotional toll that occurs when working to meet the needs of the dying person and his or her family. Providing emotional support to other caregivers can help them maintain the high level of energy needed to meet the various physical and psychosocial needs of the dying.

COMMUNICATION AT THE END OF LIFE

Effective communication is a challenge at the best of times. Communication can be even more challenging during stressful times, such as when the end of life is near. Everything takes on increased importance in this once-in-a-lifetime experience. There is no chance to do things over, so it is essential that they be done right.

One of the most important thing caregivers can do is spend more time with the dying person and encourage family members to do the same. This is not easy because demands on nurses' time are high, but when the nurse recognizes the importance of communication at the end of life, priorities can change. Most people surveyed do not want to die alone, but too many do. Studies have shown that dying people in institutional settings spend a great deal of time alone. One study done in a hospital reports that physician visits average 3 minutes, nursing personnel visits average 45 minutes, and family visits average only 13 minutes per day. These statistics mean that the dying person is alone for 23 of 24 hours. Another study revealed somewhat better, but still worrisome, results. In this study, dying patients spent 18 hours and 39 minutes alone in their rooms. Nurses and nursing assistants spent by far the greatest amount of time, 94 minutes of the day, with the dying person, but most of this time was broken into 45 short visits that were highly task-oriented. It is interesting to note that physicians spent more time than expected with patients who had "do not resuscitate" (DNR) orders and those receiving palliative care for cancer. Patients with dementia received the least time from physicians. Attention from family members varied widely based on age, availability, culture, and real or perceived proximity to death.

The basic challenge of all communication is to develop and maintain rapport. To accomplish this, the nurse needs to know as much as possible about the person receiving care. This includes the patient's religion, cultural background, values and beliefs, advance directive for health care, and past experiences that may affect decision making.

To do this, nurses need to demonstrate verbally and nonverbally that they are approachable and not detached or indifferent. A good way to start is by consistently addressing or referring to the patient by name. This shows respect and helps the dying person maintain a sense of self-worth and dignity. An empathetic word and gentle touch can demonstrate caring. Holding a hand, stroking a forehead, gentle repositioning, providing good basic hygiene, and maintaining an aesthetically pleasing environment free from odors, clutter, and the like all help communicate that the dying person is respected and valued.

Nurses need to demonstrate willingness to listen to suggestions, requests, or criticism made by the dying person or, more likely, by his or her family. Near the end of life, emotions run high, and people often think that they are at the mercy of the "system." Out of frustration or distress, they may perceive that their loved one is not getting all of the care he or she deserves. Nurses must be open and willing to listen to these criticisms without becoming defensive, whether the criticism is justified or not. Prompt response to requests or an explanation regarding why certain things cannot be done communicates that caregivers recognize the importance of the dying person's needs.

Questions should be answered honestly and directly. If the nurse does not have the information or is not at liberty to disclose it, actions should be taken so that the necessary information is obtained from the appropriate source in a timely manner. Discussions regarding end-of-life experiences and care should be clear and truthful. Dying persons and their significant others need to be supplied with all necessary information. The patient and his or her family should be informed, to the degree that it is humanly possible, about what to expect. All medical terms such as feeding tubes, ventilators, CPR, DNAR orders, and so forth should be explained in plain language using simple sentences. Even simple information or explanations can be confusing at stressful times and may need to be repeated often. The nurse should try to prevent or correct any misunderstandings or mistaken perceptions that may occur. This can be done by summarizing and restating what the nurse thinks the patient or family member said. Time for response and further clarification should be allowed if necessary.

Within culturally acceptable parameters, the patient should be actively involved in discussion regarding the plan of care. Nothing is more demeaning or frustrating to a dying person than having a nurse discuss plans with the physician or family while the one person most intimately involved is ignored. Nurses can help the patient work through fears and end-of-life decisions by spending time listening in a nonjudgmental manner. Sensitive communication cannot be hurried, and the time the patient wishes to talk cannot be scheduled like a procedure. Once upon a time, nurses provided direct care and had the opportunity to really talk with terminal patients. Too often these days, patients spend more time communicating their fears and concerns about death and dying with the nursing assistant who helps with their hygiene than with a nurse. Nurses often spend more time dealing with paperwork, passing pills, and assisting or performing procedures than they do caring for the actual person. Measures need to be developed to rectify this problem.

Reflective and open-ended statements such as "There seem to be things that are worrying you," "If you want to talk, I'll listen," or "It must be hard. Do you want me to sit with you for a while?" are often effective ways to encourage a conversation. Nurses should start communication from where the patient is and then go where the patient wishes to go. Patients should be free to discuss the things that concern them the most, not just the topics with which the nurse feels most comfortable. The nurse should be careful not to interrupt or dominate the conversation. Whenever possible, the dying person should have adequate privacy so that he or she can communicate freely and undisturbed by unnecessary noise and commotion.

Reassurance that the nurse will keep information confidential may encourage the dying person to communicate his or her fears or concerns more freely. This may also encourage dialogue, which can help dying persons begin a life review through which they can validate their life experiences and enhance their level of peace.

When death is near, one or more members of the family or significant others may wish to remain with the dying person. Most facilities encourage this and provide some accommodations for their comfort. The nurse often needs to explain what to expect as death approaches; how to best communicate with the patient; and what, if anything, loved ones can do to help to make the end of life as peaceful as possible.

After the person dies, the nurse should not be afraid to express emotion at the loss. Often, particularly in extended-care settings, the nurse and other caregivers have developed a true affection for the person and will need to grieve his or her loss. Family members usually report that seeing the nursing staff's grief actually helped them cope with the loss, because they knew that other people cared enough about their loved ones to say a prayer or shed a tear.

PSYCHOSOCIAL PERSPECTIVES, ASSESSMENTS, AND INTERVENTIONS

CULTURAL PERSPECTIVES

A person's cultural beliefs influence how he or she thinks, lives, and interacts with other people; the beliefs also affect how a person will approach death. Each person develops a unique set of beliefs and values over a lifetime, but as death approaches, many revert to the beliefs formed early in life. Understanding people and their needs would be much easier if there were predictable patterns, if all people who shared a cultural heritage thought and acted identically. Of course, this is not the case. Wide variations of beliefs and behaviors exist within any culture. A part of the nurse's responsibility is to assess each individual to determine his or her unique preferences and viewpoints so that trust can be developed and culturally sensitive care can be planned. When nurses and patients come from different cultural and religious backgrounds, the nurse must be careful not to impose his or her beliefs, but should work to understand the perspectives of others. Areas that need to be explored as part of a culturally sensitive assessment include issues such as (1) communication about death, (2) the decision-making process, (3) amount and type of intervention that will be accepted, and (4) the significance of pain and suffering.

COMMUNICATION ABOUT DEATH

The Western or European/American perspective tends to emphasize the patient's "right to know" his or her diagnosis and prognosis so that the patient can make informed decisions. This perspective differs greatly from cultures such as Asians and American Indians, who often believe that speaking about death or other bad things will decrease hope and produce bad outcomes. Asking for clarification of beliefs can enhance cultural awareness and ensure compliance with privacy issues. This can be accomplished by a statement such as, "Some people like to get information about their health directly; others prefer we speak to another family member instead. Which do you prefer?"

The nurse should ensure that the patient understands questions or information provided. When giving explanations, a "yes" or "no" response should be followed up with requests for the patient to explain what he or she understood. If there is a language barrier, a professional who speaks the language should ideally do the translating, not a family member who is emotionally involved.

DECISION-MAKING PROCESS

The dominant Western perspective tends to emphasize the right of the individual to make decisions regarding his or her own life, regardless of the views of family or significant others. This is the basis of laws governing advance directives. Yet many other cultures, including Asian Americans, African Americans, and Mexican Americans, are likely to view life and death decisions as family issues that must be discussed and decided as a group. These groups are significantly less likely to have initiated any form of advance directives (Cultural Considerations box).

🌐 Cultural Considerations

Religious Practices Regarding End of Life

- Buddhism—A person's state of mind at the time of death is of great importance. A peaceful state may be achieved by listening to friends, family, or monks, reading scriptures, and chanting mantras. Buddhists view death not as a continuation of the soul but as an awakening. Funeral rites last 49 days ending in the rebirth of the individual. Cremation is common.
- Judaism—Anything that may hasten death is forbidden. Death is viewed as a natural process in movement to a more rewarding afterlife. Extensive rituals are used to show respect for the dead and to comfort the living. After death, the body is not left alone until burial. Special washing and wrapping in a simple shroud with religious symbols is typically done by special religious volunteers. There is no viewing of he remains; a simple casket is used and the body is always buried, never cremated. In general, autopsies are discouraged unless required by law.
- American Indian (Lakota)—Death is a part of life and that after death, people enter a neutral spirit land. The spirit is believed to reside in the body and should not be disturbed, so burial is preferred over cremation. A religious celebration of the person's spirit is held a year after death.

Amount and Type of Intervention That Will Be Accepted

The dominant Western perspective focuses on helping people cope with death. Other cultures, such as African Americans, American Indians, Asians, Pacific Islanders, and Latinos, are more likely to focus on living and prolonging life. Aggressive interventions at the end of life are often desired. These groups also appear to place greater responsibility and expectations on the family, church, or social network to provide end-of-life care. To some extent, this may explain why hospice care is becoming more accepted by some cultural groups but not by others.

Significance of Pain and Suffering

The Western perspective focuses on achieving freedom from pain and suffering. Non-Western cultures are more likely to view pain as a test of faith or a preparation for the afterlife; it is something that is to be endured rather than avoided.

SPIRITUAL CONSIDERATIONS

Religion plays an important part in the lives of many individuals and may be even more important as death nears. As the end of life approaches, thoughts about the reality of death and what will occur afterward are intensified. This sometimes results in increased spiritual or religious interest and concern, even among individuals who did not express any particular interest in religion for most of their lives.

❓ Critical Thinking

Spiritual Needs of the Dying

It has been said that there are no atheists in foxholes. What connection does this statement have to meeting spiritual needs at the end of life?

There are far too many variations in spiritual beliefs and practices to adequately address them in this textbook. Religious counselors, including priests, pastors, rabbis, imams, mullahs, shamans, and other ministers, are familiar with the distinctive concerns and practices of their religion. They are usually willing to act as a resource to the nurse and other caregivers regarding ways to adapt and individualize care to incorporate specific spiritual beliefs and practices. Religious symbols or items of devotion (e.g., bibles, rosaries, and medallions) that provide comfort to the dying person should be kept readily available and treated with respect.

Although many nurses feel uncomfortable discussing spiritual topics with dying patients, they can play an important role in helping dying persons meet their spiritual needs. The following are some guidelines to remember when attempting to meet the spiritual needs of the dying person:

1. **Determine whether any specific religious beliefs or practices are important to the patient or his or her family members.**

2. **Assess whether the patient has a preferred spiritual counselor.** When no particular individual is identified, the nurse should ask the patient whether he or she wishes to receive counsel from anyone else. Spiritual counseling is very personal, and the dying person should have the right to select whomever he or she wishes.

3. **Offer choices when available.** Most hospitals or extended-care facilities maintain a listing of ministers who will visit the dying without concern to denomination or church affiliation. Not all spiritual counselors are equally sensitive to the needs of the dying. If one spiritual counselor does not meet the patient's needs, the patient should be aware that others are available.

4. **Determine whether the person wishes any spiritual counselor to be notified.** Nurses should respect the wishes of people who do not wish spiritual counsel. Spiritual counseling can be very beneficial when desired. When it is not desired, intervention can cause more problems than it solves.

5. **Demonstrate respect for the patient's religious and spiritual views.** The dying person should be allowed time for private thought, prayer, or meditation when he or she desires it. Important activities and items should be incorporated into the plan of care. The religious rituals related to dying can differ widely among cultures, and the nurse should help the family whenever possible to facilitate their practices even if this involves moving furniture to face a specific sacred direction, opening windows, or providing space for a large group of family members.

6. **Avoid imposing your own beliefs on the patient.** The nurse should keep the focus of spiritual discussions on the patient and his or her beliefs, not on the nurse's beliefs.

7. **Be present, be available, and listen.** The nurse cannot and should not attempt to solve the patient's problems, but empathy demonstrates acceptance and caring. This allows the patient to feel less alone and often decreases spiritual distress.

8. **Avoid moving beyond role and level of expertise unless you have specific ministerial or pastoral training in death and dying.**

DEPRESSION, ANXIETY, AND FEAR

An older man was heard to say, "I think that waiting to die is worse than death itself." It is one thing to know that you will die eventually; it is another to realize that you have lived most of your life and that death is likely to be a reality soon. At that point in life, individuals must decide whether they will give up and let fear,

anxiety, or depression overwhelm them or whether they will do something to remain in control of whatever time they have remaining.

Nurses can help dying people cope with emotional distress by listening to their concerns and helping them find constructive ways of dealing with these concerns. Participation in crafts, art, or other creative activities may provide distraction and an outlet for expression. Art, poetry, and other writings can provide a means for many dying patients to leave a tangible message for their family and loved ones. Physical activity, if allowed, can help reduce both physical and emotional tension. Relaxation classes or support groups designed to help people dealing with terminal conditions may help decrease social isolation.

Everyone has good days and bad days. When there are more bad days—and these bad days seem to be getting worse—professional help may be necessary. A psychological evaluation may be needed to determine the nature and severity of the problem. Counseling and use of antidepressant or antianxiety medications can help.

Anger is not uncommon, particularly soon after a terminal diagnosis is made. The nurse should accept this, allow patients the opportunity to verbalize their anger, and then help them find ways to move forward and to cope with the future. More general approaches are discussed in Chapters 11 and 13.

PHYSIOLOGIC CHANGES, ASSESSMENTS, AND INTERVENTIONS

Physicians and nurses are often asked how long it will be until a person dies. No one can say exactly when a person will die, but a pattern of physiologic changes can help predict when the end is near. Those who work with the dying must be able to recognize these physical signs of approaching death and be prepared to implement interventions that will provide the dying person with the highest level of comfort possible. Typical physiologic changes observed as death nears include fatigue, dyspnea, gastrointestinal changes (dry mouth, anorexia, nausea and vomiting, constipation), anxiety, and delirium. Pain is not always present as death nears, but when it is present, pain relief is a priority need. Effective medical and nursing interventions at the end of life require commitment, creativity, and caring. This may involve use of a variety of traditional, complementary, and technologic approaches.

PAIN

Nurses may have heard dying patients say facetiously, "A little pain is OK . . . when I hurt, I know I'm alive." However, pain is no joke. Pain is often the most significant concern of the dying person and his or her significant others. This is particularly true when the dying person suffers from a highly painful disease such as cancer. Pain at the end of life can interfere with the dying person's ability to maintain control, to cope, and to complete end-of-life tasks. Pain increases the likelihood of fatigue, depression, and loss of appetite. Most important, pain interferes with the ability of the dying person to make thoughtful decisions and to communicate effectively with loved ones at a critical time.

The goal of pain management is to reduce pain to an acceptable level while retaining an adequate level of alertness to allow the dying person to remain aware of daily activities and to interact with family and loved ones. It may not be possible to relieve all pain; however, treatment is aimed at achieving a level of control that the patient finds acceptable. No dying person should be allowed to suffer needlessly.

Relief of pain begins with careful assessment. Assessment needs to be performed early and often, because the patient's status can change dramatically in a relatively short period. Pain is what the patient says it is, but many older patients who have lived with multiple discomforts often underreport the amount of pain they are experiencing. When working with alert and responsive older adults, the nurse may need to explain or clarify the standard pain scales (i.e., 0 to 10) that are used to determine the severity or intensity of pain. The nurse needs to be patient and take an adequate amount of time to elicit from the older person the frequency, location, quality, and duration of the pain, as well as precipitating and relieving factors. A good nursing assessment helps the physician determine whether the person's condition is worsening and whether a change in the type or amount of medication is needed. All pain assessments need to be documented carefully. Special pain assessment flow sheets are effective in condensing observations so that changes in pain status can be recognized quickly. The patient or his or her family should be taught how to keep a pain log that supplements nursing assessments. This log should be simple enough that a lay person can understand it and should include all of the factors a nurse would assess. Self-reported logs are helpful because the patient and significant others are more focused and attuned to subtle changes in the individual. Pain logs often reveal important information that would otherwise be missed (Figure 15-2).

The nurse must be particularly aware of pain issues in patients who are unable to verbalize their distress.

Loss of cognitive abilities does not eliminate or diminish the ability of the person to feel pain. Although cognitively impaired older adults may not recall past pain, current reports of pain and behavioral changes are usually accurate indicators.

Alternative assessments must be used with patients who are unable to communicate verbally. When trying to determine the nature and severity of pain, the nurse should begin by reviewing whether the patient has an existing condition or has recently experienced some trauma that may cause pain. Careful head-to-toe assessment may help the nurse determine whether there are any objective data that might indicate the source of pain, such as swelling, inflammation, or bruising. During the assessment, the nurse should watch the patient carefully for any responses such as restlessness, moaning, guarding, grimacing or striking out when body parts are touched or moved. The presence of any of these responses between assessments, especially during routine activities such as repositioning, can also indicate the likelihood of pain. Family members, friends, or staff members may be aware of behaviors the patient exhibits when in pain. This information should be indicated on the plan of care so that all care providers can respond appropriately.

Good pain management is based on an understanding of the patient's needs and wishes. This involves thorough assessment of his or her physical needs, coping ability, and support network. Religious, cultural, and ethnic factors also should be considered. Specialists, including physicians, nurses, pharmacists, and counselors, have been doing considerable research on pain control and are bringing improved understanding to health care professionals and to the public. An increasing number of facilities are using this knowledge to improve the effectiveness of pain control techniques at the end of life.

The nurse or other caregiver should keep several things in mind when planning care for persons experiencing pain near the end of life:

1. **Do not give up trying to find an effective pain control regimen.** It may take several attempts to find the best combination of medication and non-pharmacologic approaches to reach a pain level that is tolerable for the patient.

2. **The likelihood of drug-drug and drug-disease interactions or adverse effects increases with the**

Date	Time	Severity of Pain	Activity at Time of Pain	Medication Given	Comfort Measures	Severity of Pain in 1 Hour
6/2/07	0800	level 6 "mostly in my back"	walking in hallway	morphine sulfate 30 mg	encouraged to rest back massage given	level 2 "not entirely gone, but I can tolerate this"

FIGURE 15-2 Sample pain management log.

addition of new medication or higher doses. Careful assessment is needed each time a change in medication is made.

3. **Changes in medication, dose, or frequency may be needed.** Good assessment reveals when the medication is no longer providing adequate pain relief. The physician should be consulted so that a more effective pain management plan can be prescribed.

4. **Various routes of administration are available for pain control.** Oral medication is the most common and accepted route for administration, but it may cause problems for older adults who have difficulty swallowing pills. Solid medications designed for sustained release should never be crushed, because this could result in too rapid absorption. When the person has difficulty swallowing, the physician should be consulted regarding a change to liquids, suppositories, or transdermal skin patches. These are often more acceptable to older patients and are easier to administer. Parenteral administration of medication is usually a last choice for an older adult unless he or she has an existing intravenous (IV) or central line, peripherally inserted central catheter (PICC), or implanted port.

5. **Timing is important.** Pain medication is most effective when taken before the pain becomes severe. Long-acting or sustained-release opioids are commonly ordered because they are effective at maintaining pain control while eliminating the need to disturb the patient frequently to administer pain medication. Even with long-acting pain control, breakthrough pain may occur. This should be treated promptly with a rapid-acting analgesic. As-needed (prn) medications should be given as soon as possible after they are requested.

6. **Pain medications should not be stopped suddenly when they have been taken for an extended period.** Withdrawal symptoms including headache, shakiness, or diaphoresis can occur if medications are stopped suddenly.

7. **Non-pharmacologic approaches should be used to supplement pharmacologic interventions in control of pain.** The nurse or other caregiver should discuss possible options and implement those that are most acceptable to the patient. Activities that may help provide relief include (1) hot or cold applications such as warm baths, showers, cool wash cloths, or ice packs; (2) comfort devices such as cushions, pillows, and pads; (3) massage, foot rubs, or reflexology; (4) relaxation breathing or other relaxation exercises; (5) imagery or visualization; (6) distractions such as socialization, listening to music, and watching television or movies; (7) biofeedback; (8) transcutaneous electrical nerve stimulation; (9) hypnosis; and (10) anything else that helps reduce stress.

Sedation using neuroleptics, benzodiazepines, barbiturates, or high doses of opioids may be ordered when the pain is severe and not relieved by using standard narcotic medications. These should be used very selectively and only when the patient has "do not resuscitate" status and all other pain relief interventions are unsuccessful. Loss of consciousness is not the ideal solution, but it may be better than allowing the dying person to suffer and experience extreme distress. Sedation is most appropriately used only after the patient, family, or health care team determine that it is in the person's best interest. The health care team should be aware of the need for ongoing communication with the family members, who may experience fear or a change of heart regarding the treatment plan. Once sedation is begun, it may be reduced if the family or health care representative requests. This, however, may result in the recurrence of physical and emotional distress for the dying patient. Many institutions have established policies regarding the use of sedation, including the types and amounts of medication that can be used. Careful documentation of all interventions is essential.

Ethical concerns may arise as to whether the use of sedation is a form of passive euthanasia, and all health care providers are not in agreement. It is important to remember that sedation is not being used to end the person's life; rather it is being used to reduce the patient's suffering. The American Medical Association and court findings have established the position that proper use of sedation is not "slow euthanasia" when the intent is reduction of pain not the hastening of death.

FATIGUE AND SLEEPINESS

Fatigue is common with both acute and chronic illness and is not specifically a sign of impending death. It may be caused by underlying disease processes, stress, anxiety, or medications. Fatigue can interfere with the dying person's ability to carry out necessary end-of-life tasks, including communicating with loved ones. Sometimes, stimulants such as caffeine or prescription drugs may help a person overcome fatigue and lethargy; however, these should be used cautiously. Reduced activity demands and planned rest periods can help reduce fatigue. Because of metabolic changes, the patient may begin to sleep more and may be difficult to awaken as the end of life nears.

CARDIOVASCULAR CHANGES

Diminished peripheral circulation already common in older adults is likely to worsen as death nears, resulting in dry, pale, or cyanotic extremities. Peripheral pulses are often weak and difficult to palpate. Blood pressure typically is decreased by 20 or more points from the normal range and may be difficult to auscultate. Body temperature may elevate significantly as death nears.

Room temperature and ventilation should be adjusted to promote comfort while avoiding chilling drafts. Comfort measures, including bed socks, shoulder wraps, and warmed blankets (never electric because of risk for burns), are appropriate. However, heavy or restrictive covers should not be used because they may increase the person's discomfort.

RESPIRATORY CHANGES

Shortness of breath, difficulty breathing (dyspnea), and Cheyne-Stokes respirations during sleep are commonly observed in older adults as death nears. As part of the plan of care, the patient needs to know that this problem may occur and know to specify how aggressively he or she wants the medical team to be in relieving this symptom.

Mild respiratory difficulty usually can be relieved by changing positioning, elevating the upper body, opening windows or using a fan to increase ventilation, or administering oxygen by nasal cannula. Both physical and emotional stress can cause muscle tension, which exacerbates respiratory problems. The patient should be encouraged to minimize stressful experiences and to alternate episodes of activity with rest periods. Excessive talking and visiting should be minimized if they cause problems. Visitors need to know that it is sometimes better to visit for shorter periods of time or to leave the room and allow the patient to have some quiet time if breathing difficulties occur. Resting in a reclining chair or elevating the head of the bed usually aids effective breathing. Listening to music and using relaxation exercises may further help reduce tension and improve breathing effort.

Severe breathing problems, such as those seen with chronic heart or lung disease, usually do not respond well to these simple measures and need treatment that is more aggressive. Patients experiencing severe shortness of breath often exhibit acute distress because of the sensation of suffocation and resulting fear or panic. When the patient does not want aggressive medical treatment, the most common method used to manage shortness of breath is administration of morphine. The patient, family, and team of caregivers need to be aware of and be comfortable with the fact that morphine, when given in a dosage that is adequate to relieve the respiratory distress, can cause drowsiness, sleep, and even loss of consciousness.

GASTROINTESTINAL CHANGES

Loss of appetite (anorexia) and muscle wasting (cachexia) are commonly observed with advanced terminal conditions, particularly some forms of cancer. Many factors contribute to poor appetite and weight loss in the terminal patient, including medications, sores in the mouth, changes in taste, nausea and vomiting, metabolic changes, absorption problems, and emotional depression. Treatment of anorexia and cachexia is difficult because many of the underlying physiologic actions are poorly understood.

The anorexic person should be encouraged but not forced to eat. Force-feeding will make the person more uncomfortable and can result in choking. Care should focus on whatever pleasures attached to food that remain. The end of life is not a time for special or restricted diets. The person should be encouraged to eat anything that appeals to him or her. Presentation of the food should be appealing and in a quantity that does not overwhelm the person. Whenever possible, meals should be served in a place free from odors associated with illness. Food is intimately attached to good times and social events. Watching a loved one waste away is very disturbing to family members. With best intentions, they may try to force a dying person to eat. Enlisting the family to bring small amounts of special foods from home may bring back pleasant memories of better times. Sharing a meal with family members can be a positive experience, even when the person consumes very little.

The issue of artificial feeding typically arises when a dying person is unable or unwilling to eat. Many people have already addressed this issue in their advance directives by specifying what forms of feeding, if any, they would permit. Inability to take food and fluids by mouth is a part of the normal progression to death. The choice to stop eating is something different, and the underlying reason should be sought. People may stop eating as a method of hastening death. This may be a conscious decision by the patient, or it may be a response to uncontrolled pain or severe depression. Nurses need to be alert to these possibilities. Adequate pain control and actions to reduce the depression may cause changes in the person's behavior. The idea of self-starvation is usually traumatic to family members and medical personnel.

Artificial feeding by either nasogastric or gastric tubes or parenteral routes is an appropriate way to solve short-term nutrition problems. Artificial forms of feeding are more likely to cause harm than good at the end of life. Tube feeding increases the incidence of nausea and vomiting, and parenteral nutrition increases the risk for infection without proven benefit to patients at or near the end of life. People can live for days without food. Prolonged fasting leads to ketosis, which depresses hunger and may even result in mood elevation or euphoria. There is no evidence that self-chosen food refusal causes suffering. Dehydration is more likely to cause death than is starvation. People can survive for only a few days without fluid. On the other hand, dehydration appears to have some benefits near the end of life. It is theorized that dehydration leads to the release of endorphins (i.e., natural chemicals that reduce pain). Dehydration also reduces fluid congestion in the lungs, making breathing easier, and reduces respiratory secretions, reducing the need for suctioning.

Dry mouth (xerostomia) and ulcerations of the mouth can be caused by many things such as advanced age, medications, and decreased fluid intake. This problem, although not unique to the dying person, causes increased distress and discomfort that can and should be avoided as the end of life nears. A humidifier or pans of water available for evaporation increases moisture in the air. Moist air helps prevent drying of the skin and mucous membranes; it may also ease breathing. Common measures used to treat dry mouth include frequent swabbing with mouth sponges, spraying the mouth with water mist from an atomizer, brushing the teeth, and sucking on hard candy or gum. Alcohol-based swabs and mouthwash should be avoided because they tend to further dry mucous membranes. Commercial lip balms or liquid vitamin E may be helpful in easing the discomfort of dry lips. Petroleum products such as Vaseline may cause respiratory problems if they are inhaled and should not be used on the mouth.

Nausea and vomiting are not signs of impending death; rather they are distressing symptoms of underlying problems such as adverse medication reactions, constipation, intestinal obstruction, or other physiologic changes. Vomiting increases the risk for aspiration, so it is best to position the patient in a side-lying or sitting (Fowler's) position rather than supine. Temporary relief from nausea and vomiting may be obtained by rectal or parenteral administration of antiemetic medications, but the underlying cause must be identified and corrected before the symptoms will go away. If a medication reaction is suspected, the physician needs to be contacted regarding a possible change in orders.

Constipation is a common and distressing problem for the terminal patient. Common causes of constipation near the end of life include disease factors such as tumor compression, calcium imbalance, adhesions, dehydration, inadequate fiber intake, pain, immobility, and medications (e.g., opioids, antidepressants, and antacids). Constipation should be prevented whenever possible. A high-fiber diet, bulk-forming supplements such as psyllium, and plenty of fluid intake may be enough to prevent problems while the patient is able and willing to eat. Stool softeners, laxatives, suppositories, or enemas may be needed to promote bowel evacuation when dietary intake is not adequate, but caution is needed to prevent electrolyte imbalance when these methods are used. As the end of life approaches and muscle tone in the rectum decreases, manual removal of fecal material may be required to decrease rectal pressure and pain. Digital removal should be done gently and carefully using adequate lubrication (K-Y Lubricating Jelly or petroleum jelly). Extreme caution should be used before performing rectal examination or digital removal when the person has thrombocytopenia.

Diarrhea is a less common problem at the end of life, but one that can have a profound effect on the quality of life. Repeated episodes of diarrhea contribute to electrolyte imbalance, dehydration, skin breakdown, fatigue, and depression. Diarrhea can be caused by numerous factors, including disease processes, psychological factors, medications, herbal remedies, bacterial or parasitic infections, and antibiotic therapy. Treatment may include increased clear fluid intake to replace electrolytes, antibiotics to treat infectious diseases, steroids to decrease bowel inflammation, medications, or bulk-forming agents to slow intestinal peristalsis. Bulk-forming agents should be used only when the person has adequate fluid intake of approximately 2000 mL/day or an obstruction may occur.

URINARY CHANGES

Oliguria is commonly observed because of decreases in fluid intake, blood pressure, and kidney perfusion. Urinary incontinence is also common. Absorbent pads or an indwelling catheter can be used to reduce the need for bed changes that may disturb the dying person.

INTEGUMENTARY CHANGES

Skin breakdown is a problem with malnourished patients near the end of life. Interventions designed to prevent skin tears or pressure sores include proper skin cleansing, careful handling of the skin, frequent turning and positioning, and measures to reduce pressure. Chapter 17 provides further information on the prevention of pressure sores.

Use of soft, nonconstricting, nonirritating (free from harsh detergents and other chemicals) clothing helps promote comfort and minimize risk for skin dryness and rashes. Comfort should take precedence over style. Older, loose, cotton clothing is often best, particularly when the person is diaphoretic. A major advantage of cotton is that it breathes, allowing perspiration to escape, which helps keep the skin dry.

SENSORY CHANGES

Vision diminishes and the visual field narrows as death nears. To compensate for this change in vision, caregivers and loved ones must come close to the dying person to be seen. Indirect lighting with minimal shadows is most restful and least disturbing. Hearing remains acute until death, even if the dying person does not respond. All caregivers and family members must remember this when they speak in the presence of a dying person. Calm, supportive, loving messages should be delivered to the person even when he or she does not respond. Negative or disturbing conversations should be avoided because they can cause the dying person to become distressed and more agitated.

CHANGES IN COGNITION

Delirium, a series of changes in mental status, is present in as many as 80% to 85% of older adults in the last days of life. As death nears, periods of delirium may be interspersed with periods of coherent thought. Assessment of the patient's behavior may reveal varying levels of disturbance. Common symptoms include decreased ability to think and process information, perceptual changes, disorientation, loss of consciousness, insomnia with daytime sleepiness, nightmares, agitation, irritability, anxiety, hypersensitivity to light and sound, fleeting illusions, visual hallucinations, delusions, mood swings, attention deficits, and memory disturbances.

Many forms of delirium are treatable if they are recognized and reported promptly. Causes of delirium include hypotension, oxygen deprivation resulting from apnea or hypoventilation, fever, neurologic changes, metabolic abnormalities such as hyperglycemia and uremia, dehydration, and other physiologic or emotional disturbances. Opioid analgesics can also contribute to delirium. Careful assessment of vital signs, oxygen saturation, and laboratory values may provide valuable information about underlying problems.

Delirium is disturbing to the patient; to his or her family and loved ones; and to physicians, nurses, and other caregivers. Some decrease in symptoms may occur with simple interventions such as calm, reassuring support. Medical treatment is aimed at restoring the patient to as close to his or her baseline cognitive level as is possible. Treatment should be individualized to meet the needs of each person. Correction of underlying physiologic or metabolic problems may bring some relief, as may discontinuation of some medications.

DEATH

Family members and significant others often wish to be present at the time of death. Planning for death differs slightly when the person is in an institutional setting instead of at home. Some families can spend only limited time with their dying loved one and wish to be called only when there is a significant change in the person's status. Others would rather be notified only after death has occurred. The nurse should discuss the family's wishes early so that appropriate notification of family, clergy, and so forth can take place. The nurse needs to know exactly who to call, how they can be reached, and whether there are any limitations regarding time of day. Nurses need to be careful not to judge the choices made by a family. Coping ability, resources, and personal factors including the age, health of older members, and work or family demands on younger members can all influence family decisions. There are advantages and disadvantages to whatever choice the family makes. This may result in situations in which the family assembles only to have the patient rally and live for an extended period of time or situations in which the patient dies before the family can reach the hospital or care facility. Other families can become so exhausted trying to keep a deathwatch that they have little physical or emotional energy left when death actually does occur.

Nurses need to rely on the assessment of physiologic changes and experience to estimate when death is approaching, but there is no way to predict the exact moment or manner of death. Some indicators of imminent death may include, but are not limited to, the following:

1. Increased sleepiness
2. Decreased responsiveness
3. Confusion in a person who has been oriented
4. Hallucinations about people (sometimes deceased family members)
5. Increased withdrawal from visitors or other social interaction
6. Loss of interest in food and fluids
7. Loss of control of bowel and bladder in a person who has been continent
8. Altered breathing patterns such as shallow breathing, Cheyne-Stokes respirations, and rattling or gurgling respirations
9. Involuntary muscle movements and diminished reflexes

Death may be quick or lingering. Some individuals experience an acute physiologic change that results in death. They are alert and talking one minute and gone the next. In other individuals, bodily function shuts down system by system, heart rate slows, respiration fades, and the individual slowly slips away. Signs of death include absence of heartbeat and respiratory activity; open eyes without blink; dilated pupils; slightly open mouth; slack jaw; and lack of responsive to touch, speech, or painful stimuli. Legal pronouncement of death is made by the physician.

If family members are present when the patient expires, they should be allowed to sit at the bedside and say farewells or grieve as long as they need. It is appropriate for the nurse to discretely remove oxygen, IV lines, or other medical devices that are visible. Cultural practices regarding grieving and preparation of the body should be respected and accommodated whenever possible. Adequate time should be given to the family, and nursing support should be available for them until they are ready to leave. This is not the time to avoid the family. A simple hug or other demonstration of sympathy by the nurse is long remembered by family members.

The body should be allowed to remain in the room if other friends or family members who were not present at the time of death wish to assemble. The body may remain in the room until the funeral director arrives, or it may be transported to the **morgue**, depending on agency policies. When death occurs in a shared room, arrangements should be made to provide privacy without unduly disturbing the surviving resident. Some facilities provide a special room for these situations.

The body should be prepared in keeping with cultural and spiritual preferences. Typical postmortem care includes removal of any soiling and application of a clean sheet or shroud according to agency policies. In most cases the head is elevated slightly to prevent discoloration. Eyes are gently closed, dentures are inserted, and a small towel is positioned to close the mouth. This will give the face a more natural appearance if a funeral visitation is desired. Most health care facilities have policies and procedures regarding the legalities pertaining to a death. The nurse in attendance needs to note and document the time of death if witnessed. When death is not witnessed, time of death needs to be approximated. The physician and funeral director specified by the family need to be notified according to agency policies. Personal belongings should be identified, listed, and bagged for return to the family.

Coordinated Care

Supervision

End-of-Life Care

- Nursing assistants who work with dying patients may have many concerns related to end-of-life care.
- Agency policies and licensed nursing personnel should provide guidance so that nursing assistants know what is expected of them.
- Some concerns that need to be addressed include (1) what information regarding changes in status they should report, (2) whether they should start CPR in light of the patient's code, (3) how they should respond to questions from the family, and (4) how to respond to abusive or difficult family members.
- Supervising nurses can work to recognize and meet the needs of their staff.
- Many nursing assistants, particularly those in long-term care settings, become attached to older patients and grieve when they die. The nursing assistants may feel unprepared and have difficulty dealing with a death. They may need reassurance if they feel guilty of doing something wrong when a patient dies after an activity such as bathing or ambulation. They may need guidance, and they may be concerned that they may have said something that upset the dying patient or the family. They may need support when they are criticized and demeaned by family members who rarely visited the patient during his or her life and who appeared only when death was near. They may need empathy when they are expected, as another task, to prepare the body of the deceased when they need an opportunity to grieve the loss.

FUNERAL ARRANGEMENTS

Many religious and cultural implications are related to burial or other disposal of the body. Most older people have given some thought to their final resting place, and many have made specific plans, issued specific directions regarding their wishes, and, in some cases, even paid for their funeral. Activities following death are easier when advanced planning has taken place. It is best when the family is not forced to make difficult choices at a time of high emotion. It is common for grieving families to commit to expensive caskets or services that place an unnecessary financial burden on the family. Some patients do not want burial, but prefer cremation.

Funeral services also are highly influenced by culture and religion. In most cultures, some type of service takes place after death to memorialize the life of the deceased and to allow the family to begin to work through some of their grief. Nurses sometimes desire to attend services for long-term patients. This is appropriate when possible and is often greatly appreciated by the family.

BEREAVEMENT

Entire books have been written on coping with death and dying. This chapter can identify some general guidelines only (Box 15-3). Nurses who deal with dying patients and their loved ones should plan to obtain some additional resources from the library or bookstore.

There is no single "good" or "right" way to feel after a person dies. Survivors often express having ambivalent feelings regarding the death. On one hand, they feel a sense of relief that the struggle is over and that the loved one is at rest. On the other hand, they seriously grieve and miss the loved one's presence. Even when death is anticipated, the initial feeling of shock and numbness typically occurs. For a few weeks after death, people describe their behavior as "being in a fog" or "going through the motions." After this initial time, the reality of the loss strikes and survivors are likely to experience signs of depression such as loss of appetite, inability to sleep, avoidance of social interaction, and uncontrolled bouts of crying. They may also be angry with the person who died and voice statements such as, "How could he do this to me?" Talking to the deceased loved one is not abnormal and may be useful for some individuals.

In normal grieving, the frequency and severity of these signs of grieving gradually decrease over time, but the loss of a loved one never goes away completely. Life goes on, but it is not the same as before. Normal life does not seem the same without the loved one. Most people who lose a loved one require at least a year to work through the most severe phase of emotional

Box 15-3 Kübler-Ross's Stages of Grief

The following stages were identified by Dr. Elizabeth Kübler-Ross in her groundbreaking book, which was the first to address grief related to death and dying. Although listed in a sequence, these stages do not necessarily follow in this specific order. A person may move in and out of the stages unpredictably and erratically.

DENIAL

Numbness protects the survivor from the intensity of the loss. This typically decreases as the individual acknowledges the reality and permanence of the loss.

ANGER

Feelings of anger are often directed at the deceased or at a deity because the survivor feels abandoned. Anger is one method for dealing with the feelings of helplessness and powerlessness. Anger tends to decrease over time.

BARGAINING

Survivors try to identify whether they could have done something different to prevent the loss. Some may make resolutions to change their behavior or lifestyle based on these reflections. Remorse and guilt that they did not do enough are common and can slow the grief process.

DEPRESSION

Feelings of emptiness, loneliness, and isolation are common after the loss of a loved one. Frequent crying spells, inability to sleep, inability to concentrate or make decisions, and loss of appetite are typical. Some survivors describe their lives as colorless and meaningless. Many people try to hide their feelings and suffer needlessly. Support from family, friends, nurses, physicians, and bereavement groups can help the survivor work through feelings of depression. Antidepressant medications are sometimes used on a short-term basis.

ACCEPTANCE

There is no set time limit for grief over the loss of a loved one. Acceptance and healing occur slowly as the person works through his or her feelings and reestablishes a meaning and pattern to life.

Data from Kübler-Ross, E. (1969). *On death and dying*. London, Routledge.

distress. Grief counselors often judge a person's responses at the first anniversary of the death as an indicator of his or her adjustment. It is common for grieving to last longer than a year, but severe adjustment problems at this point indicate the need for more aggressive help.

Nurses can help grieving individuals in several ways. They can encourage the grieving person to take time to cry and to express his or her feelings. They can listen to the grieving person talk about the loved one.

Review and reminiscence about good times may bring tears, but it gives the person opportunities to gain strength from having known the loved one. Nurses can recommend bereavement support groups, which use sharing of mutual experiences to help individuals coping with loss and grief. Nurses can help identify individuals who are experiencing severe or protracted grief and who may need a referral to a grief counselor who has special training and techniques to help the person.

Get Ready for the NCLEX® Examination!

Key Points

- Eighty percent of the deaths in the United States occur in the older-than-65 population.
- Despite increased attention by professional organizations and groups, death and end-of-life care do not receive adequate attention in nursing education or society as a whole.
- Many older adults do not desire aggressive medical intervention at the end of life, so caregivers need to be prepared to provide palliative and holistic interventions.
- Older patients and their families need to be included in planning for end-of-life care.
- Most older people state that they wish to die at home, but most deaths occur in institutional settings.
- Culture and ethnicity play a role in beliefs and expectations related to the end of life.
- Most individuals fear that they will die in pain. Nurses must work to allay this fear and provide adequate pain control for dying patients.
- Although it is not possible to predict exactly when a person will die, several physiologic changes occur as death approaches.

- The nurse needs to provide ongoing care to minimize preventable problems and discomforts.
- Family members need to be apprised of the significance of physiologic and behavioral changes that occur as death nears.
- Nurses can play an important role in helping survivors deal with grief after the death of a loved one.

Additional Learning Resources

SG Go to the Study Guide on pp. 379–397 for additional learning activities to help you master the chapter content.

evolve Go to your Evolve website (http://evolve.elsevier.com/Wold/geriatric) for the following FREE learning resources:
- Animations
- Answer Guidelines for Nursing Care Plan Critical Thinking Questions
- Answers and Rationales for Review Questions for the NCLEX® Examination
- Glossary with pronunciations in English and Spanish
- Video Clips

Review Questions for the NCLEX® Examination

1. An elderly resident in a long-term care facility asks the nurse, "What is it like to die?" The nurse's best response would be:

   1. "You're healthy, you don't want to talk about dying now."
   2. "You've been thinking about death today?"
   3. "I've seen people die and it's different for everybody."
   4. "Did the doctor tell you something at your last visit?"

2. A calorie-restricted, low-sodium diet was prescribed for a DNAR, terminally ill patient, who is diabetic and in renal failure. As death nears, they have very little appetite and pick at the food. Appropriate nursing interventions include: (Select all that apply.)

   1. Continue diet as ordered.
   2. Encourage family to bring in small amounts of food from home.
   3. Serve food in a place free from odors.
   4. Encourage the person to eat anything that appeals to him or her.
   5. Require person to eat at least one bite of each food group.
   6. Provide good oral hygeine.

3. Dyspnea, shortness of breath, and irregular breathing patterns are common as death nears. Simple measures to be taken by the nurse to help alleviate mild respiratory difficulty include: (Select all that apply.)

   1. Administering oxygen by nasal cannula
   2. Administering prn atropine sulfate
   3. Instituting measures to reduce anxiety or tension
   4. Elevating the head of the bed
   5. Administering prn morphine per physician's order
   6. Reminding visitors not to tire the client

4. List the five stages of death and dying identified by Kübler-Ross.

   1. _____
   2. _____
   3. _____
   4. _____
   5. _____

5. Pain at the time of death is:

   1. One of the greatest fears of the dying person
   2. Usually of short duration and readily treated with analgesics
   3. Normal, expected, and unavoidable
   4. Likely to require high doses of narcotic analgesics

6. Sedation, including benzodiazepines, barbiturates, and opioids, are used:

   1. As a common part of the treatment of a dying patient
   2. Only when it is in the best interest of a patient
   3. When the patient has specified its use in advance directives
   4. To calm the patient and are not likely to precipitate death

Sexuality and Aging

Objectives

1. Describe how sexuality changes with aging.
2. Discuss the effects of illness on sexual functioning.
3. Describe methods for assessing sexual functioning.
4. Identify the older persons who are most at risk for experiencing problems related to sexuality.
5. Discuss the concerns of aging lesbian, gay, bisexual, and transgender persons.
6. Identify selected nursing diagnoses related to sexuality.
7. Describe nursing interventions that are appropriate for older individuals experiencing problems with sexuality.

Key Terms

hysterectomy (hĭs-tĕr-ĔK-tō-mē) (p. 260)
intercourse (ĬN-tĕr-kŏrs) (p. 259)

masturbation (măs-tŭr-BĀ-shŭn) (p. 263)
sexuality (sĕk-shū-ĂL-ĭ-tē) (p. 259)

Sexuality is a part of life and does not cease to exist simply because a person ages. Although society may sometimes prefer to think of older adults as asexual, this is not the case. Individuals who have had an active sex life in younger years are likely to continue to do so as they age. Many older adults continue to have sexually satisfying lives well into old age.

Most women cease reproducing before 50 years of age, but medical research is pushing the limits in this area. Headlines are made when women in their late fifties—and even one woman 63 years of age—successfully give birth to a healthy child. One may question the reasons for and the ethics of considering child-bearing at an advanced age, but the fact remains that it is possible. Men remain able to father children well into their sixties and seventies without medical assistance. Although uncommon, fathering children at 80 and 90 years of age does occur. Although the ability to reproduce diminishes with age, and the frequency and form of sexual activity are likely to change, the need for sexual affection does not disappear with aging (Figure 16-1).

Sexual touching, fondling, and **intercourse** remain a part of the lives of many active older people. Sexual thoughts and feelings are normal as people age. Studies reveal that close to 40% of married couples older than 60 years of age have sexual intercourse at least once a week, and almost half of these couples have sex more frequently. A study of the sexual interests and behaviors of persons older than age 80 reveals that a significant percentage (63% of men and 30% of women) continue to participate in sexual activity. Sexuality is more than just a physical drive, it provides opportunity for the aging person to express and receive affection, connection, and emotional bonding.

FACTORS THAT AFFECT SEXUALITY OF OLDER ADULTS

Physical changes related to aging, changing health status, and loss of a sex partner all affect the sexual practices of older adults. Normal physiologic changes in sexual function may raise concerns for aging adults. In general, sexual response time slows with aging, but the ability to achieve orgasm remains throughout life.

NORMAL CHANGES IN WOMEN

Older women experience changes in the reproductive system related to the decreased levels of progesterone and estrogen. Common changes that may result in discomfort or pain during intercourse (dyspareunia) (Complementary and Alternative Therapies box for possible methods of treatment) include (1) irritation of the external genitals (pruritus vulvae), (2) thinning and dryness of the vaginal walls (atrophic vaginitis), and (3) alteration in the levels of normal microorganisms in the vagina, resulting in an increased risk for vaginal yeast infections.

In the past, hormone replacement therapy (HRT) was commonly used to reduce the incidence of these and other physiologic changes associated with aging. A study published by the National Institutes of Health (NIH) in 2000 raised serious questions about the safety of HRT, particularly for women who have preexisting cardiovascular or liver disease and those at risk for breast or endometrial cancer. Many women have made the decision to avoid or discontinue use of HRT based on this study, but some have decided to accept the risks and continue to take hormone supplements. Use of HRT is a personal decision made by each woman with guidance from her doctor. Women who continue to use HRT of any kind should be carefully monitored by their physicians and should have a yearly mammogram and Pap smear.

259

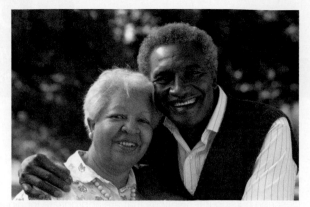

FIGURE 16-1 Love and affection are important to older adults.

Complementary and Alternative Therapies

Remedies for Postmenopausal Discomforts

1. Over-the-counter vaginal moisturizers or water-soluble lubricants may help decrease the symptoms of dryness. Vaseline or other petroleum-based products should be avoided. Very-low-dose estrogen preparations in the form of vaginal creams, gels, or rings are sometimes prescribed to reduce localized symptoms while producing minimal systemic effects.
2. Designer estrogens provide estrogen-like effects on some tissues, while blocking the effect of estrogen (acting as an antiestrogen) on other tissues. Tamoxifen and raloxifene are two designer estrogens currently in use.
3. Herbs and other "natural" remedies are sometimes used to reduce menopausal symptoms. Because the FDA has no power to oversee the quality or effectiveness of anything labeled as a dietary supplement, self-treatment with herbs may not be a safe practice. If a woman decides to try an herbal remedy, it is essential that she tell her physician what she is taking so that the physician can monitor her for any untoward effects or possible interactions with other prescription and OTC drugs. Dong quai, ginseng, black cohosh, Vitex/chasteberry, DHEA, melatonin, and St. John's wort are commonly used herbal preparations.

Other natural products include phytoestrogens and wild yams (sweet potatoes). Phytoestrogens are chemicals that act as estrogens on some parts of the body and antiestrogens on others. Soybeans are a rich source of phytoestrogens. Research in this area is still very new, and more scientific information is needed. Wild yams are thought to be helpful because they contain a chemical similar to one used for making the type of progesterone in birth control pills. Wild yam creams are considered nonhormonal and are currently being tested for effectiveness.

ERECTILE DYSFUNCTION IN MEN

Older men experience a delayed reaction to sexual stimuli. They require a longer time to achieve an erection, and the erection is often less firm than it was at a younger age. Male orgasm takes longer to achieve and has a shorter duration than at a younger age. Ejaculation is less forceful and a smaller volume of seminal fluid is released. Loss of erection occurs quickly after orgasm. In general, the time between orgasms increases, and orgasm may not occur with every episode of sexual intercourse. Diabetes, depression, and cardiovascular disease contribute to impotence in men, even at a young age. Prostatectomy (removal of excess prostate tissue) normally does not cause problems with achieving an erection because newer surgical techniques do not cause the nerve damage that was common in the past. Medications such as sildenafil citrate (Viagra) or tadalafil (Cialis) are effective for many individuals suffering from erectile dysfunction.

ILLNESS AND DECREASED SEXUAL FUNCTION

Illness of one or both partners is a common reason for decreased sexual function. Many disease processes interfere with normal sexual function, as do many of the medications taken to treat illness. Incontinence does not interfere with sexual relations but may cause some people to avoid sex because of possible embarrassment. Treatment can at least control if not completely cure incontinence problems. Joint pain resulting from arthritis can interfere with sexual activity. Cardiac problems are likely to interfere with normal sexual activity, although this is more from fear than from actual danger. The actual risk for death resulting from sexual intercourse is low, but older persons who have experienced a heart attack should discuss their concerns with a physician. Stroke need not prevent sexual activity. Sex is not likely to cause another stroke, although modification in position or use of assistive devices may be needed to compensate for any residual weakness or paralysis. Neither hysterectomy (removal of the uterus) nor mastectomy (removal of a breast) changes sexual functioning, although loss of these organs may make the woman feel less desirable or make her fear that she will be viewed that way. Counseling may be required to help women with these concerns. Depression can decrease sexual interest and lead to decreased response to intimacy.

ALCOHOL AND MEDICATIONS

Alcohol and medications affect sexual function in older adults. Excessive alcohol intake results in delayed orgasm in women and loss of the ability to achieve or maintain an erection in men. A wide range of medications and drugs (Table 16-1) is likely to cause sexual problems for both men and women. Changes in the medication or the dosage may help resolve the problem. Interestingly, some antiparkinsonian medications actually enhance sexual desire, but not necessarily the ability to perform sexually.

LOSS OF A SEX PARTNER

One of the most common reasons for decreased sexual activity in older adults is loss of the sex partner (Figure 16-2). Because single women older than 65 years of age outnumber single men of the same age

Table 16-1	Examples of Medications and Drugs Associated with Sexual Dysfunction
Antihypertensives	Diuretics; alpha and beta adrenergic blockers; ACE inhibitors; calcium channel blockers
CNS medications	Monoamine oxidase inhibitors (MAOIs); Selective serotonin reuptake inhibitors (SSRIs); tricyclic antidepressants; anxiolytics; antipsychotics; lithium carbonate, opioids
Miscellaneous	Seizure medications; cimetidine, methotrexate, estrogens, amphetamines, cholesterol-lowering drugs
OTC medications	Some antihistamines, decongestants; antiinflammatories
Street drugs	Alcohol, cocaine, heroin, tobacco, and marijuana

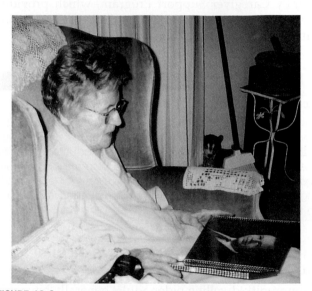

FIGURE 16-2 Loss of a loved one and sexual partner may affect the remaining person both emotionally and physically.

by 4:1, the odds for men interested in relationships are good but poor for women. Social norms may suggest to older women that interest in men, particularly sexual interest, is not socially acceptable. More elderly men voice an interest in sex while more older women express a desire for companionship and love.

MARRIAGE AND OLDER ADULTS

Most older adults think of sex within the context of marriage, but this may change as the Baby Boomers, who matured during a more sexually experimental time, age. Marriage, or remarriage, among older adults garners many different responses, particularly from the families of older adults. Some families are accepting and recognize the need for older adults to find affection and meaning in later life. Others believe that

marriage at a late age is somehow unacceptable. Children often fear that the marriage is a slap in the face of the deceased parent. Many children also fear that remarriage will displace them from their parent's affection or affect their inheritance. It should be the right of alert older persons to determine what is best for themselves. Ideally, family and friends will be supportive of the decision.

Marriage is not always an option for aging individuals. Some older people, particularly widows, stand to lose a great deal if they remarry. Pensions, insurance benefits, and other financial concerns may be contingent on the person's remaining single. For this reason, some older people choose to live together without marrying, which can be a difficult decision for both older adults and their families. Long-standing moral or religious values may result in guilt on the part of older persons who can see no alternative, and families may have a great deal of difficulty accepting this lifestyle.

CAREGIVERS AND THE SEXUALITY OF OLDER ADULTS

Sexuality is a difficult area to address at any age. Young people may not be comfortable with the thought of sexual activity among seniors, believing that it is somehow offensive or abnormal. Even health care professionals may be unaware of or uncomfortable about addressing the sexual needs of older adults. This situation is not helped by the fact that older adults are often reluctant to discuss their own sexuality. Fear, shame, or embarrassment over what younger persons may think causes many older people to hide their sexual interests and activity even from health care professionals. Physicians, nurses, and others who care for older adults must be nonjudgmental and sensitive to the values and attitudes of older individuals.

It is best for caregivers to address issues dealing with sexuality in private and to ask open-ended questions such as, "Are you concerned about how your sexuality has changed with age?" or "Are you satisfied with your sex life?" These questions allow the older person the opportunity to verbalize a range of possible concerns or questions. Caregivers need to indicate a willingness to listen and allow adequate time to discuss any concerns that arise. This reluctance by older adults to speak about sexuality may change because aging Baby Boomers who grew up during the "sexual revolution" may be more willing to participate in or even initiate conversations about sex.

SEXUAL HEALTH AND SEXUAL ORIENTATION

Other concerns must also be addressed with regard to sexual activity in older adults. Older adults often are not considered when sexually transmitted diseases are discussed, yet 10% of acquired immunodeficiency syndrome (AIDS) cases occur in people older than 50 years of age. Human immunodeficiency virus (HIV) is commonly overlooked because older adults are not considered to be at risk. All sexually active individuals, no matter what their age, should use safe sex practices. The risk for sexually transmitted disease does not disappear with age.

🌐 Cultural Considerations

HIV and Older Adults

In a study done with African-American, Chinese-American, Latino, and white participants, it appears that regardless of their cultural group, older adults tended to perceive or verbalize that HIV is a problem of someone else, not themselves. Common misconceptions were present in all groups. Although most did not think HIV actively involved them, they were in general willing to learn about it to "teach their children or grandchildren." Several older African Americans stated that they thought HIV was less of a problem now and that older adults were most likely to contract HIV through contact with doctors, dentists, and hospitals. Drug use and sexual activity were viewed as much less likely sources. Latina women had difficulty accepting that HIV occurred in older adults. Chinese Americans, though apparently knowledgeable regarding HIV, expressed views that a stable life, good diet, and exercise could prevent HIV. White participants supported the belief that HIV was a young person's disease. Older adults in all cultural groups were reluctant to discuss the use of condoms.

Sexual orientation must also be addressed. For personal or social reasons, persons who have concealed their sexual orientation in younger years may be more comfortable expressing it as they age. Health care providers must be careful to recognize the sexual needs and concerns of older lesbian, gay, and transgender people. Estimates indicate that between 1.75 and 3.5 million Americans age 60 and over are lesbian, gay, bisexual, or transgender. These numbers are likely to increase as the older population grows.

Studies show that older lesbian, gay, bisexual, and transgender (LGBT) people experience aging in much the same way as do heterosexuals. Most appear to be satisfied with their lives and express similar concerns regarding health care, housing, and social support networks that other older people typically report.

Discrimination against lesbian, gay, and transgender people is still common in society. Too often, social service and health care providers are uncomfortable discussing homosexual unions. Because of this, many aging LGBT people are reluctant to make contact with community organizations for the elderly or to access a health care system that has focused on the heterosexual population and often failed to address concerns of the homosexual community. Many express concern about accessing health care because of confidentiality concerns or fears that discrimination might result in substandard care.

LGBT people are interested in senior housing options such as retirement communities and assisted living, but currently most of these are directed at the heterosexual community and do not address the concerns of alternative lifestyles. LGBT older persons fear nursing home placement because they feel that they may be especially vulnerable if the health care staff is not sensitive to their needs. For example, they are concerned that nursing homes may not allow LGBT residents to share a room with their partner and fear that any demonstration of affection between partners will be viewed negatively. Many aging homosexuals report becoming depressed and express concern about having to deny or conceal their life choices to gain acceptance. While some aging LGBT people maintain close, supportive relationships with their family, others rely on close friends or partners for emotional, social, and sometimes physical support. This support network has been aided by the passage of the National Family Caregiver Support Program, which provides assistance to anyone caring for a frail older adult, including unrelated individuals.

🏃 Health Promotion

Health Care Directives for Nonrelated Caregivers

Lesbian, gay, bisexual, and transgender people need to be aware of the importance of completing advance care directives if they wish to have their friends, partners, or other nonfamily members participate in health care decision making. Without these directives, even long-term partners have no legal standing in decision making and may even be prohibited from visiting in some situations.

PRIVACY AND PERSONAL RIGHTS OF OLDER ADULTS

Community-dwelling older adults generally have privacy to conduct their sex lives without interference. They are free to touch, hold, and have sex whenever they choose. However, institutional placement of one or both partners can interfere with sexual expression. Obtaining adequate privacy may be difficult, even for married couples who reside in the same institution, particularly if regular medical or nursing care is necessary (Figure 16-3).

In the past, displays of sexual affection were discouraged among older adults. Fortunately, attitudes are changing as health care providers grow in awareness. Some facilities have policies that indicate respect for older residents' right to keep sexually explicit materials. Touching, handholding, and cuddling are encouraged. Unmarried older adults are allowed to form whatever relationships they desire. A closed door must be respected when privacy for intimacy is desired. Of course, special judgments are necessary when either person in a relationship suffers from

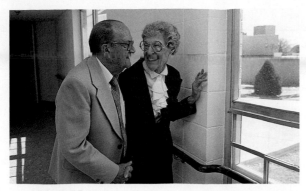

FIGURE 16-3 Much can be said with a touch.

cognitive impairment. When there is any sign of disinterest or resistance to sexual advances, the behavior is not permitted. It is important that institutions protect vulnerable older adults from undesired physical contact, but mutually agreeable physical contact should remain a right of older adults.

❖ NURSING PROCESS FOR SEXUAL DYSFUNCTION

■ Assessment/Data Collection

- Does the person have any discharge or drainage from the genitals?
- If the person is sexually active, does he or she complain of any difficulty or discomfort during sexual activity?
- Does the person have any diseases or disabilities that interfere with sexual activity?
- Are there any emotional issues, such as depression, that interfere with sexual interest or activity?
- Does the person take any medications that may interfere with sexual activity?
- What level of sexual activity does the person desire?
- Does the person have any real or perceived barriers to sexual activity?
- Does the person have adequate privacy for sexual activity?

Box 16-1 lists risk factors for sexual dysfunction in older adults.

Nursing Diagnosis

Sexual dysfunction

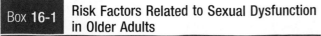

Box **16-1**	**Risk Factors Related to Sexual Dysfunction in Older Adults**

- Loss of partner
- Problems with physical mobility
- Institutional setting
- Physical illness or a reaction to therapeutic medications

Nursing Goals/Outcomes Identification

The nursing goals for older persons with sexual dysfunction are to (1) verbalize feelings about sexual identity, (2) discuss concerns regarding sexuality, and (3) describe the effects of aging and illness on sexual functioning.

Nursing Interventions/Implementation

The following nursing interventions should take place in hospitals, in extended-care facilities, and at home:

1. **Encourage verbalization of concerns.** Many older adults do not feel comfortable talking about sex to anyone, particularly a younger person. Without undue prying into the older person's privacy, nurses should communicate a willingness to discuss any concerns older adults have, including those that deal with sexuality. Nurses should allow adequate time and provide a private place for these discussions.

2. **Provide privacy.** Alert older adults who wish to court or visit should have the opportunity to do so without interference from nursing staff. Private areas should be available for dating interactions. Older residents of extended-care facilities should have the opportunity for conjugal visits in the institution or at home if they so desire. Nurses should ensure that these visits meet all federal and state regulations that pertain to residents' rights. Privacy during these visits must be carefully respected.

3. **Protect the sexual dignity of confused older adults.** Individuals who are confused may display sexually inappropriate behaviors (e.g., exposing themselves in public, masturbating, and making inappropriate sexual advances to nursing staff). Undressing in public can be decreased by modifying clothing. For men, elastic-waist pants can replace pants with zippers. For women, buttonless or back-opening tops and slacks instead of skirts can help reduce exposure. Masturbation is common and is not abnormal. Distraction is often effective at reducing the incidence of public masturbation. If distraction is not effective, the person should be taken to his or her room and provided with privacy. Restraints should not be applied to prevent masturbation. If a confused older person makes inappropriate sexual advances, nurses should attempt to distract the individual and, if necessary, stop care temporarily. Confused individuals do not realize that their behavior is inappropriate. Nurses should be careful not to overreact to the behavior because this can precipitate violent or verbally abusive episodes (Nursing Care Plan 16-1).

★ Nursing Care Plan 16-1   Sexual Dysfunction

Mr. Silver, age 89, has a history of hypertension and diabetes. Mrs. Silver, age 87, has severe osteoarthritis and congestive heart failure. Both are residents of Pine Grove Care Center. They have been married for 67 years. Because of space constraints, they have been assigned to separate rooms. Mr. Silver spends a great deal of time at Mrs. Silver's bedside, where he holds her hand and talks to her. Both often verbalize the wish to hold and touch more intimately. They both state, "I wish we just had some privacy around here."

Nursing Diagnosis
Sexual dysfunction

Defining Characteristics
- Lack of privacy
- Separation from significant other
- Altered body function related to age and disease processes

Patient Goals/Outcomes Identification
Mr. and Mrs. Silver will identify methods for satisfying their need for sexual expression.

Nursing Interventions/Implementation
1. Allow opportunities for both parties to verbalize their feelings about continuing sexual contact.
2. Attempt to arrange for a shared room, if this is agreeable to both parties.
3. Develop a method, such as hanging a "Do Not Disturb" sign, for ensuring private time for the couple, while recognizing the need for access in case of emergency.
4. Assist with hygiene needs so that both parties are physically clean and attractive.
5. Verbalize an understanding of the continued need for physical closeness throughout life.

Evaluation
Mr. and Mrs. Silver are observed spending time privately in her room with the door closed. After these visits, Mr. Silver states that "It feels good just to touch, share a kiss, and be together quietly for a while. It isn't how I thought we'd end up, but it's better than nothing." You will continue the plan of care.

Critical Thinking Questions
1. Some facilities permit or encourage married couples to share a room in long-term care facilities.
2. Do you think that this is something that should be encouraged or discouraged? Why?
3. How can the nurse provide for privacy needs if a couple is still interested in sexual activity? How can the nurse determine whether there is mutual consent to sexual activity?

Get Ready for the NCLEX® Examination!

Key Points

- Sexuality is an area that is often minimized or ignored in older adults.
- Health problems, loss of a partner, and the normal physiologic changes of aging all affect sexual practices.
- Although these changes affect the type and frequency of sexual activity, many individuals maintain an active interest in sex into old age.
- Nurses and other younger health care providers must recognize that older adults are still sexual beings, and they continue to have sexual needs.
- Older adults have the right to meet sexual needs without age bias.

Additional Learning Resources

SG Go to the Study Guide on pp. 379–397 for additional learning activities to help you master the chapter content.

ℯvolve Go to your Evolve website (http://evolve.elsevier.com/Wold/geriatric) for the following FREE learning resources:
- Animations
- Answer Guidelines for Nursing Care Plan Critical Thinking Questions
- Answers and Rationales for Review Questions for the NCLEX® Examination
- Glossary with pronunciations in English and Spanish
- Video Clips

Review Questions for the NCLEX® Examination

1. A 70-year-old married man confides to the nurse that he recently began to have difficulty achieving an erection. He states that "It wasn't much of a problem until recently." The nurse's best response would be:
   1. "That's quite normal at your age."
   2. "What do you think is wrong?"
   3. "Are you having problems in your marriage?"
   4. "Did you recently change any medications?"

2. A 69-year-old woman reports that she avoids intercourse because it is uncomfortable. She asks the nurse if she has any suggestions to relieve this problem. The nurse would:

   1. Suggest that she ask the physician for an estrogen vaginal cream.
   2. Describe herbal and natural products that have effects similar to estrogen.
   3. Clarify what she means by "uncomfortable."
   4. Explain that this is a normal and expected change of aging.

3. An elderly man who suffers from dementia often masturbates in the lounge area of a long-term care facility. Appropriate nursing interventions include: (Select all that apply.)

   1. Modify clothing to make genital exposure more difficult.
   2. Apply mitten restraints to prevent self-stimulation.
   3. Provide privacy by escorting him back to his room.
   4. Explain repeatedly that this type of behavior is not acceptable.

5. Distract him with an activity that he finds interesting.
6. Administer a prn sedative medication.

4. An elderly gay person is reluctant to move into a long-term care facility because he:

   1. Fears that he will receive substandard care.
   2. Prefers not to associate with aging heterosexuals.
   3. Understands that he will lose legal rights in the facility.
   4. Knows that most caregivers will discriminate against him.

5. When assessing the sexual practices and behavior of an older adult, it is very important that the nurse:

   1. Conduct the interview in a private setting.
   2. Ask clear and probing questions.
   3. Only address the subject when brought up by the patient.
   4. Include the spouse or sex partner in the discussion.

chapter

17

Care of Aging Skin and Mucous Membranes

Objectives

1. Discuss changes related to aging that have an effect on skin and mucous membranes.
2. Identify the older adults who are most at risk for problems related to the skin and mucous membranes.
3. Describe interventions that assist older adults in maintaining intact skin and mucous membranes.

Key Terms

alopecia (ăl-ō-PĒ-shē-ă) (p. 271)
aseptic (ā-SĔP-tĭk) (p. 277)
caries (KĂR-ēz) (p. 279))
exudate (ĔKS-ū-dāt) (p. 274)
gingivitis (jĭn-jĭ-VĪ-tĭs) (p. 279)
halitosis (hăl-Ĭ-TŌ-sĭs) (p. 279)
hyperkeratosis (hĪ-pĕr-kĕr-ă-TŌ-sĭs) (p. 273)

leukoplakia (lū-kō-PLĀ-kē-ă) (p. 280)
pigmentation (pĭg-mĕn-TĀ-shŭn) (p. 268)
pressure ulcers (p. 266)
pruritus (prū-RĪ-tŭs) (p. 266)
scabies (SKĀ-bēz) (p. 268)
xerostomia (zēr-ō-STŌ-mē-ă) (p. 280)

The skin undergoes several changes with aging that make it more susceptible to damage. Over time, the epidermal layer becomes thinner and subcutaneous padding diminishes, increasing the risk for traumatic injuries such as skin tears or **pressure ulcers**. Bruises are more common because capillary walls are more fragile. Medications used to treat various health problems can cause problems. Corticosteroids make the skin more fragile, and anticoagulants increase the risk for bleeding with even minor trauma. Decreased sebaceous secretions and circulatory changes contribute to the dry skin and scaliness of the lower extremities common with aging. Aging skin is more susceptible to inflammation, infection, and rashes. **Pruritus**, which is a common complaint in older adults, may be caused by dryness, irritation, or infection but can be related to diseases such as diabetes mellitus, kidney disease, malignancy, or anemia. Changes in the function of dermal receptor cells result in a decrease in the ability of the older person to perceive sensations such as touch and pressure, increasing the risk for pressure-related disorders. Although skin problems usually are not life threatening, they are significant because they can distress the older person and lead to decreased quality of life. Skin problems should be prevented whenever possible; in situations in which the problems are not preventable, they should be recognized, treated, and resolved in a timely manner.

AGE-RELATED CHANGES IN SKIN, HAIR, AND NAILS

Changes in the skin, hair, and nails may indicate a variety of problems related to nutritional and circulatory adequacy. Because these structures are the ones most easily observed, they can provide a great deal of information about the metabolic health of the entire body (Table 17-1).

Complete assessment of skin, hair, and nails is best done when the person is undressed so that all skin surfaces can be inspected. Skin assessment can be performed during a bath, during daily personal hygiene, at bedtime, or at any other convenient time for the older person. Independent older persons should be aware of what is normal for themselves, and they should bring any changes to the attention of the physician. In a hospital or extended-care setting, privacy must be maintained and modesty protected during the skin inspection. Assessment of the skin and ancillary structures is an important responsibility of nurses. Nursing assistants and attendant health care workers who assist with bathing or other care should be instructed to report any unusual or questionable observations promptly to a nurse for further investigation. Inspection should follow a logical order so that no pertinent observations are missed. Most nurses find that a head-to-toe progression is the most helpful, as is a body diagram on which observations are indicated (Figure 17-1).

Table 17-1   Age-Related Changes in Skin, Hair, and Nails

PARAMETERS	OBSERVABLE CHANGES	CAUSE
Skin		
Color	Paleness in white skin Brown spots (senile lentigines) Purple patches (senile purpura)	Decreased vascularity of dermis, loss of melanocytes Hyperpigmentation Blood leaking from poorly supported fragile capillaries
Moisture	Dry skin, decreased perspiration	Decreased sebaceous and sweat gland activity
Elasticity, turgor	Decreased elasticity Loose folds and wrinkles Decreased turgor	Loss of collagen and elastic fibers
Texture	Some rough areas Thin, more transparent skin	Environmental effects over time; less moisture Thinning of epidermis from decreased vascularity of dermis; loss of underlying tissue
Hair		
Color	Grayness	Decreased number of melanocytes in hair
Consistency	Thinner on head and body Coarser in noses of men	Decreased density and rate of hair growth Increased density of nasal hair
Distribution	Loss of hair on head and body Increased hair on faces of women	Decreased rate of hair growth; decreased hormones; decreased peripheral circulation Higher androgen/estrogen ratio
Nails		
	More brittle Longitudinal ridges Thickening and yellowing of toenails	Slowing of nail growth; decreased peripheral circulation

From Phipps WJ, et al: *Medical-surgical nursing: concepts and clinical practice,* ed 4, St Louis, 1991, Mosby.

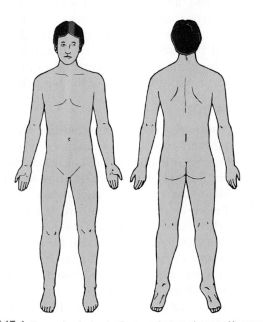

FIGURE 17-1 Example of a body diagram that can be used in assessing older patients for skin impairment.

SKIN COLOR

Skin color changes can indicate a variety of disorders. When assessing skin for color, it is important to be aware of the differences in skin pigments among ethnic groups. Examination of the skin should take place in good, preferably natural, light; one side of the body should be compared with the other; and touch should be used to determine skin temperature or the presence of rashes or irritation. Stretching the skin slightly may also help in determining the underlying tones. Color changes, including pallor, cyanosis, jaundice, or erythema, can indicate a variety of problems. The extent and location of any color changes should be recorded and reported promptly.

🌐 Cultural Considerations

Pressure Ulcers

When assessing people with dark skin tones, changes in tissue color that indicate stage I pressure ulcers can be better distinguished using a halogen light, which may reveal a purple hue. Be sure to use touch to determine changes in tissue temperature and palpate for signs of localized edema over pressure points.

DRY SKIN

Dry skin is one of the most common problems of aging. Various studies have shown that 75% to 85% of people older than 65 years of age experience some degree of problem with dry skin. Physiologic changes, excessive bathing, the use of harsh soaps, and a dry environment all contribute to problems with dry skin.

Dry skin can result in itching (pruritus), burning, and cracking of the skin (Figure 17-2). Many older people develop a habit of scratching or picking at dry or cracked skin, increasing their risk for further tissue damage and infection. Skin irritation can be severe

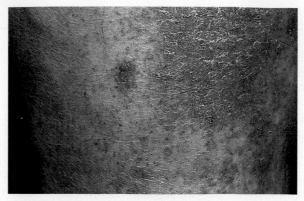

FIGURE 17-2 Dry, scaly skin commonly seen in older adults.

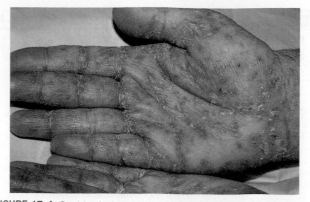

FIGURE 17-4 Scabies lesions at three different stages are evident on this patient's hand. The lesion at the far left features a well-demarcated round border surrounding a blister, whereas the sore nearest the thumb fold has already erupted and appears to be healing.

and can cause intense discomfort to older adults. In fact, it may be so distracting that affected individuals cease to participate in social activities.

RASHES AND IRRITATION

Rashes and skin irritation can be caused by factors other than dryness. Medications, communicable diseases, and contact with chemical substances are common causes of skin rashes and pruritus (Figure 17-3).

Allergic response to medications can manifest as diffuse rashes over the body. Whenever a rash develops soon after administration of new medication, an allergy should be suspected. It is appropriate to withhold that particular medication and contact the physician to report the symptom.

One communicable source of skin irritation and severe pruritus is scabies. Scabies is a superficial infection caused by a parasitic mite (*Sarcoptes scabiei* var. *hominis*) that burrows under the skin (Figure 17-4). Older adults, especially individuals who suffer from chronic illness, dementia, or a depressed immune system, are particularly vulnerable to scabies infections. Signs of scabies include intense itching and fine, dark, wavy lines at the flexor surface of the wrist or elbow, the webbed area of the fingers, the axilla, and the genitals. Recognition of scabies may be difficult in older adults because it has an asymptomatic incubation period of 4 to 6 weeks and because atypical presentations are common. When infestation is suspected, skin scrapings should be examined to determine the presence of ova or mites.

Scabies is spread from person to person by direct contact. Because recognition is difficult, treatment may be delayed, allowing the parasite to infect other people. To reduce outbreaks of scabies infection within an institution, all new residents in extended-care settings should be assessed carefully on admission. All cases must be identified and treated promptly to prevent spread or reinfestation with the parasite.

PIGMENTATION

Changes in skin pigmentation are common with aging. These changes are discussed in Chapter 3. Many of the changes are cosmetic and do not cause problems unless they are located on the face or arms, where they may be distressing to the affected person. Common conditions such as acne rosacea can be treated with topical medications, which help heal the skin and reduce redness, whereas others can be concealed by appropriate use of cosmetics. Changes in the size or pigmentation of moles are of greater significance because these changes may indicate the presence of a precancerous or cancerous condition that needs immediate medical attention.

TISSUE INTEGRITY

Breaks in tissue integrity increase the older person's risk for infection and often result in the need for costly, time-consuming treatments. These breaks can cause disfigurement and are frightening to older adults. Skin tears, abrasions, lacerations, and ulcers most often result from friction, shearing force, moisture, and pressure. Even simple incidents such as contact with furniture, sliding across bed linens, a grip during a transfer,

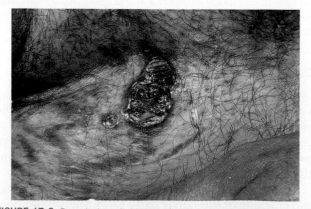

FIGURE 17-3 Drug-induced skin reactions are seen more commonly among older patients than in younger patients. Use of a potent topical corticosteroid has resulted in severe striae. The atrophy was so severe that the skin tore, forming an ulcer.

or the removal of tape may result in significant skin trauma to the older person.

PRESSURE ULCERS

Pressure ulcers are a particular risk to older adults who suffer from compromised circulation, restricted mobility, altered level of consciousness, fecal or urinary incontinence, or nutritional problems (Table 17-2). Studies estimating the occurrence of pressure ulcers vary widely, but one consistent point is that they occur in all settings. Although most studies show that the incidence of pressure ulcers has declined, there is still much work to be done. Pressure ulcers have negative effects on the overall health of an elderly person . They can lead to infection, pain, loss of function, and even death. Furthermore, incidence of pressure ulcers can leave care facilities and nurses vulnerable to lawsuits for negligence. They strain the health care system with treatment costs estimated at $11 billion per year. New Medicare rules specify that a hospital will not be reimbursed for the care of a patient who develops a pressure ulcer after being admitted to a hospital. This should be a great motivator for hospitals to institute pressure ulcer prevention programs.

Excessive pressure on tissues, particularly over bony prominences, can quickly lead to skin breakdown (Figure 17-5). Ulcer development depends on the amount of pressure, the length of time pressure is exerted, and the underlying status of the tissues

Table 17-2	Quick Guide to Prevention of Pressure Ulcers
RISK FACTOR	**NURSING INTERVENTIONS**
Immobility	Establish individualized turning schedule; reduce shear and friction by using trapeze and/or turning sheet; elevate HOB <30 degrees; provide pressure-relief surface
Inactivity	Provide assistive devices to increase activity
Incontinence	Assess the need for incontinence management; clean and dry skin after soiling
Malnutrition	Provide adequate nutritional and fluid intake; assist with snacks and meals, monitor intake and output (I & O); consult the dietitian for nutritional evaluation
Diminished sensation, decreased mental status	Assess the patient's and family's ability to provide care; educate caregivers regarding pressure ulcer prevention
Impaired skin integrity	Avoid pressure; do not use donut-shaped cushions or sheepskin; lubricate skin; apply barrier ointments to protect skin from moisture; do not massage red areas; Do not use heat lamps, heating pads, or hot water.

Modified from Catania K, et al; PUPPI—The pressure ulcer prevention protocol interventions, *Am J Nurs*, 107(4): 44–52, 2007.

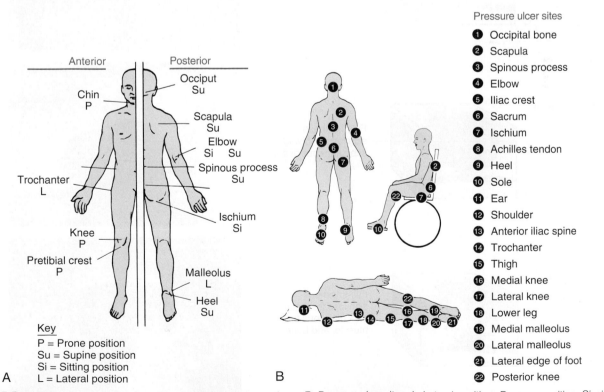

Pressure ulcer sites
1 Occipital bone
2 Scapula
3 Spinous process
4 Elbow
5 Iliac crest
6 Sacrum
7 Ischium
8 Achilles tendon
9 Heel
10 Sole
11 Ear
12 Shoulder
13 Anterior iliac spine
14 Trochanter
15 Thigh
16 Medial knee
17 Lateral knee
18 Lower leg
19 Medial malleolus
20 Lateral malleolus
21 Lateral edge of foot
22 Posterior knee

Anterior   Posterior
Chin P
Occiput Su
Scapula Su
Elbow Si Su
Spinous process Su
Trochanter L
Ischium Si
Knee P
Pretibial crest P
Malleolus L
Heel Su

Key
P = Prone position
Su = Supine position
Si = Sitting position
L = Lateral position

A   B

FIGURE 17-5 A, Bony prominences most often underlying pressure ulcers. **B,** Pressure ulcer sites. *L,* Lateral position; *P,* prone position; *Si,* sitting position; *Su,* supine position.

involved. Tissue that is subjected to excessive pressure does not receive adequate oxygen or nutrients. This can result in ischemia and increased susceptibility to breakdown. When tissue is deprived of necessary nutrients for a longer period, necrosis and tissue destruction result. Tissue that is fragile because of poor nutrition or circulation is most susceptible to breakdown. Early danger signs indicating a risk for breakdown include pale or reddened tissue. Pressure ulcers are categorized or staged based on their appearance and the depth of tissue penetration (Figure 17-6).

Individuals who have had one pressure ulcer are at greater risk for future development of additional ulcers. Additional factors that contribute to development of pressure ulcers include the following:
- Multiple coexisting diseases
- Underweight or overweight
- Poor nutritional status
- History of alcohol and tobacco use
- Bladder and/or bowel incontinence
- Restricted mobility
- Cognitive impairment

Rather than wait for skin breakdown to occur, most health care agencies perform a formal risk assessment at the time of admission and then at regular intervals. The most common tools used for

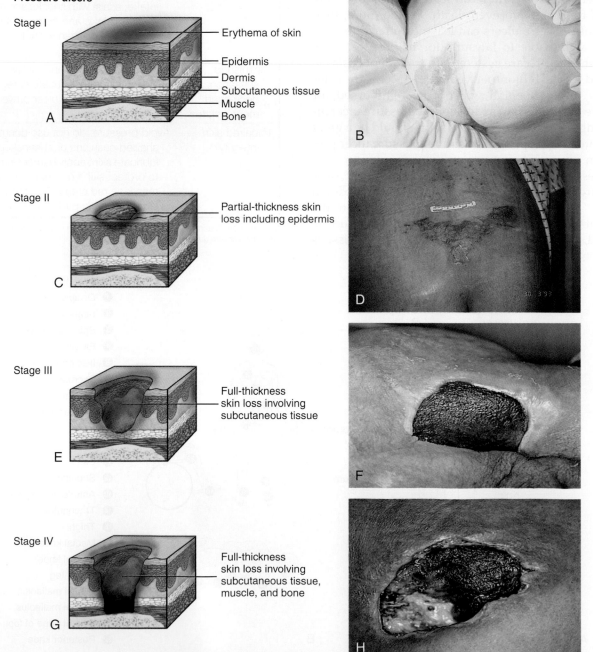

Pressure ulcers

Stage I
- Erythema of skin
- Epidermis
- Dermis
- Subcutaneous tissue
- Muscle
- Bone

A

B

Stage II
- Partial-thickness skin loss including epidermis

C

D

Stage III
- Full-thickness skin loss involving subcutaneous tissue

E

F

Stage IV
- Full-thickness skin loss involving subcutaneous tissue, muscle, and bone

G

H

FIGURE 17-6 Pressure ulcers. **A** and **B,** Stage I. **C** and **D,** Stage II. **E** and **F,** Stage III. **G** and **H,** Stage IV.

this assessment are the Braden and Norton Scales (see Tables 17-3 and 17-4). Nurses use the information from this assessment to develop a plan of care that minimizes risk factors and promotes skin integrity.

AMOUNT, DISTRIBUTION, APPEARANCE, AND CONSISTENCY OF HAIR

The amount, distribution, appearance, and consistency of the hair change with aging. The hair of both men and women typically becomes thinner and has a finer consistency with advanced age. Heredity and gender play a role in hair loss patterns. Men tend to lose more hair than do women, although some men retain a full head of hair throughout life. Male pattern baldness typically results in progressive loss of hair at the temples and back of the head. Sudden and excessive hair loss (**alopecia**) or breakage is likely to indicate a systemic problem. Abnormal hair loss can be related to high fevers, medications, nutrition problems, fungal or bacterial infections, endocrine disorders, or stress. Sudden or unusual hair loss should be reported so that the physician can determine the cause.

Table 17-3 Braden Scale for Predicting Pressure Sore Risk

ASSESSMENT TOOL	1 POINT	2 POINTS	3 POINTS	4 POINTS
Sensory Perception				
Ability to respond meaningfully to pressure-related discomfort	Completely limited: Unresponsive (does not moan, flinch, or grasp) to painful stimuli because of diminished level of consciousness or sedation *or* Limited ability to feel pain over most of body surface or discomfort over half of body	Very limited: Responds only to painful stimuli; cannot communicate discomfort except by moaning or restlessness *or* Has a sensory impairment that limits the ability to feel pain on one or two extremities	Slightly limited: Responds to verbal commands but cannot always communicate discomfort or the need to be turned *or* Has some sensory impairment, which limits ability to feel pain or discomfort	No impairment: Responds to verbal commands; has no sensory deficit that could limit ability to feel or voice pain or discomfort
Moisture				
Degree to which skin is exposed to moisture	Constantly moist: skin is kept moist almost constantly by perspiration, urine, and the like; dampness is detected every time patient is moved or turned	Very moist: Skin is often, but not always, moist; linens must be changed at least once a shift	Occasionally moist: skin is occasionally moist, requiring an extra linen change approximately once a day	Rarely moist: Skin is usually dry; linen requires changing only at routine intervals
Activity				
Degree of physical activity	Bedridden: Confined to bed	Chairfast: Ability to walk severely limited or nonexistent; cannot bear own weight and/or must be assisted into chair or wheelchair	Walks occasionally: walks occasionally during day, but for very short distances, with or without assistance; spends majority of each shift on bed or chair	Walks frequently: walks outside room at least twice a day and inside room at least once every 2 hours during waking hours
Mobility				
Ability to change and control body position	Completely immobile: does not make even slight light changes in body or extremity position without assistance	Very limited: Makes occasional slight changes in body or extremity position but is unable to make frequent or significant changes independently	Slightly limited: makes frequent although slight changes in body or extremity position independently	No limitations: makes major and frequent body position changes without assistance

Continued

Table 17-3 Braden Scale for Predicting Pressure Sore Risk—cont'd

ASSESSMENT TOOL	1 POINT	2 POINTS	3 POINTS	4 POINTS
Nutrition				
Usual food intake pattern	Very poor: Never eats complete meal; rarely eats more than one third of any food offered; eats two servings or less of protein (meat or dairy products) per day; takes fluids poorly; does not take a liquid dietary supplement *or* receives nothing by mouth and/or is maintained on clear liquids or intravenous	Probably inadequate: rarely eats a complete meal; generally eats only approximately half of any food offered; protein intake includes only three servings of meat or dairy products per day; occasionally takes a dietary supplement *or* receives less than optimal amount of liquid diet or tube feeding solutions for more than 5 days	Adequate: Eats more than half of most meals; eats a total of four servings of protein (meat or dairy products) each day; occasionally refuses a meal, but usually takes a supplement if offered *or* is on a tube feeding or total parenteral nutrition regimen that probably meets most of nutritional needs	Excellent: Eats most of every meal; never refuses meal; usually eats total of four or more servings of meat and dairy products per day; occasionally eats between meals, does not require supplements
Friction and shear				
	Problem: Requires moderate to maximal assistance in moving; complete lifting without sliding against sheets is impossible; frequently slides down in bed or chair, requiring frequent repositioning with maximal assistance; spasticity, contractions, or agitation leads to almost constant friction	Potential problem: moves feebly or requires minimal assistance; during a move, skin probably slides to some extent against sheets, chair, restraints, or other devices; maintains relatively good position in chair or bed most of the time but occasionally slides down	No apparent problem: moves in bed and in chair independently and has sufficient muscle strength to sit up completely during move; maintains good position in bed or chair at all times	

From Bergstrom N, et al: The Braden scale for predicting pressure sore risk, *Nurs Res* 36(4): 205–210, 1987. Instructions: Score patient in each of the six subscales. The maximum score of 23 has the best prognosis, and the minimum score of 6 has the worst prognosis. A patient is at risk for pressure ulcer if the score is ≤16.

Table 17-4 Norton Risk Assessment Scale

PHYSICAL CONDITION		MENTAL CONDITION		ACTIVITY		MOBILITY		INCONTINENT		TOTAL SCORE
Good	4	Alert	4	Ambulant	4	Full	4	Not	4	4
Fair	3	Apathetic	3	Walk/help	3	Slightly limited	3	Occasional	3	3
Poor	2	Confused	2	Chairbound	2	Very limited	2	Usually/Urine	2	2
Very bad	1	Stupor	1	Bed	1	Immobile	1	Doubly	1	1
Name										
Date										

From the Centre for Policy on Ageing, London, England, 1962.

The amount and distribution of body hair also change with aging. Diminished or absent hair on the lower legs or feet—particularly when combined with excessively dry, scaly, or flaky skin and weak or absent pedal pulses—indicates decreased blood supply to the lower extremities.

Tissue of the Feet

Inspection of the tissue on the feet warrants special attention in older adults. Because many aging individuals are unable to bend adequately to view the feet, a family member or friend can perform this inspection for independent older adults (Figure 17-7). In an

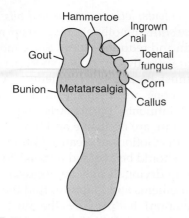

FIGURE 17-7 Common foot problems in older adults.

Labels on figure: Hammertoe, Ingrown nail, Gout, Toenail fungus, Corn, Bunion, Metatarsalgia, Callus

institutional setting, foot inspection should be performed by the nursing staff. Many older adults neglect their feet simply because they cannot see or reach them. Unless foot inspection is done on a regular schedule, severe problems can occur before anyone is aware of them.

Nails

Aging results in **hyperkeratosis** of the nails, particularly the toenails. Thick, hard nails are difficult to cut using normal foot care equipment. The strength and effort required to cut these nails may exceed the older person's abilities, resulting in overgrowth. Soaking the feet in warm water before attempting to cut them may help soften the nails and make them easier to cut. Assistance from a family member or health care provider is appropriate when there is no history of circulatory problems or diabetes. When diabetes or circulatory problems are present, care should be provided by a foot care specialist. Special heavy-duty equipment may be needed to accomplish proper nail care. Use of safety glasses is recommended during nail care to prevent eye injuries from flying nail particles.

If proper care is neglected, uncut nails confined in shoes often begin to curl under the toes, resulting in a condition called **ram's horn nails.** In this condition, the nail curls over the top of the toe and grows into the flesh on the bottom, causing pain. When the discomfort becomes severe, the older person may stop wearing shoes and decrease ambulation in an attempt to reduce the discomfort. In such severe cases, care from a podiatrist is advisable. Nail fungus is increasingly common with aging. Fungi cause the nails to become thick, brittle, misshapen and discolored. Fungal infections are more likely to affect the feet because the environment in shoes (dark, moist, and warm) supports growth of these microorganisms. Fungal infections are more common in elderly persons with diabetes or other conditions of diminished peripheral circulation. These infections need to be recognized and treated so that they do not cause more widespread problems.

Other Common Foot Problems

Other common foot problems include corns, calluses, blisters, and bunions, which usually result from years of wearing poorly fitted footwear. These conditions often cause discomfort for older adults and lead to some degree of activity restriction. Many independent older adults use commercially available foot remedies or attempt to remove corns or calluses with a knife or scissors. This practice is dangerous and significantly increases the risk for serious foot infections, which may necessitate amputation of a toe, toes, or the entire foot. Older persons with diabetes or impaired peripheral circulation are particularly prone to develop foot ulcers or infections and are at greatest risk for amputation.

❖ NURSING PROCESS FOR IMPAIRED SKIN INTEGRITY

■ Assessment/Data Collection

- What is the general appearance of the person's skin?
- Are any sores evident on the scalp?
- What is the color of the skin? Are there any signs of pallor, jaundice, cyanosis, or erythema? If so, where?
- Are there any areas of dry skin? If so, where?
- Does the person complain of itching?
- Is there any evidence of scratching?
- Are there any signs of scabies (fine, wavy, dark lines or spots at the webs of the fingers or folds of the skin)?
- Are there any rashes? If so, where are they located? What is their appearance (e.g., macular, papular, or vesicular)?
- Is there any sign of pallor or erythema over bony prominences?
- Are there any breaks in the skin integrity? If so, where? What do they look like?
- Are any abrasions (friction burns) or skin tears evident?
- Is there any change in the amount, distribution, or appearance of the hair?
- What is the appearance of the toenails? Are they thickened? Difficult to cut? Discolored?
- Are any sores or lesions evident on the feet or ankles?
- What is the person's nutritional status? Is the person overweight or underweight?
- Is the person alert and able to move freely? If not, what is the level of immobility?
- Is the person incontinent of bladder or bowel?
- Are there pedal pulses? Are these pulses easy or difficult to detect?

Box 17-1 lists risk factors for skin, hair, or nail alterations in older adults.

■ Nursing Diagnoses

Risk for impaired skin integrity
Impaired skin integrity
Impaired tissue integrity

| Box 17-1 | Risk Factors for Alterations in Skin, Hair, or Nails in Older Adults |

- Circulatory problems
- Restricted mobility
- Nutritional or fluid imbalances
- Cognitive impairments
- Exposure to irritating chemicals, including body secretions or waste products
- Exposure to communicable diseases
- Lack of adequate hygiene facilities or assistance in the home

■ Nursing Goals/Outcomes Identification

The nursing goals for older individuals with or at risk for impaired skin or tissue integrity are to (1) remain free from excessive skin dryness or skin breakdown; (2) display timely healing of wounds, lesions, and ulcerations; and (3) maintain optimal nutritional status to promote tissue integrity and healing.

■ Nursing Interventions/Implementation

The following nursing interventions should take place in hospitals or extended-care facilities:

1. **Assess the level of impairment and the contributing factors.** The nurse should perform a daily skin inspection; measure the location, size, and depth of the affected area or areas; and identify any conditions or changes that may have caused the problem. Changes in skin condition can occur rapidly in older adults. All problem areas must be measured and documented so that improvement or further breakdown can be evaluated. Nurses should explore any possible causes for the problem and institute nursing measures to prevent or reduce further tissue damage.

2. **Institute measures to reduce the risk for skin and tissue breakdown.**
   - *Reduce the frequency of complete bathing.* The type and frequency of baths or showers depend greatly on the individual. The condition of the skin and the presence of perspiration or other body wastes must be considered. Some individuals require a complete bath or shower daily; others benefit more from a complete bath on a biweekly or weekly basis. On days when total baths are not taken, partial or sponge baths of the face, axilla, and perineum provide adequate cleanliness and prevent body odors.
   - *Keep skin free from wastes and* **exudate** *by using mild nondetergent soaps.* Reducing the frequency of bathing is suggested if dryness is a problem. Use of mild, nondetergent, nonperfumed, superfatted soaps (e.g., Basis, Caress, Dove, Neutrogena) for cleansing decreases excessive skin dryness.

   - *Use emollients, lotions, creams and oils to maintain skin moisture.* Emollients help keep moisture in the skin and reduce dryness. Since most preparations are effective for only a short period of time, they must be applied frequently. A variety of preparations are available at a wide range of costs. Ointments, particularly those containing petrolatum, are occlusive and tend to be longer-lasting than lotions or creams. Lotions containing alcohol should be avoided because they can contribute to drying. It may be necessary to try various emollients and lotions to find the one (or the combination) that provides the most relief to the older individual (Box 17-2).
   - *Rinse skin carefully.* Soaps tend to dry the skin and should be rinsed off completely before drying. If a basin is being used, complete rinsing may require frequent water changes.
   - *Dry skin tissue gently and thoroughly.* To decrease skin irritation, the skin should be dried by patting rather than rubbing. If the skin is severely irritated, soft towels that have been rinsed carefully to remove all detergents may be necessary.

| Box 17-2 | Products That Help Moisturize the Skin |

All of these products are available without a prescription. Other moisturizers are also available in stores. Ask the doctor or pharmacist whether these moisturizers would work well.

CREAMS AND LOTIONS
- Cetaphil cream and lotion
- Complex 15 hand and body cream and lotion
- Curel moisturizing cream and lotion
- Eucerin cream and lotion
- EverSoft
- Keri lotion
- Lubriderm cream and lotion
- Moisturel lotion
- Nivea moisturizing lotion
- Nivea ultramoisturizing cream
- Nutraderm cream and lotion
- Purpose dry skin cream
- Shepard's cream lotion
- Shepard's skin cream

OINTMENTS
- Aquaphor natural healing ointment
- Crisco vegetable shortening
- Dermasil
- Neutrogena Norwegian Formula Emulsion
- Unibase
- Vaseline pure petroleum jelly

UREA- OR LACTIC ACID-CONTAINING CREAMS AND LOTIONS
- Aqua Care cream
- Carmol 10
- Lac-Hydrin Five
- LactiCare
- Nutraplus

- *Turn and position the person frequently, and reduce sources of pressure by keeping bed linen tight and clear of foreign objects.* Pressure over bony prominences restricts blood flow to the tissues that are being compressed (Figure 17-8). These areas are most likely to become ischemic or necrotic. Frequent position changes allow reestablishment of blood flow and reduce the risk for skin breakdown. The maximal amount of time a person is in one position should not exceed 2 hours. More frequent turning is necessary for individuals at high risk for skin problems. The frequency of position changes should be based on assessment of pressure points after the person is turned. A 30-degree lateral position (Figure 17-9) is preferred to a full lateral position. A turning schedule will help ensure that repositioning is done at appropriate times.

Pressure points over bony prominences are most susceptible to breakdown, but anything that exerts resistance against the skin can become a pressure point. Foreign objects such as large wrinkles, personal belongings (rosary or prayer beads), or needle caps trapped under the body can also contribute to skin breakdown.

Each time the person is repositioned, the skin should be inspected for signs of circulatory reduction such as blanching or hyperemia. If these signs are present, a more frequent turning schedule should be established. Reddened areas should be treated with caution and should not be massaged because massage is likely to increase the risk for ulcer formation.

- *Wash the skin and supply clean, dry linens after episodes of incontinence.* Urine and stool contain waste products that are highly irritating to the skin and must be cleansed promptly with gentle washing and rinsing. Barrier ointments can be applied to clean skin to reduce contact with body wastes. Older persons who are known to be incontinent of stool or urine must be checked frequently to reduce the chance of prolonged exposure to moisture and body wastes. Special absorbent pads or garments that wick moisture away from the skin are appropriate in some situations. Problems of incontinence are addressed in greater depth in Chapter 18.

Once the skin is thoroughly washed and dried, moisture barriers (e.g., A+D Ointment) can be applied to protect the skin. These types of preparations must be removed from the skin at regular intervals to prevent bacterial overgrowth.

- *Keep the skin dry after episodes of diaphoresis; check skin surfaces where moisture caused by normal perspiration can become trapped.* Moisture on the skin surface can cause maceration and tissue breakdown. Moisture caused by perspiration usually evaporates and causes few problems unless perspiration is excessive or is trapped between skin surfaces (e.g., under pendulous breasts). Frequent sponging with clear water and thorough drying, exposure to air, or use of a drying substance such as cornstarch helps reduce the amount of moisture and friction between skin surfaces.

- *Move and transfer the person carefully.* The skin of older individuals is thinner, less elastic, and has less subcutaneous padding than that of younger people. This makes it particularly vulnerable to shearing forces during movement. When the head of the bed is elevated, it is recommended that the elevation be kept at or below 30 degrees to reduce the shearing force that may occur when a person slides down in bed. To reduce the friction that occurs when tissue is dragged over bed linens, transfer sheets or other assistive devices should be used when turning, repositioning, or transferring a frail older person.

- *Provide appropriate pads, cushions, mattresses, or beds that are designed to reduce pressure.* Many types of beds and mattresses designed to distribute weight over a larger area and reduce pressure on body tissues are available. The advantages and disadvantages of some of these are presented in Table 17-5. Wheelchair pads made of gel or

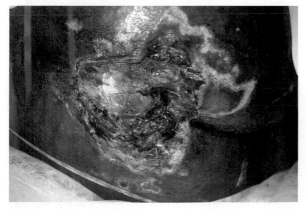

FIGURE 17-8 A stage IV pressure sore in the sacral area of an 85-year-old man. Note the sacrum (*white area*) and necrotic surrounding muscles.

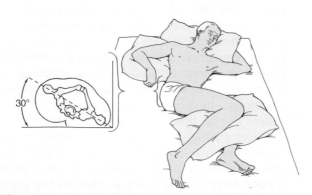

FIGURE 17-9 A 30-degree lateral position is best to avoid pressure points.

Table 17-5   Mattress Surface Types

CATEGORIES	MECHANISM OF ACTION	INDICATIONS	EXAMPLES OF MANUFACTURERS/ PRODUCT NAMES
Low-Air-Loss System			
Available in a full bed or as an overlay	Pressure redistribution device Bed: The entire surface is a powered, inflated surface with air loss Overlay: Powered surface, constant inflation and air loss at the surface; place over the bed mattress	Prevention of skin breakdown in patients who cannot be turned or have existing skin breakdown	Hill-Rom/Flexicair Eclipse Kinetic Concepts, Inc/First Step Select Crown Therapeutics/ SelectAir Mattress
Foam			
Available as an overlay or in a full mattress	Redistributes pressure and the cover (top) can reduce friction and shear Overlay: Placed on top of bed mattress Full mattress: Used in place of the usual mattress	Pressure redistribution for high-risk patients	Bio Clinic/Bio Guard BG Industries/ MaxiFloat
Static Air-Filled Overlay			
Available as an overlay	Interconnected air-filled cells, inflated to appropriate level Pressure redistribution	High-risk patients	Crown Therapeutics/ RoHo mattress Gaymar Industries/ Sof-Care
Air-Fluidized Bed			
Available as a bed	Bed frame with silicone-coated beads that become fluidized when air is pumped through the beads Pressure redistribution, antishear, antifriction surface	For patients with burns or multiple stage III or stage IV pressure ulcers, protection of new grafts and flaps	Kinetic Concpts, Inc/FluidAir Hill-Rom/Clinitron
Kinetic Therapy			
Available as a bed	Provides continuous passive motion to promote mobilization of respiratory secretions; also provides low-air-loss therapy	Patients who are at risk for or have developed atelectasis and/or pneumonia	Hill-Rom/Total Care Sport Kinetic Concepts, Inc/TriaDyne II

From Potter PA, Perry AG, Stockert PA, Hall A: *Basic nursing: essentials for practice,* ed 7, St Louis, 2011, Mosby.

inflated with air help reduce pressure on the ischial tuberosities. Only full chair cushions should be used. Inflatable "donuts" are not recommended because, although they reduce pressure on one area, they increase pressure on surrounding tissues. This can lead to more ischemia and result in extending the area of tissue damage.

3. **Institute measures to promote tissue healing.**
   - *Promote adequate nutritional intake.* Tissue regeneration occurs more slowly in older adults than in younger individuals. Increased intake of calories with emphasis on protein and vitamin C is particularly important because these nutrients are necessary for tissue repair.
   - *Encourage adequate rest.* Tissue healing uses energy and places additional physiologic stress on the aging body. Therefore, older adults may require additional rest periods during the day.
   - *Check wounds daily for signs of inflammation or infection, and obtain cultures of wound drainage if appropriate.* The typical signs of inflammation or infection may be absent or diminished in older adults; therefore, special attention should be paid to any open areas. Wound cultures are indicated if any purulent or foul-smelling drainage is observed. Infection delays healing and places additional stress on older adults.
   - *Follow aseptic technique when cleansing wounds, changing dressings, or applying medications.* When treatments are ordered for skin breakdown such as pressure ulcers, it is essential that good **aseptic** technique be used to prevent the introduction of pathogenic microorganisms into the

area. Good handwashing between patient contacts and strict adherence to body substance precautions are essential. All personnel should have their own supply of dressing materials that are kept apart from other people's supplies. Multipatient treatment carts should not be taken to the bedside. All supplies used for wound care should be protected from environmental contamination by dust, water, or other such substances.

Dead tissue is typically cleansed from a wound by being rinsed or irrigated with normal saline. Harsh cleansers, povidone-iodine, and hydrogen peroxide should be avoided because they can damage underlying healthy tissues. Excessive force during irrigation can also cause tissue damage. Clean rather than sterile dressings are used in most situations, as long as they comply with the institutional infection-control guidelines. A variety of preparations is available for wound care; the particular type selected by the physician or wound care specialist depends on the location and stage of the lesion (Table 17-6). Individuals with severely compromised immune systems may require use of sterile technique and supplies.

If a patient has more than one lesion, the most contaminated wound (e.g., one near the perineum) should be cleaned last. Dressings should be kept clean to prevent cross-contamination among lesions.

4. **Provide good foot care.** The feet of older adults are particularly susceptible to problems. Poor circulation, increased incidence of problems such as bunions, excessively thick toenails, and the results of years of wearing poorly fitted shoes all contribute to foot problems in older adults. The feet should be soaked regularly to remove old, dry skin. After a good soaking, the feet should be dried by patting rather than rough rubbing. The nurse should be sure to dry the feet thoroughly, paying careful attention to the areas between the toes. If permitted, the toenails should be cut straight across and the sharp edges filed off. The toenails of people with diabetes and other older persons with circulatory problems should be cared for by a foot specialist. Emollients should be used if the skin on the feet is very dry. When emollients are used on the feet, older adults need to be aware of the importance of wearing socks to prevent slipping. A daily change into clean socks or stockings is preferable and should be encouraged, because clean footwear reduces the risk for infection. Older persons with diabetes or circulatory impairment of the lower extremities should be encouraged to wear white cotton socks to promote cleanliness and provide early recognition of any injury or drainage. Caution should be used to ensure that the socks fit properly and do not cause excessive constriction around the ankles or calves.

Any signs of foot irritation, color change, skin breakdown or changes in the appearance of the nails should be documented and reported promptly.

The following interventions should take place in the home:

1. **Encourage adequate fluid intake and good nutrition.** Good nutrition and adequate fluid intake are needed to maintain healthy tissue. Inadequate intake of nutrients such as protein, vitamin A, and vitamin C can result in fragile tissue that is more susceptible to bruising, shearing force injuries, and breakdown. When inadequate intake is suspected, a more complete assessment (including a food and fluid diary) is appropriate. This helps nurses determine the cause or causes (e.g., depression and illness) and plan suitable interventions.

2. **Maintain adequate humidity in the environment.** Exposure to hot, dry air, whether in the desert or in overly warm living quarters, results in excessively dry skin. An excessively dry environment intensifies the tendency toward dryness, which is already a problem in older adults. The result is skin that is rough, dry, cracked, irritated, and more susceptible to breakdown and infection. Dry mucous membranes usually accompany dry skin, increasing the risk for epistaxis (nosebleeds). Living spaces should be maintained at a temperature of approximately 70° F to 72° F. Relative humidity between 40% and 60% is most comfortable and beneficial for the skin and mucous membranes. Commercial humidifiers or even open pans of water set around the house help increase the amount of moisture in the room.

3. **Avoid excessive exposure to the sun.** Older adults have fewer melanocytes, which are unevenly distributed over exposed body areas. Excessive exposure to sunlight can cause irregular, blotchy, and cosmetically unacceptable tanning. Use of sunblock is recommended when significant sun exposure is expected. Older adults are encouraged to wear loose, lightweight, light-colored clothing to prevent exposure to the ultraviolet rays in sunlight that increase the risk for skin cancer.

4. **Obtain regular professional foot care.** Older persons, particularly those living alone, often find that foot care is difficult because of the loss of flexibility. Regular appointments with a foot care specialist reduce the risk for trauma or infection. Professional foot care is essential for individuals with diabetes and those with impaired peripheral circulation.

5. **Use any appropriate interventions that are used in the institutional setting.**

Table 17-6　Treatment Options by Ulcer Stage

ULCER STAGE	ULCER STATUS	DRESSING	COMMENTS*	EXPECTED CHANGE	ADJUVANTS
I	Intact	None Film, adherent Hydrocolloid	Allows visual assessment Protects from shear May not allow visual assessment	Resolves slowly without epidermal loss over 7 to 14 days	Turning schedule Support hydration Nutritional support Silicone-based lotion to decrease shear Pressure-relief mattress or chair cushion
II	Clean	Composite film (Viasorb film, plus Telfa, Exudry) Hydrocolloid Hydrogel sheet	Limits shear Change every 7 days if occlusive seal Absorbent, requires secondary dressing of gauze or adherent film	Heals through epithelialization and epithelial budding Manages incontinence	See previous stage
III	Clean	Hydrocolloid Hydrogel foam Exudate absorbers, calcium alginate, wound pastes Gauze, fluffy Growth factors	See stage II Apply ¼ inch thick, cover with gauze or hydrocolloid Change when strikethrough is noted on secondary dressing; cover with gauze or hydrocolloid Use with normal saline Use with gauze	Heals through granulation and reepithelialization (Note: does not become stage II ulcer as it heals)	See previous stages Electrical stimulation Evaluate pressure-relief needs
IV	Clean	Hydrogel Hydrocolloid plus hydrocolloid paste/beads Calcium alginate Gauze Growth factors Adherent film	See stage III, clean See stage III, clean; critical to treat areas of undermining See stage III, clean Pack deeply undermined ulcers Use with gauze Will facilitate softening of eschar	Heals through granulation and reepithelialization Because of contraction, surface may close more rapidly than base, leaving wound cavity Eschar will lift at the edges as healing progresses; cross-hatching central area of eschar with a small blade will facilitate release from center	Surgical consult for closure See stages I, II, and III, clean See previous stages Surgical consult for debridement Enzymes covered with gauze dressing may be used to debride ulcer
	Eschar	Hydrocolloid Gauze plus ordered solution None	Will facilitate softening of eschar Absorb drainage and control odor if Dakin's is used Rarely, if eschar is dry and intact, no dressing is used, allowing eschar to act as physiologic cover		

From Potter PA, Perry AG: *Clinical nursing skills and techniques*, ed 5, St Louis, 2003, Mosby.
*As with all occlusive dressings, wounds should not be clinically infected.

AGE-RELATED CHANGES IN ORAL MUCOUS MEMBRANES

Problems in the oral cavity may render an older individual unable to chew certain foods. Inspection of the oral cavity is needed to determine the status of the individual's teeth, tongue, and oral mucous membranes. Changes in the condition of the gums and oral mucous membranes may be related to several factors.

Dental care was not readily available to many of today's older adults during their youth because of the cost and the associated discomfort. Therefore, older individuals who neglected their teeth now suffer tooth loss. Even those who maintained good dental practices are likely to experience tooth decay and loss because of the fact that preventive dental techniques were not as advanced as they are today. Water fluoridation, which started in the 1940s, has helped prevent some dental problems, resulting in a larger percentage of today's elderly who have retained at least some of their teeth. Studies show, however, that poor oral hygiene is a major problem for the older population. Reasons for this include (1) failure of the elderly to see dental care as a priority, (2) the cost of dental care, (3) restricted access due to transportation problems or inadequate availability of dental services, which is particularly a problem in rural areas, and (4) physical or cognitive limitations. Many elderly persons are unable or unwilling to maintain good oral hygiene practices. Unfortunately, nursing staff members too often place oral hygiene at a lower priority than other more visible aspects of care. The author has often told others that if she were able to perform only one assessment to determine a person's overall quality of care, she would inspect the person's oral cavity. When oral care is good, then there is a high probability that all of the care is good. Nurses need to recognize the importance of this aspect of care and give it the attention it deserves.

DENTAL CARIES

Tooth decay, loose teeth, and lost teeth are ongoing problems in the older adult population. Poor nutrition and decreased appetite in older adults can often be attributed to dental problems. Decay, or caries, is caused by the action of bacteria that penetrate through the enamel shield of the tooth and cause destruction (see Figure 17-10). If caries is not recognized early, a significant amount of the tooth structure may be destroyed. If the caries extends deep into the tooth, a nerve may be exposed, and painful neuritis (toothache) may result. Replacement of the lost tooth material with amalgam restorations (fillings) can help rebuild the tooth, but this leaves a weakened structure that remains susceptible to problems. Lost restorations leave rough edges that cause irritation of the oral mucous membranes, particularly the cheek and tongue.

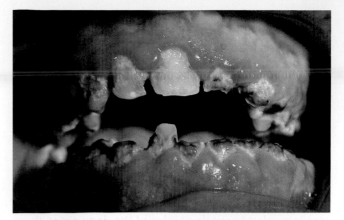

FIGURE 17-10 Extensive dental caries in an older adult.

PERIODONTAL DISEASE

Food debris and plaque build up in the mouth and on the teeth when oral hygiene is inadequate. Activity of bacteria on this debris causes halitosis, or bad breath, which is often disturbing to the older person and to anyone who has close contact. Periodontal disease is a less obvious but potentially more serious complication of poor oral care. One form of periodontal disease is gingivitis, or inflammation of the gums. Gingivitis causes gum swelling, tenderness, and bleeding and eventually leads to recession of the gum tissue away from the tooth. As the gums recede the teeth lose support, become loose in the sockets, and eventually fall out. When a tooth is lost, a gap is created. Healthy teeth shift position or move into the space, resulting in an uneven bite. Chewing becomes increasingly difficult when significant numbers of teeth, particularly the molars needed for chewing and grinding food, become loose or lost. Periodontal disease is suspected to play a role in thromboembolitic disorders, bacterial endocarditis, and myocardial infarction. Individuals who have a cardiac history are typically given prophylactic antibiotics before or following any dental work.

PAIN

Dental caries and periodontal disease are the most common reasons for oral pain, but oral lesions such as stomatitis or altered sensations in the mouth are frequently reported. Pain may be limited to the oral cavity or may affect the face and jaw. As many as 18% of older adults in one study reported oral pain within the previous year. Oral pain can cause loss of appetite and decreased food intake and can have a negative effect on the overall quality of an older person's life.

DENTURES

If only a few teeth are missing, the dentist may attempt to bridge the gaps by attaching artificial teeth to the good teeth. If too many teeth are missing, a partial plate may be required. When all of the upper or lower teeth are removed, a complete set of dentures is required. Both partial plates and dentures can cause problems for the wearer. Partial plates tend to catch particles of food and may weaken the healthy teeth to which they are attached. Complete dentures are expensive and difficult to fit.

Dentures that fit properly at one time may not fit properly if the older person loses or gains a significant amount of weight. Fit is also a problem when dentures are left out of the mouth for prolonged periods of time. Many older adults refuse to wear their dentures because of the discomfort caused by an improper fit. This is because the arch of the jaw changes to compensate for the edentulous state. Professional dental attention is needed to repair or rebuild the dentures in these cases.

Dentures can cause irritation, inflammation, and ulceration of the gums and oral mucous membranes. Older adults should inspect their mouths regularly and promptly report any problems to the dentist. Sometimes, a minor adjustment of the denture or use of a fixative agent or cushion is all that is required to prevent painful problems.

DRY MOUTH

Xerostomia, or dry mouth, is commonly observed with aging. Dryness may result from the normal age-related reduction in saliva secretion, inadequate hydration, or disease conditions such as diabetes. Medications such as diuretic agents, antidepressants, sedatives, hypnotic agents, antihistamines, and anticholinergic medications also contribute to problems with xerostomia. In turn, xerostomia makes chewing and swallowing more difficult, promotes tooth decay, and alters the sense of taste.

LEUKOPLAKIA

Inspection of the mouth can reveal a number of abnormalities. White patches in the mouth, called leukoplakia, often are precancerous and require prompt medical attention (Figure 17-11). Lesions on the posterior third or the sides of the tongue often are abnormal and should be brought to the attention of the physician.

CANCER

According to the Oral Cancer Foundation, as many as 30,000 people are diagnosed with oral or pharyngeal cancer each year. A large percentage of this group are elderly. These forms of cancer have a poor prognosis. Early recognition and treatment before the cancer has metastasized to other tissues offer the best hope. Symptoms of oral cancer include (1) leukoplakia or erythroleukoplakia, a mixture of white and red patches in the mouth, (2) sores in the mouth that do not heal, (3) oral bleeding, (4) pain or difficulty swallowing, (5) difficulty wearing dentures, (6) swollen lymph nodes in the neck, and (7) earache.

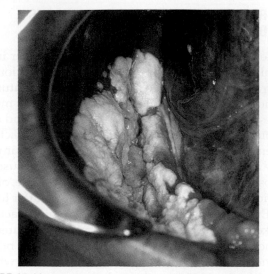

FIGURE 17-11 Leukoplakia. Note the formation of white spots, which may become malignant.

Older individuals who have a history of alcohol and tobacco use are at higher risk for developing these forms of cancer.

DISORDERS CAUSED BY VITAMIN DEFICIENCIES

Vitamin deficiencies, particularly deficiencies of riboflavin, niacin, and vitamin C, can affect the oral mucous membranes. A smooth, purplish, sore tongue may be related to riboflavin deficiency. Complaints of a burning sensation or soreness of the mouth may be related to niacin deficiency. Multiple painful ulcers of the oral mucous membranes with enlargement of the cervical lymph glands, difficulty swallowing, and foul odor may indicate Vincent's angina. Vincent's angina is a condition caused by opportunistic microorganisms that normally live in the mouth but cause infection only when the individual becomes malnourished.

SUPERINFECTIONS

Superinfections of the mouth are relatively common in older individuals who receive broad-spectrum antibiotic therapy for some other infection. Antibiotics destroy the normal mouth flora and allow opportunists or yeast colonies to become established and grow. Candidiasis, a yeast infection (also known as *thrush*), appears as white patches that adhere to the tongue, lips, and gums. Attempts to remove these patches may result in sore, bleeding tissue. A hairy tongue is the result of enlargement of the papillae on the tongue; this often follows antibiotic therapy. Black or brown discoloration on the tongue may be caused by tobacco use or by a chromogenic (color-producing) bacterium. These conditions are more commonly observed in malnourished older adults and those with poor oral hygiene practices. Yeast infections are usually treated by direct oral application or swishes of prescription medication. Hairy tongue usually resolves without medical treatment.

ALCOHOL AND TOBACCO-RELATED PROBLEMS

Alcohol and tobacco, even in small amounts, can harm the mucous membranes. Alcohol is chemically irritating and drying to the mucous membranes. Tobacco, whether smoked, chewed, or taken as snuff, increases the risk for oral cancer.

PROBLEMS CAUSED BY NEUROLOGIC CONDITIONS

Good oral hygiene practices are part of routine health maintenance, but meeting oral hygiene needs may be difficult for older individuals who have lost strength, coordination, or cognitive processes. Neurologic conditions such as stroke, multiple sclerosis, or Parkinson's disease decrease coordination and strength, making it difficult for the person to manipulate the equipment needed for oral hygiene. Individuals with severe arthritis may not only find the equipment difficult to manipulate, but they may also find it difficult to open their mouth adequately for good, thorough cleaning. Older persons who take medication for epilepsy or other seizure disorders need to use special precautions because these medications often cause hyperplasia of the gingiva. Oral hygiene with soft toothbrushes or swabs is recommended to prevent excessive trauma and bleeding from the tender, swollen tissues. Providing oral hygiene to persons with Alzheimer's disease can be a challenge because affected people do not understand the need for oral hygiene and are likely to resist care.

❖ NURSING PROCESS FOR IMPAIRED ORAL MUCOUS MEMBRANES

■ Assessment/Data Collection

- Does the person have his or her own teeth? If so, how many?
- What is the condition of the teeth?
- Are any teeth loose or decayed?
- Does the person have halitosis?
- Does the person wear dentures? If so, are they upper dentures, lower dentures, or both? Partial plates or bridges?
- Are dentures worn during meals or removed? Why?
- How do the dentures fit?
- Are there any signs of irritation in the mouth?
- Are food particles trapped under the dentures at meals?
- How good is the person's appetite? What types and consistency of food does he or she prefer to eat?
- What is the condition of the oral mucous membranes?
- Are the mucous membranes moist or dry?
- Is any residual food or debris evident in the mouth?
- What is the condition of the tongue?
- Is the tongue clean, coated, pale, red, or irritated?
- Does the person use tobacco or have a history of tobacco use?
- What medications is the person receiving?

Box 17-3	Risk Factors for Problems With Oral Mucous Membranes in Older Adults

- Impaired cognitive, neurologic, or musculoskeletal function
- Inadequate fluid intake
- Medication that affects the oral mucous membranes
- Complete or partial artificial teeth
- Tobacco use (smoking or chewing)
- Poor health-maintenance practices

- Does the person have any physical conditions that interfere with performing his or her own oral hygiene?

Box 17-3 lists risk factors for problems with oral mucous membranes in older adults.

■ Nursing Diagnosis

Impaired oral mucous membranes

■ Nursing Goals/Outcomes Identification

The nursing goals for older individuals diagnosed with impaired oral mucous membranes are to (1) obtain regular professional dental care; (2) demonstrate techniques for maintaining or restoring the integrity of the mucous membranes; (3) inspect the oral cavity regularly and seek care promptly if any symptoms occur; (4) experience no complaints such as irritation, inflammation, or ulceration; (5) ingest foods and fluids without discomfort; and (6) verbalize specific actions that promote healthy oral mucous membranes.

■ Nursing Interventions/Implementation

The following nursing interventions should take place in hospitals or extended-care facilities. In a hospital or extended-care setting, individuals who are able to provide their own oral hygiene should be encouraged to do so. When individuals are not capable of meeting their own oral hygiene needs, nurses or nursing assistants must provide the care. When performing oral hygiene, gloves and other appropriate protective devices should be worn to maintain universal precautions.

1. **Complete a thorough assessment of the oral mucous membranes.** Individuals who require intermediate or skilled nursing care are likely to have more oral hygiene problems and greater oral hygiene needs. If one wishes to judge the quality of nursing care provided in an extended-care facility, the first place to look is in the mouths of the patients or residents. For whatever reason, oral hygiene seems to be the area of hygiene that is most often neglected. This is troubling, because oral care is a very important component of nursing care. Good oral hygiene promotes comfort, enhances appetite, and fosters a sense of well-being.

2. **Initiate referral to a dentist or dental hygienist.** If any problems with the teeth or oral mucous membranes are observed, the individual should be seen

by a dentist. Hospitals may have outpatient dental clinics that will see in-house patients if necessary. If the problem is not urgent, the individual should be encouraged to make an appointment with his or her own dentist after discharge. Extended-care facilities should have a clinic or dentist on staff who sees residents on a scheduled or referral basis. If there is no dentist on the premises, transportation needs to be arranged with the family or a transport service. It is important that nurses refer individuals as soon as a problem is detected to prevent the development of more serious conditions. Patients with problems related to ill-fitting dentures should be referred to the dentist for prompt follow-up. Nurses must be sure to send the improperly fitting dentures along on the visit. Dental hygienists can perform more detailed oral assessment, provide cleanings and other preventive treatments, and assist the nurse in developing strategies for providing effective oral hygiene.

3. **Provide oral hygiene.** Thorough oral hygiene should be provided a minimum of once a day. Brushing after each meal and at bedtime is more desirable and is probably necessary for individuals suffering from halitosis, xerostomia, or gingivitis. Individuals who have poor nutritional intake because of funny tastes in the mouth should have additional oral hygiene before meals. Frequent oral hygiene is also necessary for individuals with upper respiratory infections. Excessive respiratory secretions coat the mouth and tongue, leaving a bad taste. The frequency of oral hygiene should be determined by the nurse and stated specifically in the care plan (e.g., "oral hygiene q2h and prn").

Dentures should be cleansed using warm water and a nonabrasive cleanser. The dentures should be brushed over a basin of water or a towel to prevent the possibility of breakage. Ultrasonic cleaning devices are available in some facilities and are very effective at removing particles of debris, particularly from the wire clasps on partial plates. The oral cavity should be cleaned thoroughly and inspected before dentures are reinserted.

Older denture wearers should be discouraged from removing and wrapping their dentures in paper napkins or tissue. Many dentures wrapped this way have been accidentally thrown away. It is also wise for anyone who wears dentures to have his or her name (or social security number) etched into each plate. This can prevent permanent loss of these costly items if, for some reason, the owner is separated from them. Dentures should be removed from the mouth before sleep to prevent slippage, which could result in trauma to the mouth or problems with breathing.

When performing oral hygiene on an unconscious patient, nurses must take special care to prevent aspiration. Unconscious individuals should be placed in a side-lying position, and adequate towels should be used to protect the bedding and clothes. The mouth is propped open with gauze or padded tongue blades. All surfaces of the teeth, tongue, and oral mucous membranes should be cleansed with a soft brush; damp gauze; sponge-tip swab; or clean, moistened washcloth. Special toothbrushes that attach to suction machines are available in some facilities. Lemon and glycerin swabs should be used with caution because they may be irritating to open areas on the mucous membranes and because they may ultimately cause drying (glycerin tends to draw moisture away from tissues).

Dry lips may require application of Vaseline, mineral oil, or a lip balm such as Carmex. These petroleum-based products should be used with extreme caution because of the potential for aspiration and resulting pneumonia.

4. **Promote adequate intake of nutrients and fluids.** If the individual is avoiding certain foods or fluids because of dental problems, it may be necessary to contact the physician or dietary department to obtain a change in food consistency. Soft, chopped, or puréed foods may be necessary for persons who are unable to chew because of loose teeth or improperly fitting dentures. If food tends to become trapped under the dentures, they should be removed promptly after each meal and cleansed. Excessively hot or cold foods may irritate the mucous membranes or teeth and should be avoided if they cause problems. Any temperature modification should be documented in the care plan so that consistent approaches can be used. For example, if the individual tolerates beverages at room temperature, all fluids—including the water at the bedside—should be provided this way. Fluids should be kept at the bedside and offered to the individual at planned intervals throughout the day.

5. **Provide lozenges or topical analgesics as prescribed.** If severe or painful lesions are present in the mouth, the physician may order the use of topical analgesics in lozenge or viscous form (viscous lidocaine). Drinking and eating should be avoided for 1 hour after administration of these preparations.

6. **Communicate suspected oral side effects of medication therapy to the physician and dentist.** If the nurse suspects that a drug may be causing untoward side effects on the oral mucous membranes, he or she should promptly communicate this information to the physician so that any necessary adjustments in dosage or drugs can be made.

The following interventions should take place in the home:

1. **Complete a thorough assessment of the oral mucous membranes.** A thorough assessment is necessary to detect the presence and severity of any problems. Specific interventions are based on the information gathered.

2. **Stress the importance of regular dental visits.** Dental hygiene is essential for aging individuals. Periodic dental visits should be part of ongoing health-maintenance practice, even for edentulous individuals. Those living at home should be encouraged and reminded to make and keep regular dental appointments. If cost is prohibitive, dental clinics and schools of dentistry and dental hygiene may offer care at reduced rates. Some dentists also give price reductions to older people if requested.

3. **Review the person's oral hygiene practices.** Older persons who have their own teeth should be taught to brush, floss, and irrigate the mouth at least once daily. If problems of halitosis, plaque formation, bad taste, or gingivitis are present, more frequent brushing may be required.

   Brushing is best done with a soft to moderate bristle brush. Too firm a bristle may scratch or irritate the oral cavity. Commercial fluoridated toothpastes are available at a reasonable cost. Special toothpastes such as Sensodyne are available for individuals with sensitive teeth and gums. Older individuals who have been in the habit of using salt or baking soda as a dentifrice should be counseled to avoid ingesting these products, because they are high in sodium.

   Flossing between the teeth helps remove trapped food and maintain healthy gums. If the older person has difficulty holding the floss, a loop tied at each end of the string can help provide a better grip.

   Irrigation of the mouth is best accomplished with a commercial irrigator. If a commercial irrigator is too costly, a bulb syringe can be used. Even the swish-and-swallow technique of rinsing the mouth with water is better than doing nothing. The person should also be instructed to gently brush the tongue and to inspect the entire oral cavity for signs of irritation.

   Individuals who wear dentures should also be instructed in proper oral hygiene. Dentures should be cleaned thoroughly every day. In some people, food debris tends to become trapped under the dentures. If this is a problem, the person should be instructed to remove the denture and rinse it after each meal to prevent irritation. Thorough cleansing can be done by brushing with a commercial dentifrice or by using a soaking cleanser. Some people choose to use both. Many individuals use a powder or pad to help the dentures adhere to the gums. It is important that all of the fixative be removed at each cleansing. If it is not removed, an uneven surface may result and irritate the gums. Dentures should be cleansed and stored in tepid water, because hot water may cause them to warp. When the dentures are out of the mouth, the entire oral cavity should be cleansed with a soft to moderate-bristle brush and the entire oral cavity inspected for signs of irritation. If signs of irritation from the dentures are present, the individual should see the dentist. Dentures can be reworked until they fit comfortably.

4. **Provide assistive devices as needed.** If the individual has difficulty holding the toothbrush because of arthritis or a weakened grip, modifications may be needed. Wrapping tape, aluminum foil, a small sponge, a polystyrene ball, or other padding around the handle of the brush may make it easier to grasp. Handle extenders made of a ruler or dowel rod may help those who are unable to reach the mouth easily (Figure 17-12).

5. **Obtain the assistance of family members, friends, or community agencies.** Some older adults may require the assistance of family members, friends, or transportation services in getting to dental appointments. Family and friends can also help by purchasing and setting up oral hygiene equipment. A family member or friend can be shown how to modify a toothbrush or prepare floss for use by the older person.

6. **Explain the need to avoid alcohol and tobacco use.** Because alcohol and tobacco are likely to irritate the mucous membranes and cause significant health problems, it is important that nurses stress the importance of eliminating, or at least restricting, their use.

7. **Promote adequate intake of nutrients and fluids.** Nurses should explain how nutrients, particularly vitamins, can contribute to healthy mucous membranes. Instruction about diet may be necessary if inadequacies are detected. The importance of fluid intake for saliva formation and its use as a rinse for the mucous membranes should be stressed. Older adults should be encouraged to keep a glass of water by the chair or bedside as a reminder to

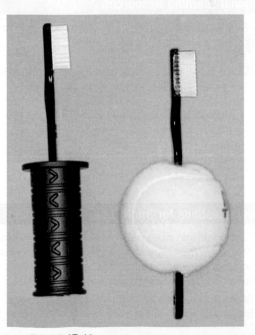

FIGURE 17-12 Adaptive aids for brushing.

drink adequate fluids. Highly sugared beverages should be avoided because they encourage tooth decay. Many older adults with altered mucous membranes prefer to avoid ice in beverages, which can stimulate toothache. If the individual has difficulty chewing food because of loose or missing teeth, a food processor, grinder, or blender can be used to change the food's consistency.

8. **Discuss the benefits of adequate moisture in the environment.** If the environment is dry or if the individual is a mouth-breather, an additional source of moisture may be needed. A freestanding humidifier or one attached to the furnace increases the moisture present in the air so that less is drawn away from the mucous membranes.

9. **Suggest use of hard candy, chewing gum, or artificial saliva to increase moisture in the mouth.** Sucking on hard candy or chewing gum stimulates the production of saliva. If a sugar-based candy or gum is used, the teeth must be brushed more frequently to prevent tooth decay. Individuals on sugar-restricted diets should use only sugar-free candy or gum. Artificial saliva preparations may be used according to package directions if there is no medical contraindication.

10. **Discuss the relationship between medications and oral hygiene.** If the individual is receiving any medications that could affect the mucous membranes, he or she should be taught any necessary observations or precautions. For example, people who are taking phenytoin (Dilantin) for epilepsy or people who are on antibiotic therapy should know the possible side effects that indicate the necessity to contact the physician.

11. **Use any appropriate interventions that are used in the institutional setting.**

Get Ready for the NCLEX® Examination!

Key Points

- Under normal conditions, the aging skin and mucous membranes are more susceptible to damage than are the comparable tissues of younger individuals. When disease factors are present, the risk for damage is even greater.
- Careful assessment allows nurses to recognize normal changes and identify any abnormalities that may indicate problems that are more serious.
- Nursing interventions are designed to reduce the risk for damage or trauma to fragile tissues.

Additional Learning Resources

SG Go to the Study Guide on pp. 379–397 for additional learning activities to help you master the chapter content.

evolve Go to your Evolve website (http://evolve.elsevier.com/Wold/geriatric) for the following FREE learning resources:
- Animations
- Answer Guidelines for Nursing Care Plan Critical Thinking Questions
- Answers and Rationales for Review Questions for the NCLEX® Examination
- Glossary with pronunciations in English and Spanish
- Video Clips

Review Questions for the NCLEX® Examination

1. A 71-year-old immobile patient has been in his wheelchair for 2 hours. When repositioning him, the nurse observes a reddened area at the base of the buttocks. This observation would best be documented as a:
   1. Stage 2 at greater trochanter
   2. Stage 1 at ischial tuberosity
   3. Stage 1 on iliac crest
   4. Stage 0 on posterior superior iliac spine

2. The most appropriate nursing diagnosis for an elderly patient who is bedridden due to progressed Parkinson's disease is:
   1. Risk for impaired skin integrity related to immobility.
   2. Immobility related to Parkinson's disease.
   3. Impaired skin integrity related to incontinence.
   4. Ischemia related to disuse syndrome.

3. An elderly female patient complains that her skin feels dry and itchy. The nurse would advise her to:
   1. Not scratch, but trim her nails so she is less likely to break the skin and get an infection
   2. Drink more fluids, use cool water when bathing, and wear cotton clothing only
   3. Ask her physician for a prescription for antihistamines to decrease the itching
   4. Bathe less often, use soap more sparingly, and apply a good skin emollient after each bath

4. The nurse notices that an elderly patient is using a large amount of denture fixative paste. The patient states this is because the denture hurts, otherwise. It is most important for the nurse to:
   1. Make a note about this practice in the patient's care plan and make a note to tell the dentist.
   2. Check that the denture does not have rough spots and that all of the old fixative has been removed.
   3. Assess the patient's oral cavity to make sure there is no irritation or breakdown.
   4. Assist the patient with oral hygiene and request an order for a topical anesthetic to reduce oral discomfort.

5. Family members are caring for their elderly mother at home. Which statement by the daughter indicates the need for further teaching?
   1. "I change Mom's diaper whenever it is really wet."
   2. "I make sure Mom eats good meals and extra snacks."
   3. "We try to change Mom's position at least every two hours."
   4. "I try to use lotion on Mom's skin every morning and evening."

6. The nurse in an older adult daycare setting assesses that many of the clients have long toenails, calluses, corns, hammertoe, and other foot problems. The most appropriate nursing action would be to:
   1. Set up a clinic in which the nurse and volunteers do foot soaks and nail cutting.
   2. Recommend that the family members do more to take care of the elder patients' needs.
   3. Make arrangements for podiatry services at the day care setting and provide literature about proper foot care.
   4. Determine which patients need to have foot care done on site, and add this intervention to their care plans.

Objectives

1. Describe the normal elimination processes.
2. Describe age-related changes in bladder and bowel elimination.
3. Discuss methods for assessing elimination practices.
4. Identify the older adults who are most at risk for problems with elimination.
5. Identify selected nursing diagnoses related to elimination problems.
6. Describe interventions used to prevent or reduce problems related to elimination.

Key Terms

catheterization (kă-thĕ-tĕr-ĭ-ZĀ-shŭn) (p. 294)
constipation (kŏn-stĭ-PĀ-shŭn) (p. 286)
defecation (dĕf-eĕ-KĀ-shŭn) (p. 286)
diarrhea (dī-ă-RĒ-ă) (p. 286)
diuretics (dī-ŭ-RĔ-tĭks) (p. 289)
enemas (ĔN-ĕ-măs) (p. 287)

fecal impaction (FĒ-kăl Ĭm-PĂK-shŭn) (p. 288)
incontinence (ĭn-KŎN-tĭ-nĕns) (p. 286)
laxatives (LĂK-să-tĭvs) (p. 287)
parasitic (păr-ă-ŠĬ-tĭk) (p. 292)
retention (rē-TĔN-shŭn) (p. 293)
sphincter (SFĬNGK-tĕr) (p. 286)

To function properly, the body must be able to rid itself of waste products effectively. The two major systems involved in waste elimination are the urinary system and the gastrointestinal (GI) system. Small amounts of urea (a by-product of protein metabolism) and sodium chloride can be eliminated through the skin, but the skin is not considered a major site of elimination.

NORMAL ELIMINATION PATTERNS

Each individual adult develops patterns for bowel and bladder elimination that are somewhat unique to himself or herself. As long as the pattern is within normal limits and is effective for the individual, no special intervention is required. Diet, fluid intake, activity, and lifestyle influence these patterns. Even in young adults, elimination patterns can be disrupted by illness, medications, or changes in daily routine.

The typical adult bowel movement consists of a moderate amount of formed, brown stool that is passed without difficulty. The normal frequency of bowel elimination varies from several stools per day to only two or three per week. Most adults experience bowel elimination every 1 to 2 days. The urge to defecate most commonly occurs 30 to 45 minutes after a meal, when the gastrocolic and defecation reflexes stimulate peristalsis. Another common time for defecation is first thing in the morning after

consumption of a warm beverage. Many people develop a daily routine or establish rituals over their lifetimes that are designed to promote normal elimination. Attempts to change these habits late in life can create problems.

Urine elimination in adults also follows patterns. The typical adult experiences the urge to urinate when the bladder contains approximately 300 mL of urine. Voluntary control of the external sphincter muscles enables healthy adults to hold larger amounts within the bladder until urination is convenient. Most adults void between 6 and 10 times per day, but this may vary greatly, depending on fluid consumption, personal habits, and emotional state.

ELIMINATION AND AGING

A large percentage of the older adult population suffers from problems with elimination. The most common elimination problems experienced by older adults are constipation, diarrhea, and incontinence of bladder and/or bowel. These problems may result from changes in the function of the GI system or the urinary system, or they may be related to changes in other body systems such as the musculoskeletal and nervous systems.

Incontinence of bladder and/or bowel is one of the most common reasons that older adults are institutionalized. Many families who can cope with other problems are unable to deal with incontinence.

CONSTIPATION

Constipation means different things to different people. It is not a disease but rather a symptom of some other problem. Constipation is defined as hard, dry stools that are difficult to pass. Because bowel elimination patterns can differ widely from person to person, the frequency of elimination is not a good measure. For some people, regularity means more than one bowel movement a day; for others, it means three bowel movements a week. Other people who were reared with the idea that a daily bowel movement is essential to health tend to spend undue amounts of time worrying about their bowels. An objective set of criteria has been developed to make the diagnosis of constipation more consistent (Box 18-1).

Constipation, both real and perceived, is a common complaint of older adults. Studies show that more than 25% of the elderly experience constipation and that it is more commonly a problem for women. The following changes related to aging or chronic illness increase the risk for constipation: decreased abdominal muscle tone, inactivity, immobility, inadequate fluid intake, inadequate dietary bulk, disease conditions, medications, dependence on laxatives or enemas, and various environmental conditions.

Peristalsis normally slows somewhat with aging. Loss of abdominal muscle tone and inadequate physical activity contribute to even slower peristalsis. Older individuals with weak abdominal muscles and those who are inactive or immobile are highly likely to become constipated.

Water is absorbed as waste products pass through the large intestine. Inadequate fluid intake or excessive fluid loss through perspiration, emesis, or wounds increases the body's need to recover as much fluid as possible. Because many older adults suffer from some degree of fluid volume deficit, their bodies attempt to reabsorb as much fluid from the stool as possible. The physiologic need to absorb water, combined with a slower rate of peristalsis, results in stools that are drier, harder, and more difficult to pass. Fluid volume deficit also leads to a decrease in urine production.

Dietary fiber plays an important role in promoting normal bowel elimination because this indigestible substance is effective at trapping moisture and providing bulk to the wastes. Foods such as whole grains, fruits, vegetables, and lean meats are high in fiber. Fiber-rich foods are often lacking in the older person's diet because these foods are more difficult to chew, particularly when teeth are loose or missing. Foods such as dairy products, eggs, refined breads, desserts, and many convenience foods consumed by older adults contain very little fiber. When the diet lacks adequate fiber, less stool is produced. This small amount moves more slowly through the intestine, further contributing to excessive dryness. The small mass of stool produced without fiber is inadequate to stimulate the normal defecation reflex, resulting in infrequent elimination with as many as 4 or more days between bowel movements.

The risk for constipation is increased with a number of disease processes, including stroke, diabetes, hypothyroidism, uremia, lupus, scleroderma, multiple sclerosis, Parkinson's disease, dementia, and depression. Cancerous tumors located in the GI tract can result in a partial or total obstruction that can be mistaken for constipation or impaction. Medications often contribute to constipation in older adults. The more medications an older person takes, the greater his or her risk is of medication-induced constipation. Medications that increase the risk for constipation include the following:

- Narcotic analgesics, particularly those containing codeine
- Anticholinergics, including many tricyclic antidepressants and antipsychotics
- Diuretics
- Iron supplements
- Calcium-channel blockers
- Antacids containing calcium or aluminum
- Anticonvulsants
- Antidepressants
- Antiparkinson's drugs
- Nonsteroidal antiinflammatory agents
- Antihypertensives, such as the angiotensin-converting enzyme (ACE) inhibitors

Many older individuals who have had problems with constipation over the years may have developed a habit of taking laxatives or enemas. It is estimated that approximately 30% of healthy older persons take laxatives regularly. Some started taking laxatives when they were quite young because absolute regularity (having a daily bowel movement) was at one time considered important for good health. Thus, some older people have been taking laxatives or enemas daily for 50 to 60 years. We now recognize that this is dangerous because the body can become dependent on laxatives and require this assistance to stimulate elimination. Reestablishing normal bowel elimination in

---

| Box **18-1** | **Rome III Criteria for Constipation** |

A diagnosis for constipation must include two or more of the following symptoms for the past 3 months. Symptoms must have an onset at least 6 months before the diagnosis.
- Straining
- Hard or lumpy stools
- Sensation of incomplete evacuation or of anorectal blockage
- Less than three defecations per week
- Loose stool rarely present without use of laxatives
- Use of manual maneuvers such as digital stimulation to facilitate defecation

Modified from Longstreath GF, et al. *Gastroenterology* 130:1480–1491, 2006.

a laxative-dependent older person is almost impossible because the body has forgotten how to work on its own.

Repeatedly ignoring the urge to defecate can lead to suppression or even extinction of the defecation reflex. Changes in neurologic sensitivity or fear of pain may cause older adults to ignore or delay defecation. Those with neurologic disorders may not be aware of the need to defecate because the strength of nerve impulses transmitted to and from the sphincter muscles is decreased. With no urge to defecate, individuals may go for many days unaware of the fact that their bowels have not emptied. Older individuals who encounter pain with defecation are more likely to avoid or deliberately delay what they know will be a painful experience. Pain can originate from the decreased production of mucus in the intestine that is typical with aging. Without the lubrication provided by mucus, the stool becomes excessively dry and irritating to the rectal tissues. The presence of hemorrhoids or anal fissures further contributes to the likelihood of pain. Delaying defecation creates a vicious circle. When defecation is delayed, the stool becomes harder, drier, and more difficult to pass. This, in turn, leads to more painful defecation, which results in further avoidance of defecation. Active interventions are needed to break this cycle. Untreated constipation can result in fecal impaction.

Delays in defecation are not always chosen by the older person. An aging person who requires assistance may need to suppress the defecation reflex while waiting for help getting to the bathroom. If this occurs repeatedly, the individual may lose sensitivity to the urge to defecate and become constipated. If unable to suppress the urge, the person runs the risk of being considered incontinent.

Environmental factors can play a role in constipation, particularly with institutionalized older adults. The aging person may be embarrassed by the sounds or odors involved with bowel elimination. Lack of privacy may cause anxiety or may result in the person's ignoring or suppressing the urge to defecate.

Difficulty assuming an anatomically suitable or comfortable position can also interfere with effective bowel elimination. Sitting upright or squatting are the preferred positions for defecation because it is easier to bear down in these positions, and gravity assists elimination when the entire body is upright. People confined to bed find that bedpans are particularly uncomfortable and difficult to use. Although they may be necessary, bedpans should be avoided whenever the use of a toilet or commode chair is possible.

FECAL IMPACTION

Fecal impaction, the presence of a mass of hardened feces that is trapped in the rectum and cannot be expelled, is a result of unrelieved constipation. In severe cases, the fecal mass may extend up into the sigmoid colon. Individuals who have a history of chronic constipation are most at risk for impaction.

Symptoms of impaction include a longer-than-usual delay in defecation. More than 3 days without a bowel movement warrants close attention. Passage of small amounts of liquid stool without any formed fecal material can also indicate impaction. This liquid stool is fecal material from higher in the colon that is able to pass around the hardened mass. It typically oozes from the rectum and differs from a diarrheal stool, which passes with normal force.

Aging persons suffering from fecal impaction are likely to complain of cramping or rectal pain. Abdominal distention and loss of appetite are common. Digital examination of the rectum typically reveals the presence of a hardened mass of feces. This procedure should be done with extreme caution because it is uncomfortable and traumatic to the rectal tissues. Particular caution must be used when examining older persons with a history of cardiac problems because rectal examination can stimulate the vagus nerve and result in a sudden decrease in heart rate, syncope, or even loss of consciousness. Some facilities require physician's orders before a digital examination of the rectum is performed. Sometimes the impacted mass is higher in the intestinal tract and cannot be detected by digital examination. In these cases, abdominal x-rays may be necessary. Before deciding that an older person has a problem with bowel elimination, nurses should thoroughly assess the total situation, including the frequency, amount, and consistency of stools. Assessment should also include identification of factors that contribute to the development of bowel elimination problems. This enables the development of a plan that promotes sound elimination patterns.

Patient Teaching

When It May Be More Than Constipation

Elderly patients should be taught to contact their physician when:

- There is severe vomiting or abdominal pain.
- The frequency of bowel movements slows dramatically.
- Blood is present with bowel movements.
- There is a continuous sensation of pressure, fullness, or pain in the rectal area, but they are unable to pass stool.
- They pass only small amounts of loose stool or leaking of stool.

❖ NURSING PROCESS FOR CONSTIPATION

■ Assessment/Data Collection

- How often does the person have a bowel movement?
- Is there any pattern to when bowel elimination occurs?

- Is the person continent or incontinent of stool?
- What is the consistency of the stool?
- What is the amount of stool?
- What is the color of the stool?
- Are blood, mucus, undigested food, or other unusual substances evident in the stool?
- Has the stool been checked for occult blood?
- Does the person have to strain to have a bowel movement?
- Is the stool expelled with excessive force, or does it ooze from the body?
- Does the person report or has the nurse observed any particular foods that affect bowel movements?
- Do these foods cause diarrhea or constipation?
- Does the person rely on any aids for bowel elimination (e.g., suppositories, laxatives, and enemas)?
- How long has the person been using this aid?
- Is the abdomen distended?
- If the person cannot speak, does he or she rub the abdomen?
- Has the person's appetite decreased?
- If the person cannot sense rectal fullness, what does a digital examination of the rectum reveal?
- Does the person's diet have adequate bulk?
- Does the person take any bulk enhancers?
- What does the person say about his or her bowel habits?
- Has the person's bowel pattern changed recently?
- Does the person report any concerns related to bowel elimination?

Box 18-2 lists risk factors for constipation in older adults.

▪ Nursing Diagnosis

Constipation

▪ Nursing Goals/Outcomes Identification

The nursing goals for older individuals diagnosed with constipation are to (1) exhibit regular patterns of bowel elimination, (2) identify behaviors that promote normal bowel functioning, and (3) modify behaviors to enhance regular bowel elimination.

Box 18-2	Risk Factors Related to Constipation in Older Adults

- Neurologic problems that decrease the ability to sense the need for elimination or to control the sphincter muscles
- Reduced mobility
- Inadequate intake of dietary bulk
- Tube feedings
- Gastrointestinal obstructions or disease (e.g., Crohn's disease and diverticulosis)
- Inadequate fluid intake
- Cognitive impairment (e.g., Alzheimer's disease and dementia)

▪ Nursing Interventions/Implementation

The following nursing interventions should take place in hospitals or extended-care facilities:

1. **Assess bowel elimination patterns and contributing factors.** It is important to determine whether the aging person actually has a problem with constipation or only perceives a problem. Because many older people cling to the idea that daily bowel elimination is necessary, they may consider themselves constipated when no real problem exists. If this is the case, nurses should explain the normal range of variation. If the person is truly experiencing constipation, the causes should be determined and the plan of care directed toward eliminating or reducing the causative factors. Aging persons with a history of constipation or risk factors for constipation must be assessed regularly to avoid fecal impaction.

2. **Increase physical activity.** Physical mobility—even as little as twisting the body, turning from side to side, flexing the trunk, or lifting the legs to the abdomen—can help stimulate peristalsis. If possible, older adults should be encouraged to participate in activities that are more vigorous such as walking, bending, and stretching.

3. **Increase intake of dietary fiber and fluids.** Adequate fluid and dietary bulk enhance the normal process of defecation. Cereal fiber is more effective at preventing constipation, and most older adults find it palatable. Some foods such as bran or prunes have bulk and a natural laxative effect. Many older adults accept these foods if they are offered as part of the breakfast meal. Some people find that other foods, such as cabbage or licorice, are helpful in stimulating bowel elimination. Adequate fluid intake reduces the risk for constipation from excessive absorption in the large intestine. Fluid intake of 2000 mL/day is recommended. More fluid is necessary during hot summer months or when illness results in excessive fluid loss. Older people who take diuretics should be encouraged to consume adequate fluids as long as their cardiovascular status is stable.

4. **Schedule or encourage toileting at times when the person's defecation urge is strongest.** If the individual suppresses the urge to defecate, he or she is at greater risk for constipation. Encouraging older adults to use the toilet (or taking them there) at a time when defecation is likely enables a healthy pattern to develop. The most likely times are early in the morning, after drinking the first warm beverage of the day, and shortly after meals. Some older persons go through established rituals that support normal elimination. The existence and nature of these rituals should be determined by talking with the person, and this information should be used in care planning.

5. **Position the person to facilitate ease of elimination.** Use of a toilet is most conducive to normal elimination. If this is not possible, a bedside commode on which the person can be seated is the next best option. Positioning a small footstool under the feet of the older person who has weak abdominal muscles increases intraabdominal pressure and may make defecation easier. A bedpan is the least desirable option. Bedpans are uncomfortable, and their use makes it difficult for the person to achieve the normal bearing-down force that is necessary for defecation.

6. **Provide privacy for elimination.** Privacy reduces the risk for constipation that results from suppressing elimination to prevent embarrassment. To prevent unpleasant odors, nurses should promptly remove soiled bedpans and supply an air freshener.

Coordinated Care
Supervision
Patient Privacy

- The supervisory nurse should ensure that all older patients are given adequate privacy for elimination and that cultural modesty standards are observed.
- This is particularly important when the nurse is assisting an incontinent patient.

7. **Administer stool softeners or bulk-forming laxatives as prescribed by the physician.** Stool softeners keep fecal material moist and reduce the chance of irritation to the anus when stool is passed. Bulk-forming substances such as psyllium (Metamucil) expand and trap moisture in the feces. Nurses must take care to administer these bulk-forming laxatives with adequate amounts of fluid. If adequate fluid is not ingested, these substances can cause constipation or bowel obstructions (Table 18-1).

8. **Administer prescribed suppositories or enemas if other methods have not been effective.** If other methods of stimulating defecation have not been effective, it may be necessary to administer suppositories or enemas. Glycerin suppositories are usually well tolerated by older adults. They enhance elimination by drawing fluid into the bowel through osmosis. Bisacodyl suppositories are fairly well tolerated but are more likely to cause cramping. Older adults are more apt to accept suppositories because they are generally less traumatic and less invasive than are enemas. Enemas should be used with caution because they can lead to damage of the rectal mucosa and contribute to electrolyte imbalance. If performed incorrectly, enemas increase the risk for rectal perforation.

9. **Perform digital rectal examination and impaction removal as ordered or according to agency**

Table 18-1 Considerations Related to Certain Laxatives

TYPE	CONSIDERATIONS
Stimulant Laxatives	
Phenolphthalein Castor oil Bisacodyl Senna	Use with caution in older adults; can cause cramping or vomiting; may lead to electrolyte imbalance, altered fat absorption, fat-soluble vitamin deficiency, and dependency; less expensive than some other forms
Bulk Laxatives	
Psyllium Calcium polycarbophil Methylcellulose	Work effectively; safe for long-term use in older adults; can cause flatulence; resistance or noncompliance is common because of taste; risk for worsened constipation or impaction if fluid intake is inadequate
Hyperosmolar Laxatives	
Lactulose Sorbitol	Safe and effective even in frail older adults
Fecal Softeners	
Docusate sodium	Do not have a laxative action so are not effective for chronic constipation; result in softer stool, allowing easier passage when straining is dangerous

policies. Provide privacy and emotional support. Verify that there are no preexisting conditions that contraindicate digital manipulation. Digital examination is done with a well-lubricated gloved hand. Some agencies use a lubricant containing a topical anesthetic to reduce discomfort. When an impaction is detected, oil-retention enemas may be ordered to soften the mass. These are followed by large-volume enemas to evacuate the mass. If this is not successful, digital removal may be necessary. With the client positioned in a side-lying position, the fecal mass is manually broken into smaller pieces and removed. Caution should be used to prevent trauma to the rectal tissues. This process may need to be done in increments to reduce the risk for damage.

The following interventions should take place in the home:

1. **Provide information regarding high-fiber foods, and encourage increased consumption of these.** Many older individuals prefer processed foods that are easy to prepare and chew. Providing information about the value of foods that are easily obtained such as cereals, whole wheat breads, bran muffins, and prunes can help older adults select foods that may reduce the incidence of constipation. If family members prepare the meals, the importance of fiber in preventing constipation should be discussed.

2. **Encourage adequate fluid intake.** Approximately 2000 mL of fluid should be taken each day. This should include approximately six glasses of water, juice, and other beverages such as tea or coffee. Some individuals drink senna tea, which has laxative properties.

3. **Encourage adequate activity and exercise.** Activity enhances peristalsis and, along with good dietary practices, is most important in preventing constipation. Walking after meals may effectively stimulate the urge to defecate. Aging persons should stay near toilet facilities so that they can act immediately when the urge arises. Suppressing the urge to defecate can increase the risk for constipation.

4. **Discuss the risks involved with the use of laxatives without medical supervision.** Many older adults are unaware of the side effects and problems related to laxative use. These concerns should be discussed, and older adults should be encouraged to discuss any bowel elimination problems with the physician before using laxatives.

5. **Use any appropriate interventions that are used in the institutional setting** (Nursing Care Plan 18-1).

DIARRHEA

Diarrhea is defined as the frequent passage of liquid, unformed stools. The stools are liquid because they pass through the large intestine too rapidly and are expelled before sufficient water can be absorbed in the large intestine. Diarrhea is a symptom and can have many causes in older adults, such as malabsorption syndromes, tumors of the GI tract, lactose intolerance, diverticulosis, and pathogenic organisms. Aging persons who receive large amounts of concentrated tube feedings often experience diarrhea.

✴ Nursing Care Plan 18-1   Constipation

Mrs. Port is an 85-year-old woman who resides at Shady Grove Nursing Home. She has mild osteoarthritis, and she prefers to sit and visit or do crafts. She can move about using a walker. When her osteoarthritis pain is severe, she takes acetaminophen combined with 30 mg of codeine.

She eats with friends in the dining room and prefers to eat meat, white bread, and desserts. She eats very little of the fruits or vegetables served, and she consumes about 1200 mL of fluid per day.

Mrs. Port reports that she has bowel movements about every 2 or 3 days. "I used to have a bowel movement every other day. Now I really have to push, and it hurts to have a BM." The nursing assistant reports that the stool is hard and dry.

Nursing Diagnosis
Constipation

Defining Characteristics
- 2 to 3 days between bowel movements
- Complaints of straining at stool
- Hard, dry stools
- Less than normal frequency of bowel movements

Patient Goals/Outcomes
Mrs. Port will have regular bowel movements at 1- to 2-day intervals, experience no difficulty passing stool, and describe diet changes that promote regular elimination.

Nursing Interventions
1. Assess bowel elimination pattern for the frequency, amount, consistency, and effort required.
2. Explain the importance and effect of adequate fluid intake on bowel elimination.
3. Design a plan for increasing fluid intake to 2000 mL per day, including beverages favored by Mrs. Port.
4. Encourage consumption of fruits, vegetables, and whole grain breads or cereals.
5. Discuss alternative measures for pain control to decrease reliance on codeine-based medication.
6. Encourage increased physical activity.

Evaluation
Mrs. Port has increased her fluid intake to 1800 mL/day. She reports eating bran cereal, whole wheat toast, and prune juice for breakfast and a fruit or vegetable with lunch and dinner. Formed, soft bowel movements have been reported every other day and documented in Mrs. Port's chart. She states, "It feels so much better when I don't have to strain." You will continue the plan of care.

Critical Thinking Questions
Mrs. Port has decided that the high-fiber foods and prune juice are upsetting her stomach and has stopped eating them. She reports that problems with elimination have returned.
1. What else could she do to help stimulate regular elimination?
2. What teaching does Mrs. Port require if she chooses to use a bulk-forming preparation such as psyllium?

Many older persons with diarrhea complain of nausea, vomiting, and abdominal cramps in addition to frequent stools. Rectal pain and skin irritation of the anus and buttocks are common because fecal material is very irritating.

Diarrhea can easily result in excessive fluid loss. This is a major concern in older adults, who are already at risk for fluid volume deficit. Because diarrhea can quickly result in dehydration, the physician should be notified promptly so that the cause can be isolated and treatment begun.

❖ NURSING PROCESS FOR DIARRHEA

■ Assessment/Data Collection

See the assessment for constipation on pages 288–289.

■ Nursing Diagnosis

Diarrhea

■ Nursing Goals/Outcomes Identification

The nursing goals for older individuals diagnosed with diarrhea are to (1) exhibit regular patterns of bowel elimination, (2) identify behaviors that promote normal bowel functioning, and (3) modify behaviors to enhance regular bowel elimination.

■ Nursing Interventions/Implementation

The following nursing interventions should take place in hospitals or extended-care facilities:

1. **Assess the elimination pattern and suspected causative factors.** Diarrhea in older adults can result from many factors. It is important that nurses pay close attention to the frequency and nature of stools. Time of day of the onset, as well as any factors that appear related to the onset of loose stools, should be assessed. For example, a loose stool that follows a meal, a tube feeding, or administration of a medication is significant and should be reported. Additional complaints such as pain, cramping, fever, and force of expulsion should be assessed. If the liquid stool seeps from the rectum, fecal impaction must be suspected. Removal of the impaction corrects this problem.

2. **Maintain adequate fluid intake.** Diarrheal stools lead to an excessive loss of body fluid. Fluid replacement to prevent dehydration is essential. In addition to simple fluid balance, electrolyte levels may be disturbed if the episodes of diarrhea are severe or prolonged. Oral fluids should be provided within dietary restrictions. Fluids that are rich in electrolytes (e.g., juices, Gatorade, and broth) are better than plain water. Fluids that are high in fiber, caffeine, and milk should be avoided because they tend to induce diarrhea. If the individual is unable to take fluids orally, intravenous infusions may be necessary. Older adults should be watched carefully for signs of dehydration, such as decreased skin turgor, postural hypotension, tachycardia, and altered laboratory values.

3. **Institute measures to maintain skin integrity.** The skin must be cleaned immediately after each episode of diarrhea. Diarrheal stool is very irritating to the skin and can rapidly lead to skin breakdown. The anal area should be washed after each stool, and a protective ointment or lotion should be applied to provide a barrier against the caustic body wastes. If the skin becomes excessively irritated and tender to touch, sitz baths followed by air drying or heat lamp treatments may help promote healing. Care must be taken to prevent further trauma to the tissue. Bed linens must be kept clean and dry at all times.

4. **Promptly report observations to the physician, and follow up on physician's orders regarding medications that decrease intestinal motility.** Diarrhea in older adults is a serious concern. Because it can have many causes, diarrhea should be reported to the physician promptly so that its origin can be determined. The physician will probably prescribe fluid maintenance, as well as medications, to decrease the rate of intestinal motility and increase water absorption. The timing for administering these medications is usually related to the frequency of diarrheal stools. It is important that nurses administer the medications as prescribed. If diarrhea persists, diagnostic tests on stool specimens may be ordered to determine whether the diarrhea is parasitic or bacterial in origin. Precautions, including gloves and proper handwashing, must be followed when obtaining or handling stool specimens.

The following interventions should take place in the home:

1. **Explain the importance of seeking medical attention if the person is experiencing diarrhea.** Many older persons become severely dehydrated from diarrhea before they seek medical attention. Nurses should stress the importance of calling a physician if diarrhea is severe or lasts more than 1 day. Any additional complaints such as abdominal pain, cramping, or fever also indicate the need to call a physician immediately. Many prescription and nonprescription medications can cause diarrhea. Because many older persons have prescriptions from more than one physician, it is important that they tell each physician all of the medications they are taking, including over-the-counter preparations.

2. **Explain the importance of proper food preparation and storage in preventing bacterial diarrhea.** Many cases of diarrhea are related to improper food preparation or storage. Many older people do not pay close attention to the length of time food sits on the table or stove. If not refrigerated, food becomes a good medium for the growth of bacteria, many of which can cause diarrhea. Nurses should stress the importance of refrigerating all dairy products, meats, and

other prepared foods immediately after purchase or after the meal. Food should not be allowed to warm up on the counter for hours before preparation.

3. **Use any appropriate interventions that are used in the institutional setting.**

BOWEL INCONTINENCE

Bowel incontinence is most common among elderly people who are unable to recognize and respond to normal sensations because of mental impairment or problems with mobility. Less frequently, colon or rectal disorders such as cancer, inflammatory bowel disease, diverticulitis, or weak rectal muscle cause or contribute to incontinence. Fecal incontinence is more common than suspected. Studies show that as many as 17% of the community-dwelling elderly and up to 54% of those residing in nursing homes experience some degree of fecal incontinence. In some cases, incontinence is slight, consisting of just a small leakage of stool. In other cases, incontinence is a daily occurrence. Frequent bowel incontinence is a significant problem because fecal wastes are very irritating to tissues and can contribute to skin breakdown. Inability to control bowel elimination is also psychologically disturbing and embarrassing for older adults. Many community-dwelling elderly are unwilling to bring up concerns regarding this problem with health caregivers. They attempt to manage the problem themselves by using incontinence pads or briefs. In severe cases, they may stop participating in social activities for fear of embarrassment. Identification of underlying health problems and planning additional preventive strategies can help affected older adults maintain a more comfortable lifestyle.

❖ NURSING PROCESS FOR BOWEL INCONTINENCE

■ Assessment/Data Collection

See assessment for constipation on pages 288–289.

■ Nursing Diagnosis

Bowel incontinence

■ Nursing Goals/Outcomes Identification

The nursing goals for older individuals diagnosed with bowel incontinence are to (1) exhibit regular patterns of bowel elimination, (2) identify behaviors that promote normal bowel functioning, and (3) modify behaviors to enhance regular bowel elimination.

■ Nursing Interventions/Implementation

The following nursing interventions should take place in hospitals or extended-care facilities:

1. **Assess patterns of elimination and causative factors.** It is important to know how often and when the individual is incontinent. If these episodes have a regular pattern, nurses can use this information to plan nursing care. For example, many individuals have a pattern of defecating 30 to 45 minutes after a meal. If the person is taken to the bathroom at that time, an episode of incontinence will be prevented. Unfortunately, not all individuals have such a regular pattern of defecation.

2. **Establish a toileting schedule.** If a defecation pattern is detected, the person should be taken to the bathroom at the time he or she is most likely to defecate. If no detectable pattern is present, the physician may order the use of digital stimulation or glycerin suppositories. When repeated daily or every other day, these measures may establish a regular pattern of defecation. When planning a toileting schedule, nurses should consider the older person's daily routines and scheduled appointments (e.g., physical therapy). To be effective, all individuals and departments that have contact with the individual should be aware of the plan and follow through with it.

3. **Take measures to prevent or reduce episodes of constipation.** It is difficult to prevent incontinence when an individual is constipated. Measures used to prevent constipation increase the likelihood of regular elimination.

4. **Use appropriate aids or garments.** It is best if episodes of incontinence are prevented by regular toileting or other methods discussed previously. If these measures are not completely successful, use of special pads or garments can reduce the embarrassment of soiling the bed or clothing. However, these aids should not be used in place of other nursing measures that promote bowel control. Recent development of anal bags to collect stool show promise as an alternative approach.

5. **Clean the person promptly after each episode of incontinence.** Incontinence can easily lead to skin breakdown. It is essential that any soiled linens or garments be removed as soon as possible to reduce skin irritation. This care should be provided tactfully to reduce damage to the self-esteem of older adults, most of whom are acutely embarrassed by their incontinence and are sensitive to any negative verbal or nonverbal communication from the nursing staff. All soiled materials should be removed from the room and put into appropriate containers to reduce environmental odors.

6. **Use any appropriate interventions that are used in the institutional setting.**

NURSING PROCESS FOR IMPAIRED URINARY ELIMINATION

URINARY RETENTION

Urinary retention is an abnormal accumulation of urine in the bladder because the bladder is unable to empty completely. Normally, no more than 50 mL of urine remain in the bladder after voiding. The person experiencing urinary retention often has several hundred milliliters remaining after voiding. Urinary retention in older adults can result from decreased muscle tone in the bladder wall, decreased fluid intake, prostate gland enlargement, trauma to the muscles of the perineum, neurologic damage, medications, or anxiety.

Symptoms of retention include a feeling of fullness, discomfort or tenderness in the bladder, restlessness, and diaphoresis. Persons experiencing urinary retention may complain of a total inability to void or of passing small amounts (between 25 and 50 mL) of urine at frequent intervals. This pattern is called **retention with overflow.** Severe retention results in bladder distention that can be detected by inspecting or palpating the area over the symphysis pubis. Treatment of urinary retention depends on the cause. If retention is caused by perineal trauma or anxiety, noninvasive measures such as medications or a sitz bath may be enough to stimulate effective voiding. If severe retention is caused by an obstruction such as an enlarged prostate, catheterization or surgery may be necessary to prevent serious bladder damage that may result from persistent or excessive bladder distention.

URINARY TRACT INFECTION

Urinary tract infections are a common problem, particularly for elderly women (see Chapter 3).

URINARY INCONTINENCE

Urinary incontinence is the involuntary loss of urine in sufficient amount or frequency to be a social or hygiene problem. Urinary incontinence is not a normal part of aging but it is a major problem in the aging population. Women are twice as likely to experience urinary incontinence as men. It is estimated that nearly 30% to 50% of independent-living elderly and 50% to 75% of institutionalized older adults have problems with incontinence (Box 18-3). The national cost of urinary incontinence currently exceeds 26 billion dollars a year and has been increasing steadily. Urinary incontinence is among the leading causes of long-term institutional placement.

Incontinence has medical, emotional, social, and economic consequences for older adults. It can result in skin irritation or breakdown and can contribute to pressure ulcers; it can lead to guilt and frustration; it can lead to social isolation; and it can be costly because

Box 18-3	Reversible Causes of Incontinence

D—Delirium
I—Infections
A—Atrophic vaginitis
P—Psychological causes (depression, psychosomatic)
P—Pharmaceutical agents
E—Endocrine conditions (particularly diabetes mellitus)
R—Restricted mobility (including environmental barriers)
S—Stool impaction

of the need to purchase expensive undergarments and replace or launder clothing more frequently. Ultimately, it can lead to the emotional, social, and economic costs of institutional care.

🏠 Home Health Considerations

Community Education Programs

Community education programs can be helpful in reducing the extent and severity of incontinence among community-dwelling elderly, particularly women. These programs should stress that incontinence is not a part of normal aging and emphasize behavioral management of incontinence, including the use of incontinence diaries, identification of dietary triggers, recognition of signs and symptoms of urinary tract infections, and performing pelvic muscle strengthening exercises.

Older adults may hesitate to discuss incontinence problems with the physician or nurse because they are embarrassed or because they think that incontinence is simply a problem of aging that they must endure. Therefore, the topic must be introduced in a sensitive manner by caregivers. In some cases, incontinence is curable using surgery, medications, or other treatments. In other cases, it can be better managed, thus allowing the older person a more normal lifestyle.

👥 Coordinated Care

Collaboration

Prevention of Incontinence

Incontinence can be reduced if there is a commitment to success rather than a defeatist attitude. Stressing the benefits to the patient and identifying the benefits to caregivers can help motivate the process. All members of the health care team are essential to reduce incontinence. The physician, nurses, nursing assistants, physical therapists, occupational therapists, and facility management need to be actively involved in the development, communication, and implementation of the plan. A staffing system designating specially trained certified nursing assistants to implement restorative interventions to prevent incontinence has been shown to be effective. However, no staff members should consider themselves "too important" to respond to the needs of patients. A successful plan can improve the self-esteem of residents and enhance the perceptions of the level of care held by family members and the community.

A number of normal age-related physiologic changes or common diseases seen with aging can cause or contribute to incontinence. Different forms of incontinence (i.e., stress, urge, overflow, functional, and total incontinence) are recognized as problems in older adults.

Stress Incontinence

Stress incontinence is leakage of urine during conditions that increase intraabdominal pressure such as exercise, lifting heavy objects, laughing, coughing, or sneezing. When a full bladder is compressed against weakened urinary sphincters, incontinence occurs. This problem is most commonly observed in women, particularly those who have weakened perineal muscles resulting from aging and childbearing. Generally, the amount of urine lost is small.

Urge Incontinence

Urge incontinence is caused by involuntary contraction of the detrusor muscle of the bladder. It is characterized by a sudden, strong urge to void. Individuals suffering from urge incontinence are often unable to hold back the urine long enough to reach a commode or toilet. Urge incontinence is often seen in older individuals who suffer from diseases that affect nerve transmission to the bladder (e.g., Parkinson's disease, multiple sclerosis, stroke, and dementia). Urge incontinence is also observed when there is increased bladder stimulation caused by lower urinary tract infections, concentrated urine, and irritating chemicals such as caffeine or alcohol. Atrophic urethritis, uterine prolapse, fecal impaction, or prostate enlargement also increases the likelihood of urge incontinence. Even healthy older individuals with no known medical problems may experience occasional episodes of urge incontinence.

The basis of urge incontinence is in the physiologic changes seen with aging. With aging, the bladder decreases in size; it can hold less volume (often 200 mL or less) and needs to be emptied more often. This results in the increased urinary frequency seen with aging. When larger volumes of urine are produced in response to excessive fluid intake or increased use of diuretics, the problem of urinary frequency is magnified. In addition, many older adults experience involuntary spasms of the muscles of the bladder wall, called **detrusor spasms.** These spasms can occur even when the bladder contains small volumes, resulting in a sense of urgency to empty the bladder. When the need to void is frequent and urgent, the result is urge incontinence.

Urge incontinence is likely to occur after the removal of an indwelling catheter. Use of an indwelling catheter results in diminished bladder capacity. Frequency, urgency, and incontinence are likely to occur when a catheter is removed suddenly without incremental clamping, which allows the bladder muscles to stretch gradually to accommodate larger volumes.

Overflow Incontinence

Overflow incontinence is defined as leakage of small amounts of urine from an overly full bladder. The bladder cannot hold the amount of urine being produced, so it overflows. Overflow incontinence is a common problem for diabetic patients suffering from loss of bladder muscle tone because of neuropathy or experiencing polyuria related to hyperglycemia. Overflow incontinence is also common in older men with benign prostate hyperplasia. Enlargement of the prostate restricts the flow of urine, so the bladder never empties completely. This contributes to overflow problems (see the section on urinary retention). Women who have an obstruction at the outlet of the bladder resulting from a prolapsed uterus, cystocele, or rectocele may experience similar problems. Those with neurologic disorders, such as multiple sclerosis or spinal cord injuries above the sacral area, are also prone to overflow incontinence. Anticholinergic medications may also cause excessive relaxation of smooth muscle.

Functional Incontinence

Functional incontinence is seen in older adults who have normal urethral and bladder function. It is caused by a poor relationship between the aging person's abilities and his or her environment. Changes in functional ability may be cognitive or physical in nature. The inability to recognize a toilet, perform simple tasks such as using a zipper or pulling down underwear, walk to the bathroom, transfer to the toilet, or ask for assistance can result in functional incontinence. Environmental factors contribute to the problem of functional incontinence and increase its likelihood. Functional incontinence is likely to occur when there are not enough toilets, when toilets are difficult to access because of their location or height, when there are not enough caregivers to provide needed assistance, and when physical restraints prevent free movement. Weakness, changes in dexterity, and decreased ability to manipulate clothing contribute to problems. Medications that interfere with cognition or mobility, alter bladder tone, and increase urine production often contribute to functional incontinence (Table 18-2).

Total Incontinence. Total incontinence is a condition in which older adults experience continuous and unpredictable loss of urine. Total incontinence can be caused by neurologic changes, bladder muscle spasms, trauma, or diseases affecting the bladder or sphincter muscles.

Some incontinent older adults appear to have more than one form of incontinence. This problem is sometimes called **mixed incontinence.** For example, many older adults report that when they have the urgent need to urinate, they cannot respond quickly enough because of decreased functional ability and environmental limitations. Incontinence can be a continuous and ongoing problem or may occur occasionally only. Careful history taking and medical examination are needed to determine the specific type of incontinence and the underlying causes so that appropriate medical treatment and nursing interventions can be initiated.

❖ NURSING PROCESS FOR IMPAIRED URINARY ELIMINATION

■ Assessment/Data Collection

- Is the person continent or incontinent?
- Is the person incontinent at any specific time of day or under any special conditions?

Table 18-2 Medications That Affect Continence

Diuretics	Cause rapid filling of the bladder resulting from the rapid increase in urine production
Anticholinergics	Interfere with normal contraction of the muscles of the bladder wall
Sedatives and hypnotics	Interfere with alertness and recognition of the need to urinate
Narcotics	Interfere with normal contraction of the muscles of the bladder wall; decrease awareness of sensations from the bladder
α-Adrenergic agonists	Increase tone of the internal sphincter muscle
α-Adrenergic antagonists	Decrease tone of the internal sphincter muscle
Calcium-channel blockers	Decrease tone of the muscles of the bladder wall

- Does the person have a history of any medical conditions that would interfere with urine elimination (neurogenic bladder)?
- Does the person have a history of any medical condition that would decrease awareness of the need to void?
- What is the volume of a typical voiding?
- How much urine is produced each day?
- What is the odor, color, and consistency of urine?
- Are there any signs of a urinary tract infection (burning, pain with urination, frequency)?
- Has a urinalysis been done recently? What are the results?
- What is the person's normal pattern of voiding?
- Does the person experience any difficulty in starting to urinate?
- Does the person experience any involuntary loss of urine when he or she coughs, laughs, or sneezes?
- Does the person complain of any pain or burning with urination?
- What is the person's pattern of fluid intake?

Box 18-4 lists risk factors for impaired urinary elimination in older adults.

■ Nursing Diagnoses

- Functional urinary incontinence
- Reflex urinary incontinence
- Stress urinary incontinence
- Urge urinary incontinence

Box 18-4 Risk Factors Related to Impaired Urinary Elimination in Older Adults

- Neurologic problems that decrease the ability to sense the need for elimination or to control the sphincter muscles
- Endocrine disorders
- Altered structures that interfere with elimination (prostate enlargement or tumors)
- Decreased mobility (especially those on bedrest)
- Inadequate or excessive fluid intake
- Cognitive impairment (Alzheimer's disease, dementia)

- Impaired urinary elimination
- Urinary retention

■ Nursing Goals/Outcomes Identification

The nursing goals for older individuals diagnosed with impaired urinary elimination are to (1) exhibit a reduction in episodes of urinary incontinence or retention, (2) urinate at acceptable times in acceptable places, (3) identify measures that reduce episodes of urinary incontinence or retention, and (4) establish a routine to reduce or prevent the occurrence of bladder elimination problems.

■ Nursing Interventions/Implementation

The following nursing interventions should take place in hospitals or extended-care facilities:

1. **Assess elimination patterns.** Older adults may experience a variety of urinary problems. Careful assessment of elimination patterns and problems enables nurses to develop a care plan that addresses the unique needs of a specific person. Nurses should determine how often the person voids and how much is voided each time. If the older person is incontinent, nurses need to know how often and when incontinence occurs. Nurses should also consider whether the person is receiving medications that affect continence. For example, if incontinence occurs only at night when the older person is receiving diuretic medications, the time of administration should be considered.

2. **Assess fluid intake patterns.** Fluid intake has a direct effect on urine elimination. Many older individuals with urination problems attempt to correct the problem by drinking less. This is likely to increase problems with incontinence because the more-concentrated urine that is produced is more likely to irritate the bladder, increasing the risk for an episode of incontinence. Fluid restriction also increases the risk for problems with fluid balance and bowel elimination. Older adults should be

encouraged to consume most of the day's fluids early in the day and to reduce fluid intake after 7 P.M. to reduce the incidence of incontinence during sleep. Fluids that irritate the bladder such as alcohol or caffeine should be avoided.

3. **Explain measures that help improve tone of the sphincter muscles.** Kegel exercises are helpful in improving the tone of the sphincter muscles (Box 18-5). These exercises include starting and stopping the stream of urine when voiding. Improved muscle tone can help the person hold the urine until he or she can reach a toilet or obtain assistance. Biofeedback has also shown promise as a method of reducing stress and urge incontinence.

4. **Modify clothing to make toileting easier.** The time that is wasted manipulating buttons or zippers may be long enough to cause incontinence.

Box 18-5 | **Modified Kegel Exercises**

The purpose of the following exercises is to strengthen the pelvic floor muscles and the squeezing action that helps hold back the flow of urine. It is important that these exercises be done faithfully for 3 to 4 months to see improvement. If no improvement is seen in this time, consultation with a urologist is suggested.

A. Follow these instructions to identify the muscles you will be exercising
   1. Sit or stand. Without tensing the muscles of your legs, buttocks, or abdomen, imagine that you are trying to hold back a bowel movement by tightening the ring of muscle around the anus. Do this exercise only until you identify the back part of the pelvic floor.
   2. When you are passing urine, try to stop the flow, then re-start it. This helps you identify the front part of the pelvic floor. Now you are ready to do the complete exercise.

B. Do this exercise for 2 minutes at least three times daily (at least 100 repetitions)
   Working from back to front, tighten the muscles while counting to four slowly, then release them. You can do this exercise anywhere—sitting or standing, while watching television, or waiting for a bus. There is no need to interrupt your normal daily activity. To feel only the pelvic muscles, do not tighten the abdominal, thigh, or buttock muscles, or cross your legs. Their movement is distinct and separate from that of the other muscles and can be checked by women while they are in the bath or shower by placing one finger inside the vagina and contracting the muscles. Men can check success only through improved urine control.

C. Do this exercise every time you urinate
   Start and stop your stream five times each time you urinate (i.e., start the flow of urine, squeeze to hold back, then let go to resume the flow). Repeat this sequence several times. Remember, do this every time you urinate. You probably will notice that you have much more control of the flow of urine in the morning than you do in the afternoon. That is because your muscles are not so tired.

From National Association For Continence (NAFC), PO Box 1019, Charleston, SC 29402

Use of Velcro closures and elastic waists with loops may speed undressing and reduce functional problems related to toileting.

5. **Reduce environmental barriers by providing grab bars in the bathroom, installing toilet risers, keeping the urinal or bedpan readily available, and providing a call signal for assistance.** Minimizing environmental barriers to safe elimination can help older adults function more effectively and will reduce the incidence of incontinence caused by mobility problems.

6. **Answer call signals promptly.** Decreased muscle tone and neurologic changes hinder the ability of many older persons to delay urination. An older person is less able to wait for assistance to the bathroom than is a younger person. Call signals or other requests for assistance with toileting must be responded to promptly, or an episode of incontinence is likely. An occurrence of incontinence caused by lack of staff response is embarrassing for the older person and frustrating to all involved because it need not happen. Routine scheduling of trips to the bathroom at regular intervals throughout the day helps reduce the need for the person to call for assistance (Table 18-3).

7. **Develop a toileting schedule.** Planning a regular toileting schedule encourages emptying of the bladder at regular intervals. This reduces the likelihood of urgency and incontinence. The schedule should be based on the individual's urinary elimination patterns; there is no absolute best time schedule. If the person is frequently incontinent, begin by scheduling toileting at 2-hour intervals. Because urine is produced at a rate of approximately 50 to 75 mL/hour and the older person's bladder capacity is approximately 150 to 200 mL, this frequency will reduce episodes of incontinence. Toileting too frequently can actually decrease the ability of the bladder to hold an adequate amount of urine, increasing the risk for incontinence. When a 2-hour schedule is successful, the time should be increased gradually to retrain the bladder to accommodate larger volumes of urine. A regular schedule of every 3 to 4 hours is desirable. Monitor the patient's response to scheduled toileting and praise successes.

8. **Familiarize older adults with the locations of bathrooms throughout the facility.** Many older persons who experience urgency or incontinence are afraid to leave their rooms because they fear being unable to reach a bathroom when necessary. This may result in isolation and withdrawal from others. Even a short distance may be too far for an older person with an urgent need to urinate. Reassurance that toilets are available can reduce these fears.

Table 18-3	**Promoting a Continence-Friendly Environment**
ASSESSMENTS	**MODIFICATIONS OR INTERVENTIONS**
Accessibility	
Are restrooms close to bedrooms and activity centers?	Schedule activities in locations with convenient restrooms.
Are restrooms clearly identified?	Use signs that contrast with walls and have large, bold, dark lettering.
Can client recognize restrooms?	Show clients where restrooms are located.
Can client read signs regarding restroom locations?	Use universal picture symbols for restrooms in addition to words.
Is the client able to ask for assistance to the restroom?	Watch for nonverbal signs of discomfort. Assist client to toilet on a 2-hour schedule.
Does the client ask for assistance to the restroom?	Assist client to restroom before start of activities. Answer call lights promptly.
Are adequate staff assistants available?	Plan to have adequate staff available based on number of clients with continence issues.
Are there any physical barriers or restraints that restrict mobility?	Minimize use of restrictive devices or other barriers to movement.
Safety	
Are the restroom equipped with call signals and grip bars?	Verify presence of safety devices. Develop plan for acquisition if not in place.
Are floors level, dry, and non-skid?	Check condition of floors regularly. Post safety signs during cleaning sessions.
Are restrooms free from clutter?	Remove all clutter from restroom floors promptly.
Is there adequate lighting in restrooms?	Use adequate wattage in restroom. Leave lights on in restroom at night.
Does the client have and wear appropriate footwear?	Remind client to wear shoes or slippers when going to restroom.
Does the client require assistive devices such as walkers or wheelchairs?	Consult with physical therapist regarding need for assistive devices. Encourage client to use recommended devices.
Does the client need help transferring from wheelchair to toilet?	Verify that client and staff are both aware of proper transfer techniques between wheelchair and toilet.
Privacy	
Does the client share a restroom with other clients?	Be aware that more than one person may need to use the restroom at the same time. Have an alternative restroom identified.
Do restrooms have doors and locks?	Doors with safety locks that can be released by staff promote a sense of privacy.
Are toileting requests handled tactfully?	Ask client tactfully if they need to use the toilet. Don't shout.
Is modesty protected during toileting?	Close curtains and doors. Make sure client is adequately dressed when moving in room or public spaces.
Comfort	
Are toilets and toilet seats in good condition, clean, and secure?	Check regularly for chips or cracks and check cleanliness on a regular basis. Report any need for cleaning or repairs promptly.
Are special needs addressed?	Consult with a physical therapist and/or occupational therapist regarding the need for seat riser or padded seat based on client needs.
Are clients assisted off of the toilet promptly?	Assist client off of toilet when finished. Excessive waiting time is uncomfortable and can result in unsafe actions.
Does the client have the opportunity to wash hands after toileting?	Assist to sink or provide washcloths or hand sanitizer after toilet use.

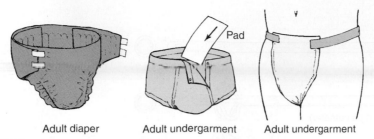

FIGURE 18-1 Disposable and reusable incontinence garments for men and women.

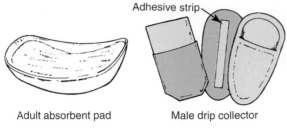

FIGURE 18-2 Disposable incontinence pads.

9. **Provide support and encouragement.** Incontinence is disturbing to alert older persons. Episodes of incontinence are embarrassing and can lead to frustration and loss of self-esteem. Even those involved in bladder training programs are likely to have accidents. It is essential to focus on successes and minimize failures.

10. **Initiate actions to maintain skin integrity.** Aging skin is particularly susceptible to damage from moisture and the waste products in urine. Wet clothing and linens must be removed immediately to prevent maceration and irritation. The skin should be thoroughly washed and dried after each episode of incontinence.

11. **Provide incontinence pads or garments when appropriate.** Incontinence pads or garments reduce the need to completely change the bed linens or clothing after an episode of incontinence (Figures 18-1 and 18-2). However, these items tend to trap moisture next to the skin and should be used with caution. Some of the newer incontinence garments are constructed with a barrier that keeps moisture away from the skin. Because newer incontinence garments are also smaller and less conspicuous, they are more acceptable to older persons than are the bulkier diaper-type garments. The newer garments allow wearers more freedom to move about without fear of embarrassing themselves. Whenever possible, however, these pads and garments should not be used as a replacement for toileting.

The cost of incontinence garments can be significant for persons with limited financial resources. When incontinence pads or garments are soiled, they should be changed promptly and disposed of properly to reduce environmental odors.

12. **Administer medications as prescribed by the physician.** Uroseptic medications, such as sulfonamides, are often used to treat urinary tract infections. Nurses should be sure to check with the individual for allergies to sulfa before administering these medications. Medications such as oxybutynin (Ditropan) or imipramine may be prescribed to reduce bladder spasms that cause incontinence. Nurses must administer these medications as prescribed and assess the patient for signs of their effectiveness. Many of the medications prescribed to treat incontinence cause side effects such as dry mouth, dry eyes, confusion, constipation, orthostatic hypotension, and tachycardia. Comfort measures and safety precautions are necessary if these side effects occur.

13. **Insert catheter as prescribed by physician.** Catheterization requires a physician's order (Figure 18-3). Insertion of an indwelling catheter is not a recommended method for treating incontinence. The risk for urinary tract infections increases dramatically with this invasive procedure. Catheters should be used only when the benefits to the patient outweigh the risks involved. It is essential that a strict sterile technique be used when inserting an indwelling catheter. When the catheter is in place, good perineal care is essential for reducing the possibility of ascending urinary tract infection. Many older persons who have had an indwelling catheter even for a limited time are at increased risk for incontinence once it is removed. When the catheter is in place, the bladder is decompressed. Once the catheter is removed, the bladder is unable to adapt to holding a significant volume of urine. Before removing the catheter, a procedure in which the catheter is clamped intermittently to increase bladder capacity can reduce this problem.

The following interventions should take place in the home:

1. **Encourage the individual to establish a pattern of urine elimination.** A pattern of voiding on awakening, after meals, before leaving home, before becoming interested in a lengthy activity, before exercise, and before bed can reduce the risk for incontinence.

2. **Stress the importance of good skin care and hygiene after episodes of incontinence.** Poor

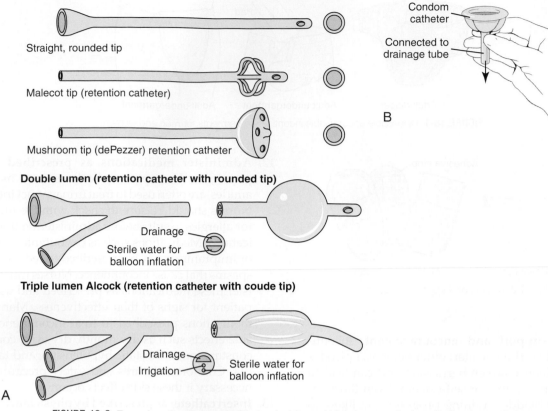

Single lumen

Straight, rounded tip

Malecot tip (retention catheter)

Mushroom tip (dePezzer) retention catheter

Double lumen (retention catheter with rounded tip)

Drainage

Sterile water for balloon inflation

Triple lumen Alcock (retention catheter with coude tip)

Drainage

Irrigation

Sterile water for balloon inflation

A

Condom catheter

Connected to drainage tube

B

FIGURE 18-3 Examples of catheters. **A,** Single, double, and triple lumen catheters. **B,** Condom catheter.

hygiene increases the risk for skin irritation or breakdown and increases the risk for urinary tract infections. The importance of changing soiled clothing promptly, careful handwashing after toileting, and (for women) proper wiping from front to back should be reinforced.

3. **Encourage discussion of concerns with the physician.** Nurses working in a home setting may be aware of urinary problems that have not been shared with the physician. Older adults should be encouraged to reveal their problems and concerns with a physician so that an appropriate diagnosis can be made and treatment initiated. All observations regarding urine elimination should be documented appropriately in the person's record and appropriate notification made to the physician.

4. **Provide encouragement during treatment for urinary problems.** Problems with urinary retention or incontinence do not usually respond quickly to treatment. Weeks or months of treatment may be required before any improvement is noticed. This can easily result in noncompliance with the plan of care. Older adults need encouragement to take medications, practice exercises, or follow through with other medical recommendations.

5. **Discuss methods for coping with incontinence.** Aging persons are more likely to become socially isolated rather than embarrass themselves in public. Developing strategies for coping (e.g., use of incontinence garments and learning the location of toilets in stores or theaters) can help prevent this.

6. **Use any appropriate interventions that are used in the institutional setting.**

Get Ready for the NCLEX® Examination!

Key Points

- Bladder and bowel elimination is essential for normal body functioning.
- Unless waste products are removed effectively from the body, serious consequences will result.
- Aging results in less effective removal of waste products, but a problem more significant to older adults is any alteration in the ability to control the elimination process.
- Problems related to elimination are serious concerns for older adults, and a great deal of physical and mental energy is devoted to dealing with changes in elimination function.

Additional Learning Resources

SG Go to the Study Guide on pp. 379–397 for additional learning activities to help you master the chapter content.

evolve Go to your Evolve website (http://evolve.elsevier.com/Wold/geriatric) for the following FREE learning resources:
- Animations
- Answer Guidelines for Nursing Care Plan Critical Thinking Questions
- Answers and Rationales for Review Questions for the NCLEX® Examination
- Glossary with pronunciations in English and Spanish
- Video Clips

Review Questions for the NCLEX® Examination

1. While caring for an elderly patient the nurse determines that further teaching regarding bowel elimination is needed when the client states:
   1. "I'll do some exercise and increase my daily fluid intake."
   2. "I'll give myself an enema if I don't have a BM every day."
   3. "I'll increase my intake of fruits and vegetables."
   4. "I'll try to eat more whole grain foods, like bran, daily."

2. An elderly patient who recently has had small watery BMs, complains of pressure in the rectal area and abdominal cramping. The most appropriate initial nursing action would be to:
   1. Administer an oil retention enema.
   2. Notify the physician of these observations.
   3. Digitally stimulate the rectal sphincter.
   4. Administer the prn laxative medication.

3. The nurse recognized that, when caring for an elderly person who has a history of cardiac problems, it is most important to institute measures to prevent:
   1. Constipation
   2. Diarrhea
   3. Urinary tract infection
   4. Bladder incontinence

4. An older woman reports leakage of urine during exercise, coughing, and sneezing. These characteristics are associated with:
   1. Urge incontinence
   2. Stress incontinence
   3. Overflow incontinence
   4. Functional incontinence

5. An elderly woman has begun to stay in her apartment, avoiding socializing with her peers in the independent living center. She states that she cannot wait when she needs to urinate. She is afraid that she will have an accident. It is most appropriate for the nurse to:
   1. Tell her not to worry because many of the other ladies have the same problem.
   2. Suggest that she begin to wear an adult incontinence garment when she goes out.
   3. Recommend that she restrict her fluid intake so the problem does not occur as often.
   4. Provide encouragement and discuss Kegel exercises and other approaches to cope with incontinence.

Activity and Exercise

Objectives

1. Describe normal activity and exercise patterns.
2. Describe how activity and exercise patterns change with aging.
3. Discuss the effects of disease processes on the ability to participate in exercise and activity.
4. Describe methods of assessing changes in the ability to participate in activity or exercise.
5. Identify the older adults who are most at risk for experiencing problems related to activity and exercise.
6. Identify selected nursing diagnoses related to activity and exercise problems.
7. Describe nursing interventions that are appropriate for older individuals experiencing problems related to activity and exercise.
8. Differentiate between a custodial focus and a rehabilitative focus in nursing care.
9. Discuss the impact of nurses' attitudes on care planning.
10. Identify the benefits of a rehabilitative focus on older adults.
11. Identify the goals of rehabilitation nursing.

Key Terms

agility (ă-JIL-ĭ-tē) (p. 303)
alignment (ă-LIN-měnt) (p. 307)
arthritis (ăhr-THRĪ-tĭs) (p. 305)
coordination (Kō-ŏr-dĭ-NĀ-shŭn) (p. 303)
custodial (kŭ-STŌ-dē-ăl) (p. 304)
dexterity (děk-STĔR-ĭ-tē) (p. 303)
diversional activities (dĭ-VŬR-zhăn-ăl) (p. 321)
dyspnea (DĬSP-nē-ă) (p. 315)
hemiparesis (hěm-ē-pă-RĒ-sĭs) (p. 307)

hemiplegia (hěm-ē-PLĒ-jä) (p. 307)
intermittent claudication (ĭn-těr-MĬT-ěnt klaw-dĭ-KĀ-shŭn) (p. 305)
isometric (ī-sō-MĔT-rĭk) (p. 307)
isotonic (ī-sō-TŎN-ĭk) (p. 307)
rehabilitation (rē-hă-bĭl-ĭ-TĀ-shŭn) (p. 305)
rehabilitative (rē-hă-bĭl-ĭ-TĀ-tĭv) (p. 304)
tachycardia (tăk-ē-KĂR-dē-ă) (p. 314)

NORMAL ACTIVITY PATTERNS

The activity-exercise health pattern deals with behaviors related to exercise, activity, leisure, and recreation. Nurses must consider the wide range of behaviors within this pattern that fall under the general term **activity.** Activity is anything that requires the expenditure of energy. Some activities require only a small expenditure of energy, whereas others require a great deal of energy.

Basic body functions such as breathing, temperature control, and metabolism expend the least amount of energy. Sitting, resting, watching television, reading, and playing cards or bingo are sedentary activities that require little energy. Activities of daily living (ADL) such as dressing, grooming, eating, bathing, and toileting require a greater expenditure of energy. Cooking, cleaning, driving, and shopping require still more effort and expend more energy. Walking can be a mild or vigorous activity, depending on the pace. Running, swimming, dancing, aerobics, and other forms of active exercise require the greatest energy expenditure. Although the amount and type of exercise an individual performs change over the life span, exercise and activity remain an essential part of life. Persons who were not physically active as young adults are not likely to become physically active as they age. A healthy pattern of activity and exercise should be established early in life to ensure that these behaviors become habitual and are carried into old age.

Exercise helps people look and feel better. Physical activity is necessary to maintain normal joint mobility and muscle tone. When people do not participate in regular activity, all body systems suffer. Preventing mobility problems is easier than trying to overcome the problems when they develop. Older individuals should be encouraged to be as active and independent as possible. Because existing medical conditions may restrict activity, nurses should be aware of any problems that may affect the individual's ability to participate in activities. Older adults should be assisted to do as much as is permitted.

Many aging individuals remain physically active. Today, it is common to see individuals in their sixties, seventies, and eighties leading active, self-sufficient lives. Aging no longer implies that a person must sit forever in a rocking chair or recliner and vegetate.

All one has to do is visit a park or shopping mall early in the morning, where many older adults can be seen walking for their health. Access to golf courses is more difficult because of the amazing number of senior citizens playing 18 holes. Activity is good for people of all ages. Aging may change the type and amount of participation, but more and more people are realizing that active participation in a variety of activities is the best way to maintain high-level function.

Physical activity requires a complex interaction of physiologic processes, primarily those of the neurologic, musculoskeletal, cardiovascular, and respiratory systems. Anything that interferes with the coordination of these systems can alter the ability to participate in physical activity.

Of major importance is the function of the nervous system, which is the primary coordinating system of the body. The brain controls the involuntary activities of the body, including metabolism, respiration, and temperature control. Areas of the brain control the high-level processes of perception and cognition. Before any voluntary activity occurs, individuals must be able to recognize that a need for action exists. Once the need is recognized, the individual must have the desire, as well as the ability, to perform that action. The brain is also the motor control center of the body, and it communicates with the somatic peripheral nervous system. Any physiologic age- or disease-related change that alters the function of the brain's motor centers or that interferes with the transmission of impulses from the brain to the musculoskeletal system can interfere with activity.

The musculoskeletal system must then be able to respond to these messages from the brain. Normal and pathologic changes in muscles or bones can interfere with normal activity. Even if the nervous and the musculoskeletal systems are intact, problems in the cardiovascular and respiratory systems can lead to alterations in activity. Muscles, including the heart muscle, require an adequate supply of oxygen and nutrients to function properly. Anything that interferes with the oxygen supply to tissues affects a person's ability to perform activity.

ACTIVITY AND AGING

With advancing age, most people experience some changes in the ability to perform or tolerate activity, and this ability varies widely among older adults. In general, the more active a person has been, the more active he or she remains with aging.

The first change noticed by most aging persons is a decrease in the rate or speed of activity. Things that could be done quickly in the past now take longer. Many older individuals complain that it takes them much longer to dress, shop, or do other simple activities than it used to. Normal aging does not interfere with the transmission of nerve impulses, but it does slow the speed of nerve transmission.

A loss of muscle mass can interfere with activities that require muscular strength. Activities such as moving furniture, lifting bags of groceries, shoveling snow, and vacuuming may be increasingly difficult.

Loss of cushioning cartilage can result in arthritic joint pain, which inhibits motion and makes a person less likely to exercise. Ligaments and tendons become more stiff, contributing to decreased joint flexibility. This can result in problems with performing ADL. Reaching for objects on shelves, dressing, bending to put on shoes, and even washing the feet or back may be difficult.

Agility, the ability to move quickly and smoothly, decreases with age. This may cause difficulty when older adults try to climb ladders or avoid hazards while walking. Dexterity, the ability to perform fine manipulative skills, is also likely to decrease with age. Gross motor skills remain intact longer than do fine motor skills. However, skills that were perfected when younger, such as playing a musical instrument or sewing, may be maintained at a high level if the skills are used regularly.

Decreased stamina is typically seen with aging. This is most often a result of a decrease in oxygen supply to body tissues. Decreased oxygen exchange may be caused by a loss of elasticity in the lungs and a smaller chest cavity. The decreased availability of oxygen may lead to frequent pauses during activity or a slower pace when performing activities.

Coordination of multiple activities is likely to decrease with aging. Activities that require simultaneous perception of many stimuli and quick physical response (such as driving) are often affected. Older individuals with impaired vision and hearing, decreased strength, slow reaction time, and decreased coordination may not be able to safely perform this type of complex activity.

Because these changes appear gradually, most older individuals learn to compensate for or cope with them. Many strategies such as pacing activities, finding alternative methods of performing activities, and simplifying activities demonstrate the capacity of older adults to adapt and adjust.

EXERCISE RECOMMENDATIONS FOR OLDER ADULTS

Regular, planned exercise is of benefit to all ages, and it is of particular benefit as we age. Scientific evidence increasingly indicates that regular physical activity can extend years of active independent life, reduce disability, and improve the quality of life for older persons. Exercise helps gain or maintain muscle mass, strength, balance, coordination, and joint flexibility. It helps decrease stress and promotes normal sleep.

Exercise does not have to be demanding to be of benefit. Current recommendations state that moderate exercise done for 30 minutes a day is more beneficial than strenuous exercise done infrequently. Because there may be medical reasons why certain activities are contraindicated, older persons should check with their physician before starting an exercise program. Physicians often refer older patients to a physical therapist, who can develop a plan specific to their needs. Elderly adults with special physical limitations will need an individualized plan developed to meet their unique needs. The proper exercise plan for a frail elderly person will be quite different from the plan most suited to a high-functioning 65-year-old. Physical therapists can recommend exercise programs designed for use by wheelchair-bound individuals or anyone with special needs. Before starting an exercise program, the older person should know the importance of acquiring good supportive footwear and clothing appropriate for the environment and type of exercise. Because elders are more at risk for thermal imbalance, they should be aware that it is wise to avoid excessive exercise during extreme weather conditions.

A 94-year-old man was interviewed at a private health club where he spends 1 hour a day, 6 days a week. He said he started coming to the club when he was in his late seventies to give his wife, who had Alzheimer's disease, some privacy while she received personal care at home. He said he thought it would help him decrease his stress and increase his physical strength so that he could help her. She has since died, but he keeps coming to the club to use the treadmill and flexibility machinery. When asked why he likes to come to the club to exercise, the man replied, "It keeps me young." He also mentioned that he likes the social atmosphere and "watching the youngsters sweat."

Specific types of exercise provide unique benefits. Aerobic or endurance exercises promote cardiovascular and respiratory function. Aerobic exercise includes activities that can be done at home, such as walking, biking, or square dancing. Many residential facilities, YMCAs, and senior centers provide additional opportunities for aerobic exercise using treadmills, rowing machines, steps, and others. Swimming is a pleasurable aerobic exercise for many seniors, and water exercises can help individuals with sore joints because the water provides support and eases movement. Even doing routine household chores and yard work can be considered aerobic if done for a long enough time. Resistance and conditioning exercise will help maintain muscle mass. These exercises can be done using exercise balls, inexpensive elastic stretch bands, or weights. More complex equipment may be available in health clubs or senior centers, but the individual must know how to use the equipment properly to avoid injury. Stretching exercises are important to promote joint flexibility. Little equipment is needed for these exercises, but caution should be used when doing standing exercises if the older person has balance problems. Balance training is particularly important for the elderly. Studies show that this training reduced falls by up to 17%. Even general exercise programs can reduce the incidence of falls by 10%.

Technologic innovations such as the Nintendo Wii and other interactive games appear to have the potential of stimulating interest in activity within the aging population.

Keeping motivated to exercise is a major problem at any age—perhaps more so as a person gets older. Nurses should educate older persons about the importance of exercise and emphasize the benefits such as weight loss, improved blood glucose control, lower blood pressure, decreased risk for falls, and others specific to the individual. Here are some guidelines that can help older adults make a regular exercise program a reality:

- **Keep it simple.** Simple exercise programs are more likely to be successful than complicated ones that are hard to remember or difficult to perform.
- **Have a plan.** Set up a weekly calendar with a planned time for exercise to keep on track.
- **Do it with a friend.** Enlisting the company of a friend or group of friends who can provide mutual encouragement and support is highly motivating. Even a pet can be your friend and exercise buddy for a walk.
- **Keep it interesting.** Join an exercise or dance class as a way to try some new form of exercise that is more interesting and motivating (see Complementary and Alternative Therapies box).
- **Try music.** Upbeat rhythms or waltzes can help coordinate your movements. Many tapes and CDs designed specifically for exercise are available at music stores or online. Exercise videos are also available, but choose one that is appropriate for your needs and abilities.
- **Get a coach.** A physical therapist, personal coach, or health club trainer can provide additional teaching and motivation.
- **Set a goal.** Goals should be realistic but challenging. Focus on small but measurable gains, such as increasing strength to walk an additional block or being able to get your shoes on more easily. Remember, anything that you can do now but had trouble with before is a gain. In fact, not losing function as you age is a significant gain in itself.

Focusing on the positive outcomes of exercise is key to maintaining a regular program. See the Nursing Process for Impaired Physical Mobility on pages 306–312 for additional benefits that can increase an older adult's motivation to continue exercising.

Complementary and Alternative Therapies

Qi Gong and Tai Chi

Qi gong and tai chi are forms of exercise from Asia that are gaining popularity because they are less stressful to the body and yet require more focus and concentration. This makes these exercises beneficial for both body and mind. While traveling in China, the author observed individuals and groups of all ages, including many elderly persons, performing tai chi. Early in the day people were exercising everywhere you looked. The major components include body posture adjustments, gentle motion, regulated breathing, meditation, and other purposeful relaxation. Some forms also include massage or hand resistance. These exercises can be done vigorously or gently, making them suitable for a wide range of individuals. They are typically performed while standing but can also be adapted for walking, sitting, or lying. These forms of exercise are inexpensive to perform because they require no special equipment or facilities. Research conducted abroad and in the United States has shown many benefits from these exercises, including the following: increased oxygen consumption, decreased blood pressure, improved flexibility, increased lower extremity strength, increased bone density, improved posture and balance, and even improved immune system function. Additional reported benefits include decreases in stress, anxiety, and depression.

These exercise practices have gained some support in the United States, but many health care providers and potential elderly participants are unaware of them or remain skeptical of their benefits. This may be due, in part, to lack of familiarity with the techniques and a perception of difficulty. In addition, there are not enough teachers who are prepared to explain the principles and skills of these exercises appropriately. Further research and dissemination of information are being funded by the Robert Wood Johnson Foundation and others. Many articles and video training materials are now available.

EFFECTS OF DISEASE PROCESSES ON ACTIVITY

If, in addition to normal changes, the aging person has health problems that affect the critical body systems, his or her ability to participate in activity is further impaired. Organic brain syndrome, Alzheimer's disease, and stroke can affect both the high-level thinking functions and the motor functions of the brain. Persons suffering from severe forms of these diseases may not recognize the need for the most basic activities such as moving, eating, dressing, bathing, or toileting. Even if they do recognize these needs, their altered motor function may prevent them from meeting basic needs.

Neurologic damage resulting from head injury, infection, degenerative disease, Parkinson's disease, or toxic drug reactions can interfere with normal nerve impulse transmission. Older persons suffering from these conditions may recognize a need and have the desire to perform an activity yet are unable to carry out the activity. The nervous system does not transmit appropriate messages to the muscles to enable them to perform the activity. Abnormal nerve transmission can result in difficulty getting started with movement or in uncoordinated muscle activity (e.g., a staggering gait), which further limits the ability to participate in normal activities.

Diseases or injury to the musculoskeletal system can interfere with the ability to perform activity. Fractures can lead to limited or extensive mobility restriction, depending on the part or parts of the body affected. Fracture of a small bone such as a finger results in limited loss of mobility. Fracture of a large bone such as the femur results in severe limitation of mobility. Not only does the fracture itself restrict mobility, but also the treatment further limits mobility. Even after surgical repair, the person with a fractured hip is not permitted to participate in certain activities (e.g., weight bearing on the extremity) until healing has occurred. While waiting for healing to occur, strength and joint mobility can be lost if preventive nursing interventions are not instituted.

Diseases such as gout and **arthritis** cause joint pain, which leads to restricted activity. A person with severe gout or arthritis is likely to avoid use of the painful joints to reduce discomfort. Unfortunately, this inactivity can lead to further loss of joint mobility and muscle strength, which even further reduces the person's ability to perform activities. Joint degeneration with aging severely restricts mobility, particularly in the weight-bearing joints in the knees and hips. Joint replacement surgery is an increasingly common option for older adults. After a period of **rehabilitation**, most older adults achieve a greatly improved activity level.

Foot conditions commonly seen in older adults (e.g., bunions, hammertoes, and calluses) may interfere with ambulation, particularly if footwear does not fit properly. Painful feet are a common reason for decreased activity in older adults.

Any disease condition that interferes with the intake or distribution of oxygen to body tissue significantly interferes with a person's ability to participate in activity and exercise. These conditions include diseases of the respiratory system that prevent adequate gas exchange in the lungs (e.g., asthma, emphysema, bronchitis, and pneumonia) and diseases of the cardiovascular system that prevent adequate distribution of oxygen to body tissues and heart muscle (e.g., myocardial infarction, congestive heart failure, heart block, arteriosclerosis, and hypertension).

Inadequate oxygenation places additional stress on the cardiovascular and respiratory systems. Pulse and respiratory rates increase in an attempt to compensate for the decreased amount of oxygen. If additional demands for oxygen occur, as they do with even moderate activity, older adults may experience additional symptoms. Fatigue with minimal activity is common with oxygen deprivation. Pain may be reported with activity. Most common are angina (when the heart muscle does not receive adequate amounts of oxygen) and **intermittent claudication** (when the tissues of the lower extremities are deprived of oxygen). Initially, this pain occurs with activity only; in severe cases of deprivation, it also occurs at rest. Severe oxygen deprivation can result in cardiac or respiratory distress.

To compensate for these symptoms, older adults spontaneously restrict their activities. Individuals may become housebound because the effort of dressing is too much for them. Some are unable to eat or perform basic hygiene because it is too exhausting. Sometimes the activity limitation is so severe that individuals are able to maneuver around the house only by placing chairs at 10-foot intervals. They move that short distance, then sit and rest until they are able to move to the next chair.

Malnourishment can also contribute to the reduced ability to perform activity. Inadequate intake of nutrients can result in muscle atrophy. Malnourished individuals lack adequate protein to build muscle tissue, an adequate supply of glucose to fuel the muscles, and adequate iron to form hemoglobin. Inadequate iron intake can result in anemia, which leads to a decrease in the oxygen available to tissues and further reduces the ability to perform activity.

Although not physiologic in origin, emotional disorders such as severe grief, anxiety, or depression can lead to decreased participation in normal activity. Individuals who are emotionally disturbed may be directing all of their energy inward and may not be willing or able to summon the energy required for physical activity. It is important to remember that these people need to continue to use their bodies to prevent loss of physical function.

❖ NURSING PROCESS FOR IMPAIRED PHYSICAL MOBILITY

Most older adults experience some changes in their ability to perform physical activities. These changes may result from the normal changes of aging or from some pathologic changes.

■ Assessment/Data Collection

- Does the individual have full range of motion in the joints?
- Does the person have any contractures or deformities?
- Does the person experience any pain or tenderness in the joints?
- Is there any particular motion that aggravates joint pain?
- What relieves discomfort?
- How is the muscle tone of the arms and legs?
- Is muscle strength equal on both sides of the body?
- Is there any muscle tenderness?
- Is the person bedridden, wheelchair-bound, or ambulatory?
- If ambulatory, what is the pattern of the gait? Steady? Shuffling? Ataxic? Slow? Rapid?
- Is the person able to lift his or her feet when walking, or does the person shuffle?

- Does the person maintain an upright posture when walking?
- Do both sides of the body move evenly?
- How well can the person maintain balance?
- What kind of footwear does the person wear for walking?
- Does the person have any foot problems (e.g., bunions and calluses) that interfere with walking?
- How far can the person ambulate without discomfort?
- Does the person require any assistive devices (walkers or canes) for ambulation?
- Does the person know how to use these assistive devices properly?
- Does the person feel comfortable and confident using these aids?
- Does the person require the assistance of another person to ambulate?
- If the person is not ambulatory, what is his or her activity level?
- Does the person use a wheelchair?
- Can the person operate the wheelchair himself or herself?
- Does the person receive passive range-of-motion exercises?
- Is the environment safe for the individual?

Box 19-1 lists risk factors for impaired physical mobility in older adults.

■ Nursing Diagnosis

Impaired physical mobility

■ Nursing Goals/Outcomes Identification

The nursing goals for individuals with impaired physical mobility are to (1) increase participation in physical activities that maintain strength and mobility, (2) maintain normal anatomic position and function in all joints, (3) remain free from joint contractures and foot drop, and (4) maintain or increase strength and mobility using assistive devices.

■ Nursing Interventions/Implementation

The following nursing interventions should take place in hospitals or extended-care facilities:

1. **Identify the prescribed activity level.** The activity level is established by the physician based on the

---

Box 19-1	Risk Factors Related to Impaired Physical Mobility in Older Adults

- Intolerance of physical activity because of medical conditions that decrease endurance or strength
- Pain
- Neuromuscular or musculoskeletal conditions
- Cognitive impairment (Alzheimer's disease or dementia)
- Severe anxiety or depression
- Prescribed bed rest
- Restrictive devices (restraints, casts, splints, and immobilizers)

older person's overall health status. It is important that the patient be as active as possible yet not exceed the prescribed activity level. It is particularly important that the nurse be aware of any weight-bearing restrictions related to fractures or joint replacements. Failure to take proper precautions can lead to serious and permanent harm.

2. **Continue to assess strength and joint mobility.** Strength and joint mobility are not always consistent in older adults. Changes may be caused by something as simple as a change in the weather, or they may be an early indication of a change in the older person's health status. Nurses should pay special attention to mobility if the older person has experienced weakness or falls. Significant changes such as one-sided weakness or severe pain should be reported promptly to the physician.

3. **Perform physical mobility activities in conjunction with daily care.** Passive range-of-motion exercise can be provided in conjunction with the bath. Active exercise can become part of dressing, meals, grooming, toileting, and other ADL. Even minimal participation in ADL can increase physical mobility. Any exercise performed by the older individual during bathing, hair combing, and oral hygiene that uses the joints and muscles can be beneficial.

4. **Provide good body alignment and frequent position changes.** Bedridden older adults are at high risk for loss of joint mobility. Poor alignment can result in muscle fatigue, which enhances the likelihood of contractures. Flexion contractures of the hip, knee, and foot occur when the stronger flexor muscles dominate. These contractures can result in permanent loss of the ability to stand or ambulate. To prevent this, good alignment and positioning are important. Positioning devices (pillows, trochanter rolls, and foot supports) should be used when needed to maintain proper alignment.

5. **Avoid unnecessary restraint that limits physical mobility.** By definition, restraints limit mobility. Any device that restricts mobility is a restraint, including vests, wheelchair tables, foot pedals, and safety bars. Many of these devices that historically have been used to protect older adults from falls have actually increased the likelihood of injury. An older person who is prevented by these devices from using joints and muscles loses strength and function and becomes increasingly susceptible to injury. Nurses must ensure that splints or other devices do not unnecessarily restrict joint movement.

6. **Consult with the physical therapist to determine a suitable activity/exercise plan that maintains muscle strength and joint mobility.** The physical therapist may be able to suggest exercises that will benefit a specific individual. These exercises should become part of the nursing care plan and be included in the day's activities (Figure 19-1). Passive range-of-motion exercises help keep the joints flexible, but they do little to maintain muscle strength. Passive range of motion should be provided a minimum of twice a day for immobile older individuals. Active range of motion helps with both joint flexibility and muscle toning. Older persons with hemiplegia or hemiparesis can be taught to use the stronger side of the body to exercise the weaker extremities. Many facilities provide exercise programs that are adapted to meet the ability levels of the residents. Exercise is often done to music because the rhythm encourages motion. Isometric exercises, such as alternately tightening and relaxing the muscles of the arms, abdomen, or buttocks, may benefit some older adults by helping them maintain the strength of the abdominal and gluteal muscles and quadriceps. Isometric exercise does not affect the joints. Isotonic exercise, which helps improve muscle strength, muscle tone, and joint mobility, includes such movements as lifting the body off of the bed with a trapeze (Figure 19-2), pressing against a footboard, or pushing against the bed to lift the buttocks off the mattress. Isometric and isotonic exercises should be used with caution by persons with cardiac problems because these exercises increase stress on the cardiovascular system. They may result in elevation of the blood pressure and use of the Valsalva maneuver, which can lead to cardiac overload or cardiac arrest. To prevent this problem, older adults should be instructed to breathe through the mouth while exercising.

7. **Verify that the individual is suitably dressed for activity and that he or she has the proper footwear.** Proper clothing and footwear should be selected for exercise. Clothing should be nonconstricting (to allow freedom of movement) and suitable to the environment. Many older adults choose comfortable footwear over footwear that provides proper support. Most slippers do not provide adequate support and are intended for rest periods, not ambulation. Shoes should be worn whenever possible. Shoes should fit well and support the foot to decrease the likelihood of falls. If the individual has foot problems, special footwear may be necessary. Gait changes, particularly the inability to lift the feet freely, increase the risk for falls. If footwear is too loose or is not supportive, the risk for falls increases. Shoes should fit snugly enough that they do not slip off the heel when walking. Older women, particularly those with kyphosis, should be encouraged to wear low heels when walking to provide better balance.

8. **Provide pain medication in a timely manner so that maximal benefits from the medication occur**

LYING DOWN

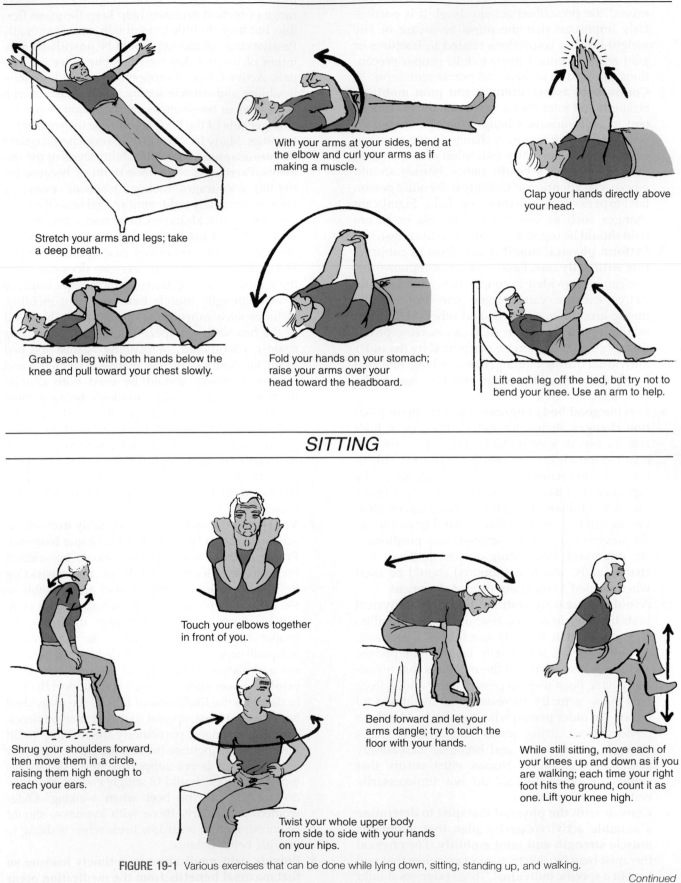

Stretch your arms and legs; take a deep breath.

With your arms at your sides, bend at the elbow and curl your arms as if making a muscle.

Clap your hands directly above your head.

Grab each leg with both hands below the knee and pull toward your chest slowly.

Fold your hands on your stomach; raise your arms over your head toward the headboard.

Lift each leg off the bed, but try not to bend your knee. Use an arm to help.

SITTING

Touch your elbows together in front of you.

Shrug your shoulders forward, then move them in a circle, raising them high enough to reach your ears.

Twist your whole upper body from side to side with your hands on your hips.

Bend forward and let your arms dangle; try to touch the floor with your hands.

While still sitting, move each of your knees up and down as if you are walking; each time your right foot hits the ground, count it as one. Lift your knee high.

FIGURE 19-1 Various exercises that can be done while lying down, sitting, standing up, and walking.

Continued

STANDING UP

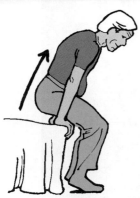

Using your arms, push off from the bed and stand up; if you get dizzy, sit down and try again.

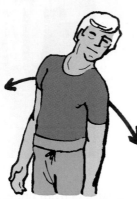

Hold your arms out and turn them in big circles.

With hands at your side, bend at the waist as far as you can to the right side, then to the left.

Keep your feet planted on the ground and twist your upper body at the waist from side to side with your arms swinging; when you twist to the right, count it as one.

While holding onto the edge of the bed or back of a chair, bend your knees slightly.

WALKING PLACES

Walking is good exercise. It helps in toning muscles and maintaining flexibility of joints. It also is good exercise for the heart and circulatory system. Walking briskly for 20 minutes a day, 3 times a week can be as effective a heart conditioner as jogging, but it does take a longer time to achieve the same effect as jogging. For those who cannot walk rapidly for long periods, walking to the point of muscular fatigue also helps maintain good muscle tone.

Your body may give you signs to indicate you are overdoing exercise. Stop, rest, and if necessary, call your physician if you experience any of these symptoms:

- SEVERE SHORTNESS OF BREATH
- CHEST PAIN
- SEVERE JOINT PAIN
- DIZZINESS OR FAINT FEELING
- HEART FLUTTERS

In all walking exercises, go only as fast as you are able to walk and still carry on a conversation. If you cannot, slow down.

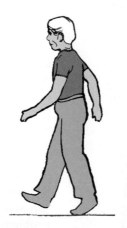

INSIDE

It is important to maintain walking ability. Determine how far you can walk and each day walk to 3/4 of that distance, building endurance. Wear supportive shoes and use whatever aids are necessary.

OUTSIDE

Wear soft-soled shoes with good support, (i.e., jogging shoes). When walking, push off from your toes and land on your heels. Swing arms loosely at your sides. Begin with 10-minute walks and build to 20 to 30 minutes.

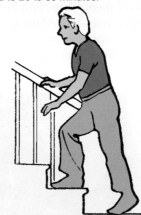

Walking up stairs requires effort. Place one foot flat on a step, push off with the other and shift your weight. Use a railing for balance if necessary.

FIGURE 19-1—CONT'D

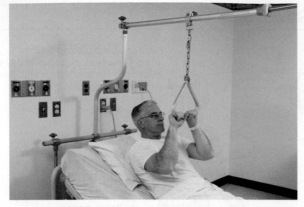

FIGURE 19-2 Patient using a trapeze bar.

when greatest physical effort is expected. Pain is a common reason for decreased physical mobility. Nurses should be aware of particular activities that intensify or relieve an individual's pain. Pain increases with fatigue; therefore, activities should be paced so that they do not overly fatigue the individual. Antiinflammatory medications or analgesics should be administered so that the older person is as comfortable as possible when physical activity is scheduled.

9. **Verify that the individual knows the correct method for using assistive devices and that he or she does, in fact, use them for activity. Explain proper use if needed.** If assistive devices such as wheelchairs, walkers, or canes are needed, nurses should verify that older adults know how to use them properly (Figures 19-3 and 19-4). Nurses must verify that the older person knows how to use the walker, particularly when climbing stairs. The nurse should also verify that the person holds the cane in the correct hand when walking. To prevent falls, older adults should be reminded to lock the wheels of their wheelchair before sitting down. In addition, nurses should ensure that the assistive devices are kept nearby so that they are easily available to the older person. If the individual

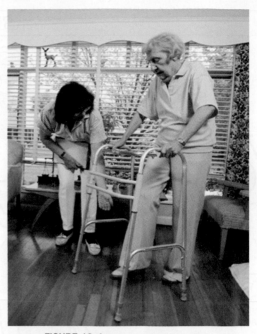

FIGURE 19-4 Patient using a walker.

suffers from one-sided weakness, the device must be placed on the stronger side. Nurses must remember that many older adults do not like to use these devices because they are cumbersome and because they are constant reminders of failing health. Nurses must continue to stress the importance of using the devices if they are needed for safety.

10. **Encourage wheelchair-bound patients to move by using their arms or feet whenever possible.** If they are unable to walk, older adults may still be able to move about in a wheelchair, which involves using either the arms to turn the wheels or the legs and feet to propel the chair.

11. **Provide adequate assistance during ambulation.** Gait belts and the assistance of one or two helpers may be needed to provide safety and a sense of security. The loss of balance seen in some older persons increases the risk for falls. A gait belt should be used when an unsteady person is being assisted. Gait belts that are properly secured around the person's waist allow the caregiver to prevent injury to the individual. The belt is near the person's center of gravity; thus the caregiver can sense subtle balance changes and anticipate problems (Figure 19-5). If the belt is too loose, it may slide up under the rib cage and cause injury. Regular belts on trousers or dresses may be used, but only with caution, because they are usually narrower and may not fasten as securely as a proper gait belt. Holding the arm of the older person to provide support is inadequate in most cases and should be avoided. If the older person starts to fall, the caregiver could dislocate the shoulder or cause other severe trauma to the older person.

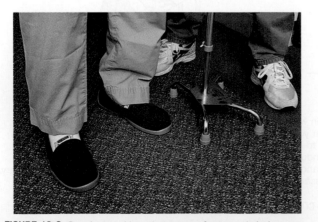

FIGURE 19-3 Quad cane. Note that proper footwear is being worn.

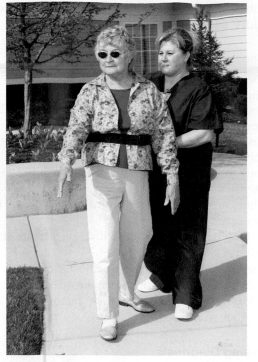

FIGURE 19-5 Assist with ambulation by walking at the person's side. Use a gait belt for the person's safety.

The following interventions should take place in the home:

1. **Teach or reinforce the benefits of regular activity and exercise.** Many articles in senior citizen magazines and the popular press address the benefits of exercise (Box 19-2). Sedentary older adults may need to be reminded or encouraged to take this information to heart. Important information to communicate to older adults includes the fact that moderate or higher levels of physical activity are associated with lower mortality rates. Physical activity has been associated with many beneficial physiologic effects, including improved cardiovascular status, decreased risk for colon cancer, beneficial effects on noninsulin-dependent diabetes

mellitus, maintenance of normal muscle strength and joint function, reduced risk for falling, and decreased incidence of obesity. Activity also has psychologic benefits, including a decreased incidence of depression, improved mood, and an enhanced sense of well-being.

2. **Assess the home for safety hazards or conditions that may interfere with mobility.** The home may present conditions that interfere with mobility or increase the risk for falls. Modifications of the environment may be required to prevent accidents or injury. Chapter 9 addresses assessment of home safety in greater detail.

3. **Help older adults develop a schedule for regular physical activity that is appropriate for their prescribed activity level.** The physician should be consulted before an older person who has a chronic disease or has lived a sedentary lifestyle starts an exercise program. Once an appropriate target level is established, the individual should be taught to start slowly and build up to the optimal level over time.

Active older persons should be encouraged to participate in regular physical activity. Exercise should be planned into the day's activities. If exercise is not viewed as important enough to plan for, it will not be done. Three 20- to 30-minute sessions a week on nonconsecutive days are good; daily exercise is even better. Midmorning is a good time for exercise, but afternoon and early evening are also good times. Much of the timing depends on the individual's peak energy time. Blood supply may be diverted to digestion for up to 2 hours after large meals; therefore, intense physical activity should not be scheduled immediately after meals. Walking is one of the best exercises for older adults. Swimming and cycling are also recommended (Figure 19-6). Exercise programs, including aerobics classes, are sponsored by many senior citizen centers. Before joining this type of exercise program, older adults should see their physicians to ensure that the

---

Box 19-2 Benefits of Exercise for Older Adults

- Maintain independence
- Retain mobility
- Prevent or reduce depression
- Encourage sleep
- Improve self-esteem
- Improve appetite
- Improve cardiovascular status
- Maintain or improve musculoskeletal function
- Prevent obesity
- Decrease stress level
- Expand social network
- Enhance appreciation for life

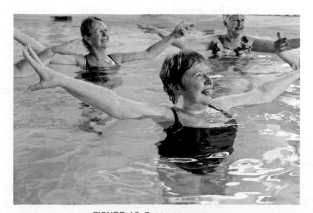

FIGURE 19-6 Healthy aging.

program is appropriate and safe for them. In addition to providing exercise, these programs provide an opportunity for social interaction. Exercising with others provides motivation and makes the effort more worthwhile and pleasant.

4. **Explain the importance of warm-up and cool-down exercise.** Before starting an exercise session, the individual should warm up for approximately 5 minutes. Simple exercises that make the joints limber and slowly stretch the muscles are recommended. Exercises that do not put undue stress on bones and joints are tolerated better by older adults. Older adults must also be aware of the importance of a cool-down period after exercise. Five minutes of slower activities (similar to the warm-up activities) help blood return from the muscles to the central circulation. If an older person stops exercise too suddenly, he or she may experience fainting (syncope) because of inadequate blood flow to brain tissue.

5. **Explain the importance of proper dress for environmental conditions and proper footwear for safety.** Environmental conditions, including heat, cold, high humidity, and air pollution, must be considered when planning activity. Older persons should try to minimize exercise on excessively hot or cold days. On very hot days, activity is best planned for early in the day or later in the evening when the temperature is cooler. Some large cities experience ozone alerts because of excessive air pollution. On ozone alert days, it is wise for all individuals, particularly older adults, to minimize their activity. On warm days, lightweight, loose clothing should be worn to allow the body to cool through evaporation. On extremely cold days, it is wise for older adults to exercise indoors. Cold weather can be extremely stressful for individuals with cardiac or respiratory conditions. If older adults must go outside in cold weather, clothing should be layered to trap heat. A mask or scarf worn over the face and mouth helps warm the air before it enters the respiratory tract.

6. **Review signs and symptoms that necessitate contacting the physician.** Older adults should be aware that any new or unusual pain, weakness, or other untoward symptoms that are experienced during activity should be reported promptly to the physician.

7. **Use any appropriate interventions that are used in the institutional setting** (Nursing Care Plan 19-1).

❖ NURSING PROCESS FOR ACTIVITY INTOLERANCE

Activity intolerance is a state in which the aging individual has insufficient physiologic or psychological energy to accomplish necessary or desired daily activities. Activity intolerance is a common problem for older adults who live a sedentary lifestyle.

▪ Assessment/Data Collection

* Does the person complain of shortness of breath, fatigue, or weakness?
* How much exertion can the person tolerate before shortness of breath or fatigue is noticed?
* Has the person's participation in normal or routine activities decreased?
* Does the person complain of decreased interest in activities?
* What are the person's pulse rate and blood pressure?
* Do the vital signs remain within normal limits with activity?
* Does the person experience orthostatic hypotension?
* Is the person's nutritional intake adequate?

See Box 19-3 for a list of risk factors for activity intolerance in older adults.

▪ Nursing Diagnosis

Activity intolerance

▪ Nursing Goals/Outcomes Identification

The nursing goals for older individuals with activity intolerance are to (1) demonstrate an increased ability to tolerate activity and (2) identify factors that contribute to activity intolerance.

▪ Nursing Interventions/Implementation

The following nursing interventions should take place in hospitals or extended-care facilities:

1. **Identify factors that contribute to activity intolerance.** People stop participating in physical activity for a variety of reasons. The approach that nurses should use depends on the nature of the problem. For example, an older person who stops participating in activities because of depression after the death of a spouse has a very different problem from that of the person who is physically unable to tolerate activity because of cardiac problems. Some aging persons have no real reason for declining activity level other than a belief that it is expected and accepted with old age. As they age, older adults become increasingly sedentary and consequently lose functional abilities. Nurses should be aware of the specific concerns and problems experienced by the individual so that an effective plan of care can be developed.

2. **Identify the activities that older adults view as essential or desirable.** The activities that nurses think are important are often different from those that older adults value. Older adults should be consulted and included in the planning and

Nursing Care Plan 19-1 | Impaired Physical Mobility

Mrs. King is a 73-year-old woman who lives at Poplar Bluff Nursing Home. She was diagnosed 3 years ago with Parkinson's disease. She has bilateral tremors in both arms. She is able to walk but does so very slowly with a rigid, flexed posture. Her coordination and balance are poor. She has experienced occasional falls when ambulating in the hall. She states, "I get tired so easily. My bones and muscles ache all of the time, and recently I've noticed that my fingers and toes tingle." The physician has ordered physical therapy three times a week to maintain her strength and flexibility. Mrs. King participated in pottery activities until recently. She states that these activities are "just too hard for me now."

Nursing Diagnosis
Impaired physical mobility

Defining Characteristics
- Impaired coordination and balance
- Muscle rigidity
- Altered posture
- Slowed movements
- Tremors

Patient Goals/Outcomes Identification
Mrs. King will participate in mobility activities and exercises and maintain mobility at the highest level possible.

Nursing Interventions/Implementation
1. Provide passive range-of-motion exercises twice daily.
2. Encourage Mrs. King to perform active range-of-motion exercises whenever possible.
3. Encourage participation in activities of daily living.
4. Consult with occupational therapy regarding assistive devices for feeding and dressing.
5. Discuss the exercise program with the physical therapist so that exercises can be incorporated into the daily routine on the nursing unit.
6. Have Mrs. King ambulate with the help of an assistant using a gait belt.
7. Provide massage for tight muscles.
8. Schedule daily or every-other-day tub baths for muscle relaxation.
9. Provide adequate periods of rest on a scheduled basis.
10. Encourage continued participation in activities such as music therapy or other relaxing pastimes.
11. Provide positive encouragement for successes.

Evaluation
Slight tremors are still noted in both arms, and Mrs. King moves slowly but with slightly less rigidity than noted previously. No falls have been reported in the past 2 weeks. She states, "I feel stronger since I've been getting the therapy and doing exercises. I even helped get myself dressed today." You will continue the current plan of care.

Critical Thinking Questions
1. What other activities can you identify that are appropriate for Mrs. King?
2. What modifications in the plan of care are likely to be necessary as the disease process progresses?

Box 19-3 | Risk Factors Related to Activity Intolerance in Older Adults

- Sedentary lifestyle
- Decreased sense of self-worth, self-esteem, or independence
- Generalized weakness, immobility, restriction to bed rest
- Problems related to oxygenation
- Cognitive impairment (Alzheimer's disease or dementia)
- Malnourishment

structuring of activities. It is easier to motivate people to work toward goals or activities that they consider important.

3. **Plan activities so that older adults progress from easier activities to those that are more demanding.** Activities should build from the least strenuous toward those requiring a greater amount of physical exertion. Those who are unable to tolerate low levels of activity need to progress slowly, because progression that is too rapid leads to exhaustion, a feeling of failure, and loss of motivation. Once mild activities are tolerated, then activities that are more physically

demanding can be attempted. The pace at which activities are introduced depends on the specific needs and abilities of the individual. Some older adults are able to resume near-normal levels of activity; others always experience some amount of activity intolerance.

4. **Encourage older adults to pace activities throughout the day, alternating periods of activity with periods of rest.** Attempting to do too much in too short a period of time is a common cause of activity intolerance in older adults. Most older adults benefit from a planned approach to activity that includes periods of activity and periods of rest. By pacing activities, the individual usually finds that he or she can accomplish more and feel better.

5. **Monitor vital signs to assess the physiologic response to activity.** Vital signs are good indicators of the older person's ability to tolerate activity. Individuals who have been immobile or sedentary may experience significant changes in vital signs as they increase their activity. Tachycardia is a common occurrence when an activity program is begun. Once the pulse of an aging individual is elevated, it takes longer for it to resume its normal rate than it does in a younger person. Changes in blood pressure, particularly orthostatic hypotension, may pose safety risks to older adults. Those who are sedentary and those who have been on bed rest often experience dizziness or lightheadedness when changing position. This may result in falls if the person is not careful. Changing position more slowly and waiting after each position change helps prevent injuries or falls.

6. **Teach methods of conserving energy.** Simple modifications in activity can help the aging person conserve energy. Sitting while dressing requires less energy than does standing. Dressing in clothing with Velcro grips and zippers is less exhausting than dressing in clothing with small buttons or other difficult fasteners. Slip-on shoes require less energy than do laced shoes. Occupational therapists can provide assistance in modifying the environment so that a maximal amount of activity can be performed with a minimal amount of exertion.

7. **Teach older adults and their families methods of reducing stress.** Both psychological stress and physiologic stress place extra demands on the body and decrease the older person's ability to tolerate activity. Methods for reducing stress are discussed in Chapter 13.

The following interventions should take place in the home:

1. **Modify the environment to reduce energy expenditure and promote safety.** All frequently used objects should be easily accessible. Remote controls for the television, stereo, or lights are desirable. Furniture should be arranged to provide easy access to resting places. Care should be taken to ensure that the environment is safe. Hazards such as throw rugs and other clutter on the floor should be removed.

2. **Identify family or community resources to assist with energy-intensive activities.** The family should be encouraged to assist the aging person in energy-intensive activities such as cleaning, cooking, and laundry. If this is not possible, service agencies such as Meals on Wheels may be available.

3. **Use any appropriate interventions that are used in the institutional setting** (See Nursing Care Plan 19-1).

❖ NURSING PROCESS FOR PROBLEMS OF OXYGENATION

To survive, body tissues and organs must have an adequate supply of oxygen. The respiratory and cardiovascular systems work together to meet the oxygen needs of the body. If either system functions inadequately, a variety of physiologic changes are observed.

In general, the aging heart and lungs are able to meet the demands of a normal activity level. However, under conditions of emotional or physical stress, they may not be able to supply the physiologic needs of the body.

■ Assessment/Data Collection

- Does the person experience excessive fatigue?
- What level of activity causes this fatigue?
- Does the person have any complaints of nausea, vomiting, or anorexia?
- Does the person complain of dyspnea? Is this worse at any specific time of day, such as during the night?
- Does the person complain of chest pain?
- Is the person experiencing tachycardia?
- What is the person's respiratory rate?
- Is the person's breathing silent and effortless? If not, describe.
- Does the person's chest expand evenly with respiration?
- Is breathing deep or shallow?
- Does the person adopt a posture that is more comfortable for breathing?
- Does the person have a cough? If so, is the cough productive?
- What is the appearance of the sputum?
- Does the person have an order for supplemental oxygen?
- Does the person have a history of exposure to air pollution?
- Does (or did) the person smoke?
- Are any signs of cyanosis present? Cold, clammy skin? Diaphoresis?
- Is the skin cool to the touch?

- Are the jugular veins distended? At what angle (30 degrees, 45 degrees)?
- Are the peripheral pulses palpable? Are pulses equal on both sides of the body?
- What color are the nail beds and fingers?
- What is the capillary refill time?
- Does the person have a normal amount of body hair over the feet and lower legs?
- Does the person experience any leg pain with ambulation? If so, how severe is the pain? Is it relieved by rest?
- Does the person complain of cold hands and feet?
- Are signs of peripheral edema present?
- Is the person's urinary output low despite normal fluid intake?
- Has the person had a rapid weight gain of more than 10 pounds?
- Has the person shown signs of confusion?
- Does the person complain of anxiety, loss of ability to concentrate, or insomnia?
- Are there any changes in relevant laboratory values (e.g., hemoglobin, hematocrit, cardiac enzymes, and electrolytes)?
- If an electrocardiogram was done, are there any changes?
- If chest radiography was done, are there any signs of heart enlargement or congestion?

Box 19-4 lists risk factors for problems related to decreased cardiac output in older adults.

■ Nursing Diagnoses

Decreased cardiac output
Impaired gas exchange
Ineffective airway clearance
Ineffective breathing pattern

■ Nursing Goals/Outcomes Identification

The nursing goals for older individuals with gas exchange problems are to (1) maintain an open, patent airway; (2) exhibit an effective respiratory pattern; (3) experience fewer episodes of dyspnea, angina, and cyanosis; (4) demonstrate an increased ability to tolerate activity; (5) identify methods to reduce physical and psychological stress; and (6) manifest signs of improved cardiac function (e.g., stable vital signs, adequate urinary output, and adequate tissue perfusion).

Box 19-4	Risk Factors Related to Decreased Cardiac Output in Older Adults

- Arteriosclerotic changes in the blood vessels
- Congestive heart failure
- Myocardial infarction
- Obstructive pulmonary disease
- Increased physiologic or psychological stress, including anxiety and pain
- Severe anemia

■ Nursing Interventions/Implementation

The following nursing interventions should take place in hospitals or extended-care facilities:

1. **Assess pulse and respiration before, during, and after activity.** Vital signs are good indicators of the ability to tolerate activity. These should be assessed while the individual participates in various levels of activity to determine which specific activities cause the greatest problems. Tachycardia is a common sign of decreased cardiac output. To compensate for the decreased volume, the heart beats more rapidly. This increased rate places increased stress on the heart muscle and can make the problem worse. Once elevated, it takes longer for the heartbeat of older adults to return to a normal resting rate. Consistent tachycardia or an excessive delay in return to a normal rate indicates serious cardiac problems. The respiratory rate is likely to increase with the heart rate because the body is attempting to meet oxygen needs. With severe cardiac problems, fluid may build up in the lungs, interfere with oxygenation, and further stress the heart.

2. **Monitor laboratory values, radiograph reports, and other diagnostic studies.** Laboratory tests, including hematocrit and arterial blood gases, provide information regarding the oxygen-carrying capability of the blood. Results of cardiac enzyme studies (e.g., elevated levels of creatinine phosphokinase and lactate dehydrogenase) can indicate cardiac damage from a myocardial infarction. Electrolyte levels should be evaluated, particularly if the person is receiving diuretics. Chest radiographs can reveal the presence of pulmonary congestion, which could indicate respiratory tract infection or pulmonary edema.

   Other diagnostic tests (e.g., electrocardiography) may reveal pathologic conditions of the heart before other symptoms are obvious. Any abnormal test results should be reported immediately to the physician.

3. **Observe respiratory effort, including the use of accessory muscles.** An individual who has difficulty breathing appears to labor when breathing. Use of the accessory muscles of the abdomen and shoulders is an indication that the individual is working harder than normal to breathe.

4. **Evaluate oxygenation by observing for signs of cyanosis and by checking capillary refill time.** To meet the life-sustaining needs of the body, blood flow to the extremities may be reduced. This results in cold, clammy skin; slow capillary refill time; pallor; and cyanosis. These changes are most often observed in the lips and fingertips. Delayed capillary refill time indicates that blood supply to the extremities is restricted.

5. **Assess the peripheral pulses, particularly in the lower extremities.** Assessment of peripheral pulses reveals any areas of the body that are not receiving adequate oxygen. The lower extremities are most at risk because of the arteriosclerotic changes of aging.

   Inadequate oxygen can result in ischemia and necrosis. Mild ischemia can result in hair loss from the lower extremities. Severe ischemia may result in stasis ulcers and in necrosis of the toes, which often necessitates amputation.

6. **Position the person to maximize chest expansion, and encourage frequent changes of position.** Age-related changes tend to reduce the size of the chest cavity. To maximize oxygen exchange, the person should be encouraged to stand or sit in a position that is as upright as possible. Bedridden individuals should change position frequently to prevent stasis and pooling of respiratory secretions within the lungs.

7. **Clear secretions and teach effective coughing.** Older adults may find it difficult to cough effectively because of loss of muscle strength and tone. The inability to remove secretions from the respiratory tract can increase the risk for respiratory tract infections. If the older person is very weak and unable to remove secretions, suction may be necessary. When suctioning is done, care should be used to avoid excessive stimulation of the respiratory tract, which increases production of secretions.

8. **Administer medication as ordered to promote cardiovascular and respiratory function.** Medications such as cardiotonics may be ordered to strengthen the pumping ability of the heart. Mucolytics, bronchodilators, and expectorants may be ordered to enhance the person's ability to remove respiratory secretions. All precautions regarding these medications must be observed, particularly careful monitoring of vital signs.

9. **Administer supplemental oxygen as ordered.** Increasing the amount of available oxygen by using supplemental oxygen may make breathing easier. Oxygen should be prescribed by the physician and administered at the prescribed rate. Low doses are normally used because high oxygen concentrations decrease respiratory effort. Supplemental oxygen is most commonly administered through a nasal cannula (Figure 19-7). When oxygen is being administered, good care of the nasal passages is essential. The nares should be kept free of secretions, and the skin should be inspected regularly for breakdown where the plastic tubing presses at the nares and over the ears. Safety precautions such as posting of No Smoking signs are important when oxygen is in use.

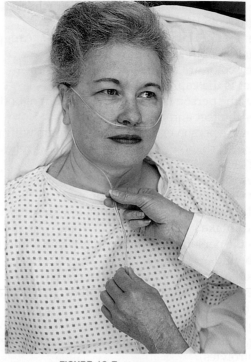

FIGURE 19-7 Nasal cannula.

10. **Use spirometers to improve ventilation.** Spirometers are often ordered by the physician to improve respiratory effort. Many older persons are unfamiliar with these devices and need clear explanations regarding their use. Many older adults find these devices unpleasant and therefore avoid using them. Nurses should continue to reinforce the importance of these devices and encourage the patient to use them at regular intervals.

11. **Assess for the presence, location, and duration of pain.** Pain that occurs during activity should be assessed and reported. Its location and severity, as well as whether it radiates or stays in one area, should be determined. It is important to know whether the pain occurs during an activity or afterward. Anginal pain originates in the heart and occurs when the heart muscle is deprived of oxygen because of coronary artery narrowing or increased oxygen demand. This pain classically starts in the upper left chest and radiates down the left arm. In some individuals, the pain is referred to the jaw. Coronary vasodilators such as nitroglycerin are used to improve blood flow and decrease the pain.

    Intermittent claudication is a specific type of pain that is described by some as cramping, tightness, or aching. This pain is most commonly in the foot or calf, but it may extend to the thigh or buttock. It typically occurs during activity and disappears with rest. Intermittent claudication is an indication of inadequate oxygen supply to the tissues of the leg, and the pain is a result of ischemia. Most physicians recommend daily walking for 60 minutes, pausing when pain occurs. Any activity that causes vasoconstriction (e.g., smoking) must be stopped. Cold environments should also be avoided because cold further aggravates the condition.

12. **Administer sedatives and painkillers with caution.** Many sedatives and analgesics affect the rate or depth of respiration. Respiratory rate and depth should be assessed before these medications are administered to verify that the initial rate is adequate for safety. Respirations should be assessed again after administration.

13. **Maintain a calm, restful environment and provide emotional support.** Stress places additional oxygen demands on the body. A calm, restful environment decreases the effects of stress. Decreasing the number of interruptions, closing doors, playing soft music, or making other environmental changes may benefit an individual who is experiencing stress. If the stress is severe or if it is made worse by interaction with unpleasant roommates, a private room may be medically indicated. Time spent listening to the concerns of older adults is beneficial in reducing their stress.

14. **Explain stress-reduction techniques.** Stress can be controlled by means of nonmedical interventions, including meditation, guided imagery, biofeedback, and relaxation techniques. These techniques are particularly helpful to older adults because they enable the individuals to control their own behavior and lack the side effects of antianxiety medications.

15. **Promote good fluid and nutritional intake within medical restrictions.** Adequate fluid intake keeps respiratory secretions liquefied, making them easier to expectorate. If the older person has congestive heart failure or other disease processes that lead to fluid retention, it is important to give fluids with caution and assess for signs of fluid overload. Adequate nutrition, particularly adequate iron intake, is essential for production of adequate hemoglobin, which is necessary for oxygen transport.

The following interventions should take place in the home:

1. **Explain how to use oxygen equipment safely.** Nurses must ensure that the older person and his or her family know how to operate the equipment. If oxygen is required, the family should be taught safety precautions related to its use. Teaching should include the reasons that smoking and open flames are dangerous. All persons having contact with the oxygen should know the proper precautions to use when handling oxygen tanks and equipment (Figure 19-8). They should know how to verify that adequate oxygen is available and whom to call if any equipment problems arise (Table 19-1).

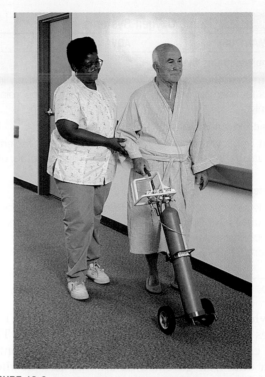

FIGURE 19-8 Portable oxygen cylinder used during ambulation.

A power outage may present a problem to individuals who use an oxygen concentrator. It is wise to keep a backup tank of oxygen for use in such an emergency. It is also wise to notify the power company in advance that the resident needs power returned quickly. Persons needing oxygen or other medical equipment are usually a priority for power companies.

2. **Explain the signs and symptoms of possible complications and the measures to take if these occur.** Older adults and their families should be aware of the signs and symptoms of a change in condition that may indicate complications. The telephone number of the physician and emergency services should be prominently displayed next to the telephone so that help can be summoned rapidly if needed.

3. **Use any appropriate interventions that are used in the institutional setting.**

❖ NURSING PROCESS FOR SELF-CARE DEFICITS

When a person is partially or totally restricted in his or her ability to perform the most basic ADL (i.e., bathing, dressing, grooming, eating, and toileting), a self-care deficit is present. With advanced age or the onset of disease, many individuals experience some degree of problem with self-care. Problems related to self-care can be devastating to older adults because of their effect on self-esteem. People who cannot meet these needs become dependent on others and lose much control over the most basic elements of their lives. Older adults who cannot feed themselves must

Table 19-1	Home Oxygen Systems		
PRIMARY USE	ADVANTAGES	DISADVANTAGES	
Compressed Gas Cylinders			
Intermittent therapy, such as for exercise or sleep only	100% oxygen, relatively inexpensive, no loss of gas during storage, relatively portable, delivery of up to 15 L/min	Bulky, possibly unsightly, frequent refilling necessary with continuous use	
Liquid Oxygen Systems			
High-liter flows for active patients	100% oxygen, conveniently portable, portable units refilled at home, delivery of up to 6 L/min	Usually weekly delivery necessary for refill, evaporates if not used, potential for frostbite at connections and if spilled	
Concentrators			
Moderate-liter flows for patients with limited mobility inside or outside home	Fixed monthly cost, minimal interruption of household by supplier, no refills of main tank, most units with delivery of up to 4 or 5 L/min	Oxygen concentration decreases as liter flow increases (usually 85% to 90%), power supply necessary, increased cost of electricity, second system for portability necessary (usually gas cylinders)	

From Dettenmeier PA: *Pulmonary nursing care,* St Louis, 1992, Mosby.

eat what they are fed. Those who cannot dress themselves must wear what another person chooses. Those who cannot bathe or groom themselves are only as clean and well groomed as another person allows. Those who cannot go to the bathroom alone are likely to become incontinent. Nurses must be able to recognize the individual's specific difficulties and degree of limitation with self-care so that appropriate nursing interventions can be planned. These interventions should be directed toward maintaining the individual's functioning at the highest possible level. The previously discussed concepts of rehabilitation form the basis for working with older individuals with self-care deficits.

■ Assessment/Data Collection

- Can the person feed himself or herself? If not, what level of assistance is required (0-4)?
  0 = Completely independent
  1 = Requires devices or equipment
  2 = Requires help, supervision, or teaching from another person
  3 = Requires devices and help from another person
  4 = Totally dependent
- Can the person toilet himself or herself? If not, what level of assistance is required (0-4)?
- Can the person bathe himself or herself? If not, what level of assistance is required (0-4)?
- Can the person dress himself or herself? If not, what level of assistance is required (0-4)?

Box 19-5 lists risk factors for self-care deficits in older adults.

■ Nursing Diagnoses

Feeding self-care deficit
Bathing/hygiene self-care deficit
Dressing/grooming self-care deficit
Toileting self-care deficit

Box 19-5	Risk Factors Related to Self-Care Deficits in Older Adults

- Decreased strength or endurance resulting from respiratory or cardiovascular changes
- Altered neuromuscular or musculoskeletal function related to disease or aging
- Pain
- Cognitive or perceptual problems (Alzheimer's disease or dementia)
- Severe anxiety or depression
- Impaired mobility

■ Nursing Goals/Outcomes Identification

The nursing goals for older individuals with self-care deficits are to (1) perform self-care at the highest possible level within limitations, (2) demonstrate the use of modified techniques and assistive devices to accomplish self-care, (3) verbalize improved self-esteem related to self-care abilities, and (4) identify resources that are available to provide assistance.

■ Nursing Interventions/Implementation

The following nursing interventions should take place in hospitals or extended-care facilities:

1. **Assess the individual to determine the factors that cause or contribute to the deficit such as age-related changes, disease processes, medications, and cognitive or perceptual changes.** Each aging individual presents a unique set of problems to which nurses must respond when planning care. Unless the specific needs of each person are identified, the plan of care is meaningless. Some individuals are able to regain many skills and become less dependent; others remain at lower levels of function. A good assessment covers the person's strengths and limitations so that the most appropriate care plan can be developed.

2. **Include older adults in problem identification and care planning.** A plan that does not include the individual is likely to fail. Overcoming a self-care deficit requires the person's total commitment and cooperation. The only way nurses can hope to ensure this level of commitment is by including the older person in the entire process. If the aging individual is unable to communicate verbally, nurses should observe nonverbal communication. Many individuals who cannot express their needs verbally will respond to simple directions and positive encouragement.

3. **Allow adequate time for completion of activities.** With aging, even healthy, active persons require more time than do younger individuals to accomplish a task. Those experiencing self-care deficits require even more time than do older adults who are well. Most facilities and nurses are geared toward getting things done as quickly as possible. In many facilities, older individuals who are perfectly capable of completing self-care activities are not allowed to do so because it takes too long. This practice is in opposition to those of the rehabilitative focus. Encouraging and allowing older adults to perform self-care does take more time than having the care provided by the nursing staff. This fact must be taken into consideration when assignments are made so that adequate time is available. If these adjustments are not made, the staff can actively undermine any chance of success.

4. **Develop a plan that moves in stages toward the highest possible level of function, and give positive feedback to reinforce positive changes.** The plan to increase self-care ability should be structured in stages so that the individual achieves some successes. If too much is expected, the individual may become frustrated and give up. It is better to work toward and build on small successes. For example, if the person has not been doing any personal hygiene, successfully washing the face is a major accomplishment. Success of this nature should not be ignored but should be reinforced by a comment such as, "You did a good job washing your face." A simple checklist that enables the person to see that he or she is making progress may be helpful. Reinforcing the positives and minimizing the negatives is the best way to achieve the desired goals and increase motivation.

5. **Consult with occupational and physical therapists to identify alternative methods and equipment that would most benefit the individual.** Occupational and physical therapists are specialists in rehabilitation. They have extensive knowledge of the techniques and equipment available to improve self-care ability. Modification of an activity (such as sitting instead of standing) may enable an individual to perform self-care activities (Figure 19-9). Modified clothing or eating utensils may mean the difference between complete dependence and independence.

6. **Modify the environment with assistive devices designed to meet the specific needs of the individual.** Once the need for special assistive devices is identified, nurses should ensure the availability of these devices (Figures 19-10 and 19-11). Identifying the need for a toilet riser, grip rail, or special spoon does no good if the item is not available. The staff may have to wash special eating utensils so that they are not lost. Residents sharing a bathroom may have to adjust to the presence of a toilet riser. They must either use the riser or be willing and able to remove and replace it when they use the toilet. In some situations, modification of the environment with assistive devices may necessitate room changes so that individuals with common needs are grouped together.

The following interventions should take place in the home:

1. **Assess the ability of the family or significant others to provide safe care.** Many totally dependent older adults are being cared for today in the home setting. Nurses may make regular visits, but much of the responsibility for care falls on spouses or other family members. These caregivers may have little or no training for the tasks involved. Often, the caregiver is elderly or infirm. Nurses are responsible for ensuring that no harm comes from the home care situation. If the care needs exceed the ability of the caregivers, nurses may have to contact other family members or social services to ensure the older individual's safety. If the caregiver is capable of providing care, he or she will probably need additional teaching related to providing care.

2. **Assess the home environment to determine safety and the need for modifications such as grip rails, bath chairs, or toilet risers.** Depending on the level of self-care deficit, the home may require major modification. Individuals with minimal self-care deficits may require only a few assistive devices to function adequately (Figure 19-12). Those with serious self-care deficits require more modifications.

3. **Identify community resources available to help obtain the necessary equipment.** Special assistive devices can be costly and may require special skill for installation. Many communities have agencies or volunteer groups that help provide the necessary assistance.

4. **Inform the families or significant others of the necessity to allow older adults to do as much as possible for themselves.** Family members often are too helpful and do not expect the older individual to do anything for himself or herself, which can lead to a loss of functional ability. Nurses should

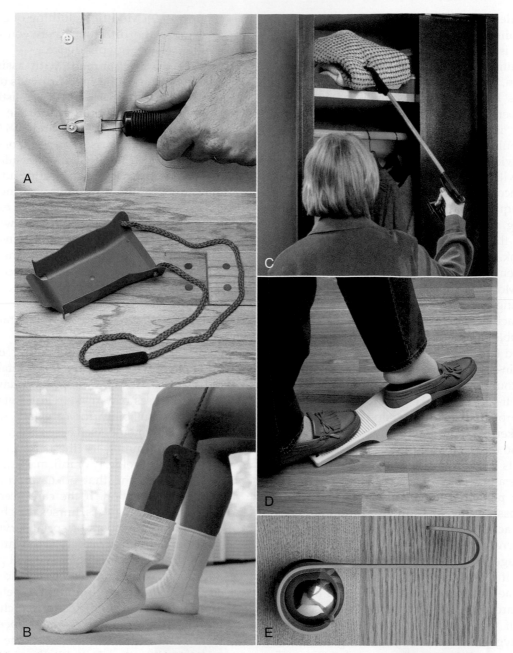

FIGURE 19-9 A, A button hook is used to button and zip clothing. **B,** A sock assist is used to pull on socks and stockings. **C,** "Reachers" are helpful to remove items from high shelves. **D,** A shoe remover is used to take off shoes. **E,** A door knob turner increases leverage to help turn the knob.

explain the importance of allowing and encouraging the aging individual to do as much as possible. Nurses should stress that this is the best thing caregivers can do for their loved ones, and that they are not being thoughtless or neglectful.

5. **Discuss respite care and other options with caregivers.** Anyone who provides long-term care in the home places himself or herself at risk. Home care is often exhausting for the caregivers. It is advisable for nurses to discuss the possibility of some form of respite care so that caregivers are able to maintain their own health and mental well-being.

6. **Assist the family with arrangements for hospitalization or extended-care placement.** When the aging individual becomes completely dependent, the spouse or family may have to consider alternative methods of providing care. This is a very difficult topic, both financially and emotionally. Nurses may be able to provide some guidance or may be able to contact other social service agencies that can help the family through this difficult process.

7. **Use any appropriate interventions that are used in the institutional setting.** (see Nursing Care Plan 19-1).

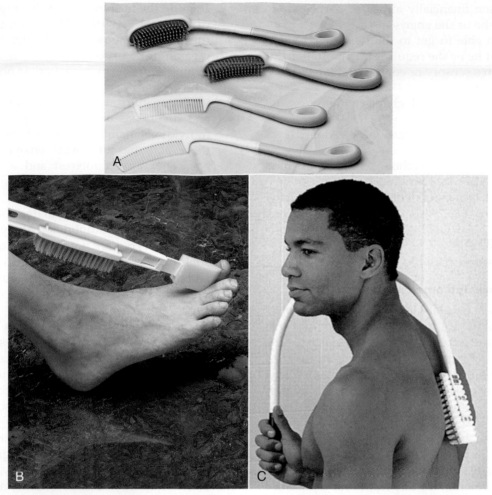

FIGURE 19-10 **A,** Long-handled combs and brushes for hair care. **B,** Long-handled brushes for bathing. **C,** Brush with a curved handle.

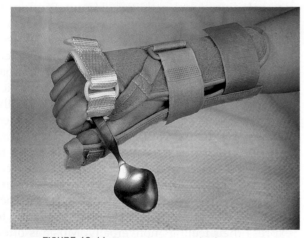

FIGURE 19-11 Eating device attached to a splint.

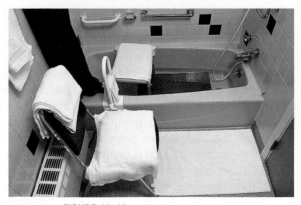

FIGURE 19-12 Bathtub with grab bars.

❖ NURSING PROCESS FOR DEFICIENT DIVERSIONAL ACTIVITY

Diversional activities play an important role in the lives of older adults. Diversional activities can help fill time and provide creative outlets, particularly when they are meaningful to the older person.

■ Assessment/Data Collection

- What activities does the person enjoy?
- How often does the person participate in these activities?
- Does the person prefer solitary or social activities?
- How much time does the person spend alone?
- Does the person interact with other individuals? Who? How often?
- What is the nature of these interactions?

- Can the person financially afford to participate in the activities he or she enjoys?
- Is the person able to get to the desired activities, particularly if he or she requires transportation?
- Do the person's sensory or cognitive changes interfere with interests?
- Do the person's physical changes interfere with interests?
- Is the person napping because of boredom? If so, how often?
- What is the person's psychological state of mind (e.g., depressed)?

Box 19-6 lists risk factors for deficient diversional activity in older adults.

▪ Nursing Diagnosis

Deficient diversional activity

▪ Nursing Goals/Outcomes Identification

The nursing goals for older individuals with deficient diversional activity are to (1) identify activities that might be of interest, (2) express interest in participating in diversional activities, (3) participate in selected diversional activities, and (4) demonstrate socially acceptable behaviors while participating in activities.

▪ Nursing Interventions/Implementation

The following nursing interventions should take place in hospitals and extended-care facilities:

1. **Assess current and past hobbies, activities, and interests.** The best way to prepare for a good old age is to have as many interests as possible when you are young. Young people are so busy raising families and working that they often neglect to develop hobbies or interests outside of family and work. Individuals who have developed a wide range of interests seem to adjust to aging better than do individuals with few interests. After their families have grown and they have retired from work, many men and women finally get the opportunity to participate in hobbies and other activities that they desire. Some older persons have a steady stream of activities that keep their days full. Others complain that there is nothing to do and that they are bored. Lack of interests and diversions makes time seem to pass slowly and may lead to depression and social isolation.

Box 19-6	**Risk Factors Related to Deficient Diversional Activities in Older Adults**

- Restricted mobility
- An environment with limited activities
- Anxiety, depression, or grief
- Limited financial or transportation resources
- Cognitive or perceptual problems

---

2. **Include the individual in selecting and planning diversional activities.** Older adults should have the right to choose the activities they find most meaningful. Purposeful activity is good for maintaining self-esteem; busywork is not. Older adults who reside in extended-care facilities because of illness or infirmity may have fewer opportunities and diversions available. Nurses can help these individuals maintain active interests by exploring those activities that were enjoyed at an earlier age. The nurse's interest and a little creativity can go a long way toward meeting the social and diversional needs of older adults.

3. **Provide suitable reading materials such as large-print books or audiobooks.** Many older persons enjoy books but are not able to read because of visual changes. Books with large print may be usable and are available through most libraries. If visual impairments are severe, audiobooks on tapes or CDs are also available.

4. **Focus on what the individual can do rather than on what he or she cannot do.** Successes, even small ones, are likely to lead to more successes. It is often depressing to older adults to focus on activities that they can no longer do. Directing attention to accomplishments helps the person maintain a more positive attitude.

5. **Suggest activities that are occurring in the facility, such as music or discussion groups, occupational therapy, activity therapy, or religious activities.** Many older persons are not able to leave the care setting to participate in certain activities. Physical or economic changes may interfere with normal diversional activities. Hospitalization or change of living accommodations can lead to a variety of restrictions and inconveniences. Nurses can help individuals maintain social contacts and interests by exploring other activities. Occupational and activity therapists may suggest activities and provide assistance in learning new skills. Activity and occupational therapy are provided in most residential care settings. Therapists can help individuals learn new activities or ways to modify existing interests. For example, if physical changes make knitting too difficult, lap weaving may be possible. Music therapy provides another form of diversion and allows individuals to express their feelings nonverbally. Music is often combined with exercise because rhythm seems to enhance activity.

6. **Work with the activities department to plan new or different activities based on patient input.** Many facilities tend to fall into habits or patterns of repeating the same activities. Many older adults are very creative and should have input into decision making. Some facilities are progressive and offer a variety of activities; others do not. Nurses

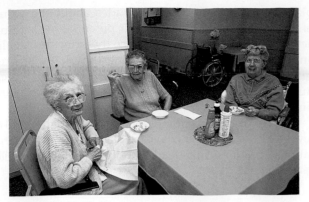

FIGURE 19-13 Residents enjoying an ice cream social.

play a more important role in extended-care facilities and home care than they do in acute care settings.

7. **Encourage social interaction among residents with similar interests.** People of all ages find shared activities enjoyable. Those who share common interests are more likely to want to spend time together (Figure 19-13).

8. **Spend time with individuals to demonstrate interest in their personal interests.** We all need to know that we are special. Even a few minutes spent with an older person will help nurses know that person better and will elicit responses that are more personal. Commenting on clients' latest craft projects or asking how they are enjoying a television show demonstrates interest and caring.

9. **Change the physical environment to increase stimulation and interest (e.g., use of bulletin boards of currently scheduled activities, seasonal themes, and flyers about topics of interest).** Lack of stimulation can lead to loss of interest and disengagement from others. Any device that helps maintain interest and contact with the rest of society will help the aging person remain alert and interested.

10. **Enlist the help of volunteers to read, play games, or just talk with residents.** There is not enough time for nursing staff to meet the needs of all the patients in an institution. Many groups such as Scouts, social clubs, and school groups are interested in providing community service. Volunteering to work with older adults is a very rewarding activity. The resulting intergenerational mix can be a learning experience for both old and young.

11. **Display the results of residents' activities in a prominent place and give recognition to all participants.** Displaying what residents have created (e.g., craft work, creative writing, and other achievements) recognizes their positive accomplishments and enables the staff and visitors to realize that creativity and productivity do not end with old age.

12. **Explore the possibility of new activities such as pet therapy to stimulate interest of withdrawn individuals.** Pet therapy is becoming increasingly common. The benefits of association with animals have been documented in many studies. Older individuals who have pets are healthier and live longer than do those without pets. Institutionalized individuals—even those who have isolated themselves from most human contact—seem to respond to the unquestioning affection given by animals. Some residential care centers have pets that live in the home (Figure 19-14).

13. **Ensure that physical needs are met before and during diversional activities. Make sure assistance is available for toileting, snacks, and transfers.** Many older adults with physical deficits are reluctant to leave their rooms or care units because of fear. Many are afraid that they will not get to a bathroom in time and will embarrass themselves. Others are afraid that no one will be available to help them move from place to place or meet other physical challenges. Nurses should ensure that there is adequate help to meet physical care needs before and during activities. Aging persons should be given the opportunity to use the toilet before leaving the care unit and at regular intervals during the activities. Even diversional activities require increased energy expenditure, so snacks that are in keeping with the prescribed diets should be made available.

The following interventions should take place in the home:

1. **Provide information regarding community resources for older adults, including senior citizen centers, libraries, museums, and volunteer activities.** Many senior citizen centers offer a variety of craft programs, including painting, weaving, woodworking, and pottery. Participation in these activities may provide exposure to crafts that the individual never had the opportunity to try before. Some individuals find real talents that they never suspected they had. Travelogs, movies, or speakers

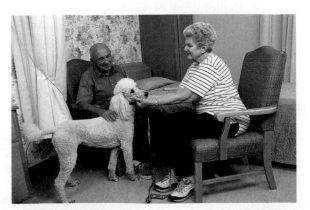

FIGURE 19-14 Pets can be a great comfort to older adults.

on topics of current interest help older adults maintain interest in world events. Activity centers can provide an opportunity for social interaction that reduces the sense of isolation. Aging individuals whose friends have died or moved often find new friends at these centers.

Some senior citizen centers also offer classes in subjects such as foreign languages, history, and even computers. Some colleges allow senior citizens to audit classes on a space-available basis. The senior citizen benefits from the stimulation of the course, and the younger students benefit from the different perspective of the older individual. Elder Hostel is a program through which older adults can travel around the world by staying in hostels and expanding their knowledge. Some older adults are interested in volunteer activities such as foster grandparenting or literacy programs.

2. **Identify community resources that provide transportation to desired activities. Lack of transportation is a common cause for social isolation and failure to participate in activities.** Many communities have special programs that provide buses or vans to transport older adults to shopping centers or activities for a nominal fee. Older adults should be made aware of these services and be assisted with making contact if they are hesitant to call for help.

3. **Explore and identify options for meaningful use of time.** Many older persons look only at the things that they are unable to do and do not consider all of the options available. Spending time exploring interests and possible activities can help expand their outlook.

4. **Encourage participation in new and meaningful activities.** Many older persons need encouragement to seek diversional activities. Many are interested in participating in new activities but are afraid to try because of their age. They often fear that others will not accept them or will laugh at their inexperience. Information that familiarizes the person with the activity can be provided beforehand. Knowledge about the activity can reduce fear of the unknown. Exploration of past successes in facing new or different challenges may provide the necessary encouragement to try something new.

5. **Use any appropriate interventions that are used in the institutional setting.**

REHABILITATION

Our attitudes affect our expectations, and our expectations affect our plans. If caregivers do not expect much from older adults, they will not get much; if caregivers keep their expectations high, much is possible.

The attitudes held by nurses regarding aging and older adults have a significant impact on their planning of nursing care. Attitudes about the value of older persons and about their potential for leading active, meaningful lives influence the priorities, goals, and interventions selected during the planning process. Attitudes also influence the extent to which nurses include and involve older adults in the planning process.

Low expectations for older adults lead to a low-level, or custodial, focus in care planning. High expectations of older adults lead to a high-level, or rehabilitative, focus.

▪ Negative Attitudes: The Controlling or Custodial Focus

Nurses who take a negative view of aging see aging as a process of deterioration and loss. With this negative perspective, older adults are viewed as helpless, passive, dependent, and incapable of making decisions regarding their own care. Nurses who have these negative attitudes generally see little potential for improvement in older adults. Although this may be true for a small percentage of older adults, it is not the norm.

If nurses have predetermined that older adults are incapable of making their wishes known or that they are not interested in what happens, then the nurses will not consider older adults' input important or necessary for care planning. Preferences or desires often go unnoticed merely because the nurse chose not to listen to verbal or nonverbal communication.

Once nurses predict or anticipate little potential for improvement, their expectations are kept low. With a negative attitude toward aging and older adults, priority is given to slowing the process of physical deterioration. Maintenance of function is supported, but no improvement or higher level of functioning is expected or encouraged. Little, if any, attempt is made to reverse or undo any functional losses. Goals are limited to maintaining the existing level of function, or the status quo.

With maintenance as the goal, the care plan is often limited to physiologic and safety concerns. In general, interventions address the lowest level of needs, according to Maslow. Older adults are kept clean, groomed, clothed, and fed. Basic elimination needs are met. Accommodations are clean and reasonably comfortable. Medications are administered, and treatments are performed. However, higher-level needs such as security, love, and a sense of belonging are minimized or ignored.

Nurses then control all aspects of the planning process and take total responsibility for determining what is best for the older person. The care plan requires the nurse to be active and the older adult to be passive. By its very nature, this type of care plan promotes helplessness, loss of function, and dependence on nurses and other caregivers. Little is expected; even less is achieved. A few older persons are severely impaired and have experienced a profound loss of mental and physical capabilities because of aging and disease. Some are so severely affected that they are truly unable to communicate their wishes or do anything for themselves. However, it is amazing how much even severely impaired persons can and will communicate about their care, often nonverbally, if nurses pay attention.

If functional losses are so severe that the person is unaware of reality or is absolutely unable to function, then and only then should all needs be anticipated and provided by nurses or other caregivers. However, this determination should not be made quickly. Many seemingly hopeless and helpless older adults have more ability and potential than we give them credit for. Often, the potential remains hidden because we do not expect to find it.

Negative attitudes that older adults themselves have may lead to declining function. They may feel helpless, hopeless, or afraid to try. If nurses reinforce these negative feelings, nothing positive will occur. Older persons who have potential for improvement but are given only custodial care are likely to lose hope. Loss of the will to fight and of the ability to strive for something better is the most destructive attitude.

■ Positive Attitudes: The Rehabilitative Focus

When nurses have a positive attitude toward aging and believe that older adults are able and willing to participate in their care, the outcome is very different. These nurses recognize that, as older adults experience the normal physiologic changes of aging or the impact of disease, they are more likely to require nursing care. This care may be given in the home, in the hospital, or in an extended-care facility. Nurses who have a positive attitude toward aging recognize that most older people have a great deal of unused and often unrecognized potential. Nurses with a positive attitude toward aging recognize that most aging persons want to retain control of their lives. A rehabilitative care focus addresses both the actual and potential problems older adults are likely to experience. A rehabilitative focus does not wait until problems occur. It is a proactive approach to nursing care planning that deals with the prevention of problems, not just reactions to them.

Most aging persons benefit from a rehabilitative focus in care planning. To plan care with a rehabilitative focus, nurses must (1) acknowledge that older adults have intrinsic worth that exceeds their limitations; (2) accept that older adults have the right to make informed decisions regarding their care; (3) recognize that loss of function or disability has a serious impact on older adults, as well as on their families and significant others; and (4) recognize that older adults, their families, and significant others are important members of the health team and that all should play a role in decision making whenever possible.

The long-term goal of rehabilitative nursing care is to help older adults achieve and maintain maximal physical, psychosocial, and spiritual health. When planning care with a focus on rehabilitation, nurses must (1) attempt to prevent complications of physical disability, restore optimal functioning, and help the individual adjust to alterations in lifestyle; (2) attempt to minimize the impact of physical changes or disease processes that interrupt or alter functioning and life satisfaction; (3) focus on maintaining the highest achievable level of independent function; (4) provide for comfort needs and adjustments in lifestyle that are conducive to health; (5) support the ability of older adults to adapt to change; (6) help aging persons reestablish and maintain control over their lives; and (7) work to reduce the impact of societal factors that restrict the older person's ability to maintain independence.

Under these guiding principles, nurses work with older adults and establish priorities based not on the nurse's values, but on the older adult's values. Goals that are challenging yet realistic are established with the aging patient. The nursing interventions most likely to help these persons achieve their goals are then selected and communicated as the plan of care.

When planning care with a rehabilitative focus, nurses look beyond the nursing interventions and act as coordinators for all of the various disciplines that enable the aging person to achieve the highest level of physical, mental, psychosocial, and spiritual functioning. Nurses seek input from a wide range of specialists, including physicians, pharmacists, dietitians, physical therapists, occupational therapists, speech therapists, activity therapists, dentists, podiatrists, chaplains, and social workers. For older individuals residing in their own homes, nurses consider the environmental impact of the surroundings and the community services available.

All of these specialists, along with the older adult and his or her family, should have input into the development of the care plan. When a formal meeting is held in a hospital or extended-care facility, it is commonly referred to as a *staffing*. Regular reviews of the plan of care should be scheduled to determine whether any modifications are necessary. Information should be shared by all concerned parties and communicated clearly. Interventions should be spelled out in enough detail that all parties are aware of their roles. Older adults should be reminded of their rights to change or modify the plan of care.

A rehabilitation focus is not limited to the care provided in institutional settings. Rehabilitation is also directed toward improving or maintaining the capability of disabled older adults to function in society. Like other healthy, capable adults, nurses are often unaware of environmental barriers that prevent the disabled from accessing goods and services. Box 19-7 provides a good way of assessing the world through the eyes of a disabled person. Nurses who believe that older adults have the desire and ability to maintain high-level function at home and in the community must become social activists and work to make others aware of the needs of the disabled. Much work is needed to make the everyday world accessible to them.

Box **19-7**	Accessibility of Public Places

The term *accessible* means that public transportation and public places (as well as objects therein) are approachable and *usable* by someone with a physical disability. The list of questions below can be used as a guideline to determine accessibility.

- Does public transportation allow entry and appropriate space for people who use wheelchairs?
- Do streets have crosswalk signals for people with vision loss?
- Does the facility have access to someone who can use sign language?
- Are there parking spaces reserved for the disabled? If so, are these parking spaces clearly marked? Are they near the entrance?
- Are there any steps or curbs between the parking area and the front door? If so, how many?
- If the front door is not at ground level, are there:
  - Alternative entrances (e.g., ramp, side door at ground level)?
  - Alternative methods of entry (e.g., restaurant personnel willing and able to assist)?
- Are doorways to public areas at least 28 inches wide (32 inches for an electric wheelchair)?
- Is the doorway threshold no higher than half an inch?
- How many doors are at the entrance? The restroom entrance? If there are consecutive sets of doors, how much space is between them?
- Are entrance doors easily opened (automated, opened with a button or levered handles and a minimum of force)?
- Are reception areas well-marked and lit with desk space available at a suitable height for wheelchair users?
- Are steps leading to the restrooms? Are restroom doors at least 28 (32) inches wide? Is there a wider stall (3 ft × 5 ft)? Are grab bars installed?

- Are walkways and hallways at least 36″ wide and free of obstacles?
- Do directional signs and menus use large print and/or Braille?
- Are any ramped or steep areas sloped 1:10-1:12 with handrails on either side?
- Are drinking fountains no higher than 48 inches from the floor? If not, are drinking cups provided?
- Do elevator doors open at least 28 (32) inches wide? What are the internal dimensions of the elevator? Are elevator buttons set lower? Are there Braille elevator buttons?
- Are public telephones set lower?
- Are there clear routes to emergency exits?
- Are alarm and alert systems both audible and visible?
- Are specially adapted hotel rooms available for the disabled? If yes, how many?*
- If no specially adapted hotel rooms are available, ask the following:
  - Are the doorways to rooms at least 28 (32) inches wide?
  - Is there a sill or step at the door entering the room?
  - At the door entering the bathroom?
  - Are bathroom doors at least 28 (32) inches wide?
  - Does the bathroom door swing in or out? If the door swings in, does it block any of the pluming?
  - Does the room have a bathtub or shower stall? If there is a shower stall, what is its width and depth?
  - Are there grab bars by the toilet, tub, and shower?
  - Are there handheld showerheads?
  - Can a wheelchair fit under the bathroom sink (at least 29 inches of clear space is necessary)?
  - Are telephones no higher than 48″ from the floor and equipped with sound amplifiers?
  - Is there a teletypewriter or teletype display reservations system?
  - Are guide dogs allowed?

*Because of the number of questions involved in checking a hotel's accessibility, you may want to call or email ahead if time permits. Share this checklist with travel agents and others who may make travel arrangements for you. It will increase accessibility awareness and let others know what features are required to meet your needs. Data from Centers for Disease Control and Prevention. (March 30, 2011). "Accessibility." *Disability and health.* Retrieved from www.cdc.gov/ncbddd/disabilityandhealth/accessibility.html; Hampton, C., White, G., & Nary, D. (n.d.). "Increasing access for people with physical disabilities." *The Community Tool Box.* Retrieved from http://ctb.ku.edu/en/tablecontents/sub_section_tools_1223.aspx#tool3; and Sacred Heart Rehabilitation Institute at Columbia St. Mary's (Milwaukee, Wisconsin).

Get Ready for the NCLEX® Examination!

Key Points

- The ability to perform activity and exercise requires that the musculoskeletal, respiratory, cardiovascular, and nervous systems work together effectively.
- Age- and disease-related changes in these systems contribute to the decreased level of activity that is common with aging.

- Any problems with activity and exercise can result in lifestyle changes for older adults.
- Careful assessment and prompt initiation of appropriate nursing interventions help older adults achieve and maintain the highest level of function possible.

Additional Learning Resources

SG Go to the Study Guide on pp. 379–397 for additional learning activities to help you master the chapter content.

evolve Go to your Evolve website (http://evolve.elsevier.com/Wold/geriatric) for the following FREE learning resources:

- Animations
- Answer Guidelines for Nursing Care Plan Critical Thinking Questions
- Answers and Rationales for Review Questions for the NCLEX® Examination
- Glossary with pronunciations in English and Spanish
- Video Clips

Review Questions for the NCLEX® Examination

1. The nurse would recommend the following activities as appropriate for an elderly patient with no serious medical problems: (Select all that apply.)

    1. Swimming three times per week
    2. Jogging every other day
    3. Ballroom dancing weekly
    4. Tai chi every day
    5. Walking three or four times per week
    6. Stretching exercise daily
    7. Step aerobics weekly

2. Identify five benefits of exercise for older adults.

    1. _____
    2. _____
    3. _____
    4. _____
    5. _____

3. The nurse is caring for a patient with a history of severe cardiac problems. The goal is to use exercise to maintain the highest level of function possible. To prevent hypertension or use of the Valsalva maneuver, precautionary teaching should include directions to:

    1. Breathe through your mouth while exercising.
    2. Start slowly and work up until you feel short of breath.
    3. Limit exercises to range of motion and stretching.
    4. Perform isotonic and isometric exercise frequently.

4. A diagnosis of activity intolerance related to oxygenation problems was made. The nurse knows the client needs more teaching when he or she states:

    1. "I'll need to rest if my pulse rate gets too fast."
    2. "I need to do my activities quickly to get everything done."
    3. "I need to work on strategies that reduce my stress."
    4. "I'll use my oxygen so I can breathe easier."

5. An elderly client residing in a community-based residential facility, CBRF, states "I just don't know what to do except sleep. I worked hard all my life, I never had the time or money to do lots of things." The most appropriate nursing intervention would be to:

    1. Schedule the patient to join a museum trip with the local senior center.
    2. Select books and videos from the library to occupy his time.
    3. Refer him to occupational therapy for evaluation.
    4. Explore the variety of activities that are now available to him.

Sleep and Rest

Objectives

1. Describe normal sleep and rest patterns.
2. Describe how sleep and rest patterns change with aging.
3. Discuss the effects of disease processes on sleep.
4. Describe methods of assessing changes in sleep and rest patterns.
5. Identify older adults who are most at risk for experiencing disturbed sleep patterns.
6. Identify selected nursing diagnoses related to sleep or rest problems.
7. Describe nursing interventions that are appropriate for older individuals experiencing problems related to disturbed sleep patterns.

Key Terms

apnea (ĂP-nē-ă) (p. 330)
boredom (p. 334)
circadian (sĭr-KĀ-dē-ăn) (p. 328)
diurnal (dī-ŬR-năl) (p. 328)
fatigue (p. 328)

hypnotic (hĭp-NŎT-ĭk) (p. 334)
insomnia (ĭn-SŎM-nē-ă) (p. 329)
nocturnal (nŏ-TŬR-năl) (p. 330)
sedative (SĔD-ă-tĭv) (p. 334)

SLEEP-REST HEALTH PATTERN

The sleep-rest health pattern describes the patterns of sleep, rest, and relaxation that are exhibited throughout the 24-hour day. Individual perceptions, rituals, and aids used to promote sleep and rest are included.

No one knows exactly why we sleep, but it is a fact that we all require sleep to function normally. Sleep apparently allows the body time to rejuvenate and to respond to the stresses of daily living. Lack of adequate sleep can affect health and behavior. Studies have connected sleep deprivation and insomnia to altered appetite; fatigue; decreased ability to perform tasks that require high-level coordination; increased traffic accidents, home accidents, falls, and irritability; emotional instability; difficulty with concentration; and impaired judgment.

Many older people experience problems related to sleep. It is estimated that as many as half of all independent-living older adults and two-thirds of institutionalized older adults have sleep disturbances. Sleep-related problems can be troubling to the aging individual and often are the basis of visits to the physician and complaints to the nurse. Some of these problems result from changes that normally occur with aging; others may be caused or aggravated by acute or chronic health problems. Nurses must understand normal sleep patterns and be able to identify common age-related changes in sleep patterns and common sleep disorders to assess, plan, and intervene appropriately and effectively.

NORMAL SLEEP AND REST

Periods of sleep and wakefulness occur in regular and somewhat predictable cycles. Most humans develop a pattern that repeats approximately every 24 hours. This cycle occurs in response to the day-night cycle of the sun and is referred to as circadian (from the Latin word meaning "about a day") or diurnal (from the Latin word meaning "daily") rhythm. Within this cycle, individuals develop their own unique patterns for waking and sleeping.

The usual times that people go to bed and rise differ widely among individuals. Some go to sleep at 10 p.m. and rise at 6 a.m.; others go to sleep at midnight and rise at 8 a.m. These sleep-wake patterns can be disturbed by shift work, time-zone changes, illness, emotional stress, medications, and numerous other factors. The amount of sleep needed also varies widely among individuals. Some individuals function normally with less than 6 hours of sleep, whereas others require 9 hours of sleep or more to feel rested. The average amount of sleep required for people ages 20 to 60 years is 7.5 hours per day.

Sleep is under the control of the central nervous system. Current research indicates that wakefulness is regulated by the neurotransmitter norepinephrine. Sleep appears to be controlled by the release of serotonin within the brainstem. Melatonin, which is produced by the pineal gland, is released when the level of light decreases. Levels of cortisol and growth hormone also affect sleep. Sleep is not a uniform state of unconsciousness; rather, it is divided into a series of cycles of lighter and deeper stages of sleep. Immediately before falling asleep, most adults experience a stage of increased relaxation and drowsiness that typically lasts from 10 to 30 minutes. This is followed by four to six complete sleep cycles lasting between 1 and 2 hours each. Each cycle consists of four non-rapid eye movement (NREM) stages and one rapid eye movement (REM) stage (Box 20-1 and Figure 20-1). As the night's sleep progresses, REM periods increase in length and NREM periods decrease in length. If sleep is

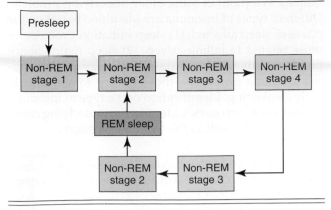

FIGURE 20-1 The adult sleep cycle.

interrupted at any time, the individual goes back to stage 1 of NREM sleep and begins a new cycle.

SLEEP AND AGING

As a person ages, the levels of hormones associated with sleep change. Decreases in melatonin (which regulates the sleep-wake cycle) and growth hormone (which promotes sleep) lead to a shifting in circadian rhythm, causing many elderly people to feel sleepy earlier in the evening and to awake earlier in the morning.

Because sleep efficiency decreases as age increases, many older adults complain that they do not feel refreshed after sleep. Although the amount of time spent in bed may increase with age, the amount of time actually spent sleeping decreases. The average 70-year-old sleeps only 6 hours per night, which is 1.5 hours less than most younger adults sleep. A decreased amount of time is spent sleeping, and the nature of the sleep changes. Older individuals experience more stage 1 and fewer stages 3 and 4 of NREM sleep and somewhat less REM sleep. REM sleep occurs earlier in the sleep cycle than seen in younger adults. These changes result in less deep restorative and refreshing sleep. Circadian rhythm also appears to change with age, resulting in earlier bedtime and earlier rising. It is suspected that this alteration in circadian rhythm is a result of earlier drop in core body temperature, decreased light exposure, or even genetic factors. In addition, sleep interruption and nocturnal awakening are increasingly common because older adults are more easily aroused by environmental noise or stimuli.

SLEEP DISORDERS

Insomnia

The risk for sleep disorders increases with age. Studies show that up to 40% of older individuals report experiencing sleep difficulties at least a few nights each month. The most commonly reported sleep disorder is **insomnia**, which is defined as difficulty falling asleep or remaining asleep or the belief that one is not getting enough sleep. Insomnia is not a disease in itself but

---

Box 20-1   **Stages of Sleep Cycle**

STAGE 1: NREM
Stage includes lightest level of sleep.
Stage lasts a few minutes.
Decreased physiologic activity begins with gradual fall in vital signs and metabolism.
Person is easily aroused by sensory stimuli such as noise.
Awakened, person feels as though daydreaming has occurred.

STAGE 2: NREM
Stage is period of sound sleep.
Relaxation progresses.
Arousal is still relatively easy.
Stage lasts 10 to 20 minutes.
Body functions continue to slow.

STAGE 3: NREM
Stage involves initial phases of deep sleep.
Sleeper is difficult to arouse and rarely moves.
Muscles are completely relaxed.
Vital signs decline but remain regular.
Stage lasts 15 to 30 minutes.

STAGE 4: NREM
This is deepest stage of sleep.
It is very difficult to arouse sleeper.
If sleep loss has occurred, sleeper will spend considerable portion of night in this stage.
Vital signs are significantly lower than during waking hours.
Stage lasts approximately 15 to 30 minutes.
Sleepwalking and enuresis may occur.

REM SLEEP
Vivid, full-color dreaming may occur. Less vivid dreaming may occur in other stages.
Stage usually begins about 90 minutes after sleep has begun.
It is typified by autonomic response of rapidly moving eyes, fluctuating heart and respiratory rates, and increased or fluctuating blood pressure.
Loss of skeletal muscle tone occurs.
Gastric secretions increase.
It is very difficult to arouse sleeper.
Duration of REM sleep increases with each cycle and lasts an average of 20 minutes.

rather a symptom of some other underlying problem. Different types of insomnia are identified based on the phase of sleep affected: (1) sleep initiation problems—those related to falling asleep, (2) sleep maintenance problems—those related to staying asleep, or (3) terminal insomnia problems—those related to abnormally early awakening. Identification of the type of insomnia problem can help nurses identify the underlying cause or causes and result in the best interventions.

Baby Boomers have been found to be chronically sleep-deprived with more than half of adults over age 50 reporting that they get less than 7 hours of sleep per night. According to a study done by the Institute of Medicine, 50 to 70 million Americans suffer from sleep disorders, which have been associated with a wide range of deleterious health conditions, including increased risk for hypertension, diabetes, obesity, depression, heart attack, and stroke. The magnitude of problems reported does not bode well for the future, as Baby Boomers continue to age.

Older individuals with existing health problems are more likely to experience sleep problems than those who report themselves to be in good health. Insomnia can be related to a variety of medical conditions, medications, and psychological, behavioral, or environmental factors. Medical conditions that cause pain, interfere with breathing, or cause frequent bladder or bowel elimination can contribute to frequent awakening. Common medical problems that may lead to insomnia include arthritis, bursitis, gastroesophageal reflux, chronic obstructive pulmonary disease (COPD), congestive heart failure, sleep apnea, prostatic problems, cystitis, and others. Nocturnal movement disorders, including restless leg syndrome (RLS), which is an irresistible urge to move the lower extremities, or nocturnal myoclonus, which causes sudden repetitive jerking or kicking movements of the lower extremities, can also contribute to insomnia in older adults.

Anxiety is likely to be related to difficulty falling asleep and interrupted sleep. Depression is most likely to be associated with early awakening but may also be related to hypersomnia (excessive sleepiness at a time of normal wakefulness). People with dementia often experience abnormal sleep cycles and are prone to waking and wandering during the night. Both prescription and over-the-counter (OTC) medications are likely to affect sleep in older adults (Table 20-1). Some medications make falling asleep more difficult, whereas others cause frequent awakening (Box 20-2). A few medications can result in hypersomnolent responses.

Behaviors that contribute to sleep problems include physical inactivity, poor sleep routines, late-night eating or exercise, the use of tobacco, and consumption of alcohol or caffeine. Environmental factors such as excessive noise, light, activity, or other distracting stimuli can also contribute to the problem. Afternoon sleepiness is common with aging. Naps may adversely affect nighttime sleeping, particularly if the nap is taken too late in the afternoon or lasts too long. Occasional naps of less than 30 minutes are usually not a problem. Box 20-3 lists risk factors for problems related to sleep or rest in older adults.

Table 20-1 Characteristics of Selected Medications Used to Promote Sleep

CLASSIFICATION	EXAMPLES	PRECAUTIONS
Sedative/hypnotics GABA receptor agents	Zolpidem tartrate	May cause morning drowsiness, headache, hangover, dizziness, or paradoxic excitement
Benzodiazepines	Flurazepam, temazepam, estazolam, lorazepam, clonazepam	Likely to cause daytime sedation and short-term memory impairment in older adults, particularly with long-acting forms; associated with increased risk for falls; paradoxic excitement may occur; must be avoided in individuals with sleep apnea; legislation restricts use in nursing home settings
Tricyclic	Diphenhydramine	May result in agitation, confusion, orthostatic hypotension, urinary retention, and arrhythmias; can make the quality of sleep less restful; not preferred for older adults
Antidepressants	Amitriptyline, desipramine, nortriptyline	Potential side effects include urinary retention, constipation, orthostatic hypotension, and confusion; risk for cardiac arrhythmias, fatigue, headache, blood dyscrasias, altered blood glucose readings, nausea, and photosensitivity
Antidepressants SSRI, MAOI	Imipramine, Fluoxetine, Buspirone	Affect amount (increase or decrease) of REM sleep; danger of overdose; daytime hangover;
Others	Chloral hydrate Barbiturates such as phenobarbital	Sedation with hangover effects; severe interaction with other sedatives; gastrointestinal toxicity. Addictions; loss of effectiveness with chronic use; low lethal dose

GABA, gamma-amino butyric acid; MAOI, monoamine oxidase inhibitor; REM, rapid eye movement; SSRI, selective serotonin reuptake inhibitor.
Modified from Pagel JF and Parnes BL: *Medications for the treatment of sleep disorders,* Primary Care Companion J Clin Psychiatry, 3(3), 2001.

Box 20-2	Drugs That Contribute to Sleep Disorders

- Caffeine
- Alcohol
- Xanthine derivatives—theophylline
- Bronchodilators—terbutaline, albuterol, metaproterenol, etc.
- Decongestants—pseudoephedrine, phenylpropanolamine
- Hormones—cortisone, thyroxine, progesterone
- Diuretics—furosemide
- Neuroleptics—phenytoin, levodopa, methylphenidate, etc.
- Antidepressants—SSRIs, MAOIs, bupropion, etc.
- Antihypertensives—clonidine, propranolol, atenolol, methyldopa, reserpine
- Antineoplastics—interferon, medroxyprogesterone, pentostatin, etc.
- Anticholinergics—ipratropium bromide
- Antihistamines (paradoxic reactions)
- Benzodiazepines (paradoxic reactions)

MAOI, monoamine oxidase inhibitor; SSRI, selective serotonin reuptake inhibitor

Box 20-3	Risk Factors Related to Sleep or Rest Problems in Older Adults

- Pain
- Chronic respiratory or cardiovascular problems
- Frequent elimination
- Nocturnal movement disorders
- Anxiety, depression, or delirium
- Drugs likely to interfere with sleep
- Excessive environmental stimuli
- Excessive caffeine, alcohol, or tobacco use
- Sedentary lifestyle

Occasional problems with insomnia are experienced by individuals of all ages, but these random, acute episodes are likely to result in chronic insomnia if not properly addressed. Chronic insomnia can result in daytime sleepiness, irritability, decreased ability to concentrate, and other problems related to sleep deprivation. Daytime sleepiness is often ignored or excused as a normal change of aging rather than viewed as a symptom of sleep deprivation.

Health Promotion

Teaching to Promote Adequate Sleep

- Establish a regular bedtime and wake-up time, and follow this schedule as closely as possible.
- Develop a daily exercise program, preferably early in the day and outdoors.
- Avoid naps or limit them to no more than 30 minutes and no later than early afternoon.
- Avoid beverages containing caffeine such as coffee, cola, tea, hot chocolate, etc.

- Avoid use of alcohol and tobacco, particularly in the evening.
- Avoid eating large meals late at night.
- Try taking a warm bath or shower.
- Use relaxation breathing or meditation techniques. Try listening to audiotapes with relaxing music.
- Establish a restful sleep environment with a comfortable bed, good pillow and covers, shades or curtain to block out light, comfortable temperature, etc.
- If you cannot fall asleep after 30 minutes, do not get upset. Get up. Read, watch TV, or do something relaxing until you feel tired. Then go back to bed.

Treatment of insomnia includes both nonpharmacologic and pharmacologic approaches. Nonpharmacologic approaches include sleep hygiene education, relaxation therapies, cognitive-behavioral therapy, and other behavioral interventions. Pharmacologic approaches include the use of drugs such as antihistamines, antidepressant agents (most often benzodiazepines), and hypnotic agents. These medications are usually prescribed for limited periods and only when other approaches are not effective. Sleep-inducing medications are likely to have deleterious effects on older adults, such as urinary retention, drowsiness, fatigue, confusion, and disturbed coordination, which increases the risk for falls. Newer drugs with fewer side effects are under study.

Complementary and Alternative Therapies

Insomnia

The herb valerian has been reported to have positive effects on sleep. However, the results of clinical trials of this substance have not conclusively shown benefits. Studies of OTC preparations of melatonin have shown mixed effectiveness for the treatment of insomnia in older adults. Because OTC melatonin is not regulated by the FDA, concerns exist in the medical community regarding the purity and consistency of this product. There are also questions regarding the safety of melatonin because in vitro studies have shown it to be associated with coronary vasoconstriction.

Sleep Apnea

Sleep apnea, also called *sleep disordered breathing*, is a common problem with aging. Studies report that as many as 45% to 65% of the elderly population are suspected to have some breathing problem that disturbs sleep. Obstructive sleep apnea caused by a collapse of the airways is the most common problem experienced. Men are more likely to experience sleep apnea, but obesity, hypertension, and diabetes have also been correlated to its occurrence. Sleep apnea has been found to be more common and more severe in African Americans than in Caucasians. Signs of sleep apnea include excessively loud snoring interspersed with periods of apnea lasting 10 to 30 seconds. Lack of oxygen causes the person to awaken frequently throughout the night, although the person may not be aware of it. This cycle repeats hundreds of times each night. Recurrent disturbance of sleep results in daytime sleepiness. Individuals experiencing obstructive sleep apnea are also at increased risk for developing cardiovascular complications, including hypertension, arrhythmias, myocardial infarctions, and stroke. People experiencing sleep apnea should try to lose weight and avoid alcohol, sedatives, and muscle relaxants, which can worsen the condition. Sleeping in the supine position may also make the condition worse, so a side-lying position is recommended. Mechanical oral or dental devices that prevent relaxation of tissues may help some individuals. Continuous positive airway pressure (CPAP) devices are another common treatment. Occasionally, surgery is recommended. Many individuals need a combination of interventions to control the problem.

REM Sleep Behavior Disorder

REM sleep behavior disorder is a less common problem seen most often in men in their sixties and seventies. Muscle activity is normally inhibited during REM, so little or no gross muscle activity occurs during dreams. However, when a person experiences REM sleep behavior disorder, this protective mechanism does not operate effectively, and the older individuals may thrash around in bed, jump or fall out of bed, or sustain an injury as they attempt to protect themselves from vivid or violent dreams. Manifestation of this disorder may be a predecessor to the development of Parkinson's disease or dementia. Long-acting benzodiazepines are frequently used to treat this disorder.

❖ NURSING PROCESS FOR DISTURBED SLEEP PATTERN

When assessing sleep patterns in older adults, nurses must use a combination of objective and subjective data. Simply because an older individual's eyes are closed during nighttime checks does not mean that the person is asleep. Nurses should watch closely for signs of fatigue and decreased participation in activities and should ask older adults how they feel about the adequacy of their sleep and rest.

■ Assessment/Data Collection

- Does the person feel rested after a night's sleep?
- What time does the person normally go to bed and rise?
- Is the person allowed to choose the time he or she goes to bed, or is the time chosen by someone else?
- Does the person sleep continuously through the night, or does he or she have interrupted sleep?
- Does the caregiver or bed partner report any abnormal breathing pattern, excessive snoring, or unusual movement during sleep?

- What causes the person to awaken? Pain? Noise? Other factors?
- Does the person have difficulty falling asleep?
- Does the person awaken early?
- Does the person nap or sleep during the day?
- Does the person ever fall asleep during activities?
- Has the person's behavior changed? Is the person increasingly irritable, disoriented, or lethargic?
- Does the person appear to be tired?
- Have any signs such as yawning or dark circles under the eyes been observed?
- Does the person complain of feeling tired? When?

■ Nursing Diagnosis

Disturbed sleep pattern

■ Nursing Goals/Outcomes Identification

The nursing goals for older individuals diagnosed with disturbed sleep pattern are to (1) verbalize an understanding of sleep changes associated with aging, (2) verbalize appropriate interventions to promote sleep, and (3) report feeling rested and refreshed on rising.

■ Nursing Interventions/Implementation

The following interventions should take place in hospitals and extended-care facilities:

1. **Identify the factors that contribute to sleep disturbance.** Nurses must identify the cause of sleep disturbance so that the most appropriate interventions can be selected. Various internal and external factors can interfere with sleep. Pain, whether it is chronic or acute, interrupts or prevents sleep. The causes of pain must be identified and measures taken to make the older person as comfortable as possible. Medical conditions and the medications taken to treat them can affect sleep. Older persons with cardiovascular disease are likely to experience anginal pain during REM sleep that causes them to awaken. Patients with ulcers secrete excessive amounts of acid during REM sleep, causing pain and awakening. Individuals with COPD may experience dyspnea related to lying down during sleep. This may result in oxygen hunger and anxiety and may interfere with sleep. Anxiety and depression often result in early-morning rising and an inability to return to sleep once awakened. Medications for hypertension commonly cause altered sleep patterns. Environmental factors, including lighting, noise, and temperature change, also should be considered.
2. **Schedule nursing interventions to allow for adequate undisturbed sleep.** Nursing and medical interventions can interfere with sleep. Medication administration, dressing changes, or toileting can interrupt sleep. Although nurses do not have total control over the scheduling of medications and treatments, they should attempt to formulate a

plan that causes the least interference with sleep. For example, if diuretic medications are given close to bedtime, urinary frequency may prevent the individual from getting continuous sleep. A schedule change that involves giving the diuretic agent early in the morning will decrease this problem. If a procedure is not essential for the well-being of an individual, it should not be scheduled during the night. Many treatments and medications are now specifically ordered to be given to the patient while he or she is awake to eliminate any confusion or concern regarding interpretation of the order. The benefits to the patient must be weighed against the risks of sleep deprivation.

Clinical Situation

Sleep and Rest

Mrs. Jones, age 79, had some problems with incontinence but no difficulty participating in her activities of daily living until she was placed on a toileting schedule in which she was reminded to use the bathroom every 3 hours—day and night. After being awakened 5 nights in a row, she began to display an inability to dress and feed herself. Staff members began to search for symptoms of illness or disease to account for this change, but they found none. Nursing notes indicated that Mrs. Jones was attending fewer activities, and she was observed napping in her room on several occasions. On the sixth night of toileting, Mrs. Jones remarked, "If you would just let me sleep, I'd feel better."

The nurse put these pieces of information together and realized that, although the toileting schedule reduced problems with incontinence, it caused other problems related to sleep. After a discussion with Mrs. Jones, her physician, and her family, it was determined that using incontinence briefs during the night would be the lesser of the evils. After three nights of uninterrupted sleep, Mrs. Jones began to dress and feed herself again and to participate in social activities instead of napping.

3. **Plan bedtimes and wake-up times to meet the individual's needs and desires rather than the institution's.** Although a regular bedtime schedule is advisable, this time should be chosen with input from the aging person. The fact that an older person resides in an institutional setting does not mean that sleep patterns established over a lifetime should change to fit the institution. The institution should allow for individual preferences. Many older persons find that they cannot sleep once they have gone to bed. They often lie awake and become increasingly anxious. This anxiety further interferes with their ability to fall asleep. If the person is unable to sleep after 20 to 30 minutes, he or she should be encouraged to get up and quietly watch television, read, or listen to music. A lounge should be available so that this activity does not disturb the sleep of others. When the individual

is tired, he or she should then return to bed. This supports the mental connection that bed is a place for sleep.

4. **Allow the individual to maintain rituals that help induce sleep.** Many older persons have rituals that help them sleep. These presleep rituals are highly individual and include hygiene activities, the use of special pillows, praying, and a variety of other activities. Nurses should discuss individual preferences and incorporate these into the plan of care.

5. **Assist in providing an environment that is conducive to sleep.** To prevent awakening roommates, nurses should use the minimum amount of light necessary and make as little noise as possible when checking patients or performing required treatments. Ideally, individuals sharing a room should have similar sleep schedules. A schedule for routine rounds should be established so that even if nightly sleep is interrupted, it is at the same time each night. If possible, place individuals who have sleep difficulties in rooms away from noisy telephones, workrooms, and other loud areas. Noise that goes unnoticed during the day, particularly conversation near the nurses' station and unanswered call systems, can disturb sleep at night. Because of changes in circulation, many older individuals need an extra blanket for comfort at night. A warm, light blanket that does not feel heavy is preferred by many aging individuals.

Coordinated Care

Supervision

Minimizing Disturbances at Night

The supervising nurse should schedule activities such as treatments and medications so that they minimize the number of times a patient will be disturbed during the night. In addition, the nurse needs to communicate to other staff members that excessive noise from conversations or equipment use should be minimized because it can easily disturb the sleep of elderly patients who already may have difficulty sleeping.

6. **Modify lighting through the day to imitate normal daily patterns.** Most institutions do not provide adequate light during the day to allow the body to maintain normal circadian rhythm. Bright lighting should be provided during the daytime, particularly during winter months. Dark rooms are best for sleep, but this may not be feasible in institutional settings. Lighting that allows for safety but does not interfere with sleep should be provided. Curtains and doors should be positioned to avoid undesired light. Some individuals can sleep only if there is a night-light; others are disturbed by any light.

7. **Provide comfort measures to promote sleep.** A comfortable environment promotes sleep. The bed linens should be clean, dry, and free of

wrinkles. Top linens should be tightened or loosened to provide the greatest comfort. Sleepwear should be nonrestricting and of the type preferred by the individual (see Figure 20-2). Oral hygiene should be encouraged or provided. Older adults should be encouraged to empty the bladder before going to bed to avoid the need to get up once they become sleepy. Nocturia occurs most commonly within a few hours of going to sleep. In addition, if the older person is left wet, sleep is disturbed for several hours. Awakening the person and changing wet clothes usually results in a return to normal sleep.

8. **Administer sleep medications (sedatives and hypnotics) as ordered.** Nurses should assess their patients or residents for desired effects and untoward effects of sleep medications. Because many medications that are used to promote sleep can cause orthostatic hypotension, individuals should be observed for dizziness, position changes should be made slowly, and assistance should be provided during ambulation to reduce the risk for falls or other injuries.

   Medications to promote sleep should be a last resort because many sedative and hypnotic drugs can leave older adults with lingering or hangover effects and can contribute to insomnia. These drugs can actually lead to disturbed sleep because they alter the nature and quality of sleep. Long-acting drugs can be retained in the body for an excessive amount of time, potentially leading to confusion, disorientation, and daytime sleepiness. Medications that affect respiration should be used with extreme caution in older adults. Low doses of drugs with short half-lives are best tolerated by older adults.

9. **Provide nutritional supplements that aid sleep.** A light snack or beverage before bed is commonly requested. Caffeinated beverages such as coffee should be discouraged, because caffeine can interfere with sleep. Decaffeinated coffee, herbal tea, and milk are good choices. Milk is often

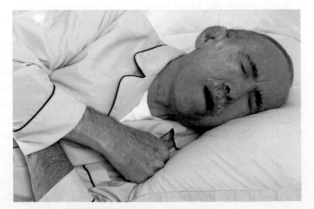

FIGURE 20-2 Nonrestricting sleepwear.

suggested because it contains tryptophan, which has sleep-inducing properties. Heavy meals put extra stress on the body and should be avoided near bedtime. Alcoholic beverages should also be discouraged because they may interfere with the normal sleep cycles and may lead to awakening because of diuresis.

10. **Promote emotional comfort by spending time listening to concerns.** Anxiety and depression interfere with sleep. A back rub or a few minutes of quiet conversation at bedtime may help relieve the concerns of the day and promote sleep in older adults. Relaxation training or other stress management techniques may be appropriate for some individuals.

11. **Observe patients for patterns of fatigue or napping throughout the day.** Excessive napping or fatigue during the day can interfere with nighttime sleep. Nurses should assess for daytime behaviors that affect sleep. If individuals spend too much time napping, nurses should determine the reason. If boredom is the cause, diversional activities should be increased. If the individual is too fatigued or stimulated by the day's activities, then more frequent rest periods should be encouraged.

   The following interventions should take place in the home:

1. **Use a journal to assess sleep and rest patterns.** Many older individuals who complain of sleep problems are unaware of their daily routines. Keeping a journal to record naps, bedtimes, periods of awakening, and time of rising in the morning often yields important information. If the individual cannot do this alone, a spouse or relative may assist. Any information that may be relevant (e.g., pain and nocturia) should be noted. Loud snoring and apnea are more likely to be noticed by a close family member than by the affected party. Reports of these behaviors should be referred to the physician for follow-up.

2. **Explain the importance of adequate activity and exercise throughout the day.** Adequate exercise and activity help promote good sleep. Excessive activity should be avoided within 2 hours of bedtime because such activity may raise body temperature and actually interfere with sleep.

3. **Assist older adults in establishing an environment that promotes rest and sleep.** Nurses should verify that the conditions in the home promote rest and sleep and that the older individual has an adequate bed and suitable covers. They should also make sure heating is adequate. If noise from neighbors or traffic is a problem, possible ways of dealing with this should be discussed.

4. **Discuss limiting fluid intake at night if nocturia is a problem.** If nocturia is interrupting sleep, older adults should be encouraged to decrease fluid

intake for 1 to 2 hours preceding bedtime. However, it is important that adequate fluid be consumed earlier in the day to prevent fluid balance problems.

5. **Encourage the use of relaxation exercises, creative visualization, self-hypnosis, or other relaxation techniques.** Many techniques that promote relaxation can be used to help induce sleep. Numerous audiotapes and books are available to describe these techniques, many of which could benefit older adults and are unlikely to cause the problems that are caused by medications.

6. **Use any appropriate interventions that are used in the institutional setting** (Nursing Care Plan 20-1.)

★ Nursing Care Plan 20-1 | Disturbed Sleep Pattern

Mrs. Star, age 83, lives at Larkspur Court Residence Center. Her room is near the nurses' station. She is frequently observed to be awake during the night. She often does not want to get up for breakfast, stating, "I'm too tired." She yawns often during the day and takes frequent naps in her room. She complains, "I can't get comfortable. There is just too much noise around here."

Nursing Diagnosis
Disturbed sleep pattern

Defining Characteristics
- Observed periods of awakening at night
- Frequent yawning and napping
- Complaints of fatigue

Patient Goals/Outcomes Identification
Mrs. Star will report feeling adequately rested.

Nursing Interventions/Implementation
1. Identify specific factors that make sleep difficult for Mrs. Star.
2. Ask Mrs. Star whether she can identify any changes that would help her sleep.
3. Consider a room change if possible.
4. Close her door to reduce extraneous noise.
5. Discourage daytime napping.
6. Encourage daytime physical activities.
7. Recommend that she avoid caffeine after dinner.
8. Teach relaxation techniques.
9. Provide comfort measures at bedtime.
10. Assess the need for further sleeping aids.

Evaluation
Mrs. Star now states, "I really like my new room. It's much quieter, so I don't have trouble sleeping at night. In fact, I've even started going to more activities now that I'm feeling more rested during the day." She is observed to be sleeping soundly when checked at night. Fewer daytime naps are documented in her chart. You will continue the plan of care.

Critical Thinking Questions
A new resident who calls out loudly day and night was admitted to the room next door. Mrs. Star states to another resident, "I just started getting a good night's sleep, and now he's keeping me awake again."
1. What would your most appropriate response be to Mrs. Star's concerns?
2. How could you resolve this problem for her and other residents who may be disturbed?

Get Ready for the NCLEX® Examination!

Key Points

- Changes related to sleep are a major concern for many older persons.
- Because sleep problems can result from normal age-related changes or other problems, concerns about sleep should not be taken lightly.
- A thorough assessment of sleep behaviors and appropriate interventions help older adults achieve the rest and sleep they require to function at the highest possible level.

Additional Learning Resources

SG Go to the Study Guide on pp. 379–397 for additional learning activities to help you master the chapter content.

eVolve Go to your Evolve website (http://evolve.elsevier.com/Wold/geriatric) for the following FREE learning resources:

- Animations
- Answer Guidelines for Nursing Care Plan Critical Thinking Questions
- Answers and Rationales for Review Questions for the NCLEX® Examination
- Glossary with pronunciations in English and Spanish
- Video Clips

Review Questions for the NCLEX® Examination

1. When teaching an elderly client about ways to improve sleep habits, the nurse takes into consideration that many elders:

    1. Feel sleepy later and sleep later in the morning
    2. Feel tired earlier and need more hours of sleep
    3. Go to bed earlier and rise earlier
    4. Spend more time sleeping than younger adults

2. List four factors that are likely to cause sleep problems in older adults.

    1. _____
    2. _____
    3. _____
    4. _____

3. The wife of an elderly patient reports that her husband snores very loudly then stops breathing several times each night. In addition to recommending a physician's visit, the nurse would suggest that the husband:

    1. Have a glass of wine at bedtime to promote relaxation.
    2. Use an OTC decongestant to open the respiratory passages.
    3. Sleep in the supine position with two pillows to open the airway.
    4. Lose weight and sleep in a side-lying position to facilitate breathing.

4. An elderly patient requests an evening snack. The most appropriate food to facilitate sleep would be:

    1. Graham cracker with banana and milk.
    2. Cheese, toast, and hot chocolate.
    3. Slice of cake and hot tea.
    4. Fruit, cheese, and a glass of wine.

5. An elderly patient has just started taking diphenhydramine (Benadryl) as a sleep aid. The nursing care plan should be modified to include: (Select all that apply.)

    1. Monitor for orthostatic hypotension.
    2. Assess for urinary retention.
    3. Observe for paradoxic excitement.
    4. Stand and change position slowly.
    5. Monitor blood glucose readings.
    6. Check for cardiac arrhythmias.

6. An older client tells the nurse that she has used phenobarbital to promote sleep for 6 months since her husband died. Which statement indicates a knowledge deficit related to phenobarbital?

    1. "Phenobarbital is a barbiturate."
    2. "Phenobarbital has a low lethal dose."
    3. "Phenobarbital can be addictive."
    4. "Phenobarbital's effectiveness will increase with chronic use."

Laboratory Values for Older Adults

TEST NAME	ADULT NORMALS	OLDER ADULT NORMALS	SIGNIFICANCE OF DEVIATIONS
Hematology			
Red blood cells (RBCs)	M 4.7–6.1 F 4.2–5.4 million/unit	Unchanged with aging	Low: hemorrhage, anemia, chronic illness, renal failure, pernicious anemia High: high altitude, polycythemia, dehydration
Hemoglobin	M 14–18 g/dL F 12–16 g/dL	Values may be slightly decreased	Low: anemia, cancer, nutritional deficiency, kidney disease High: polycythemia, CHF, chronic obstructive pulmonary disease (COPD), high altitudes, dehydration
Hematocrit	M 42%–52% F 37%–47%	Values may be slightly decreased	Low: anemia, cirrhosis, hemorrhage, malnutrition, rheumatoid arthritis High: polycythemia, severe dehydration, severe diarrhea, COPD
White blood cells (WBCs) (total)	5.0–10.0 thousand/mm^3	Unchanged with aging	Low: drug toxicity, infections, autoimmune disease, dietary deficiency High: infection, trauma, stress, inflammation
Neutrophils	55%–70%	Unchanged with aging	Low: dietary deficiency, overwhelming bacterial infection, viral infections, drug therapy High: physical and emotional stress, trauma, inflammatory disorders
Eosinophils	1%–4%	Unchanged with aging	Low: increased adrenosteroid production High: parasitic infections, allergic reactions, autoimmune disorders
Basophils	0.5%–1%	Unchanged with aging	Low: acute allergic reactions, stress reactions High: myeloproliferative disease
Monocytes	2%–8%	Unchanged with aging	Low: drug therapy (predisposition) High: chronic inflammatory disorders, tuberculosis, chronic ulcerative colitis
Lymphocytes	20%–40%	Unchanged with aging	Low: leukemia, sepsis, systemic lupus erythematosus, chemotherapy, radiation High: chronic bacterial infection, viral infections, radiation, infectious hepatitis
Folic acid	5–25 ng/mL	Unchanged with aging	Low: malnutrition, folic acid anemia, hemolytic anemia, alcoholism, liver disease, chronic renal disease High: pernicious anemia
Vitamin B_{12}	160–950 pg/mL	Unchanged with aging	
Total iron binding	250–460 mcg/dL	Unchanged with aging	Low: hypoproteinemia, cirrhosis, hemolytic capacity (TIBC) anemia, pernicious anemia High: polycythemia, iron-deficiency anemia
Iron (Fe)	M 80–180 mcg/dL F 60–160 mcg/dL	Unchanged with aging	Low: insufficient dietary iron, chronic blood loss, inadequate absorption of iron High: hemochromocytosis, hemolytic anemia, hepatitis, iron poisoning
Uric acid	M 4.0–8.5 mg/dL F 2.7–7.3 mg/dL	May be slightly increased	Low: lead poisoning High: gout, increased ingestion of purines, chronic renal disease, hypothyroidism

Continued

TEST NAME	ADULT NORMALS	OLDER ADULT NORMALS	SIGNIFICANCE OF DEVIATIONS
Prothrombin time (PT)	11–12.5 sec	Unchanged with aging	High: liver disease, vitamin K deficiency, warfarin ingestion, bile duct obstruction, salicylate intoxication
Partial thromboplastin time (PTT) Partial thromboplastin time activated (APTT)	60–70 sec 30–40 sec	Unchanged with aging	Low: early stages of disseminated intravascular coagulation, metastatic cancer High: coagulation factor deficiency, cirrhosis, vitamin K deficiency, heparin administration
Platelets	150,000–400,000/mm^3	Unchanged with aging	Low: hemorrhage, thrombocytopenia, systemic lupus erythematosus, pernicious anemia, chemotherapy, infection High: malignancy, polycythemia, rheumatoid arthritis, iron-deficiency anemia
Blood Chemistry			
Sodium	136–145 mEq/L	Unchanged with aging	Low: decreased intake, diarrhea, vomiting, diuretic administration, chronic renal failure, CHF, peripheral edema, ascites High: increased intake, Cushing's syndrome, extensive thermal burns
Potassium	3.5–5.0 mEq/L	Unchanged with aging	Low: deficient intake, burns, diuretics, Cushing's syndrome, insulin administration, ascites High: excessive dietary intake, renal failure, infection, acidosis, dehydration
Chloride	98–106 mEq/L	Unchanged with aging	Low: overhydration, CHF, vomiting, chronic gastric suction, chronic respiratory acidosis, hypokalemia, diuretic therapy High: dehydration, Cushing's syndrome, kidney dysfunction, metabolic acidosis, hyperventilation
Calcium	9.0–10.5 mg/dL	Tends to stay the same or decrease	Low: renal failure, vitamin D deficiency, osteomalacia, malabsorption High: Paget's disease of the bone, prolonged immobilization, lymphoma
Phosphate	3.0–4.5 mg/dL	Slightly lower	Low: inadequate dietary ingestion, chronic antacid ingestion, hypercalcemia, alcoholism, osteomalacia, malnutrition High: renal failure, increased dietary intake, hypocalcemia, liver disease
Magnesium	1.3–2.1 mEq/L	Decreases 15% between third and eighth decade	Low: malnutrition, malabsorption, alcoholism, chronic renal disease High: renal insufficiency, ingestion of magnesium-containing antacids or salts, hypothyroidism
Glucose, fasting (FBS)	70–110 mg/dL	Increase in normal range after age 50	Low: hypothyroidism, liver disease, insulin overdose, starvation High: diabetes mellitus, acute stress response, diuretic therapy, corticosteroid therapy
Glucose, postprandial	Less than 140 mg/dL 2 hr after meal	Less than 160 mg/dL 2 hr after meal	Low: hypothyroidism, insulin overdose, malabsorption High: diabetes mellitus, malnutrition, Cushing's syndrome, chronic renal failure, diuretic therapy, corticosteroid therapy
Amylase	60–120 Somogyi units/dL	Slightly increased in elderly	High: acute pancreatitis, perforated bowel, acute cholecystitis, diabetic ketoacidosis
Glycosylated hemoglobin (Hgb A$_{1c}$)	4.0%–5.9%	Unchanged with aging	Low: hemolytic anemia, chronic renal failure High: newly diagnosed diabetes, poorly controlled diabetes, nondiabetic hyperglycemia

Continued

TEST NAME	ADULT NORMALS	OLDER ADULT NORMALS	SIGNIFICANCE OF DEVIATIONS
Total protein	6.4–8.3 g/dL	Unchanged with aging	Low: liver disease, malnutrition, ascites High: hemoconcentration
Albumin	3.5–5 g/dL	Decrease slightly with aging	Low: malnutrition, liver disease, overhydration High: dehydration
Blood urea nitrogen (BUN)	10–20 mg/dL	May be slightly higher	Low: liver failure, overhydration, malnutrition High: hypovolemia, dehydration, alimentary tube feeding, renal disease
Creatinine	M 0.6–1.2 mg/dL F 0.5–1.1 mg/dL	Decrease in muscle mass may cause decreased values	Low: debilitation, decreased muscle mass High: reduced renal blood flow, diabetic neuropathy, urinary tract obstruction
Creatinine clearance	M 107–139 mL/min F 87–107 mL/min	Values decrease 6.5 ml/min/decade of life after age 20 due to a decline in GFR	Low: impaired kidney function, CHF, cirrhosis High: high cardiac output syndromes
Cholesterol (total)	<200 mg/dL	Increase until about middle age but decrease there after (or can increase abruptly in women)	Low: malabsorption, malnutrition, cholesterol-lowering medication, pernicious anemia, liver disease, hyperthyroidism High: hypercholesteremia, hyperlipidemia, hypothyroidism, uncontrolled diabetes mellitus, hypertension, stress
High-density lipoprotein (HDL)	M >45 mg/dL F > 55 mg/dL	Unchanged with aging	Low: familial low HDL, liver disease, hypoproteinemia High: familial HDL lipoproteinemia, excessive exercise
Low-density lipoprotein (LDL)	<130 mg/dL	Increase with aging after menopause	Low: hypolipoproteinemia High: hypothyroidism, alcohol consumption, chronic liver disease, Cushing's syndrome
Alkaline phosphatase	30–120 units/L	Slightly higher	Low: hypothyroidism, malnutrition, pernicious anemia High: cirrhosis, healing fracture, Paget's disease
Acid phosphatase	0.13–0.63 units/L	Unchanged with aging	Low: thrombosis High: heparin administration, cirrhosis, prostate cancer
Aspartate transaminase (AST)	0–35 units/L	Values slightly higher	Low: acute renal disease, diabetic ketoacidosis, chronic renal dialysis High: myopathy, hepatitis, cirrhosis, multiple trauma, acute hemolytic anemia
Creatinine kinase (CK)	M 55–170 units/L F 30–235 units/L	Unchanged with aging	High: diseases or injury affecting heart muscle, skeletal muscle, and brain
Thyroid Testing			
Thyroxine (T_4) - total	4–12 mcg/dL	Slightly decreased	Low: hypothyroidism, malnutrition, renal failure, cirrhosis High: hyperthyroidism, hepatitis
Triiodothyronine (T_3) Age 20–50 >50	70–205 ng/dL 40–180	Slightly decreased	Low: hypothyroidism, pituitary insufficiency, protein malnutrition, renal failure, liver diseases, Cushing's syndrome High: hyperthyroidism, hepatitis, hypoproteinemia
Thyroid-stimulating hormone (TSH)	2–10 μU/mL	Unchanged with aging	Low: pituitary dysfunction, hyperthyroidism High: primary hypothyroidism
Urine Chemistry			
Color	Yellow; amber	Same	Straw-colored urine indicates dilution.
Appearance	Clear	Same	Cloudy urine may indicate presence of pus, casts, blood, and bacteria.

Continued

TEST NAME	ADULT NORMALS	OLDER ADULT NORMALS	SIGNIFICANCE OF DEVIATIONS
Specific gravity	1.005–1.030	Values decrease with aging	Low: overhydration, renal failure, diuresis, hypothermia High: dehydration, water restriction, vomiting, diarrhea
pH	4.6–8.0	Same	Acidic urine: diarrhea, metabolic acidosis, diabetes mellitus, respiratory acidosis, emphysema Alkaline urine: respiratory alkalosis, metabolic alkalosis, vomiting, gastric suctioning, diuretic therapy, UTI
Protein	0–8 mg/mL	Same	Positive: diabetes mellitus, CHF, systemic lupus erythematosus, malignant hypertension
Glucose	Negative	Same	Positive: diabetes mellitus, Cushing's syndrome, severe stress, infection, drug therapy
Ketones	Negative	Same	Positive: uncontrolled diabetes mellitus, starvation, excessive aspirin ingestion, high-protein diet, dehydration
Blood	Negative	Same	Positive: renal trauma, renal stones, cystitis, prostatitis
Leukocyte esterase	Negative	Same	Positive: possible UTI
Bacteria	Negative	May be seen in older adults without symptoms; evaluate for pyuria and symptoms	Positive: UTI
Arterial Blood Gases			
pH	7.35–7.45	Same	Low: respiratory or metabolic acidosis High: respiratory or metabolic alkalosis
Po_2	80–100 mm Hg	Decrease 25% between 30 and 80 years old	Low: cardiac or respiratory disease
Pco_2	35–45 mm Hg	Same	Low: respiratory alkalosis High: respiratory acidosis
O_2 saturation	95%–100%	95%	Low: impaired gas exchange
HCO_3	21–28 mEq/L	Same	Low: metabolic acidosis High: metabolic acidosis

Adapted from Pagana KD, Pagana TJ: *Diagnostic and laboratory test reference,* ed 10, St Louis, 2011, Mosby; and Pagana KD, Pagana TJ: *Manual of diagnostic and laboratory tests,* ed 4, St Louis, 2010, Mosby.

The Geriatric Depression Scale (GDS)

by Lenore Kurlowicz, PhD, RN, CS

The Geriatric Depression Scale (GDS) was developed as a basic screening tool for depression in older adults and is used in the clinical setting. It is a short questionnaire that requires a *yes* or *no* response from the participant, based on how the person feels on the day the tool is administered.

GERIATRIC DEPRESSION SCALE

Patient _____ Examiner _____ Date _____

Directions to Patient: Please choose the best answer for how you have felt over the past week.
Directions to Examiner: Present questions VERBALLY. Circle answer given by patient. Do not show to patient.

1. Are you basically satisfied with your life?.. yes **no (1)**
2. Have you dropped many of your activities and interests?........................... **yes (1)** no
3. Do you feel that your life is empty?... **yes (1)** no
4. Do you often get bored?.. **yes (1)** no
5. Are you hopeful about the future?... yes **no (1)**
6. Are you bothered by thoughts you can't get out of your head?.................... **yes (1)** no
7. Are you in good spirits most of the time?... yes **no (1)**
8. Are you afraid that something bad is going to happen to you?..................... **yes (1)** no
9. Do you feel happy most of the time?... yes **no (1)**
10. Do you often feel helpless?... **yes (1)** no
11. Do you often get restless and fidgety?.. **yes (1)** no
12. Do you prefer to stay at home rather than go out and do things?................ **yes (1)** no
13. Do you frequently worry about the future?... **yes (1)** no
14. Do you feel you have more problems with memory than most?................... **yes (1)** no
15. Do you think it is wonderful to be alive now?... yes **no (1)**
16. Do you feel downhearted and blue?... **yes (1)** no
17. Do you feel pretty worthless the way you are now?................................. **yes (1)** no
18. Do you worry a lot about the past?... **yes (1)** no
19. Do you find life very exciting?... yes **no (1)**
20. Is it hard for you to get started on new projects?.................................... **yes (1)** no
21. Do you feel full of energy?.. yes **no (1)**
22. Do you feel that your situation is hopeless?... **yes (1)** no
23. Do you think that most people are better off than you are?....................... **yes (1)** no
24. Do you frequently get upset over little things?.. **yes (1)** no
25. Do you frequently feel like crying?... **yes (1)** no
26. Do you have trouble concentrating?... **yes (1)** no
27. Do you enjoy getting up in the morning?... yes **no (1)**
28. Do you prefer to avoid social occasions?... **yes (1)** no
29. Is it easy for you to make decisions?.. yes **no (1)**
30. Is your mind as clear as it used to be?.. yes **no (1)**

TOTAL: Please sum all bolded answers (worth one point) for a total score. _____

Scores: 0-9 Normal 0-19 Mild Depressive 0-30 Severe Depressive

Source: www.stanford.edu/~yesavage

| | RDA[1] OR AI* | | TOLERABLE UPPER INTAKE |
	MEN	WOMEN	LEVELS (MEN AND WOMEN)
Vitamins, Elements, Electrolytes			
Biotin (ug) (mcg)	30*	30*	ND
Boron (mg)	ND	ND	20
Calcium (mg)	1200*	1200*	2500
Chloride (g)	2.0* (age 51-70) 1.8* (age 70+)	2.0* (age 51-70) 1.8* (age 70+)	3.6
Choline (mg)	550*	425*	3500
Chromium (mcg)	30*	20*	ND
Copper (mcg)	**900**	**900**	10,000
Fluoride (mg)	4*	3*	10
Folate (mcg)	**400**	**400**	1000
Iodine (mcg)	**150**	**150**	1100
Iron (mg)	**8**	**8**	45
Magnesium (mg)	**420**	**320**	350
Manganese (mg)	2.3*	1.8*	11
Molybdenum (mg)	**45**	**45**	2000
Niacin (mg)	**16**	**14**	35
Nickel (mg)	ND	ND	1
Pantothenic Acid (mg)	5*	5*	ND
Phosphorus (mg)	**700**	**700**	4000 (age 51-70) 3000 (age 70+)
Potassium (g)	4.7	4.7	
Riboflavin (mg)	**1.3**	**1.1**	ND
Selenium (mcg)	**55**	**55**	400
Sodium (g)	1.3*(age 51-70) 1.2* (age 70+)	1.3* (age 51-70) 1.2* (age 70+)	2.3
Thiamin (mg)	**1.2**	**1.1**	ND
Vanadium (mg)	ND	ND	1.8
Vitamin A (mcg)	**900**	**700**	3000
Vitamin B$_6$ (mg)	**1.7**	**1.5**	100
Vitamin B$_{12}$ (mcg)	**2.4**	**2.4**	ND
Vitamin C (mg)	**90**	**75**	2000
Vitamin D (mcg)	10* (age 51-70) 15* (age 70+)	10* (age 51-70) 15* (age 70+)	50
Vitamin E (mg)	**15**	**15**	1000
Vitamin K (mcg)	120*	90*	ND
Zinc (mg)	**11**	**8**	40

Continued

	RDA[1] OR AI*	
	MEN	**WOMEN**
Macronutrients, Fiber, Water		
Energy[2] (Kcal)	2204 (age 51-70)	1978 (age 51-70)
	2054 (age 70+)	1873 (age 70+)
Protein[3] (g) (10-35% AMDR)	**56**	**46**
Carbohydrates[4] (g) (45-65% AMDR)	**130**	**130**
Total Fat[5,6] (% Kcal) (20-35% AMDR)	20-35	20-35
n-6 PUFA (g) (5-10% AMDR)	14*	11*
n-3 PUFA (g) (0.6-1.2% AMDR)	1.6*	1.1*
Total Fiber	30*	21*
Drinking water, beverages, water in food (L)	3.7* (age 51-70)	2.7* (age 51-70)
	2.6* (age 70+)	2.1* (age 70+)

ND, not determined.

AMDR, Acceptable Macronutrient Distribution Range for intakes of carbohydrates, proteins, and fats expressed as % of total calories.

For more information, go to http://nutritionandaging.fiu.edu/DRI_and_DGs/DRI_and_RDAs.asp.

*Adequate intakes (*AIs*).

[1]Recommended dietary allowances (RDAs) are in **bold.**

[2]Values are based on Table 5-22 Estimated Energy Requirements (EER) for Men and Women 30 Years of Age. Used height of 5′7″ and "low active" physical activity level (PAL) and calculated the median BMI and calorie level for men and women. Caloric values based on age were calculated by subtracting 10 kcal/day for males (from 2504 kcal) and 7 kcal/day for females (from 2188 kcal) for each year of age above 30. For ages 51-70, calculated for 60 years old, for 70+, calculated for 75 years old. 80-year-old male calculated to require 2004 kcal, female 1838 kcal.

[3]The RDA for protein equilibrium in adults is a minimum of 0.8 gm/kg body weight for reference body weight.

[4]The RDA for carbohydrate is the minimum adequate to maintain brain function in adults.

[5]Because % of energy consumed as fat can vary greatly and still meet energy needs, an AMDR is provided in absence of AI, EAR, or RDA for adults.

[6]Values for mono- and saturated fats and cholesterol not established as "they have no role in preventing chronic disease, thus not required in the diet."

Modified from the National Policy and Resource Center on Nutrition and Aging, Florida International University, Revised 3/19/04. Data compiled from the Institute of Medicine, *Dietary Reference Intakes: Applications in Dietary Assessment,* 2000; *Dietary Reference Intakes for Energy, Carbohydrates, Fiber, Fat, Protein and Amino Acids (Macronutrients)* 2002; and *Dietary Reference Intakes: Water, Potassium, Sodium, Chloride, and Sulfate,* 2004.

Resources for Older Adults

ORGANIZATIONS

Administration on Aging
One Massachusetts Avenue NW
Washington, DC 20201
(202) 619-0724
FAX (202) 357-3555
http://www.aoa.gov/
E-mail: aoainfo@aoa.hhs.gov

Alzheimer's Association
225 N. Michigan Ave., Fl. 17
Chicago, IL 60601-7633
(312) 335-8700
TDD (312) 335-5886
FAX (866) 699-1246
http://www.alz.org

American Geriatrics Society
The Empire State Building
350 Fifth Avenue, Suite 801
New York, NY 10118
(212) 308-1414
FAX (212) 832-8646
E-mail: info@americangeriatrics.org

American Society on Aging
71 Stevenson Street
Suite 1450
San Francisco, CA 94105-2938 USA
(415) 974-9600
FAX (415) 974-0300
http://www.asaging.org/index.cfm
E-mail: info@asaging.org

Clearinghouse on Abuse and Neglect of the Elderly
College of Human Resources
University of Delaware
Newark, DE 19716
(302) 831-3525
E-mail: CANE-UD@udel.edu

Disabled American Veterans
807 Maine Avenue SW
Washington, DC 20024
(202) 554-3501
http://www.dav.org/about/Default.aspx

National Senior Citizens Law Center
1444 Eye St., NW Suite 1100
Washington, DC 20005
(202) 289-6976
FAX (202) 289-7224

National Indian Council on Aging
10501 Montgomery Blvd NE
Suite 210
Albuquerque, NM 87111
(505) 292-2001
FAX (505) 292-1922
E-mail: info@nicoa.org

National Institute on Aging
Public Information Office
Building 31, Room 5C27
31 Center Drive MSC 2292
Bethesda, MD 20892-2292
(301) 496-1752
FAX (301) 496-1072

National Council on the Aging
1901 L Street, NW, 4th Floor
Washington, D.C. 20036
(202) 479-1200

National Long-Term Care Resource Center
Institute for Health Services Research
University of Minnesota School of Public Health
420 Delaware SE
D-527 Mayo, MMC 197
Minneapolis, MN 55455
(612) 624-5171
FAX (612) 624-5434

AGING ASSOCIATIONS AND SOCIETIES

Alzheimer's Association
www.alz.org/

American Association of Retired Persons
www.aarp.org/

American Geriatrics Society
www.americangeriatrics.org/

American Society on Aging
www.asaging.org/

Gerontological Society of America
www.geron.org/

National Council on Aging
www.ncoa.org/

National Gerontological Nursing Association
www.ngna.org/

GERONTOLOGY CENTERS/EDUCATION CENTERS/ INSTITUTES

Brookdale Center on Aging
www.brookdale.org/

Consortium of New York Geriatric Education Centers
www.nygec.org/

Gerontological Nursing Interventions Research Center
www.nursing.uiowa.edu/excellence/
nursing_interventions/

Hartford Institute for Geriatric Nursing
www.hartfordign.org/

National Association of Geriatric Education Centers
www.nagec.org/

Reynolds Center on Aging
http://aging.uams.edu/

Wayne State University Institute of Gerontology
www.iog.wayne.edu/

STATISTICS AND GOVERNMENT SITES

Administration on Aging
www.aoa.gov/aoaroot/aging_statistics/index.aspx

Department of Health and Human Services (CMS/ AHRQ)
www.hhs.gov/

Fastats
www.cdc.gov/nchs/fastats/Default.htm

National Institute on Aging
www.nia.nih.gov/

JOURNALS/PERIODICALS

Generations
www.asaging.org/

Geriatric Nursing
www.sciencedirect.com/science/journal/01974572

The Gerontologist
www.geron.org/

Journal of Gerontological Nursing
www.slackinc.com/jgn.htm

Journals of the Gerontological Society of America
www.gerontologyjournals.org/

EDUCATIONAL RESOURCES

American Association of Colleges of Nursing
www.aacn.nche.edu/Education/gercomp.htm

GeroNet Health & Aging Resources for Higher Education
www.ph.ucla.edu/sph/geronet.html

National Gerontological Nursing Association
www.ngna.org/

INFORMATION ON EXERCISE

Active Aging Partnership
www.agingblueprint.org/tips.cfm

American Association of Family Practitioners
www.aafp.org/afp/2010/0101/p60.html

American Heart Association
www.heart.org

International Council on Active Aging
www.icaa.cc

International Society for Aging and Physical Activity
www.isapa.org

JAMA—Fitness for Older Adults
http://jama.ama-assn.org/content/300/9/1104.full.pdf+html

National Institute on Aging
www.nia.nih.gov/HealthInformation/Publications/ExerciseGuide/

National Institute of Diabetes and Digestive and Kidney Diseases
http://win.niddk.nih.gov/publications/young_heart.htm

President's Council on Fitness, Sports & Nutrition
www.fitness.gov

Robert Wood Johnson Foundation
www.rwjf.org

Bibliography and Reader References

CHAPTER 1

Aged care campaign: Nurse led innovation in aged care leads to top award, *Aust Nurs J* 17(4):6–7, 2009.

Aging in place: *Seniorresource.com,* 2010. www.seniorresource.com/house.htm Accessed May 5, 2001.

Aging into the 21st century, 2009. http://www.aoa.gov/AoARoot/Aging_Statistics/future_growth/aging21/preface.aspx.

Allen S: Collaborating to improve health outcomes for older people, *Aust Nurs J* 17(9):47, 2009.

American Psychological Association: *Elder abuse and neglect: in search of solutions,* 2010. www.apa.org.

AOL News: *Social Security turns 75: how healthy is it?* 2010. AOL Inc. www.aolnews.com.

Associated Press: *Trustees: Medicare hospital fund extended 12 years,* 2010. www.salon.com.

Bailey R: Accidents, murders, preemies, fat, and U.S. life expectancy, *Reason Magazine* 2008. www.reason.com.

Barringer F: Where many elderly live, signs of the future, *NY Times* March 7, 1993. www.nytimes.com/1993.

Barry P: A user's guide to health care reform, *AARP Bull* May 2010. www.bulletin.aarp.org.

Bhushan S: Aging in place: why the "high-rise" concept might be the answer, *LTL Magazine* 20–23, January 2010. www.ltlmagazine.com.

Bihari M: Understanding the Medicare Part D donut hole, *About.com* April 2010. www.healthinsurance.about.com.

Birmingham K: Age appropriate, *Nurs Older People* 18(5):12–14, 2006.

Bobbye: Nursing homes without walls, PACE provide alternative care for seniors, *Associated Content* 2010. www.associatedcontent.com.

Boissonnault P: Look out! Here come the boomers: ageism and the apocalyptic demographic, *Transformative Dialogues* 1(3), 2003. www.kwantlen.ca/academicgrowth/td/issue1-3/boomers.html.

Brandon E: 10 ways baby boomers will reinvent retirement, *US News* February 16, 2010. www.money.usnews.com.

Brown D: Life expectancy hits record high in the United States, *Washington Post* June 12, 2008. www.washingtonpost.com.

CBO projects Medicare spending at $1,038 billion by 2020, *Medicare Update* January 26, 2010. www.medicareupdate.typepad.com.

CBS News, 60 Minutes: *The cost of dying,* 2009. www.cbsnews.com.

Centers for Disease Control and Prevention: Older persons' health, January 2010. www.cdc.gov/nchs/fastats/older_americans.html.

Chaplain Mike: Health care in America—what to do at the end of life? *Internetmonk.com* August 4, 2010. www.intenetmonk.com.

Chow D: Study suggests that elderly people who use the Internet could live longer, *NY Daily News* June 30, 2009. www.nydailynews.com.

Correia E: It is time to rethink end-of-life health care, *Washington Business Journal* August 14, 2009. www.washington.bizjournals.com.

Crane M: House passes 6-month delay in Medicare pay cut, *WebMD* 2010. www.medscape.com.

CRS Report for Congress (RL23697): *Income and poverty among older Americans in 2007,* updated October 3, Patrick Purcell. www.benefitslink.com/articles/guests/RL32697...pdf.

Dartmouth Atlas of Health Care: *End-of-life care,* 2010. Dartmouth College. www.darthmouthatlas.org.

Demographics of aging and implications for U.S. health care. www.agsexhibit.frycomm.com/pdf/AGS_Prosp_Demog.pdf.

Demographics of aging, 2009. Transgenerational Design Matters. www.transgenerational.org/aging/demographics.htm.

Demographics of an aging population: module 2, 2010. www.ageworks.com.

Demographics: searching for anti-aging information and medical news in demographics within the longevity and age management section, 2011. Worldhealth.netwww.worldhealth.net/list/news/demographics/.

Derse AR: Choosing how you die so others can't, *Milwaukee J Sentinel* October 25, 2009. www.jsonline.com/opinon.

DeVaney SA, Chiremba ST: Comparing the retirement savings of baby boomers and other cohorts, *U.S. Bureau of Labor Statistics* March 2005. www.bls.gov.

Dickson DM: U.S. health plans have history of cost overruns, *The Washington Times* November 18, 2009. www.washingtontimes.com.

Diemer T: *Health care law still unpopular with 56% of Americans, poll finds,* August 8 2010. www.politicaldaily.com.

Dillon D, Ailor D, Amato S: We're not just playing games: into aging—an aging simulation game, *Rehab Nurs* 34(6):248–249, 2009.

Drea: 9 pros and cons of the new health-care reform bill, *Economy, Government, Politics* March 2010. www.businesspundit.com.

Elder advocate: the meeting place for elder care concerns, August 2006. www.myelderadvocate.typepad.com.

Federal Interagency Forum on Aging: Older Americans 2010: key indicators of well-being, 2010. www.agingstats.gov.

Fewer elderly U.S. residents live in nursing homes: U.S. census reports, *Medical News Today* October 2007. www.medicalnewstoday.com/articles/83967.php.

Francis DR: Will retirement be golden for boomers? *Christian Sci Monitor* 2005. www.csmonitor.com.

Fulmer T, Greenberg S: Elder mistreatment and abuse, *GeronurseOnline.com* 2010. www.consultgerirn.org.

Fulmer T: Screening for mistreatment of older adults, *AJN* 108(12):52–59, 2008.

Future of human life expectancy: have we reached the ceiling or is the sky the limit? *Res Highlights* March 8, 2006.

Gorman MO: *Get gammy online!,* 2009. www.rodale.com/print/2792.

Guilloton S: CMS report shows healthcare spending grew by a record amount in 2009, *Examiner.com* February 4, 2010. www.examiner.com.

Health care reform: *NY Times* July 1, 2010. www.topics.nytimes.com.

Hendrick B: *World population grows older, but at a cost: global population aging faster than ever, posing financial and social challenges,* July 2009. www.rxlist.com.

Historical experience of three cohorts of older Americans: a timeline of selected events 1923–2008. www.aoa.gov/agingstatsdotnet/Main_Site/Data/2006_Documents/Timeline.pdf.

Hussain A, Rivers PA: Confronting the challenges of long-term health care crisis in the United States, *J Health Care Finance* 36 (6):71–82, 2009.

Kaiser Family Foundation: *e-Health and the elderly: how seniors use the Internet for health information*, 2005. www.kff.org.

Kaiser Family Foundation: *Fact sheet: Medicare spending and financing*, September 2008. www.kff.org.

Kaiser Family Foundation: *Trends in health care costs and spending*, March 2009. www.kff.org.

Kanaskie ML, Tringali CA: Promoting quality of life for geriatric oncology patients in acute care and critical care settings, *Crit Care Nurs Q* 31(1):2–11, 2008.

Landau E: Doctor-patient talk could cut costs, ethicists say, *CNN.com* July 2009. www.cnn.com.

Levine JM: *Geriatrics by legislation: the trend of the future?* September 2010. www.jeffreymlevinemd.com.

Levine JM: *Long-term care update: resident assessment radically changes with MDS 3.0*, August 2010. www.jeffreymlevinemd.com.

Life expectancy in the U.S. not nearly the highest, *LifeInsuranceRate* 2010. www.lifeinsurancerate.com.

Liu L, Rettenmaier AJ, Wang Z: *The rising burden of health spending on seniors*, 2007, National Center for Policy Analysis. www.ncpa.org.

Longley R: *Census offers statistics on older Americans*, 2010. www.usgovinfo.about.com.

Marcy J: Doctors see benefit in end-of-life controversy, *MSNBC.com* August 14, 2009. www.msnbc.msn.com.

Mayo Clinic Staff: *Living wills and advance directives for medical decisions*, HA00014, July 2009. www.mayoclinic.com.

Mayo Clinic Staff: *Long-term care: early planning pays off*, HA00054, January 2010. www.mayoclinic.com.

Medicare and Social Security face large deficits, 2007. Wikimedia.org. www.upload.wikimedia.org.

Medscape Medical News: *Study finds elderly Americans spend 19% of income on healthcare*, 2000. www.medscape.com.

Messecar D: *Family caregiving: nursing standard of preference protocol: family caregiving*, January 2008. www.consultgerirn.org.

Miller S: *Social Security averages just 40% of elderly income*, 2010. www.shrm.org.

Mitchell T: Unclear about Medicare? *USA Weekend* December 4–6, 2009.

Monsivais PM: Health care reform bill 101: what does it mean for seniors? *CSmonitor.com* March 22, 2010. www.csmonitor.com.

Mosocco D: Managed care for the frail older adult, *Home Healthcare Nurs* 27(7):423–428, 2009.

Murphy T: Wave of health reform provisions coming next month, *Salon.com* August 3, 2010. www.salon.com.

Nation baby boomers, here's what's coming next, *AOL News* 2009. www.sphere.com.

New health care bill pros and cons: Obama health care plan explained, *Worldcorrespondents.com* 2010. www.worldcorrespondents.com.

O'Brien S: How baby boomers will change retirement. Part 1: Many baby boomers plan to mix work and play, *About.com Senior Living* 2010. www.seniorliving.about.com.

Obama's senior moment, *Wall St J* August 14, 2009. www.online.wsj.com.

Obamacare screwing of the elderly and disabled begins, *Economic Policy Journal* 2010. www.economicpolicyjournal.com.

Ohlemacher S: U.S. slipping in life expectancy rankings, *Washington Post* August 12, 2007. www.washingtonpost.com.

Olshansky SJ, Passaro DJ, Hershow DC, et al: A potential decline in life expectancy in the United States in the 21st century, *N Engl J Med* 352:1138–1140, 2005.

Oretag I, Weinberger D: Healthcare reform—could history repeat itself? *Onenewsnow.com* November 24, 2009. www.onenewsnow.com.

Orlov L: *Internet use cuts depression in 55+ elderly—what's it mean?* November 2009. www.ageinplacetech.com.

Palmore E: *Ageism*, 2009. www.sociologyindex.com/ageism.htm.

Palmore E: The ageism survey: first findings, *Gerontologist* 41(2):572–575, 2001.

Pear R, Calmes J: Medicare stronger, Social Security worse in short run, report finds, *NY Times* August 5, 2010. www.nytimes.com.

Pearlstein M: *Taxpayers should view reform's spending projections with a healthy distrust, Center of the American Experiment*, August 31, 2009. www.americanexperiment.org.

Pipes S: How real reform is different from Obamacare, *The Examiner* August 4, 2010. www.printthis.clickability.com.

Pipes S: Obamacare will cost you your retirement, *The Examiner* August 2, 2010. www.printthis.clickability.com.

Pipes S: Seniors will suffer under Obamacare, *The Examiner* August 3, 2010. www.printthis.clickability.com.

Postma S, Flikkema ME: The next generation of geriatric nurse specialists, *J Gerontol Nurs* 36(1):49–52, 2010.

Program of all inclusive care for the elderly (PACE): 2002. www.seniorhealth.about.com.

Ramirez E: Ageism in the media is seen as harmful to health of the elderly, *LA Times* September 5, 2002. www.globalaging.org.

Raphael C, Cornwell JL: Influencing support for caregivers, *AJN* 108(Suppl 9):78–82, 2008.

Rathbone-McCuan E: Self-neglect in the elderly: knowing when and how to intervene, *Aging* spring: 1996. www.findarticles.com.

Renold C: *Housing problems and options for the elderly: Gero 500: perspectives in aging*, University of Southern California. www.usc.edu/dept/gero/AgeWorks/online-education/courses/500.shtml.

Riedl BM: A guide to fixing Social Security, Medicare, and Medicaid, *Backgrounder* 2114, 2008. www.heritage.org.

Roan S: Using the Internet might improve brain function, *Los Angeles Times* 2008. www.latimesblogs.latimes.com.

Sebelius K: *Medicare and the new health care law—what it means for you*, 2010, Centers for Medicare & Medicaid Services, CMS Product No. 11467.

Sims M: Race, end-of-life choices correlated, study finds, *The Dartmouth* June 1, 2009. www.thedartmouth.com.

Statistical profile of American Indian and Native Alaskan elderly, 2008. www.aoa.gov.

Statistical profile of Asian older Americans aged 65+, 2008. www.aoa.gov.

Statistical profile of black older Americans aged 65+, January 2010. www.aoa.gov.

Statistical profile of Hispanic older Americans aged 65+, January 2010. www.aoa.gov.

Stokowski LA: *Forensic issues for nurses—elder abuse*, August 2008. www.cme.medscape.com.

Tariman JD: Half of patients with cancer are older than 65: do you know how to care for older adults? *ONS Connect* December, 7–9, 2009.

Trumbull M: New health care bill pros and cons: will it cut costs? *Christian Sci Monitor* March 22, 2010. http//:www.csmonitor.com.

United Nations: population division: life expectancy at birth. In *Charting the progress of populations*, (chap VII). www.un.org/esa/population/publications/charting.

University of Missouri: *Center on Aging Studies Without Walls. Distinguishing between abuse, neglect, and self-neglect*. www.cas.umkc.edu.

U.S. Administration on Aging: A profile of older Americans, 2009, U.S, *Administration on Aging* 2010. www.aoa.gov.

U.S. Centers for Medicare & Medicaid Services: *Medicare & you, 2010*, 2009, U.S. Government Printing Office.

U.S. Central Intelligence Agency: *The world fact book: country comparison: life expectancy at birth*, 2011. https://www.cia.gov.

U.S. Department of Health & Human Services: HHS proposes $737 billion budget for fiscal year 2009, *HHS.gov* February 2008. www.hhs.gov.

U.S. National Center for Health Statistics: *Health, United States, 2009: in brief*. www.cdc.gov/nchs/hus.htm.

U.S. National Center on Elder Abuse: *Elder abuse prevalence and incidence*, 2005. www.ncea.gov.

U.S. National Committee for the Prevention of Elder Abuse: *What is elder abuse?* 2008. www.preventelderabuse.org.

U.S. National Institute on Aging: *why population aging matters: a global perspective*, March 2007. NIA publication no. 07-6134.

U.S. Social Security Online: *Life expectancy for Social Security*, 2011. www.ssa.gov.

USA Today: *Debate surrounds end-of-life care costs*, October 19, 2006. www.usatoday.com.

Webster J, Hayes N: Facing the future, *Nurs Older People* 21(10):11, 2009.

What healthcare reform means for caregivers and elderly parents, *AgingCare.com* 2010. www.agingcare.com.

Whitlatch C: Informal caregivers: communication and decision making, *AJN* 108(9):73–77, 2008.

Wikipedia: *Life expectancy*, 2011. www.en.wikipedia.org.

Will the elderly dominate the Internet someday? 2009. http://www.evancarmichael.com/women-entrepreneurs.

Woolf LM: *Elder abuse and neglect*, 1998, Webster University. www.webster.edu.

World Health Organization: *What is "active ageing"?* 2010. www.who.int.

World life expectancy map, 2009. www.worldlifeexpectancy.com/world-life-expectancy-map.

Your Elder Experts: *Elderly housing options*, 2010. www.yourelderexperts.com.

CHAPTER 2

American Federation for Aging Research: How do we age? In *HealthandAge, Medical Articles and News for Health in Aging Live Well, Live Longer*, 2010. www.healthandage.com.

American Federation for Aging Research: Why and how we age? In *The Infoaging Guide to Theories of Aging*, 2006. www.afar.org.

de Magalhães JP: Damage-based theories of aging. In *Integrative Genomics of Aging Group*, 2008. www.sensence.info/causes.html.

Grossman S, Lange J: Theories of aging as basis for assessment, *Medsurg Nurs* 15(2):2006.

Health-cares.net: Theories of aging. In *Women's Health—Anti-aging, Menopause, Breast Enhancement, Pregnancy, Infertility*, July 2005. www.womens-health.health-cares.net.

IAS: *Theories of aging*. In *International Antiaging Systems*, 2011. www.antiaging-systems.com.

Stadtman E: *Modern theories of aging*, April 2002. www.macwilliam.net.

Stibich M: The hormone theory of aging. In *Longevity, Anti-Aging and You—Healthy Aging, Longevity, and Anti Aging*, July 2007. www.longevity.about.com.

Stibich M: *The immune system theory of aging*. In *Longevity, Anti-Aging and You—Healthy Aging, Longevity, and Anti Aging*, March 2007. www.longevity.about.com.

Transgenerational.org: Age and ability. In *Home of Transgenerational Design Matters*, 2007. www.transgenerational.org/aging/ability.htm.

Transgenerational.org: Myths of aging. In *Home of Transgenerational Design Matters*, 2009. www.transgenerational.org/aging/myths-of-Age.htm.

Viña J, Borrás C, Miquel J: Critical review: theories of aging, *Life* 59:4–5, 2007.

Wadensten B: An analysis of psychosocial theories of ageing and their relevance to practical gerontological nursing in Sweden, *Scand J Caring Sci* 20:347–354, 2006.

Wikipedia: Reliability theory of aging and longevity. In *Wikipedia, the Free Encyclopedia*, December 2009. www.en.wikipedia.org.

CHAPTER 3

2009 focused update: ACCF/AHA guidelines for the diagnosis and management of heart failure in adults: a report of the American College of Cardiology Foundation/American Heart Association Task Force on Practice Guidelines, *Circulation* 119:1977–2016, 2009.

Braman SS: Asthma in the elderly, Lovelace Respiratory Research Institute Annual Respiratory Symposium: Mechanisms of Respiratory Diseases in the Elderly, *Exper Lung Res* 31(6):6–7, 2005.

Cacchione PZ: Sensory changes, *Hartford Inst Geriatric Nursing* February 2005. www.consultgerirn.org/topics/sensory_changes.

Chau D, Edelman SV: Clinical management of diabetes in the elderly, *Clin Diabetes* 19(4):2001.

Chau DL, Shumaker N, Plodkowski RA: Complications of type 2 diabetes in the elderly, *Geriatric Times* 4(2):2003. www.cmellc.com/geriatrictimes…html.

Chisolm TH, Willott JF, Lister JJ: The aging auditory system: anatomic and physiologic changes and implications for rehabilitation, *Int J Audiol* 42:2S3–2S10, 2003.

Elderly and diabetes, *Diabetes* February 2010. www.dlife.com/diabetes/information//daily_living/seniors/.

Emory University: *Diabetes in the elderly: prospective study (MNElderly)*, May 2010. www.clinicaltrials.gov/NCT01131052.

Faster diagnosis of deadly melanoma skin cancers may come from infrared system, Feb 2010. www.seniorjournal.com./NEWS.

Fiore K: Biomarker trio detects Alzheimer's, *MedPage Today* August 2010. www.medpagetoday.com.

Garcia-Rio F, Dorgham A, Pino JM, et al: Lung volume reference values for women and men 65 to 85 years of age, *Am J Respir Crit Care Med* 180:1083–1091, 2009.

Gregg EW, Engelgau MM, Narayan V: Complications of diabetes in elderly people: underappreciated problems include cognitive decline and physical disability, *BMJ* 26(10):916–917, 2002.

Harvey J, Berry JA: Andropause in the aging male, *JNP* March 2009. www.npjournal.org.

Is a lack of DHEA-S accelerating your aging? *Wellsphere* January 2010. www.wellsphere.com.

Kaufman KS: DHEA a multi-functional antiaging hormone, *Antiaging-systems* 2011. www.antiaging-systems.com.

Mayo Clinic Staff: Basal cell carcinoma. In *Mayo Foundation for Medical Education and Research*, 2009. www.mayoclinic.com.

Mayo Clinic Staff: melanoma. In *Mayo Foundation for Medical Education and Research*, 2010. www.mayoclinic.com/health/melanoma/DS00439.

Meneilly G: Pathophysiology of diabetes in the elderly, *Clin Geriatrics* 18(4):25–28, 2010.

Moser M: Hypertension treatment and the prevention of coronary heart disease in the elderly, *Am Family Phys* March 1999. www.aafp.org.

Most melanoma skin cancers found by physicians are on male senior citizens, April 2009. www.seniorjournal.com.

New test predicts whether memory problems will lead to Alzheimer's, *Real-Time Health News* October 2010. www.aolhealth.com.

Panjari M, Bell RJ, Jane F, et al: The safety of 52 weeks of oral DHEA therapy for postmenopausal women, *Maturitas* 63(July):240–245, 2009. www.nursingconsult.com.

Psychological aspects of aging, *Aging and Long-Term Care* (chap 2), April 2009. www.speedyceus.com.

RelayHealth: *DHEA*, 2010. www.nursingconsult.com.

Rhone M, Basu A: Phytochemicals and age-related eye diseases, *Nutr Rev* 66:465–472, 2008.

Riegal B, Dickson VV, Cameron J, et al: Symptom recognition in elders with heart failure, *J Nurs Scholarship* 42:92–100, 2010.

Sara: *New study from Archives of Neurology finds spinal fluid test may predict Alzheimer's*, August 2010. www.healthcentral. com.

Schwanke J: Skin cancer & aging, *Dermatol Times* November 2009.

Schwartz JB: *Cardiovascular function and disease in the elderly*, June 1999. Northwestern University. www.galter.northwestern. edu.

Seniors and diabetes: *dLife for Your Diabetes Life!* February 2010. www.dlife.com/diabetes/information/system.modules/ com.gto.

Shars-Hopko NC, Glynn-Milley C: Primary open-angle glaucoma: catching and treating the "sneak thief of sight, *AJN* 109(2):40–47, 2009.

Smith CM, Cotter VT: Normal aging changes: nursing standards of practice protocol: age-related changes in health. In *Geriatric Nursing Resources for the Care of Older Adults.* www.consultgerirn.org.

Spinal tap test may offer early Alzheimer's detection, August 2010. www.foxnews.com.

Stephenson R: Hormone replacement and anti-aging, *Access* 11:36–47, 2009.

Stibich M: DHEA: do DHEA supplements slow aging? Anti aging and DHEA. In *Longevity, Anti-Aging and You—Healthy Aging, Longevity, and Anti Aging*, May 2009. www.longevity. about.com/od/researchandmedicine/a/DHEA.htm.

Studies find increases in non-melanoma, melanoma skin cancers, March 2010. http://www.seniorjournal.com/NEWS.

US DHEA and DHEAS: *An introduction to their function and measurement*, 2008. www.salimetrics.com.

US DHEA: *Vanderbilt University, Nashville, Tennessee.* www. vanderbilt.edu/ans/psychology/health_psychology/Dhea. htm.

Vigoritio C, Incalzi RA, Acabfora D, et al: Gruppo Italiano di Cardiologica Riabilitativa e Preventiva: Recommendations for cardiovascular rehabilitation in the very elderly [Article in Italian], *Monaldi Arch Chest Dis* 60(1):25–39, 2003.

Wenger NK: Cardiovascular disease in the elderly, *Curr Probl Cardiol* 17(10):609–690, 1992.

Whalen KL, Mansour H: Pharmacotherapy of diabetes in the elderly, *US Pharm* 43(7):44–48, 2009.

Young JS: Age-related eye diseases: a review of current treatment and recommendations for low-vision aids, *Home Healthcare Nurs* 26(8):464–471, 2008.

CHAPTER 4

American Federation for Aging Research: Healthy aging center, *Infoaging.org.* www.websites.afar.org.

Anti-aging, from head to toe: *Consumer Reports on Health* 22(3):3–5, 2010.

Facts for life: *Aging and Disability Resource Center of Ozaukee County*, August 2010.

Facts for seniors: *Aging and Disability Resource Center of Ozaukee County*, 1(4), 2009.

Hyer K, Brown LM: The impact of event scale—revised: a quick measure of a patient's response to trauma, *AJN* 108(11):60–68, 2008.

Kim JL: Assessment of safe living for seniors, *JNP* 5(7):542–543, 2009.

Manne DS: Celebrate healthy aging!! Guest editorial, *Access* 11:2, 2009.

Phillips EM, Davidoff DA: Normal and successful aging: what happens to function as we age, *Primary Psychiatr.* www. primarypsychiatry.com.

Schumacher K, Beck CA, Marren JM: Family caregivers: caring for older adults, working with their families, *AJN* 106 (8):40–49, 2006.

Segal-Gidan F: Elder care: immunizations schedules and screening after age 65 years, *JAAPA* 23(1):2010. www.jaapa. com.

Transgenerational Design Matters: *The aging process*, 2009. www.transgenerational.org/aging/aging-process.html.

US CDC: *A word of physical activity, advanced directives, and fresh fruits and vegetables.* www.healthyaging-list@listserv.cdc.gov.

Walker C, Hogstel MO, Curry LC: Hospital discharge of older adults: how nurses can ease the transition, *AJN* 107 (6):60–70, 2007.

Wells K: *Pros and cons of the shingles vaccine: should seniors get the herpes zoster vaccination?*, July 2009. www.senior-health-medicare.suite101.com.

Wells K: *Recommended vaccines for seniors: immunizations may prevent infections in older adults*, July 2009. www.senior-health-medicare.suite101.com.

CHAPTER 5

Webb S: Overcoming communication issues between doctors, seniors, and their caregivers, *Intentional Caregiver.com* 2010. www.ezinearticles.com.

Miller CA: Communication difficulties in hospitalized older adults with dementia: try these techniques to make communicating with patients easier and more effective, *AJN* 108 (3):58–66, 2008.

Tips for improving communication skills for caregivers, 2007. www. workingcaregiver.com.

Mayo Clinic Staff: *Communicating effectively with a person who has Alzheimer's*, AZ00004, September 2009. www.mayoclinic.com.

Elliott-Smith S: Communicating with older patients, *Access* 11:24–30, 2009.

CHAPTER 6

Adams NE, Bowie AJ, Simmance N, et al: Recognition by medical and nursing professionals of malnutrition and risk of malnutrition in elderly hospitalized patients, *Nutr Dietetics* 65:144–150, 2008.

Adiposity associated with longer survival in older adults, *Medscape Med News* 2010. www.medscape.com.

Are ages in your food aging you? *Tufts Univ Health Nutr Lett* March 2010. www.tuftshealthletter.com.

Baker H: Nutrition in the elderly: diet pitfalls and nutrition advice, *Geriatrics* 62(10):24–26, 2007.

Candy B, Sampson EL, Jones L: Enteral tube feeding in older people with advanced dementia: findings from a Cochrane systematic review, *Int J Palliative Nurs* 15 (8):396–404, 2009.

Chen H, Guo X: Obesity and functional disability in elderly Americans, *JAGS* 56:689–694, 2008.

Denny A: An overview of the role of diet during the ageing process, *Br J Community Nurs* 13(2):58–67, 2008.

DiMaria-Ghalili RA, Amella E: Nutrition in older adults: intervention and assessment can help curb the growing threat of malnutrition, *AJN* 105(3):40–50, 2005.

DiMaria-Ghalili RA: *Nutrition in the elderly: nursing standard of practice protocol: nursing in aging*, 2010. www.consultgerirn. org.

Gaillard C, Alix E, Boirie Y, et al: Are elderly hospitalized patients getting enough protein? *JAGS* 56:1045–1049, 2008.

Holmén MS, Robertsson B, Wijk H: Tools to assess the nutritional status of acutely ill older adults, *Nurs Older People* 18(5):31–35, 2006.

Johansson Y, Backrach-Lindström M, Carstensen J, et al: Malnutrition in home-living older population: prevalence, incidence and risk factors: a prospective study, *J Clin Nutr* 18:1354–1364, 2008.

Kuwabara A, Himeno M, Tsugawa N, et al: Hypovitaminosis D and K are highly prevalent and independent of overall malnutrition in the institutionalized elderly, *Asia Pac J Clin Nutr* 19(1):49–56, 2010.

Martin CT, Kayser-Jones J, Stotts NA, et al: Risk for low weight in community-dwelling older adults, *Clin Nurs Specialist* 21 (4):203–211, 2007.

Mayo Clinic Staff: Senior health: how to detect and prevent malnutrition, *MayoClinic.com* HA00066. www.mayoclinic.com.

Mentes J: Oral hydration in older adults, *AJN* 106(6):40–49, 2006.

O'Neill PS, Wellman NS, Himburg SP, et al: Aging in community nutrition, diet therapy, and nutrition and aging textbooks, *Gerontol Geriatr Educ* 25(3):65–83, 2005.

Palmer JL, Metheny NA: Preventing aspiration in older adults with dysphagia, *AJN* 108(2):40–48, 2008.

Palmer S: Food for thought: smart nutrition tips to protect the aging brain, *Environ Nutr* 32(11):3–5, 2009. www.environmentalnutrition.com.

Reuben DB: Quality indicators for the care of undernutrition in vulnerable adults, *JAGS* 55:S438–S442, 2007.

Scott TM, Peter I, Tucker KA, et al: The nutrition, aging, and memory of elders (NAME) study: design and methods for a study of micronutrients and cognitive function in a home-bound elderly population, *Int J Geriatr Psychiatr* 21:519–528, 2006.

Shepherd A: Nutrition through the life span. Part 3: adults aged 65 years and over, *Br J Nurs* 18.5:301–307, 2009.

Skates JJ, Anthony P: The mini nutritional assessment, *AJN* 108 (2):50–59, 2008.

Skates JJ, Anthony P: The mini nutritional assessment—an integral part of geriatric assessment, *Nutr Today* 44 (1):21–28, 2009.

Söderhamn U, Bachrach-Lindström M, Ek A-C: Nutritional screening and perceived health in a group of geriatric rehabilitation patients, *J Clin Nurs* 16:1997–2006, 2006.

Stockdell R, Amella EJ: The Edinburgh feeding evaluation in dementia scale, *AJN* 108(8):46–54, 2008.

Suominen MH, Sandelin E, Soini H, et al: How well do nurses recognize malnutrition in elderly patients? *Eur J Clin Nutr* 63:292–296, 2009.

Tsang MF: Is there adequate feeding assistance for the hospitalized elderly who are unable to feed themselves? *Nutr Dietetic* 65:222–228, 2008.

Vitamin D may prevent falls, *Harvard Health Lett* 2010. www.health.harvard.edu.

Webster J, Healy J, Maud R: Nutrition in hospitalized patients, *Nurs Older People* 21(10):31–37, 2009.

CHAPTER 7

Alzheimer's Disease Education and Referral Center: *Alzheimer's disease medications fact sheet*, 2008, Alzheimer's Disease Education and Referral Center, NIH pub no. 08-3431. www.nia.nih.gov.

Beers MH: Age-related changes as a risk factor for medication-related problems, *Generations* 24(4):22–27, 2000.

Beizer JL: Medications and the aging body: alteration as a function of age, *Generations* 18(2):13–17, 1994. www.web.ebscohost.com.

Cohen H, Shastay AD: Getting to the root of medication errors, *Nursing* 12:39–47, 2008. www.nursing.com.

Cohen H, Shastay AD: Getting to the root of medication errors, *Plast Surg Nurs* 24(4):247–256, 2009.

Conry M: Polypharmacology: Pandora's medicine chest? *Geriatr Times* 1, 2000. www.cmelc.com.

Drug therapy with older adults—module 8, 2007, Mosby.

Keefer A: How to prevent adverse drug effects in older adults, *eHow.com* 2010. www.ehow.com.

Leigh-Pemberton RA, von Moltke LL, Greenblatt DJ: Psycho-pharmacology in the elderly with cardiovascular disease, *Ann Long-Term Care* 14:34–45, 2006.

Mager DD, Madigan EA: Medication use in older adults in a home care study, *Home Healthcare Nurs* 28(1):15–21, 2010.

Molony S: Where's the evidence?—more psychometric properties of the Beers criteria, *AJN* 109(1):68–78, 2009.

Molony SL: Monitoring medication use in older adults, *AJN* 109 (1):68–78, 2009.

Moquin B, Blackman MR, Mitty E, et al: Complementary and alternative medicine (CAM), *Geriatr Nurs* 30(3):196–203, 2009.

Pham CB, Dickman RL: Minimizing adverse drug events in older patients, *Am Fam Physician* 76:1837–1844, 2007.

Razzi CC: Incorporating the Beers criteria may reduce ED visits in elderly persons, *J Emerg Nurs* 35(5):453–454, 2009.

Wilhelm M, Ruscin JM: The use of OTC medications in older adults, *US Pharmacist* 34(6):44–47, 2009.

Woodruff K: Preventing polypharmacy in older adults, *Am Nurse Today* 5(10):2010. www.medscape.com.

Wooten J, Galavis J: Polypharmacology: keeping the elderly safe, *Modern Med* August 2005. www.rn.modernmedicine.com.

Zurakowski T: The practicalities and pitfalls of polypharmacology, *Nurs Practitioner* 34(4):36–41, 2009.

Zwicker D, Fulmer T: *Medication: nursing standard practice protocol: reducing adverse drug events*, April 2008. www.consultgerirn.org.

CHAPTER 8

Amella EJ: Presentation of illness in older adults, *AJN* 104 (10):40–51, 2004.

Arora RC, Rockwood K: *Surgery in elderly people*, 2010. www.novelguide.com.

Basic geriatric gynecologic examination, 2010. Medscape CME Family Medicine. www.cme.medscape.com.

Basic geriatric respiratory examination, 2009. Medscape CME Family Medicine. www.cme.medscape.com.

Demers K: *Hearing screening in older adults: a brief hearing loss screener*, 2007, Hartford Institute for Geriatric Nursing. www.hartfordign.org.

Friedland R: *Emergency checklist for seniors and their caregivers*, 2010. www.care.com.

Fulmer T: Fulmer SPICES: a framework of six "marker conditions" can help focus assessment of hospitalized older patients, *AJN* 107(10):40–48, 2007.

Fulmer T: Screening for mistreatment of older adults, *AJN* 108 (12):52–59, 2008.

Graf CL: The hospital admission risk profile, *AJN* 108(8):62–71, 2008.

Hendrich A: Predicting patient falls, *AJN* 107(11):50–58, 2007.

Hyer K, Brown LM: The impact of event scale—revised, *AJN* 108 (11):60–68, 2008.

Kagan SH: Revisiting interdisciplinary teamwork in geriatric acute care, *Geriatr Nurs* 31(2):133–136, 2010.

Kennedy GJ, Smyth CA: Screening older adults for executive dysfunction, *AJN* 108(12):62–71, 2008.

Mayo Clinic Staff: Aging parents: 10 things to know for an emergency, *Mayoclinic.com* HA00029, 2008. www.mayoclinic.com.

Mayo Clinic Staff: Aging parents: 5 warning signs of health problems, *Mayoclinic.com* HA00082, 2009. www.mayoclinic.com.

MDS 3.0 for nursing and swing bed providers, 2010. https://www.cms.gov/NursingHomeQualityInits/25_NHQIMDS30.asp.

Messecar D, Powers A, Nagel CL: The family preferences index, *AJN* 108(9):52–59, 2008.

Montgomery J, Mitty E, Flores S: Resident condition change: should I call 911? *Geriatr Nurs* 29(1):15–26, 2008.

Naegle MA: Screening for alcohol use and misuse in older adults, *AJN* 108(11):50–58, 2008.

Preparing for MDS 3.0: *Information you can use from the draft MDS 3.0*, 2010. www.keanecare.com.

Rogers D: The increasing geriatric population and overcrowding in the emergency department: one hospital's approach, *J Emerg Nurs* 35(5), 2009. www.nursingconsut.com.

Skates JJ, Anthony P: The mini-nutritional assessment—an integral part of geriatric assessment, *Nutr Today* 44(1):21–28, 2009.

Talley HC, Talley CH: Evaluation of older adults, *AANA J* 77(6):451–460, 2009.

Wallace M, Shelkey M: Monitoring functional status in hospitalized older adults, *AJN* 108(4):64–71, 2008.

Watters JM: Surgery in the elderly, *J Canad Chirurg* 45(2):104–108, 2002.

Wikipedia: *OPQEST*, August 2010. www.en.wikipedia.org.

Wofford JJ: The role of emergency services in health care for the elderly: a review, *J Emerg Med* 11(3):317–326, 1993.

CHAPTER 9

Administration on Aging: *Coping with the heat*, 2010. www.aoa.gov/aoaroot.

Alarming increase in falls by elderly prompts national education campaign, *SeniorJournal.com* 2005. www.seniorjournal.com.

American Medical Association: Safety and the older driver with functional or medical impairments. Chap 1: Physician's guide to assessing and counseling senior driver safety, 2010. www.elderguru.com.

AOL Discover: *Sharpen your driving skills and have fun doing it*, 2010. www.daol.aol.com/articles/sharpen-your-driving-skills.

Barclay L: *Vitamin D may reduce falls in elderly nursing home residents*, 2010. www.cme.medscape.com.

Brennan M, Su Y-P, Horowitz A: Longitudinal associations between dual sensory impairment and everyday competence among older adults, *JRRD* 43(5):777–792, 2006.

Campbell VA, Crews JE, Moriarty DG, et al: Surveillance for sensory impairment, activity limitation, and health-related quality of life among older adults—United States, 1993–1997, *MMWR* 48(SS08):131–156, 1999.

Daniel KM, Carson CL, Ferrell S: Emergency technologies to enhance the safety of older people in their homes, *Geriatr Nurs* 30(6):384–389, 2009.

Dannemiller Memorial Educational Foundation: *Guide to the prevention and management of falls in the elderly*, 2003. McMahon Publishing Group.

Elderly falls injury prevention legislation and statutes, 2010. National Conference of State Legislatures. www.ncsl.org.

Evans LK, Cotter VT: Avoiding restraints in patients with dementia, *AJN* 108(3):40–49, 2008.

Goodwin J: *For elderly, giving up driving can be tough*, 2010. www.medicinenet.com.

Graf C: The Lawton instrumental activities of daily living scale, *AJN* 108(4):52–62, 2008.

Gray-Micelli D: Falls: nursing standard of practice protocol: fall prevention, *ConsultGeriRN.org* 2008. www.consultgerirn.org.

Heat related mortality, *Nurs Older People* 22(3):13, 2010.

Holohan E: *Driving with early Alzheimer's may be ill-advised*, 2010. www.medicinenet.com.

Horowitz A, Brennan M, Su Y-P: *Dual sensory impairment among the elderly*, 2000, Lighthouse International. www.lighthouse.org.

Marottoli RA: Assessing senior patients' ability to drive safely, *Virtual Mentor* 10(6):365–369, 2008.

New York: Bureau of Injury Prevention: *what you can do to prevent falls*, 2009. www.health.state.ny.us/publications/0640.pdf.

Older drivers, elderly driving, seniors at the wheel, *Smartmotorist.com* 2008. www.smartmotorist.com.

Radziewicz RM, Amato S, Bradas C, et al: Use of physical restraints with elderly patients, *ConsultGeriRN.org* 2009. www.consultgerirn.org.

Rowe M: Wandering in hospitalized older adults, *AJN* 108(10):62–70, 2008.

Saunders GH, Echt KV: An overview of dual sensory impairment in older adults: perspectives for rehabilitation, *Trends Amplif* 11:243–258, 2007. www.tia.sagepub.com.

Senior citizens to die in car crashes at higher rate, *SeniorJournal.com* 2006. www.seniorjournal.com.

Senior Solutions of America: *Elderly drivers: is your loved one driving safely?* 2007. www.agingsolutions.info.

Su Y-P, Brennan M: *Behavioral risk factors and dual sensory impairment*, 2003. Lighthouse International. www.lighthouse.org.

Temple University: *College of Health Professions: in home safety check, Fall Prevention Project*, 1999. www.temple.edu.

White M, Russell D, Saisan J, et al: *Senior driving: safety tips, warning signs, and knowing when to stop*, 2009. www.helpguide.org.

CHAPTER 10

Allaire JC, Gamaldo A, Ayotte BJ, et al: Mild cognitive impairment and objective instrumental everyday functioning: the everyday cognition battery memory test, *JAGS* 57:120–125, 2009.

Allen D: Tipping into forgetfulness, *Nurs Older People* 18(5):38, 2006.

Allen J, Close J: The NICHE geriatric resource nurse model: improving the care of older adults with Alzheimer's disease and other dementias, *Geriatr Nurs* 31(2):128–132, 2010.

Alzheimer's Association: *Dementia with Lewy bodies*, 2010. www.alz.org.

Alzheimer's Disease Education and Referral Center: *Alzheimer's disease medications fact sheet*, 2010. www.nia.nih.gov/Alzheimers.

Arends D, Frick S: Without warning: lessons learned in the development and implementation of an early-onset Alzheimer's disease, *Alzheimer's Care Today* 10(1):31–38, 2009.

Bond SM: Delirium at home, *Home Healthcare Nurs* 27(1):24–34, 2009.

Brennan M, Su Y-P, Horowitz A: Longitudinal associations between dual sensory impairment and everyday competence among older adults, *JRRD* 43(6):777–792, 2006.

Cadden KA: Better pain management, *Nurs Manag* 38(8):35–36, 2007.

California Workgroup on Guidelines for Alzheimer's Disease Management: Guidelines for Alzheimer's disease management, *Athealth.com* 2002. www.athealth.com.

Chaves EHB, de Barros ALBL: Aging as a related factor of nursing diagnosis impaired memory: content validation, *Int J Nurs Terminol Classif* 21(1):14–20, 2010.

Cutilli CC: Teaching the geriatric patient: making the most of "cognitive resources" and "gains," *Orthopaed Nurs* 27(3):195–198, 2008.

D'Arcy Y: Overturning barriers to pain relief in older adults, *Nursing* 39(10):32–38, 2009.

D'Arcy Y: Pain in the older adult, *Nurs Pract* 33(3):18–24, 2008. www.tnpj.com.

Delirium: *FreeDictionary.com* 2010. www.medical-dictionary.thefreedictionary.com/.

Delirium: delirium and dementia. In *Merck Manual Home Health Handbook*, 2010. www.merckmanuals.com/.

Dinsdale P: The pain problem, *Nurs Older People* 18(5):19–21, 2006.

Doerflinger DMC: The mini-cog, *AJN* 107(12):62–71, 2007.

Doheny K: New recommendations for Alzheimer's diagnosis, *MedicineNet.com* 2010. www.medicinenet.com.

Doyle E: Strategies to diagnose delirium in hospitalized patients, *Today's Hospitalist* 2004. www.todayshospitalist.com.

Evans LK, Cotter VT: Avoiding restraints in patients with dementia: understanding, prevention, and management are keys, *AJN* 108(3):40–49, 2008.

Fick DM, Mion LC: Delirium superimposed on dementia, *AJN* 108(1):52–60, 2008.

Flaherty E: Using pain-rating scales with older adults, *AJN* 108(6):40–47, 2008.

Gleason OC: delirium, *Am Fam Physician* 67(5):1027–1034, 2003.

Groves N: Research explores why aging predisposes eye to glaucoma, *Ophthalmol Times* 15(March):26, 2010.

Gupta GM: Evaluation of hearing loss in the elderly and its management, *J Indian Acad Geriatr* 4:115–122, 2008.

Harris PB: Intimacy, sexuality, and early-stage dementia: the changing marital relationship, *Alzheimer's Care Today* 10(2):63–77, 2009.

Horgas A, Miller L: Pain assessment in people with dementia, *AJN* 108(7):62–70, 2008.

Horgas AL: Assessing pain in older adults with dementia, *try this* D2, 2007. www.hartfordign.org.

Johnson EJ: Obesity, lutein metabolism, and age-related macular degeneration: a web of connections, *Nutr Rev* 63(1):9–15, 2005.

Kennes B: Pain in geriatrics, *Rev Med Brux* 22(4):A330–A337, 2001.

Ko JY: Presbycusis and its management, *Br J Nurs* 19(3):160–165, 2010.

Logsdon RG, McCurry SM, Teri L: Evidence-based interventions to improve quality of life for individuals with dementia, *Alzheimer's Care Today* 8(4):309–318, 2007.

Lyketsos CG: The interface between depression and dementia: where are we with this important frontier? *Am J Geriatr Psychiatr* 18(2):95–116, 2010.

Mann AR: Manage the power of pain, *Men Nurs* 1(4):20–28, 2006.

Mann D: Emotions may be blunted in Alzheimer's patients, *MedicineNet.com* 2010. www.medicinenet.com.

Mann D: Spinal fluid test may diagnose Alzheimer's, *MedicineNet.com* 2010. www.medicinenet.com.

Maslow K, Mezey M: Recognition of dementia in hospitalized older adults, *AJN* 108(1):40–49, 2008.

Mayo Clinic Staff: *Alzheimer's care: practical tips*, HO00125, 2009. www.mayoclinic.com.

Mayo Clinic Staff: *Alzheimer's disease*, DS00161, 2009. www.mayoclinic.com.

Mayo Clinic Staff: *Alzheimer's drugs slow progression of disease*, AZ00015, 2009. www.mayoclinic.com.

Mayo Clinic Staff: *Alzheimer's: dealing with daily changes*, AZ00026, 2009. www.mayoclinic.com.

Mayo Clinic Staff: *Alzheimer's: is it in your genes?* AZ00047, 2008. www.mayoclinic.com.

Mayo Clinic Staff: *Alzheimer's: mementos help preserve memories*, AZ00020, 2009. www.mayoclinic.com.

Mayo Clinic Staff: *Alzheimer's: understand and control wandering*, HQ00218, 2010. www.mayoclinic.com.

Mayo Clinic Staff: *Diabetes and Alzheimer's linked*, AZ00050, 2008. www.mayoclinic.com.

Melatonin: treating Alzheimer's symptoms with melatonin, 2007. www.alzheimers.about.com.

Merck Manual of Geriatrics: *delirium*, 2010. www.merck.com/mkgr/mmg/sec5/ch39/ch39a.jsp.

Montgomery J, Mitty E: Resident condition change: should I call 911? *Geriatr Nurs* 29(1):15–26, 2008.

New York Memory Services: *ABCs of aging, Alzheimer's, estrogen and memory*, 2005. www.nymemory.org.

Redmond N, While A: Age-related macular degeneration: visual impairment with advancing age, *Br J Commun Nurs* 13(2):68–75, 2008.

Sherman FT: Functional assessment: easy-to-use screening tools speed initial office work-up, *Geriatrics* 56(8):36–40, 2001.

Spencer P: Medications used to treat Alzheimer's, *Caring.com* 2010. www.caring.com.

Stokoe BD: Caring for people with end-stage dementia, *Nurs Older People* 22(2):31–36, 2010.

Stokowski LA: Cognitive health for an aging population, *Medscape Public Health & Prevention* 2009. www.medscape.com.

Vance DE: Speed of processing in older adults: a cognitive overview of nursing, *J Neurosci Nurs* 41(6):290–297, 2009.

Wallhagen MI, Pettengill E, Whiteside M: Sensory impairment in older adults: part 1: hearing loss, *AJN* 106(10):40–48, 2006.

Wallhagen MI, Pettengill E, Whiteside M: Sensory impairment in older adults: part 2: vision loss, *AJN* 106(11):52–61, 2006.

WebMD: *Alzheimer's disease health center: dementia medications*, 2007. www.webmd.com.

Yueh B, Shekelle P: Quality indicators for the care of hearing loss in vulnerable elders, *JAGS* 55:S335–S339, 2007.

CHAPTER 11

5 Ways to relieve the self-esteem effects of aging, 2008. www.agingparentsauthority.com.

Agarwal A: *Rebuilding self-esteem among the elderly—helping them regain their lost self-esteem*, 2008. www.ezinarticles.com.

Aging baby boomers, 2010. www.wikinvest.com.

Bayridge Anxiety & Depression Treatment Center: Statistics: depression/anxiety… get the facts, 2007. www.bayridgetreatmentcenter.com.

Block S: *Elder care shifting away from nursing homes*, 2007. www.usatoday.com/…/…/eldercare/2007_06-24.

Boyer JM: Understanding the context for arts and aging programs. In *Creativity Matters: The Arts and Aging Toolkit*, chap 1, 2010. www.artsandaging.org.

Chao Sy, Liu HY, Wu Cy, et al: The effects of group reminiscence therapy on depression, self-esteem, and life satisfaction of elderly nursing home residents, *J Nurs Res* 14(1):36–45, 2006.

Davidson AL: *Effects of ageism*, 2002. www.essortment.com.

Depression and elderly—depression and older adults: what it is and how to get help, 2010. www.depression-guide.com.

Depression statistics, 2010. www.indepression.com.

Dotinga R: *Aging & geriatrics: levels of self-esteem may fluctuate over time*, 2010. www/mentalhelp.net.

Filipp S-H: *Motivation—social motivation and self-esteem in old age*, 2010. www.medicine.jrank.org/pages/1180/Motivation-Social-motivation-self-esteem-in-old-age.html.

Graf C: The Lawton instrumental activities of daily living scale, *AJN* 108(4):52–62, 2008.

Happiness and self-esteem in age, 2006. www.medrounds.org/encyclopedia-of-aging.

Happiness and self-esteem in age, 2006. www.medrounds.org/encyclopedia-of-aging/2006.

Lill S: *Reminiscence therapy: therapy shown to unlock memory of individuals with Alzheimer's disease*, 2008. www.nursing.advanceweb.com.

Myths and facts about depression in the elderly, 2010. www.agingcare.com.

Older adults: depression and suicide facts (fact sheet), 2010. NIH publ: 4593. www.nimh.nih.gov.

Perceptions of aging, 2009. www.transgenerational.org.

President's Council on Bioethics: the aging self, *The New Atlantis* 10:101–113, 2005. www.thenewatlantis.com.

Price B: Older woman's body image, *Nurs Older People* 22(1):31–36, 2010.

Schoenstadt A: *Depression in the elderly*, 2010. www.depression.emedtv.com.

Self-esteem in older adults, 1998. www.theonlinepeople.com.

Smith M, Segal R, Segal J: *Depression in older adults and the elderly: recognizing the signs and getting help*, 2010. www.helpguide. org/mental/depression_elderly.htm.

U.S. National Institute on Aging: *Study finds improved cognitive health among older Americans*, 2008. www.nia.nih.gov/.../ PR20080225coghealth.htm.

CHAPTER 12

Baby boomer "retirement" facts: *What's Next in Your Life?* 2008. www.whatsnextinyourlife.com.

Bradway C, Hirschman KB: How to try this: working with families of hospitalized older adults with dementia, *AJN* 108(10):52–60, 2008.

Center for Aging Studies Without Walls: 2010. UMKC. www. cas.umkc.edu/casww/sa/relationships.htm.

Center on Aging, University of Hawaii: *Growing old in a new age*, 2008. www.growingold.hawaii.edu.

Cornett S: *The effects of aging on health literacy*, 2008. www. medicine.osu.edu/sitetool/sites/pdfs/ahecpublic/ HL_Module_Elderly.pdf.

Damron-Rodriguez J: Developing competence for nurses and social workers, *AJN* 108(Suppl 9):40–46, 2008.

Davidson AL: *The effects of ageism*, 2002. www.essortment.com/ all/ageismeffectss_rnxj.htm.

Given B, Sherwood PR, Given CW: What knowledge and skills do caregivers need? *AJN* 108(Suppl 9):28–34, 108(9):62–69, 2008.

Hansen JC: Community and in-home models, *AJN* 108 (Suppl 9):69–72, 2008.

Jenko M, Gonzalez L, Seymour MJ: Life review with the terminally ill, *J Hospital Palliative Nurs* 9(3):159–167, 2007.

Kaplan M: *Ah, to be old and fragging: roles for the elderly in video games*, 2009. www.gamecritics.com.

Lindley SE, Harper R, Sellen A: Designing for elders: exploring the complexity of relationships in later life, *Proc 22nd Ann Conf Br HCI Group* HCI, 1:77–86, 2008.

Messecar D, Powers BA, Nagel CL: How to try this: the family preferences index: helping family members who want to participate in the care of hospitalized older adults, *AJN* 108 (9):52–59, 2010.

Messecar D, Powers BA, Nagel CL: How to try this: the family preferences index, *AJN* 108(9):52–59, 2008.

Murphy F: Loneliness: a challenge for nurses caring for older people, *Nurs Older People* 18(5):22–25, 2006.

New concept for boomer retirement: freedom to work, 2007. www. ocregister.com.

O'Brien S: *How baby boomers will change retirement. Part 1: many baby boomers plan to mix work and play*, 2010. www.seniorliving. about.com.

Onega LL: How to try this: helping those who help others: the modified caregiver strain index, *AJN* 108(9):62–69, 2008.

Peterson JW: Age of wisdom: elderly black women in family and church. In Sokolovsky J, editor: *Culture Context of Aging: Worldwide Perspectives*, ed 3, chap 25, Westport, CT, 2009, Greenwood Press. www.stpt.usf.edu/~jsokolov.

Powell L: Theorising social gerontology: the case of social philosophies of age. In *Understanding Social Gerontology: the Case of Social Theory*. www.sincronia.cucsh.udg.mx/ powell.htm.

Schulz R, Sherwood PR: Physical and mental health effects of family caregiving, *AJN* 108(Suppl 9):23–27, 2008.

Zarit S, Femia E: Behavioral and psychosocial interventions for family caregivers, *AJN* 108(Suppl 9):47–53, 2008.

Zunzunegui M-V, Béland F, Sanchez M-T, et al: Longevity and relationships with children: the importance of the parental role, *BMC Publ Health* 9:351, 2009. www. biomedcentral.com.

CHAPTER 13

Aldwin CM: Does age affect the stress and coping process? Implications of age differences in perceived control, *J Gerontol* 46(4):174–180, 1991.

Aldwin CM: The role of stress in aging and adult development, APA Division 20, *Cutting Edge* 1995. www.apadiv20.phhp. ufl.edu/aldwin.htm.

Cho LM, Chau DL: Pain management in the elderly, *FPRonline* 29(9):19–26, 2007.

Elder Response Team, Elder issues: 2010. www.elderresponseteam. org/elder%20issues.htm.

Elderly depression, 2010. www.seniors.lovetoknow.com/ elderly_depression.

Ferszt GG, Leveille M: Psych review: telling the difference between grief and depression, *LPN* 5(3):12–13, 2009.

Hicks LE, Wood N: Depression and suicide risks in older adults: a case study, *Home Healthcare Nurs* 27(8):482–487, 2009.

Hunter IR, Gillen MC: Stress coping mechanisms in elderly adults: an initial study of recreational and other coping behaviors in nursing home patients, *Adultspan J* 2009. www.highbeam.com.

Husanini BA, Moore ST, Castor RS, et al: Social density, stressors, and depression: gender differences among the black elderly, *J Gerontol* 46(5):236–242, 1991.

Lau BWK: Stress, coping and aging, *J Hong Kong Coll Psychiatr* 4(SP2):39–44, 1994.

McCrae RR: Age differences and changes in the use of coping mechanisms, *J Gerontol* 44(6):161–169, 1989.

McHolm F: Rx for compassion, *JCN* 23(4):12–19, 2006.

Mehta KM, Yaffe K, Brenes GA, et al: Anxiety symptoms and decline in physical function over 5 years in health, aging and body composition study, *JAGS* 55:265–270, 2007.

Merck Manuals: Geriatrics. Intimacy: social issues in the elderly, 2009. www.merckmanuals.com/professional/sec23/ch344/ ch344g.html.

Murphy K: Unlocking the mystery of depression and anxiety, *LPN* 4(5):34–42, 2008.

Naegle MA: How to try this: screening for alcohol use and misuse in older adults, *AJN* 108(11):50–58, 2008.

Naylor M, Keating SA: Transitional care: moving patients from one care setting to another, *AJN* 108(Suppl 9):58–63, 2008.

Ronningen M: *Aging, coping with stress*, January 2010. www. examiner.com.

Sander R: Journal scan, *Nurs Older People* 22(2):15, 2010.

Smith M: *Depression in older adults and the elderly*, 2010. www. helpguide.org/mental/depression_elderly.htm.

Stress coping strategies for the elderly, www.everyday-wisdom.com. Accessed October 2010.

Sudak HS: Predicting suicide rates in the elderly, *Am J Psychiatr* 167(1):102, 2010.

US CDC: *CDC promotes public health approach to address depression among older adults*, 2009. www.cdc.gov/aging/pdf/ CIB_mental_health.pdf.

Wright PM, Hogan NS: Grief theories and models: applications to hospice nursing practice, *J Hospice Palliative Nurs* 10 (6):350–356, 2008.

Zarit S, Femia E: Behavioral and psychosocial interventions for family caregivers, *AJN* 108(Suppl 9):47–53, 2008.

CHAPTER 14

Anderson K: Baby boomerangs, *LeadershipU* 1994. www.leaderu. com/orgs/probe/docs/boomer.html.

Baby boomer generation [born 1946–1964], *ValueOptions. com* 2010. www.valueoptions.com/spotlight_YIW/baby_ boomers.htm.

Bernstein A: *Spirituality and aging: looking at the big picture*, 2010. www.agingwellmag.com.

Center on Aging Studies Without Walls: *spirituality and aging,* 2010. www.cas.umkc.edu/casww/sa/spirituality.htm.

Creel E, Tillman K: The meaning of spirituality among non-religious persons with chronic illness, *Holist Nurs Pract* 22(6):303–309, 2008.

Klaessy S: Research and trends: baby boomer values give insight into buying decisions, ISC, *Manag Market Leasing Today* 2005. www.icsc.org/srch/education/newsletter/clsmNews1005/article13.pdf.

Lynn D: *Psychotherapy, spirituality, and aging,* 2002. www.articlesfactory.com.

National Oceanographic and Atmosphere Association, Office of Diversity: *Tips to improve interaction among the generations: traditionalists, boomers, x'ers and nexters,* Honolulu, 2010, Community College, University of Hawaii. www.honolulu.hawaii.edu/intranet/committees/FacDevCom/guidebk/teachtip/intergencomm.htm.

Poitou N: *Spiritual crisis,* 2007. www.goodtherapy.org/blog/spiritual-crisis.

Retirement or senior stage of life, 2009. www.webmd.com/healthy-aging/guide/retirement-or-senior-stage-of-life.

Roof WC: *Spiritual marketplace: baby boomers and the remaking of American religion,* 2001, Princeton Univ Press.

Simmons PD: *Spirituality and successful aging: twelve rules for the road,* 2009. www.journal.oates.org.

Sinnamon SE: *Spirituality and aging,* 2010. www.go60.com/spirituality-aging.html.

Spirituality, aging, and health, (Interview with Dr. James Griffin). *Chapster,* 2002. www.elderhope.com.

Stinson CK: Structured group reminiscence: an intervention for older adults, *J Cont Educ Nurs* 40(11):521–528, 2009.

Vitale A: An integrative review of Reiki touch therapy research, *Holist Nurs Pract* 21(4):167–179, 2007.

CHAPTER 15

5 Tips on helping prevent elderly suicide, *AgingCare.com* 2010. www.agingcare.com/news/135805.

Allen CH: Providing compassionate end-of-life care, *LPN* 5(4):19–25, 2009.

Allen CH: Providing compassionate end-of-life care, *Nursing Made Incredibly Easy!* 6(4):46–53, 2008.

Authers D: *How to deal with an elderly parent's fear of dying,* 2010. www.agingcare.com/featured-stories/138570/dealing-with-elderly-parents-.

Browning AM: Incorporating spiritual beliefs into end-of-life care, *JCN* 26(1):11–17, 2009.

Coviello JS, Tadel PM: Palliative care in heart failure: a case study of collaborative practice, *Home Healthcare Nurs* 27(1):12–16, 2009. www.homehealthcarenurseonline.com.

Death and dying, 2006. www.efmoody.com/miscellaneous/dying.html.

Durham E, Weiss L: How patients die, *AJN* 97(12):41–46, 1997.

Greenwald B: *Death and dying,* 2010. www.uic.edu/orgs/convening/deathdyi.htm.

Heyman JC, Gutheil IA: Older Latino's attitudes toward and comfort with end-of-life planning, *Health Soc Work* 35(1):17–26, 2010.

How to take great care of elders, *Wings of Success* 2009. www.wingsofsuccess.info/.

Muller LS, Flarey DL: Right to die [Legal and ethical forum], *Case Manag Legal/Ethical* 10(5):224–231, 2005.

Schwarz JK: Stopping eating and drinking, *AJN* 109(9):53–61, 2009.

Turis M: Nursing homes may be only option for palliative care, *Canad Nurs Home* 17(2):4–10, 2006.

USC-Davis, School of Gerontology: Death and dying, 2010. www.usc.edu/dept/gero/AgeWorks/core_courses/gero500_core/death_lecture.

Waller E: *Lesson thirteen—death and dying process. Gerontology 130: working with the frail elderly,* 2001, Coastline Community College, University of South California. www.cvc3.coastline.edu/modelcvc3courses/elliswaller/lesson13.htm.

CHAPTER 16

Abernathy M: *Gay and gray,* October 27, 2006. www.popmatters.com.

For elderly, sex doesn't have to get old, *Reuters* August 13, 2008. www.reuters.com/article/idUSN1248113920080813.

Gross J: Aging and gay, and facing prejudice in twilight, *NY Times* October 9, 2007. www.nytimes.com.

Harris PB: Intimacy, sexuality, and early-stage dementia: the changing marital relationship, *Alzheimer's Care Today* 10(2):63–77, 2009.

Male sexual dysfunction, *Merck Manual Professional* 2007. www.merck.com/mmpe.

Medications that affect sexual function, *Cleveland Clinic* 2009, #9124. www.my.clevelandclinic.org/disorders.

Parker-Pope T: More sex for today's seniors, *NY Times* July 22, 2008. www.well.blogs.nytimes.com/2008/07/22.

Riley A: Loss of sexual desire, March 10, 2010. www.pulsetoday.co.uk.

Sexual dysfunction among older Americans tied to experiences, health, demographics, August 19, 2008. www.seniorjournal.com.

Sexual lives of older women more likely hindered by physical problems than older men's, September 25, 2008. www.seniorjournal.com.

Thornhill TH: Aging and sexuality, *US Pharm* 32(6):HS5–HS18, 2007.

Wallace MA: Assessment of sexual health in older adults, *AJN* 108(7):52–60, 2008.

Women may live longer than men but don't enjoy, engage in sex as long, March 11, 2010. www.seniorjournal.com.

Woolf LM: *Gay and lesbian aging,* 1998, Webster University. www.webster.edu/~woolflm/oldergay.html.

CHAPTER 17

Aging mouth—and how to keep it younger, *Harvard Health Lett* January 2010. www.health.harvard.edu.

Avon turns to experimental medicine to brighten skin, *Stylelist* 2010. www.stylelist.com.

Baranoski S, Ayello EA: *Wound care essentials: practice principles,* ed 2, Philadelphia, 2007, Lippincott.

Baranoski S: How to prevent and manage skin tears, *Adv Skin Wound Care* 16(5):268–270, 2003.

Baranoski S: Skin tears: the enemy of frail skin, *Adv Skin Wound Care* May/June 2000. www.findarticles.com/p/articles/mi_qa39977/is_200004/ai_n8894280.

Barr JE: Impaired skin integrity in the elderly, *Ostomy Wound Manag* 52(2):2008. www.o-wm.com/article/5635.

Beckrich K, Aronovitch SA: Hospital-acquired pressure ulcers: a comparison of costs in medical vs. Surgical patients, *Nurs Economy* September 1999. www.findarticles.com/p/mi_m0FSW/is_5_17/ai_n18609011.

Burnett CT, Ozog DM: Aging gracefully, *Dermatol Nurs* 2010. www.medscape.com/viewarticle/725083.

Campbell KE: A new model to identify shared risk factors for pressure ulcers and frailty in older adults, *Rehab Nurs* 34(6):242–247, 2009.

Catania K, Huang C, James P, et al: PUPPI: The pressure ulcer prevention protocol interventions, *AJN* 107(4):44–52, 2007.

Center for Medicare & Medicaid Services, Nursing Home Quality Initiatives: Section M: skin conditions, In *CMS's RAI Version 3.0 Manual.* www.cms.gov/NursingHomeQualityInits/45_NHQIMDS30TrainingMaterials.asp.

Columbia Univ Medical Center, Dept of Surgery: Wound healing, *Healthpoints* 2007. www.cumc.columbia.edu/dept/cs/cli/wound/.

Gender A: Pressure ulcer prevention and management, *ARNNetwork* 8–9, Oct/Nov 2008.

Gist S, Tio-Matos I, Falzgraf S, et al: Wound care in the geriatric client, *Clin Interven Aging* 2009(4):269–287, 2009.

Grupp K, Albert M: Teaching wound care in the home, *Home Health Care Qrtly* 11(3&4):157–195, 1990.

Harris CL, Fraser C: Malnutrition in the institutionalized elderly: the effect on wound healing, *Ostomy Wound Manag* 50(10) 2008. www.o-wm.com/article/3182.

Hurd TA: Nutrition and wound-care management/prevention, *Wound Care Can* 2(2):20–24, 2004.

Institute for Healthcare Improvement: *Relieve the pressure and reduce harm*, 2007. www.ihi.org/IHI/Topics/PatientSafety/SafetyGeneral/ImprovementStories/FSRelievethePressureandReduceHarm.htm.

Jackson R: Elderly patients during bath time: neat and clean, *Associated Content* April 13, 2005. www.associatedcontent.com/article/1130/elderly_patients_during_bath_time.html.

Koh-Knox CP, Sussman G: Wound care in an aging population: special considerations, *Pharm Times* 2007. www.secure.pharmacytimes.com/lessons/200404-02.asp.

Levine JM: *Dr. Gene Cohen: creative aging, and geriatric psychiatry*, December 2009. www.jeffreymlevinemd.com.

Marren JM, Harrington C, Kluger M: Nursing counts: focus on improving safety and outcomes in home care, *AJN* 106 (1):37–38, 2006.

Mayo Clinic Staff: Bedsores (pressure sores), *Mayo Clinic* DS00570, 2009. www.mayoclinic.com.

Meehan M: Prevalence of wounds among the frail elderly: a look at its value, *Wounds* April 2005. www.woundsresearch.com/article/3949.

Nelzén O, Bergqvist D, Lindhagen A, et al: Chronic leg ulcers: an underestimated problem in primary health care among elderly patients, *J Epidemiol Commun Health* 45:184–187, 1991.

Rader J, Barrick AL, Hoeffer B, et al: Bathing of older adults with dementia, *AJN* 106(4):40–48, 2006.

Risk factors for pressure ulcers identified, *News, Medscape Medical News* September 2001. www.medscape.com.

Salcido R, Popescu A: Pressure ulcers and wound care, *eMedicine* 2009. www.emedicine.medscape.com/article/319284.

Shawnee Mission Medical Center: *Wound care quick reference guide*, August 2008. www.premierinc.com/safety/topics/pressure-ulcer/pressure-ulcer-downloads/WoundCareGuide-082008.pdf.

Stein PS, Henry RG: Poor oral hygiene in long-term care, *AJN* 109(6):44–50, 2009.

Stotts NA, Gunningberg L: Predicting pressure ulcer risk, *AJN* 107(11):40–48, 2007.

Takahashi PY, Kiemele LJ, Jones JP: Wound care for elderly patients: advances and clinical applications for practicing physicians, *Mayo Clin Proc* 79:26–267, 2004.

Thomas DR: Prevention and treatment of pressure ulcers: what works? What doesn't? *Cleveland Clin J Med* 68(6):704–722, 2001.

Whittington K: Pay-4-prevention: CMS guidelines focus on prevention of pressure ulcers, *Adv Nurs* 2008. www.nursing.advanceweb.com.

Why are pressure ulcers being classified as "never events"? 2008. www.woundeducators.com/wordpress/are_you_ready_for_october_2008.

CHAPTER 18

A Place for Mom: *Elderly urinary tract infections*, 2010. www.nursing-homes.aplaceformom.com/articles/elderly-urinary-tract-infection.

Basson MC: constipation, *eMed Gastroentero* 2010. www.emedicine.medscape.com/article/184704.

Bouras EP, Tangalos EG: Chronic constipation in the elderly, *Gastroenterol Clin North Am* 38(3):463–480, 2009.

Digestive Disorders Health Center: *The basics of constipation*, 2007. www.webmd.com/digestive-disorders/digestive-diseases-constipation.

Dowling-Castronovo A, Specht JK: Assessment of transient urinary incontinence in older adults, *AJN* 109(2):62–71, 2009.

Fecal impaction removal. In Krapp K, editor: *Encyclopedia of Nursing & Allied Health*, 2002, Gale Cengage, *eNotes.com*, 2006. www.enotes.com/nursing-encyclopedia/fecal-impaction-removal.

Ginsberg DA, Phillips SF, Wallace J, et al: Evaluating and managing constipation in the elderly, *Urol Nurs* 27(3):191–200, 212, 2007.

Grover ML, Bracamonte JD, Kanodia AK, et al: Urinary tract infection in women over the age of 65: is age alone a marker of complications? *J Am Board Fam Med* 22(3):266–271, 2009.

Hill R: Don't let constipation stop you up, *Nursing Made Incredibly Easy* 5(5):47–48, 58, 2007. www.journals.lww.com/nursingmadeincrediblyeasy/Citation/2007/09000/.

Kalish VB, Loven B: What is the best treatment for chronic constipation in the elderly? *J Fam Practice* 56(12):1050–1052, 2007.

Lembo AJ: Best practices in chronic constipation in the elderly, *Intern Med News* 2010. www.internalmedicinenews.com/fileadmin/content_pdf/imn/supplement_pdf/wxvc289z_BP_Supplement2.pdf.

Leung FW: Fecal incontinence in the elderly, *Gastroenterol Clin North Am* 38(3):503–511, 2009.

Monti M: Prevalence and risk factors of constipation among the elderly in nursing homes, *G Gerontol* 57(2):78–86, 2009.

Rao SSC, Go JT: Update on the management of constipation in the elderly: new treatment options, *Clin Interv Aging* 2010 (5):163–171, 2010.

Serafin J: *Why are urinary tract infections in elderly women so common?* www.caring.com/questions/elderly-women-urinary-tract-infections. Accessed November 20, 2010.

Spinzi G, Amato A, Imperiali G, et al: Constipation in the elderly: management strategies, *Drugs Aging* 26 (6):469–474, 2009.

Stewart E: Overactive bladder syndrome in the older woman: conservative treatment, *Br J Community Nurs* 14 (11):466–473, 2009.

CHAPTER 19

American Heart Association: Exercise (physical activity) for older people and those with disabilities, 2010. www.americanheart>org/print_presenter.jtml.

Cyarto EV, Brown WJ, Marshall AL, et al: Comparison of the effects of home-based and group-based resistance training program on functional ability in older adults, *Am J Health Promotion* 23(1):13–17, 2008.

Deep down exercise helps keep you young, *Tufts Univ Health Nutr Lett* 2010. www.tuftshealthletter.com.

Gordon C: Physical activity for older adults: exercise for life! In *Live Well, Live Long: Steps to Better Health Series*, 2005, American Society on Aging. www.asaging.org/cdc/module6/home.cfm.

Huang AR: Getting a grip on aging, *CMAJ* 182(5):423, 2010.

Jennrich J: Activity ideas for elderly senior citizens, *Suite101.com* 2007. www.suite101.com/content/fun-activities-for-senior-citizens-a27665.

More studies find that regular exercise helps protect aging brains, *Harvard Women's Health Watch* April 2010. www.health.harvard.edu.

National Institute on Aging: *Exercise & physical activity: your everyday guide*, 2010. www.nia.nih.gov/HealthInformation/Publications/ExerciseGuide.

Shubert TE: The use of commercial health video games to promote physical activity in older adults, *Ann Long-Term Care* 18(5):27–32, 2010.

Sollitto M: *Exercise for the elderly, Agingcare.com* 2010. www.agingcare.com/featured-stories/95383.

Thompson PD, Buchner D, Piña IL, et al: Exercise and physical activity in the prevention and treatment of atherosclerotic cardiovascular disease: a statement from the Council on Clinical Cardiology, *Circulation* 107:3109–3116, 2003.

Traywick L: *Increasing physical activity as we age: exercise recommendations*, 2006. Univ of Arkansas, Division of Agriculture, FSFCS30. www.uaex.edu/Other_Areas/publications/PDF/FSFCS30.pdf.

U.S. Department of Agriculture: Elderly improve with exercise, too, *ScienceDaily* www.sciencedaily.com/releases/2008/03/080321123721.htm. 2008.

U.S. National Institute on Aging: Exercise and physical activity: getting fit for life, 2010. www.nia.nih.gov/healthinformation/publications/exercise.htm.

CHAPTER 20

Cole C, Richards K: Sleep disruption in older adults, *AJN* 107 (5):40–49, 2007.

de Benedictis T, Larson H, Kemp G, et al: Sleeping well as you age: health sleep habits for seniors, *Helpguide.org* 2008. www.helpguide.org/life/sleep_aging.htm.

Fisher D, Valente S: Evaluating and managing insomnia, *Nurs Practitioner* 34(8):21–26, 2009.

Freedman L: Tired of Ambien? Meet the sleep medications of the near future, *health.com* 2008. www.health.com/health.

Geriatric Mental Health Foundation: *Sleeping well as we age: insomnia is not a normal part of aging*, 2008. www.gmhfonline.org/gmhf/.../hlthage_sleep.html.

Hoffman S: Sleep in older adults: implications for nurses, *Geriatr Nurs* 24(4):210–216, 2003.

Hulisz D, Duff C: Assisting seniors with insomnia: a comprehensive approach, *US Pharm* 34(6):38–43, 2009.

Kouch M: End-of-life-care: helping patients rest easily, *LPN* 3 (4):39–45, 2007.

Mayo Clinic Staff: Alzheimer's: managing sleep problems, *Mayo Clinic* AZ00030, 2009. www.mayoclinic.com.

National Sleep Foundation: *Aging and sleep*, 2009. www.sleepfoundation.org/.../aging-and-sleep.

Neubauer DN: Sleep problems in the elderly, *Am Acad Family Physicians* 1999. www.aafp.org/afp/990501ap.

Pagel JF, Parnes BL: Medications for the treatment of sleep disorders: an overview, *Primary Care Companion J Clin Psychiatr* 3:118–125, 2001.

Sleep disorders guide: drugs to treat insomnia, *webmd.com* 2010. www.webmd.com/sleep-disorders/guide.

Sleep disorders in the elderly overview, *NY Times* January 23, 2009. www.health.nytimes.com/health/guides/disease/sleep-disorder.

Smyth C: *The Epworth sleepiness scale (ESS), Best Practice Information on Care of Older Adults* 6(2):2007. www.ConsultGeriRN.org.

Smyth CA: Evaluating sleep quality in older adults, *AJN* 108 (5):42–50, 2008.

Subramanian S, Surani S: Sleep disorders in the elderly, *Geriatrics* 62(12):10–32, 2007.

Umlauf MG, Williams LL, Chasen ER: Sleep: nursing standard practice protocol: excessive sleepiness, *Hartford Institute for Geriatric Nursing* 2008. www.ConsultGeriRN.org/topics/sleep/.

U.S. National Institute on Aging: *A good night's sleep*, 2009. www.nia.nih.gov/healthinformation/publications/sleep.htm.

U.S. National Institute on Aging: *Sleep & growing older quiz*, 2010. www.sleepeducation.com.

U.S. National Institute on Aging: *Sleep & growing older*, 2010. www.sleepeducation.com.

U.S. NINDS: Brain basics: understanding sleep, *NINDS* 2007. www.ninds.nih.gov/disorders/brain_basics.

Wolkove N, Elkholy O, Baltzan M, et al: Sleep and aging: 2. Management of sleep disorders in older people, *CMAJ* 176 (10):1449–1454, 2007.

Glossary

A

Absorption As in drug absorption, the process whereby a drug moves from the muscle, digestive tract, or other site of entry into the body toward the circulatory system.

Abuse Intentional or unintentional mistreatment or harm—physical, psychological, emotional, or financial—of another person.

Agility Ability to move quickly and smoothly.

Alignment The placing or maintaining of body structures in their proper anatomic positions.

Alopecia Partial or complete lack of hair resulting from normal aging, endocrine disorder, drug reaction, anticancer medication, or skin disease.

Anemia A hematologic disorder marked by a decrease in hemoglobin in the blood to abnormally low levels, caused by a decrease in red blood cell production, an increase in red blood cell destruction, or a loss of blood. Iron-deficiency anemia results from inadequate intake of dietary iron, and pernicious anemia results from a deficiency in intrinsic factor secreted by the stomach.

Anorexia Lack or loss of appetite, resulting in the inability to eat.

Antioxidants Chemicals or other agents that retard or inhibit oxidation of a substance to which they are added. Examples are vitamins, carotenoids, selenium, and phytochemicals.

Anxiety A vague, uneasy feeling, the source of which is often nonspecific or unknown to the individual.

Aphasia Abnormal neurologic condition in which language function is disordered or absent because of an injury to certain areas of the cerebral cortex. May be a result of a stroke.

Apnea An absence of spontaneous breathing or respiration.

Arthritis Any inflammatory condition of the joints, characterized by pain, swelling, heat, redness, or limitation of movement.

Aseptic Free of living pathogenic organisms or infected material.

Assessment In medicine and nursing, an evaluation or appraisal of a condition or the process of making such an evaluation, including the patient's subjective report of the symptoms and the examiner's objective findings of data obtained through laboratory tests, physical examination, and medical history.

Auscultation A technique of assessment that uses the sense of hearing to detect sounds produced within the body, such as heart, lung, and bowel sounds.

B

Basal metabolic rate Rate at which the body uses calories.

Biologic Pertaining to organisms; biologic aging views aging from a genetic perspective.

Blood urea nitrogen A measure of the amount of urea, the end product of protein metabolism, in the blood.

Body image A person's concept of his or her physical appearance.

Boredom The state of being made weary by dullness, tedium, repetitiveness.

C

Cachexia General ill health and malnutrition, marked by weakness and emaciation, usually associated with severe disease, such as tuberculosis or cancer.

Calorie Unit of heat that is used to measure the available energy in consumed food.

Carbohydrates Sugars and starches that constitute the main source of energy for all body functions, particularly brain functions, and that are necessary for the metabolism of other nutrients.

Carcinoma Malignant epithelial neoplasm that tends to invade surrounding tissue and to metastasize to distant regions of the body.

Cardiomegaly Enlargement of the heart, often related to congestive heart failure.

Caries As in dental caries, a tooth disease caused by the complex interaction of food, especially starches and sugars, with the bacteria that form dental plaque; cavities.

Cataract Clouding of the lens of the eye, developing over time and resulting in progressive, painless loss of vision.

Catastrophic reactions Excessively emotional responses.

Catheterization Introduction of a catheter (a hollow flexible tube) into a body cavity or organ to inject or remove a fluid.

Cheyne-Stokes As in respirations, an abnormal pattern of respirations, characterized by alternating periods of apnea and deep, rapid breathing.

Chronologic age The number of years a person has lived.

Circadian As in circadian rhythm, a pattern based on a 24-hour cycle, especially the repetition of certain physiologic phenomena such as sleeping and eating.

Cognitive Pertaining to the mental processes of comprehension, judgment, memory, and reasoning, as contrasted with emotional processes.

Cohort Term used by demographers to describe a group of people born within a specified time period.

Confrontation A communication technique used when there are inconsistencies in information or when verbal and nonverbal messages appear contradictory.

Confusion A mental state characterized by disorientation regarding time, place, or person that leads to bewilderment, perplexity, lack of orderly thought, and the inability to choose or act decisively and to perform activities of daily living.

Constipation Difficulty in passing stools or incomplete or infrequent passage of hard stools.

Coordination Harmonious functioning of muscles or groups of muscles in the execution of movements.

Coping Process by which a person deals with stress, solves problems, and makes decisions.

Creatinine A substance formed from the metabolism of creatine, commonly found in blood. It is measured in blood and urine tests as an indicator of kidney function.

Custodial focus As in custodial care, services and care of a nonmedical nature provided on a long-term basis, usually for convalescent and chronically ill individuals.

D

Defecation The elimination of feces from the digestive tract through the rectum.

Delirium A mental disorder characterized by disturbances in cognition, attention, memory, and perception. Symptoms include confusion, disorientation, restlessness, clouding of consciousness, incoherence, fear, anxiety, and excitement. It is also often characterized by illusions; hallucinations, usually of visual origin; and at times, delusions.

Dementia A general term for a permanent or progressive organic mental disorder, characterized by personality changes, confusion, disorientation, and deterioration of intellectual functioning and by impaired control of memory, judgment, and impulses.

Demographics The statistical study of human populations.

Depression A mental state of depressed mood characterized by feelings of sadness, despair, and discouragement, ranging from normal feelings of "the blues" all the way to major clinical depression. Resembling the grief and mourning that follow bereavement, the symptoms of depression include feelings of low self-esteem, guilt, and self-reproach; withdrawal from interpersonal contact; and somatic symptoms such as eating and sleep disorders.

Dexterity Skillfulness in the use of one's hands or body; the ability to perform fine, manipulative skills.

Diarrhea The frequent passage of loose, watery stools.

Distress An emotional or physical state of pain, sorrow, misery, suffering, or discomfort.

Distribution As in drug distribution, the pattern of distribution of drug molecules by various tissues after the chemical enters the circulatory system.

Diuretics Drugs that promote the formation and excretion of urine.

Diurnal Occurring daily, as sleeping and eating.

Diversional As in diversional activity, stimulation from or interest or engagement in recreational or leisure activities.

Diverticulosis The presence of pouchlike herniations (diverticula) throughout the muscular layer of the colon, which develop because of weaknesses in the intestinal mucosa.

Dysarthria Difficult, poorly articulated speech, resulting from interference in the control and execution over the muscles of speech, usually caused by neurologic damage.

Dysfunctional Unable to function normally.

Dysphasia See *aphasia*.

Dyspnea A distressful sensation of uncomfortable breathing that may be caused by certain heart conditions, strenuous exercise, or anxiety.

E

Edema The abnormal accumulation of fluid in the interstitial spaces of tissues, caused by increased capillary fluid pressure.

Electrocardiogram (ECG) A graphic record produced by an electrocardiograph, a device for recording electrical conduction through the heart.

Electrolyte An element or compound that, when melted or dissolved in water or another solvent, dissociates into ions and is able to conduct an electric current.

Empathy The willingness to attempt to understand the unique world of another person; the ability to put oneself in another person's place and to understand what he or she is feeling and thinking in various situations.

Enema The introduction of a solution into the rectum for cleansing or therapeutic purposes.

Ethical dilemmas Questions or problems related to moral values or principles.

Excretion As in drug excretion, the process of eliminating, shedding, or getting rid of a drug by body organs or tissues as part of natural metabolic activity.

Exudate Fluid, cell, or other substance that has been slowly discharged from cells or blood vessels through small pores or breaks in cell membranes.

F

Fatigue A state of exhaustion or a loss of strength or endurance, such as may follow strenuous physical activity.

Fear A response to a perceived threat that is consciously recognized as a danger.

Fecal impaction An accumulation of hardened feces in the rectum or sigmoid colon that the individual is unable to move or pass.

Feedback Information produced by a receiver and perceived by a sender that informs the sender of the receiver's reaction to the message.

Free radical Unstable molecule produced by the body during the normal processes of respiration and metabolism or following exposure to radiation and pollution. Free radicals are suspected of causing damage to the cells, DNA, and immune system.

G

Geriatrics The branch of medicine dealing with the physiologic characteristics of aging and the diagnosis and treatment of diseases affecting the aged.

Geropharmacology The study of how older adults respond to medication.

Gingivitis Inflammation of the gingiva (gums), with symptoms that may include redness, swelling, and bleeding.

Glaucoma Disease characterized by increased fluid pressure (intraocular pressure) within the eye that may result in damage to the retina.

Grief A combination of sorrow, loss, and confusion that comes when someone or something of value is lost.

H

Half-life The amount of time required to reduce a drug level to half of its initial value.

Halitosis Offensive bad breath, resulting from poor oral hygiene, dental or oral infections, ingestion of certain foods, tobacco use, or some systemic diseases such as the odor of acetone in diabetes.

Health maintenance A systemic program planned to prevent illness, to maintain maximal function, and to promote health.

Health promotion Lifestyle and health care practices that improve overall health and quality of life.

Heatstroke Resulting condition that occurs if heat exhaustion, a gradually developing condition caused by water or sodium depletion, is not recognized and treated.

Helplessness A feeling of a loss of control or ability, usually after repeated failures, or of being immobilized or frozen by circumstances beyond one's control, with the result that one is unable to make autonomous choices.

Hematocrit A measure of the packed cell volume of red blood cells, expressed as a percentage of the total blood volume.

Hemiparesis Muscular weakness of one side of the body.

Hemiplegia Paralysis of one side of the body.

Hemoglobin A complex protein-iron molecule that is responsible for the transport of oxygen and carbon dioxide within the bloodstream.

Heterogeneous As in a heterogeneous society, a more complex one in which the members of many diverse cultures with different historical and cultural experiences interact.

Homogeneous As in a homogeneous society, a simple one in which all members share a common historical and cultural experience.

Hopelessness A state in which an individual sees limited or no alternatives or personal choices available and is unable to mobilize energy on his or her own behalf.

Hospice A multidisciplinary system of family-centered care designed to assist the terminally ill person to be comfortable and to maintain a satisfactory lifestyle through the phases of dying.

Hyperkeratosis Overgrowth of the epithelial layer of the skin.

Hyperthermia A much higher than normal body temperature.

Hypnotics A class of drugs often used as sedatives.

Hypothermia A core body temperature of 95° F or lower.

Hypothyroidism Reduced function of the thyroid gland. Symptoms include cold intolerance, dry skin, dry and thin body hair, constipation, depression, and lack of energy.

Hysterectomy Surgical removal of the uterus, to treat fibroid tumors, pelvic inflammatory disease, severe recurrent endometrial hyperplasia, uterine hemorrhage, and precancerous and cancerous conditions of the uterus.

I

Imaging Formation of a mental picture or representation of someone or something using the imagination.

Immunologic Related to the immune system. The immunologic theory of aging proposes that aging is a function of changes in the immune system, which weakens over time to make an aging person more susceptible to disease.

Incontinence Inability to control urination or defecation.

Insomnia Chronic inability to sleep or to remain asleep throughout the night; wakefulness; sleeplessness.

Inspection The most commonly used method of physical assessment in which the senses of vision, smell, and hearing are used to collect data.

Intelligence The potential ability and capacity to acquire, retain, and apply experience, understanding, knowledge, reasoning, and judgment in coping with new experiences and in solving problems.

Intercourse Sexual intercourse between individuals; coitus.

Intermittent claudication Cramplike pains in the calves caused by poor circulation of the blood to the leg muscles, commonly associated with atherosclerosis (the tissues of the lower extremities are deprived of oxygen); manifested only at certain times, usually after walking; and relieved by rest.

Interstitial Pertaining to the space between cells, as in interstitial fluid, or between organs.

Intracellular Pertaining to the interior of a cell; as in intracellular fluid, a fluid within cell membranes throughout most of the body, containing dissolved solutes that are essential to electrolytic balance and healthy metabolism.

Intravascular Pertaining to the inside of a blood vessel.

Ischemic Related to a decreased supply of oxygenated blood, as in ischemic heart disease, a pathologic condition caused by lack of oxygen in cells of the myocardium.

Isometric As in isometric exercise, a form of active exercise in which muscle tension is increased while pressure is applied against stable resistance.

Isotonic As in isotonic exercise, a form of active exercise in which muscles contract and cause movement. Because there is no significant change in resistance throughout the movement, the force of contraction remains constant.

L

Laxatives Laxative agents that promote bowel evacuation by increasing the bulk of the feces, softening the stool, or lubricating the intestinal wall.

Leukoplakia A precancerous, slowly developing change in a mucous membrane, characterized by white, thickened, firmly attached patches that are slightly raised and sharply circumscribed.

M

Malnutrition Any disorder of nutrition, resulting from an unbalanced, insufficient, or excessive diet or from impaired absorption, assimilation, or use of foods.

Mantra From Hinduism; a sacred verbal formula repeated in prayer, meditation, or incantation, such as an invocation of a god, a magic spell, or a syllable or portion of scripture containing mystic potentialities.

Masturbation Sexual self-gratification; sexual activity in which the penis or clitoris is stimulated, usually to orgasm, by means other than intercourse.

Meditation A state of consciousness in which the individual eliminates environmental stimuli from awareness so that the mind has a single focus, producing a state of relaxation and relief from stress.

Memory The mental faculty or power that enables one to retain and to recall, through unconscious associative processes, previously experienced sensations, impressions, ideas, concepts, and all information that has been consciously learned.

Metabolism As in drug metabolism, the transformation of a drug by the body tissues into a metabolite as the body readies the agent for elimination.

Minerals Inorganic chemical elements that are required in many of the body's functions.

Morgue A unit of a hospital with facilities for the storage and autopsy of the dead.

N

Nasogastric Pertaining to the nose and stomach, as in nasogastric intubation, the placement of a nasogastric tube through the nose into the stomach to relieve gastric distention by removing gas, gastric secretions, or food; to instill medication, food, or fluids; or to obtain a specimen for laboratory analysis.

Neglect Passive form of abuse in which caregivers fail to provide for the needs of the person under their care.

Nocturnal Pertaining to or occurring during the night.

Noncompliance Failure of a patient to follow through with recommended health practices.

Nystagmus Rapid, involuntary eye movement.

O

Orthodox Adhering to the accepted and traditional or established faith, especially in religion.

Orthostatic hypotension Condition that occurs because the circulation does not respond quickly to postural changes.

Osteoporosis Disorder characterized by porous, brittle, fragile bones that are susceptible to breakage, caused by excessive loss of calcium from bone combined with insufficient replacement.

Otosclerosis A hereditary condition of the bony labyrinth of the ear, in which there is formation of spongy bone, resulting in hearing loss.

P

Palliative As in palliative treatment, therapy designed to relieve or reduce intensity of uncomfortable symptoms but not to produce a cure, such as narcotics to relieve pain.

Palpation A method of physical assessment that uses the sense of touch in the fingers and hands to obtain data.

Parasitic Of an organism living in or on and obtaining nourishment from another organism.

Perception The conscious recognition and interpretation of sensory stimuli that serve as a basis for understanding, learning, and knowing or for motivating a particular action or reaction.

Percussion A technique of physical assessment in which the size, position, and density of structures under the skin are assessed by tapping the area and listening to the resonance of the sound. Depending on the amount of vibration (sound) heard, the presence of masses, fluid, or air can be determined.

Pharmacokinetics The study of the action of drugs within the body, including the mechanisms of absorption, distribution, metabolism, and excretion; onset of action; duration of effect; biotransformation; and effects and routes of excretion of the metabolites of the drug.

Pigmentation Organic color produced in the body, such as melanin.

Polypharmacy The prescription, administration, or use of more medications than are clinically indicated, a common problem among older adults.

Powerlessness A perceived lack of control over a current situation or problem and the person's perception that any action he or she takes will not affect the outcome of the particular situation.

Presbycusis Hearing loss associated with aging, particularly of higher-pitched sounds.

Presbyopia Found in older people, farsightedness resulting from a loss of elasticity of the lens of the eye and resulting in a decrease in the power of accommodation.

Pressure ulcers Inflammations, sores, or ulcers in the skin over a body prominence occurring most commonly on the sacrum, elbows, heels, outer ankles, inner knees, hips, shoulder blades, and occipital bones of high-risk patients, most often aged, debilitated, immobilized, or cachectic patients.

Prophylactic Preventing the spread of disease.

Prostate-specific antigen (PSA) test A blood test used to measure the level of prostate-specific antigen, which may be present at elevated levels in patients with cancer or other diseases of the prostate, and to monitor the patient's response to therapy.

Protein Any of a large group of naturally occurring complex organic compounds, composed of amino acids, essential for tissue repair and healing.

Proxemics Study of the use of personal space in communication.

Pruritus Itching; an uncomfortable sensation leading to the urge to scratch, which may result in a secondary infection.

Psychosocial Pertaining to a combination of psychological and social factors. The psychosocial theories of aging attempt to explain why older adults have different responses to the aging process.

R

Rapport Atmosphere of mutual respect and understanding.

Rehabilitation The restoration of an individual or a part to normal or near normal function after a disabling disease or injury.

Rehabilitative focus The result of high expectations and high-level focus in planning care.

Relationships Connections formed by the dynamic interaction of individuals who play interrelated roles.

Relaxation As in relaxation therapy, treatment in which patients are taught to perform breathing and relaxation exercises and to concentrate on a pleasant situation.

Religious Having belief in or reverence for God or a deity.

Respite As in respite care; allows the primary caregiver to have time away from the constant demands of caregiving, thereby decreasing caregiver stress and the risk for abuse.

Retention The inability to urinate or defecate.

Ritual The prescribed order of a religious ceremony.

Role A socially accepted behavior pattern.

S

Scabies Contagious disease caused by a mite, characterized by intense itching of the skin and excoriation from scratching.

Screenings As in health screenings, which are done to identify older people who are in need of further, more in-depth assessment. Examples are screenings for high blood pressure, hearing problems, foot problems, and problems with activities of daily living.

Seborrheic dermatitis An unsightly skin disorder characterized by yellow, waxy crusts that can be either dry or moist, which is caused by sebum production and occurs on the scalp, eyebrows, eyelids, ears, axilla, breasts, groin, and gluteal folds.

Seborrheic keratosis Skin disorder in which lesions ranging in color from light tan to black appear as slightly raised, wartlike macules with distinct edges.

Sedative An agent that decreases functional activity, diminishes irritability, and allays excitement.

Self-esteem The degree of worth and competence one attributes to oneself.

Self-hypnosis Process of putting oneself into a trancelike state by autosuggestion, such as concentration on a single thought or object.

Senile lentigo Skin disorder whereby clusters of melanocytes form areas of deepened pigmentation; often called *age spots* or *liver spots.*

Senile purpura Red, purple, or brown areas commonly seen on the legs and arms, resulting from hemorrhaging as the walls of the capillaries become increasingly fragile with age.

Sexuality The sum of the physical, functional, and psychological attributes that are expressed by one's gender identity and sexual behavior, regardless of the relationship to the sex organs or to procreation.

Social isolation A condition in which a feeling of aloneness is experienced, which the person acknowledges as a negative or threatening state imposed by others.

Sphincter A circular band of muscle fibers that constricts a passage or closes a natural opening in the body, such as the external anal sphincter, which closes the anus, or the hepatic sphincter in the muscular coat of the hepatic veins near their union with the superior vena cava.

Spiritual Of or relating to the nature of spirit; not tangible or material.

Stimuli Things that excite or incite an organism or part to function, become active, or respond.

Stress Any emotional, physical, social, economic, or other factor that requires a response or change.

Sundowning A condition in which persons with cognitive impairment (e.g., people with Alzheimer's disease) and older people tend to become confused or disoriented at the end of the day, exhibiting such behaviors as wandering, combativeness, suspiciousness, hallucinations, and delusions.

Supplement As in nutritional supplement, which is added to complete, make up for a deficiency, and extend or strengthen the diet.

Symbol An object, action, or other stimulus that represents something else by conscious association, convention, or another relationship.

T

Tachycardia A common sign of decreased cardiac output, when the heart beats more rapidly to compensate for the decreased volume.

Theory An abstract statement formulated to predict, explain, or describe the relationships among concepts, constructs, or events.

Thermoregulation The ability to maintain body temperature in a safe range, controlled by the hypothalamus.

Trace element An element essential to nutrition or physiologic processes, found in such minute quantities that analysis yields the presence of only trace amounts.

V

Vitamins Organic compounds found naturally in foods or produced synthetically.

X

Xerosis Dry skin caused by a decrease in the function of sebaceous and sweat gland secretion.

Xerostomia Dryness of the mouth caused by cessation of normal salivary secretion.

Illustration Credits

CHAPTER 1

1-1, **1-2**, **1-3**, From Central Intelligence Agency. *World factbook*. Available at https://www.cia.gov/library/publications/the-world-factbook/index.html. **1-4**, From Congressional Research Service (CRS) analysis of the March 2008 *Current Population Survey*. **1-5**, From US Census Bureau, Current Population Survey, Annual Social and Economic Supplement, 2009. **1-6**, Courtesy of Elness Swenson Graham Architects, Inc., Minneapolis, Minnesota. **1-8**, © 2010 Photos. com, a division of Getty Images. All rights reserved. Item #: 56528719.

CHAPTER 3

3-1A, **3-2**, **3-4**, From White GM, Cox NH: *Diseases of the skin: a color atlas and text*, ed 2, Philadelphia, 2006, Mosby. **3-1B**, **3-6**, From White GM, Cox NH: *Diseases of the skin: a color atlas and text*, St Louis, 2000, Mosby. **3-3**, *A-B*, From Ignatavicius DD, Workman ML: *Medical-surgical nursing: critical thinking for collaborative care*, ed 5, Philadelphia, 2006, Saunders. **3-5**, In White GM, Cox NH: *Diseases of the skin, A color atlas and text*, ed 2, Philadelphia, 2006, Mosby. (Courtesy of O. Dale Collins III). **3-7**, *A-F*, From Tate P, Seeley RR, Stephens TD: *Understanding the human body*, St Louis, 1994, Mosby. **3-8**, *A-B*, From Phipps WJ et al: *Medical-surgical nursing: health and illness perspectives*, ed 7, St Louis, 2003, Mosby. **3-9**, From Feldman H, Gracon S: Alzheimer's disease: symptomatic drugs under development. In Gauthier S, editor: *Clinical diagnosis and management of Alzheimer's disease*, London, England, 1996, Martin Dunitz Ltd. **3-10**, From Yanoff M, Fine BS: *Ocular pathology*, St Louis, 2002, Mosby.

CHAPTER 4

4-1, From Linton A: *Introduction to medical-surgical nursing*, ed 3, Philadelphia, 2002, Saunders. **4-2**, *A*, From Sorrentino SA, Gorek B: *Mosby's textbook for long-term care*, ed 4, St Louis, 2003, Mosby. **4-2**, *B*, **4-3**, From Leahy JM, Kizilay PE: *Foundations of nursing practice: a nursing process approach*, Philadelphia, 1998, Saunders.

CHAPTER 5

5-1, From Sorrentino SA: *Mosby's textbook for nursing assistants*, ed 6, St Louis, 2004, Mosby. **5-2**, From deWit SC: *Fundamental concepts and skills for nursing*, ed 3, Philadelphia, 2009, Saunders. **5-3**, From Lewis SM et al: *Medical-surgical nursing: assessment and management of clinical problems*, ed 6, St Louis, 2004, Mosby.

CHAPTER 6

6-1, From the US Department of Agriculture. Available at www.mypyramid.gov/. **6-2**, Adapted from the Nutritional Screening Initiative, Washington, DC. **6-4**, © 2010 Meals on Wheels Association of America. **6-5**, Ebersole: Toward Healthy Aging: Human Needs and Nursing Response, ed 7, St Louis, 2008, Mosby. **6-7**, From Sorrentino SA: *Mosby's textbook for nursing assistants*, ed 6, St Louis, 2004, Mosby. **6-8**, **6-9**, From Sorrentino SA: *Mosby's textbook for nursing assistants*, ed 7, 2008, St. Louis, Mosby.

CHAPTER 7

7-1, From deWit SC: *Fundamental concepts and skills for nursing*, ed 3, Philadelphia, 2009, Saunders. **7-2**, From Sorrentino SA: *Mosby's textbook for nursing assistants*, ed 6, St Louis, 2004, Mosby.

CHAPTER 8

8-1, **8-3**, From deWit SC: *Fundamental concepts and skills for nursing*, ed 2, Philadelphia, 2005, Saunders. **8-2**, From Sorrentino SA, Gorek B: *Mosby's textbook for long-term care assistants*, ed 4, St Louis, 2003, Mosby. **8-4**, Reproduced by special permission of the Publisher, Psychological Assessment Resources, Inc., 16204 North Florida Avenue, Lutz, Florida 33549, from the Mini Mental State Examination, by Marshal Folstein and Susan Folstein, Copyright 1975, 1998, 2001 by Mini Mental LLC, Inc. Published 2001 by Psychological Assessment Resources, Inc. Further reproduction is prohibited without permission of PAR, Inc. The MMSE can be purchased from PAR, Inc. by calling (813) 968-3003. **8-5**, Briggs Corporation, Des Moines, Iowa 50306, Phone 800-307-1744.

CHAPTER 9

9-1, *A-B* From Sorrentino SA: *Mosby's textbook for nursing assistants*, ed 7, 2008, St. Louis, Mosby. **9-2**, From Sorrentino SA: *Mosby's textbook for long-term care nursing assistants*, ed 6, St Louis, Mosby, 2011.

CHAPTER 10

10-1, From Swartz M, *Textbook of physical diagnosis*, ed 5, Philadelphia, 2006, Saunders. **10-2, 10-3, 10-4, 10-6**, From Sorrentino SA: *Mosby's textbook for nursing assistants*, ed 7, 2008, St. Louis, Mosby. **10-5**, Perry AG, Potter PA: *Clinical nursing skills & techniques*, ed 7, St Louis, 2010, Mosby. **10-7**, A, From Pasero, C, & McCaffery, M. *Pain assessment and pharmacologic management*, p. 55, St Louis, Mosby © 2011, Pasero C, McCaffery M. The scale is in the public domain. May be duplicated for use in clinical practice. **10-7**, B, Hockenberry MJ, Wilson D: *Wong's essentials of pediatric nursing*, ed 8, St Louis, 2009, Mosby. Used with Permission. Copyright Mosby.

CHAPTER 11

11-1, 11-2, From Sorrentino SA: *Mosby's textbook for nursing assistants,* ed 6, St Louis, 2004, Mosby. **11-3**, © 2010 Photos.com, a division of Getty Images. All rights reserved. Item #: 87823635, **11-4**, © 2010 Photos.com, a division of Getty Images. All rights reserved. Item #: #87470466. **11-5**, © 2010 Photos.com, a division of Getty Images. All rights reserved. Item #: 87663523

CHAPTER 12

12-1, © 2010 Photos.com, a division of Getty Images. All rights reserved. Item #: 88097027. **12-2**, © 2010 Photos.com, a division of Getty Images. All rights reserved. Item #: 87519943. 12-3, From Sorrentino SA: *Mosby's Textbook for Long-Term Care Nursing Assistants*, 6th edition, Mosby, 2011.

CHAPTER 13

13-1, © 2010 Photos.com, a division of Getty Images. All rights reserved. Item #: 57563853-Photos.com. **13-2**, Christensen BL, Kockrow EO: *Foundations of nursing,* ed 5, St Louis, 2006, Mosby.

CHAPTER 14

14-1, From Sorrentino SA: Mosby's textbook for long-term care nursing assistants, ed 6, 2011. **14-3**, From deWit SC: *Fundamental concepts and skills for nursing,* ed 3, Philadelphia, 2009, Saunders.

CHAPTER 15

15-1, From Harkreader H, Hogan MA: *Fundamentals of nursing: care and clinical judgment,* ed 3, St Louis, 2007, Mosby.

CHAPTER 16

16-1, © 2010 Photos.com, a division of Getty Images. All rights reserved. Item #: 87548911. **16-2**, From Black JM, Hawks JH: *Medical surgical nursing,* ed 7, St Louis, 2005, Saunders. **16-3**, From Sorrentino SA: *Mosby's textbook for nursing assistants,* ed 7, St Louis, 2011, Mosby.

CHAPTER 17

17-1, From Sorrentino SA: *Mosby's textbook for nursing assistants,* ed 6, St Louis, 2004, Mosby. **17-2, 17-3, 17-4**, From White GM, Cox NH: *Diseases of the skin: a color atlas and text,* ed 2, St Louis, 2006, Mosby. **17-5, A-B**, From Trelease CC: Developing standards for wound care, *Ostomy Wound Manage* 26:50, 1988. **17-6, A-H**, Modified from Ignatavicius DD, Workman ML: *Medical-surgical nursing: critical thinking for collaborative care,* ed 4, Philadelphia, 2002, Saunders. **17-7**, From Ebersole P, Hess P: *Toward healthy aging: human needs and nursing experience,* ed 7, St Louis, 2008, Mosby. **17-8**, From Swartz MH: *Textbook of physical diagnosis: history and examination,* ed 5, Philadelphia, 2006, Elsevier. **17-9**, From Bryant RA et al: Pressure ulcers. In Bryant RA, ed: *Acute and chronic wounds nursing management,* St Louis, 1992, Mosby. 17-10, In Fillit: *Brocklehurst's textbook of geriatric medicine and gerontology,* ed 7, Philadelphia, 2010, Saunders. *(Reprinted with the permission of Mirriam Robbins, DDS, New York University College of Dentistry.)* **17-11**, From White GM, Cox NH: *Diseases of the skin: a color atlas and text,* St Louis, 2000, Mosby. **17-12**, From Daniel: *Mosby's Dental Hygiene,* ed 2, St Louis, 2008, Mosby.

CHAPTER 18

18-1, 18-2, From Gray M: *Genitourinary disorders,* St Louis, 1992, Mosby. **18-3**, From deWit SC: *Fundamental concepts and skills for nursing,* ed 3, Philadelphia, 2009, Saunders.

CHAPTER 19

19-1, From Johnson-Paulson JE, Kosher R: *Geriatric Nursing,* 322, 1985. **19-2, 19-5, 19-8, 19-11, 19-14**, Sorrentino SA: *Mosby's textbook for long-term care nursing assistants,* ed 6, St Louis, 2011, Mosby. **19-3**, From Perry AG, Potter PA: *Clinical nursing skills and techniques,* ed 7, St Louis, 2010, Mosby. **19-4**, From Potter PA, Perry AG: *Basic nursing: theory and practice,* ed 7, St Louis, 2011, Mosby. **19-6**, © 2010 Photos.com, a division of Getty Images. All rights reserved. Item #: 87802412. **19-7**, From Perry AG, Potter PA: *Clinical nursing skills and techniques,* ed 7, St Louis, 2010, Mosby. **19-9, A-C, E**, Courtesy Northcoast Medical Inc, Morgan Hill, Calif. **19-9, D**, Courtesy AbilityOne Corporation,

Germantown, Wisc. **19-10,** *A-B,* Courtesy Northcoast Medical Inc, Morgan Hill, Calif. **19-10,** *C,* Courtesy Sammons Preston: An AbilityOne Company, Bollingbrook, Ill. **19-12, 19-13,** From Sorrentino SA, Gorek B: *Mosby's textbook for long-term care assistants,* ed 4, St Louis, 2003, Mosby.

CHAPTER 20

20-1, From Potter PA, Perry AG: *Basic nursing: theory and practice,* ed 7, St Louis, 2011, Mosby. **20-2,** © 2010 Photos.com, a division of Getty Images. All rights reserved. Item #: 55847085.

Index

Note: Page numbers followed by *b* indicate boxes, *f* indicate figures and *t* indicate tables.

A

AARP (American Association of Retired Persons), 12
Abandonment, 24
Abdominal aortic aneurysm, 48
Absorption
  of drugs, 132, 132*t*
  of nutrients, 51
Abuse, 22–25, 24*b*, 25*b*, 26*b*
Acceptance
  in communication, 93–94
  of death and dying, 257
Access checklist for physically disabled, 326*b*
Accessibility, and health promotion and maintenance, 80–81
Accessory muscles with oxygenation problems, 315
Accidents. *See* Safety problems
Accommodation, 63
Acetylcholine, 56–57
Acquired immunodeficiency syndrome (AIDS), 261–262, 262*b*
"Acting out" behavior, with disturbed thought processes, 191, 191*b*
Active listening, 94
Active range-of-motion exercises, 307
Activities department for deficient diversional activities, 322
Activities of daily living (ADL) with disturbed thought processes, 190, 190*f*
Activity(ies), 302–326
  and aging, 303–304
  for deficient diversional activities, 322
  defined, 302
  effects of disease processes on, 305–324
  negative attitudes about, 324–325
  normal patterns of, 302–303
  pacing of, 314
  positive attitudes about, 325–326
  and sleep disorders, 334
  voluntary, 303
Activity intolerance, 312–314, 313*b*
Activity theory, 30
Acute abdomen, "silent,", 155*t*
Adalat (nifedipine), 135*t*
Adaptive devices. *See* Assistive devices.
Address in communication, 93–94, 153
Adenosine triphosphate (ATP), 38
Adequate intakes (AIs), 104
Adipose tissue, 33, 39
  muscle mass and, 39
Adrenal cortex, 68
Adrenal glands, 68
Adrenal medulla, 68
Advance directives, 19, 19*b*, 244–245, 257*b*
Adventitious lung sounds, 160*b*
Aerobic exercises, 38, 304
AF267B in Alzheimer's disease, 60
African Americans
  food patterns of, 117*b*
  preventive screenings for, 152*t*
  and spirituality, 235*b*

Age discrimination, 5–6
Age spots, 33
Ageism, 5–6, 202
Age-related macular degeneration (AMD), 64–65
Aggregate income, 10, 11*f*
Agility, 303
Aging
  alternative and complementary therapies to slow or reverse, 29*b*
  attitudes toward, 3–6, 3*b*
  current knowledge about, 4*b*
  economics of, 10–13, 10*f*, 11*f*, 12*t*, 13*b*, 20
  fear of, 5–6, 5*b*
  historical perspective on study of, 1–2
  myths about, 5*b*
  perceptions of, 202
  process of, 2
  tasks of, 30
  theories of, 28–30, 29*b*
  values about, 3*b*
Aging family members, impact on family of, 19–26, 20*b*, 20*f*, 20*t*
Aging population
  categorization of, 2–3, 2*t*
  demographics of, 6–8, 7*f*, 8*b*, 9*f*
AIDS (acquired immunodeficiency syndrome), 261–262, 262*b*
Air exchange, 41
Air fluidized surfaces, 276*t*
Air overlay surfaces, 276*t*
Albumin, 48–49, 108*t*
Alcohol abuse in response to stress, 226
Alcohol consumption
  and health promotion and maintenance, 75–76
  and medications, 139–140
  and sexual function, 260
Alcoholism and nutrition, 110–111
Alcohol-related problems, 229*f*, 281
Aldomet (methyldopa), 135*t*, 141*t*
Aldoril (methyldopa-hydrochlorothiazide), 135*t*
Aldosterone, 68
Aleve (naproxen), 135*t*, 141*t*
Alignment, 307
Allergic dermatitis, 36, 36*f*
Alopecia, 271
α cells, 68
Alprazolam (Xanax), 135*t*
Alternative and complementary therapies. *See* Complementary and alternative therapies.
Aluminum hydroxide, 141*t*
Alveolus(i), 41
Alzheimer's disease, 59–60
  and activity, 305
  assistive sensory devices, 189
  causes of, 59–60
  defined, 59
  diagnosis of, 60
  epidemiology of, 59
  ethnic differences in, 59*b*

Alzheimer's disease (*Continued*)
  facts about, 187*b*
  financial and social costs of, 59
  nursing process for, 185–192, 187*t*, 189*b*, 190*b*, 191*b*
  progression of, 59, 59*f*
  risk factors for, 59–60
  treatment for, 60
Ambulation, assistance during, 310, 311*f*
American Association of Retired Persons (AARP), 12
American Indians
  food patterns of, 117*b*
  preventive screenings for, 152*t*
  religious practices regarding end of life among, 249
  and spirituality, 235*b*
Amino acids, 104
Amiodarone (Cordarone), 135*t*
Amitriptyline (Elavil), 135*t*, 330*t*
Amphetamines, 135*t*
Anaprox (naproxen), 135*t*, 141*t*
Android (methyltestosterone), 135*t*
Anemia, 50, 113
  folic acid–deficiency, 50
  iron-deficiency, 50, 108
  pernicious, 50, 109
  due to vitamin B$_{12}$ deficiency, 106–107
Aneurysm, 48
Anger related to death and dying, 257
Angina pectoris, 46
Anginal pain with oxygenation problems, 316
Anorexia
  during dying, 253
  potentially inappropriate medication use with, 138*t*
Anorexic agents, 135*t*
Anterior cavity, of eye, 62
Anterior pituitary, 67
Antianxiety agents, 141*t*
Antibodies, 49
Anticholinergics, 135*t*
Antidepressants, 141*t*, 330*t*
Antidiuretic hormone, 67
Antihistamines, 135*t*, 330*t*
Antihypertensives, 141*t*, 261*t*
Antiinfectives, 141*t*
Antioxidant(s), 29
Antioxidant therapy, 29
Antioxidant vitamins, 106
Antipsychotics, 141*t*
Antispasmodics, 135*t*
Antiulcer medications, 141*t*
Anxiety, 208–209
  about dying, 250
  nursing process for, 208–209, 209*f*
  and sleep disorders, 330
Aorta, 44
Aortic valve, 44
Aphasia, 92, 95, 193, 193*t*
Apical pulse, 157
Apnea, sleep, 331–332
Apolipoprotein E (ApoE), 59–60

Study Guide

CRITICAL THINKING AND APPLICATION

Case Study 1

Rev. WR is a 94-year-old African-American man. He is a retired Protestant minister who, until recently, resided independently in a large senior citizen facility called The Oaks. He regularly went to the dining room and socialized with many other residents, getting around the building on a motorized scooter. He is mentally alert and very aware of current events. Rev. WR is an avid reader and enjoys watching sports, news, history, and travel shows on television. He has been widowed twice and has three living children who are approaching retirement age and live in the same community. Other extended family members are spread around the country. He has many friends and acquaintances. Rev. WR receives Social Security and a pension, which have been adequate to meet his needs, but he has minimal savings. Until recently, he was able to maintain a significant degree of autonomy with help from his family and daily visits from a home health aide, who helped with activities of daily living.

One afternoon while moving about his apartment without his walker, Rev. WR fell. The emergency call device provided by his family was on a dresser in another room, and the wall pull alarms were too far away for him to reach. After lying on the floor for more than an hour, his health aide arrived and found him in a great deal of pain. Help was summoned, and he was transported by ambulance to the local emergency department.

Once in the ED, Rev. WR continued to experience severe pain, calling out loudly when anyone tried to reposition him or move his arms or shoulders to start an IV. Vicodin was administered, but he stated that it provided little relief of the pain. Once an IV was established, morphine was administered, which provided some relief. X-rays revealed a severe comminuted fracture of the left femur immediately above an artificial knee joint. The fracture was stabilized in a cast from hip to toes because the patient was deemed to be a poor surgical risk because of preexisting medical conditions, including pulmonary fibrosis, type 2 diabetes, prostate cancer, congestive heart failure, and severe osteoarthritis of the shoulders and hips. An indwelling catheter was inserted to minimize the need for further movement and to prevent damage to the cast. The leg was elevated and placed in a cradle. Rev. WR was kept in the hospital 3 days for stabilization and pain control with IV morphine; he was then transferred to a long-term care facility. He describes needing to go into long-term care as his "worst nightmare." He states, "I wish that I could go back home, but the doctors say that will never happen. The best I can hope for is a brace instead of this cast. I will need care for the rest of my life."

Physical assessment: An alert, oriented man with soft, slightly unclear speech. He is hard of hearing and uses hearing aids in both ears. Some repetition of questions needed. Responds in full sentences. He wears glasses for reading. Height is reported at 5 feet 6 inches, and pre-cast weight at approximately 136 pounds. Apical pulse 70, BP 134/82, R 16 and shallow. Lung sounds reveal some crackles. Thin hair and warm, medium-brown skin with small darker areas visible on the hands and arms. He has a full left leg cast, which is clean and intact. His toes are pink and slightly warm to the touch. Faint pedal pulses are present in both feet. Toenails long and thick. States, "I'll never stand on that leg again. I don't know how I'll do anything. My back hurts, and my shoulders are weak and very, very painful if touched or moved. They hurt me badly just moving me into this bed. I told them not to use my arms, but they did it anyway. They just don't know how bad it is. Even the pills don't help much, and I have to wait too long for them when I ask." Little arm strength is observed, but he is able to feed himself slowly. He reports he has little appetite or interest in food. States, "I have to eat slowly and chew well or I choke and inhale food." He reports that he has been losing weight for some time and that the doctor stopped the medication for his diabetes since his blood sugar levels were staying low. Blood glucose obtained by fingerstick is 102. No abdominal distention is observed. He states, "I have difficulty moving my bowels because of the pain medications." The catheter remains in place draining dark amber urine with a strong odor.

Psychosocial assessment: He states, "Why do I have to suffer this? Why is God doing this to me? I buried two wonderful wives and I'm still here. I'm the last of nine children in my family. I have a son and two daughters who live in the area and visit often, but they have busy lives. I also have two grandchildren and two great grandchildren nearby. The rest of my family lives all around the country. I like to keep my phone handy to keep in touch with them. I used to use my computer to keep in touch with the young ones. I really miss being able to see a lot of my friends at the The Oaks and my church friends. It's hard for them to get here to see me because most of them don't drive anymore. The pastor from church used to visit me often, and I really like seeing him. He really helped me during hard times, and this is the worst. I get lonely during the day when nobody visits. They don't get me up and out of this room very often; probably just as well since most of the people here are confused anyway." He also reports, "It's hard to sleep when all I do is stay in bed. I just lie here in the dark and think. When things really get bad, I try to put them in the hands of the Lord and hope he comes for me soon."

The family reports that Rev. WR is not happy with the way the staff talks to him. They state that he feels it is disrespectful when staff calls him by his first name and when they talk to him as though he was confused. Further, they report that he is often frustrated and upset when he cannot reach his phone or call light because they were left out of reach.

Medical orders: General diet and snacks, bed rest with leg elevated in cradle, up in special w/c prn with L leg elevated, replace indwelling catheter prn, digoxin 0.125 mg daily, albuterol 2.5 mg by nebulizer tid, hydrocodone/acetaminophen (Vicodin) tab 1 or 2q4h prn, milk of magnesia 1 oz at bedtime prn.

Questions and Activities

1. Was housing in independent living appropriate before this patient's fall?

2. What, if anything, could have been done to reduce the risk or prevent this fall?

3. What financial impact is this event likely to have on the elderly person?

4. What concerns are the family likely to have related to institutional placement?

5. Are appropriate communications skills by the staff evident? How could these be improved?

6. How might cultural factors influence his perceptions or affect the care he receives?

7. Group the data into functional health patterns using the following format, and identify appropriate nursing diagnoses:

Health Pattern Data
(Objective and Subjective)   **Nursing Diagnoses**

Cognition–Perception

Self-Perception–Self-Concept

Roles–Relationships

Coping–Stress

Values–Beliefs

Sexuality

Nutritional–Fluid Needs

Skin–Mucous Membranes

Health Pattern Data
(Objective and Subjective)   **Nursing Diagnoses**

Elimination

Activity–Exercise

Sleep–Rest

8. What additional data would you like to collect?

9. How would you prioritize the top five diagnoses?
   1.
   2.
   3.
   4.
   5.

10. What interventions are most appropriate for each high-priority diagnosis? (Identify assessments, specific actions, teaching, and referrals.)

Nursing Diagnosis   **Nursing Interventions**

11. How do the prescribed medications correlate to the patient's condition? What nursing assessments, care modifications, and teaching are necessary?

12. What concerns need to be addressed with the physician?

13. What end-of-life issues may need to be addressed in this situation?

Case Study 2

Mrs. EH is an 87-year-old woman who has recently moved into a community-based residential facility for patients with Alzheimer's disease and other cognitive disorders. She spent her entire adult life as a wife and homemaker. She is a widow who receives Social Security payments and has a moderate amount of savings in the bank. She was an avid baker who also enjoyed gardening, reading, doing word puzzles, socializing with friends, and playing with her grandchildren. Over the past 8 years since she was widowed, Mrs. EH's family has noticed increased forgetfulness and significant changes in her ability to function independently. She underwent physical and psychological testing at a community hospital before the diagnosis of dementia, Alzheimer's type, was made. For 5 years her children worked to keep her in a home setting by arranging full-time supervision either in her home or by taking her to one of their homes. Changes in her behavior and needs, particularly increased nighttime wandering and frequent episodes of incontinence, necessitated a reevaluation by the family. After serious discussion, it was decided that more extensive care was required. The family also felt that Mrs. EH's socialization needs could better be met in an environment that allowed for more interaction with a variety of people. The family found a facility that had a homelike atmosphere providing a private room, community social areas, and meals cooked and served family style in a dining room. Savings from the sale of her home are being used to pay for her care. Her children have power of attorney for both health care and finances. Mrs. EH signed DNR forms before determination of incompetence.

Other than dementia, Mrs. EH had surgery for colon cancer 10 years ago with no recurrence of the disease. Cardioneurogenic syncope was diagnosed 8 years ago after episodes of dizziness and falls. She also has hypothyroidism and osteoarthritis predominantly in her R knee.

Physical assessment: An alert, smiling woman who makes faces at people in the room and frequently smiles or hugs visitors and caregivers. Her speech is clear but very repetitive and often meaningless. No obvious hearing problems; she has glasses for reading, which are seldom worn. She has partial dentures, which were taken home by the family after being "misplaced" several time in other resident's rooms. She is 5 feet tall and weighs 176 pounds, up 25 pounds since admission. Her appetite is always good, and she eats whatever she is served. P 76, R 14, BP 116/72. Pedal pulses strong in both lower extremities. Lungs clear to auscultation. Skin is intact, pale, and dry. Hair gray and "frizzy" because she frequently runs her finger through it after combing. She wears a protective garment for urinary and bowel incontinence, but she can use the toilet when supervised and reminded. She has a history of urinary tract infections. These are typically detected by changes in behavior; she becomes agitated and may strike out at caregivers. She frequently wanders the hallways, using her walker, most of the time without reminder. She has been found on the floor next to her bed on two instances, unable to report what happened. Her right knee is slightly swollen, and she has hammer toes on both feet. There is a small irritated area on the top two toes, but soft nylon shoes with Velcro closures are worn most of the time she is up. She dresses casually in slacks and cotton tops and wears a sweater when cold. She often goes into other residents' rooms and rummages through the drawers, sometimes getting irritated comments, which do not appear to disturb her. She frequently has difficulty falling asleep and sometimes spends the entire night awake playing with her doll or stuffed toys. When this occurs, she often falls asleep in a lounge chair during the following day. She requires assistance with bathing and dressing. Occasional episodes of masturbation have been observed.

Psychosocial assessment: She has a son and daughter who visit several times a week. Grandchildren and great-grandchildren visit less frequently. She often says "I love you" to them, but if asked to identify who they are, she looks totally confused. Her family usually brings pictures or magazines to look at with her. They all appear comfortable giving her hugs and kisses during each visit. She has a family picture board in her room, and several personal decorations are on the walls and tables. She participates in some of the activities provided by the facility, such as coloring or ball toss, but she spends a large percentage of time sitting in the TV room dozing on and off. Staff reports that she seems happiest when she is allowed to help cook. She is still able to measure ingredients and make cookie dough, which has amazed the staff.

Medical orders: General diet, activity as tolerated, atenolol 25 mg po daily; levothyroxine 0.05 mg po daily; citalopram 40 mg po daily; zolpidem 6.25 mg po at bedtime prn for sleep; Aricept 10 mg po daily.

Questions and Activities

1. Was the family right to make arrangement for this type of care, or would Mrs. EH be better cared for in a different setting?

2. What emotional issues might the family members be experiencing?

3. Are finances likely to be of concern in this situation? Is there any way of ensuring that her family is using her financial resources responsibly? What will happen if her financial resources are used up and a need for care continues?

4. Group the data presented into functional health patterns using the following format, and identify the appropriate nursing diagnoses:

Health Pattern Data

(Objective and Subjective)	Nursing Diagnoses
Cognition–Perception	
Self-Perception–Self-Concept	
Roles–Relationships	

Health Pattern Data
(Objective and Subjective)
Nursing Diagnoses

Coping–Stress

Values–Beliefs

Sexuality

Nutritional–Fluid Needs

Skin–Mucous Membranes

Elimination

Activity–Exercise

Sleep–Rest

5. What additional data would you like to collect?

6. How would you prioritize the top five diagnoses?
   1.
   2.
   3.
   4.
   5.

7. What interventions are most appropriate for each high-priority diagnosis? (Identify assessments, specific actions, teaching, and referrals.)

Nursing Diagnosis   **Nursing Interventions**

Nursing Diagnosis   **Nursing Interventions**

8. How do the prescribed medications correlate to the patient's condition? What nursing assessments, care modifications, and teaching are necessary?

9. What concerns need to be addressed with the physician?

Case Study 3

Ms. RG is a 65-year-old Hispanic woman who recently retired from a factory job. She lives with her retired husband and an unmarried daughter in their privately owned home. They live on Social Security and money contributed by the daughter, who is employed at a local business. Ms. RG speaks and reads both Spanish and English, but she tends to revert to Spanish when dealing with emotional issues. She considers herself Catholic and attends church weekly with her daughter. Her husband is not a regular churchgoer. Four other children, all sons, are married and live in the same community. She frequently cares for her many grandchildren and states that this is the best part of "getting older." She finally has lots of time to be with and love the grandkids, but can send them home when she wants to do something else. She and her husband had talked about finally doing some traveling and enjoying retirement.

Ms. RG reports that she was feeling fine, but started to lose her appetite, which resulted in weight loss. She states that she didn't think this was a problem at first because she always considered herself a little more than "pleasingly plump." When the problem persisted, she consulted a curandero, who suggested some herbal remedies and rituals to improve her appetite. However, when she had lost more than 40 pounds and started to notice that her skin was becoming yellow and itchy, she contacted a physician. She underwent a series of diagnostic tests, including an ultrasound, CT, and ERCP. She found these tests quite frightening, even though her family was with her at the hospital. After these tests were finished, she states that the physician came to her room and told her that she had pancreatic cancer and that it was inoperable but that treatment with radiation and chemotherapy might slow the disease. She reports that he also told her that it was unlikely she would live longer than 6 months, even with treatment.

Ms. RG reports that at first she felt overwhelmed, confused, and scared. Then she became angry that this was happening to her. She cries freely and emotionally while speaking of her condition. Her family members have spent a great deal of time with her since the diagnosis was made, but they feel angry and frustrated because they don't know what they can do to help. She is unsure whether she should undergo treatment because she had a friend who had chemotherapy and was miserable. She further says that the physician suggested she be placed in home hospice care, but she isn't sure what this means.

Questions and Activities

1. How could the nurse address the issue of aggressive medical treatment with Ms. RG?

2. How would the nurse explain home hospice to her and her family?

3. How might an understanding of cultural beliefs and practice affect interaction with this patient?

4. What community resources or services might be of benefit to this patient?

5. What types of grief response might be expected from the patient? From her family?

6. What end-of-life issues will need to be addressed? (Include legal, spiritual, family, etc.)

SELECTED ACTIVITIES BY CHAPTER

Chapter 1   TRENDS AND ISSUES

1. Describe three types of aging:
   a.
   b.
   c.

2. An abnormal fear of aging or older persons is called _____. An extreme example of this fear is called _____. When this fear results in differing treatment of older adults, _____ exists.

3. The statistical study of human populations is referred to as _____. The measurements obtained from these studies are commonly called _____.

4. Vital statistics include records of:
   a.
   b.
   c.
   d.
   e.
   f.

5. The most significant demographic group is called the _____. These individuals were born between _____ and _____. This group is significant because it makes up _____ of all Americans today.

6. Today's older-than-65 population composes _____% of the population. It is projected that this group will compose more than _____% of the population by 2030.

7. More than 75% of the older adult population live in _____ areas.

8. The major sources of income for older adults include:
   a.
   b.
   c.
   d.

9. Approximately _____% of older adults live independently; _____% live in modified housing settings; and only _____% are institutionalized.

10. Alternative forms of housing for older adults include:
    a.
    b.
    c.
    d.

11. The government program that provides health care for older adults is called _____. Inpatient hospital care is covered by _____ of this plan, whereas _____% of the costs for physician services are covered by _____. Supplemental financial assistance is available for the most needy older adults through Title 19, which is also known as _____.

12. Two legal documents used to guide families and health care providers regarding the type and amount of health care desired by older adults are:
    a.
    b.

13. Identify some of the stressors that affect members of the "sandwich" generation.
    a.
    b.
    c.

14. The most significant change affecting older adults and their children is the loss of _____.

15. Signs of self-neglect include:
    a.
    b.
    c.
    d.
    e.
    f.
    g.

16. Failure to provide necessary care is called
_____. Deliberate harm or mistreatment of
another person is called _____.

17. Different forms of abuse include:
    a.
    b.
    c.

18. Ways that may help decrease stress and the likelihood of
abuse in an institutional setting include:
    a.
    b.
    c.
    d.
    e.

19. The proper term to describe desertion of a dependent
older person is _____.

20. _____ care is one method of providing
release time for family caregivers to meet their own
needs.

21. Culture affects _____ and
_____. Cultural values have an impact on
the family's willingness to accept _____.

Chapter 2   THEORIES OF AGING

Match the theory in column 1 with the description in
column 2.

Column 1 (Theories)	Column 2 (Descriptions)
1. _____ programmed	a. cells wear out because of internal and external stressors
2. _____ run out of program	b. errors in protein synthesis result in biologic decline
3. _____ gene	c. cellular DNA or tissue interacts with free radicals, decreasing the body's ability to replace itself
4. _____ error	d. harmful genes limit the life span
5. _____ free radical	e. the body's "biologic clock" runs out
6. _____ crosslink	f. the immune system loses the ability to distinguish self
7. _____ wear and tear	g. the limited amount of genetic material is used up
8. _____ immunologic	h. DNA is damaged by exposure to the environment
9. _____ somatic mutation	i. substances produced during metabolism are not eliminated, resulting in cell damage

10. Alternative therapies involving replacement of
_____ have not been shown effective and
may, in fact, cause additional health problems in older
adults.

11. The withdrawal from society that is observed in some older
people is called _____.

12. According to Havighurst, the major task of aging is to
maintain _____. Failure to achieve this task
results in _____ or _____.

Chapter 3   PHYSIOLOGIC CHANGES

INTEGUMENTARY SYSTEM

1. With aging, the _____ becomes
increasingly fragile and subject to damage.

2. Clusters of _____ cause age spots.
The medical term for these is _____.

3. Loss of _____ results in wrinkles.

4. Dry skin, or _____, is likely to result in
itching, or _____.

5. Common skin disorders in older adults include:
    a.
    b.
    c.
    d.
    e.
    f.

6. Loss of subcutaneous tissue can reduce the ability of
older adults to regulate body temperature, leading to an
increased risk for _____.

MUSCULOSKELETAL SYSTEM

7. Aging bones tend to show loss of the mineral
_____.

8. Shrinkage of intervertebral disks leads to a condition
called _____, which results in a hunchback
appearance.

9. Muscle mass and tone typically _____ with
age, but this effect can be reduced by regular
_____.

10. Excessive loss of calcium results in _____,
which is characterized by _____,
_____, _____ bones that are
susceptible to _____.

11. Three forms of arthritis that are seen in the aging
population are _____, _____,
and _____.

RESPIRATORY SYSTEM

12. The _____ and _____ of the
chest cavity change with aging.

13. Common respiratory disorders observed with aging include:
    a.
    b.
    c.
    d.
    e.

CARDIOVASCULAR SYSTEM

14. Changes in the blood vessels with aging increase the risk for low blood pressure with position changes. This is called _____.

15. Chest pain caused by reduced blood flow to the heart muscle is known as _____.

16. Heart _____ become less pliant with age, resulting in _____ sealing of the valves during heart beat.

17. Loss of heart pumping effectiveness, called _____ or _____, is a common cardiac problem in older adults. This condition can be characterized as _____ or _____.

18. Cardiomegaly, or _____ of the heart, is commonly observed with congestive heart failure.

19. Arteriosclerosis results in loss of _____ in the blood vessels.

20. Plaque formation is enhanced by lifestyle factors that include:
    a.
    b.
    c.

21. Hypertension affects more than _____% of individuals older than 65 years of age.

HEMATOPOIETIC AND LYMPHATIC SYSTEMS

22. Blood values for erythrocytes, leukocytes, and platelets generally remain _____ with aging.

23. Changes in T cells result in a _____ immune response, leading to modified signs of _____.

24. Changes in the signs of infection seen with aging include:
    a.
    b.

GASTROINTESTINAL SYSTEM

25. A protrusion of the stomach into the thoracic cavity, known as a _____, is commonly seen with aging. Gastroesophageal reflux disease, or _____, results in movement of stomach contents into the _____, increasing the risk for _____.

26. Drugs that increase the risk for ulcer formation in older adults include:
    a.
    b.
    c.

27. Weakness of the intestinal mucosa leads to the formation of _____.

28. The incidence of colon cancer peaks between _____ and _____ years of age.

URINARY SYSTEM

29. The kidneys lose approximately _____ of their efficiency by age 70, resulting in less _____ urine.

30. Many older adults experience the urge to urinate when only _____ ml of urine is present in the bladder.

31. Urinary retention increases the risk for _____ in older adults. Aging men with _____ are at risk for this problem.

NERVOUS SYSTEM

32. Motor responses take _____ to occur in older adults. This can result in a slowing of simple everyday activities such as _____ and _____.

33. A decreased level of the neurotransmitter _____ results in Parkinson's disease.

34. Common symptoms of Parkinson's disease include:
    a.
    b.
    c.
    d.
    e.

35. Drugs commonly used to treat Parkinson's disease include:
    a.
    b.
    c.
    d.

36. _____ is a general term used to describe a permanent or progressive organic mental disorder. A common form of this disorder seen in individuals older than 60 years of age is _____ disease.

37. Behavior changes seen with dementia include:
    a.
    b.
    c.
    d.
    e.

38. A cerebrovascular accident to the right side of the brain affects the _____ side of the body. One occurring in the left side of the brain affects the _____ side of the body.

39. Farsightedness that occurs with aging is called _____.

40. Changes in the aging eye make it difficult to see in _____ or _____ environments. A severe form of this problem can cause _____.

41. Fluid secretion in the eyes decreases with aging, resulting in decreased _____ production, leading to _____, _____, or _____ eyes.

42. A clouding of the lens, called _____, is common with aging. By age 85, _____% of older adults develop this condition.

43. Glaucoma is characterized by increased _____ pressure, which will cause _____ if not treated.

44. Hearing changes with aging are likely to result in loss of the _____-pitched frequencies. This condition, called _____, is more commonly observed in _____.

45. Older adults often comment on changes in the taste of food. This may be caused by decreased sensory _____ or may be a side effect of _____.

ENDOCRINE SYSTEM

46. Decreased amounts of thyroid-stimulating hormone can lead to a decrease in the basal _____ rate.

47. Altered function of the _____ cells of the pancreas leads to a disease called _____. The incidence of this disorder _____ with each decade of life. Approximately _____% of persons older than 70 years of age have altered glucose metabolism.

48. Classic signs and symptoms of diabetes mellitus include:
    a.
    b.
    c.

49. Reduced thyroid function results in decreased _____ function.

50. Signs and symptoms of hypothyroidism that are often mistaken as signs of aging include:
    a.
    b.
    c.
    d.
    e.

Chapter 4   HEALTH PROMOTION, HEALTH MAINTENANCE, AND HOME HEALTH CONSIDERATIONS

1. It is estimated that _____% of older adults live with some chronic health condition.

2. _____ and _____ contribute to disparities in health throughout the United States. Hypertension is a major problem in the _____ community; diabetes is a more common problem for _____ and _____ people, and stomach and cervical cancer are more common in the _____ population.

3. Health promotion is (more/less) expensive than treatment of health problems.

4. Recommended health practices for older adults include:
   a.
   b.
   c.
   d.
   e.
   f.
   g.

5. Medic alert devices are most important for individuals who have _____, _____, or _____.

6. Older persons with _____, _____, and _____ limitations, in addition to those who have lost their _____ because of grief or hopelessness, are at increased risk for ineffective health maintenance.

7. A person is said to be _____ when he or she fails to follow through with recommended health practices.

8. When a person does not follow through with recommended health practices, it is most important to determine the _____ for noncompliance.

9. Nurses must remain _____ when working with noncompliant individuals.

Chapter 5   COMMUNICATING WITH OLDER ADULTS

1. Effective communication requires a climate of mutual respect and understanding, which is known as _____.

2. _____ is the willingness to attempt to understand the unique world of others.

3. When communicating with others, particularly older adults, nurses must pay special attention to _____ changes, _____ changes, _____, and _____.

4. Nonverbal methods of communication include:
   a.
   b.
   o.
   d.
   e.
   f.
   g.
   h.
   i.
   j.
   k.

5. It is most appropriate to address older persons using their _____. Baby talk names are _____ and _____ to older adults.

6. When the nurse is attempting to obtain specific information quickly, it is most appropriate to use _____ questions.

7. _____ questions help clarify feelings and fears and establish an empathetic climate.

8. Even in a crisis, people from diverse cultures may prefer to proceed _____ and may need to establish _____ through small talk before addressing more serious concerns.

9. Inconsistent information or contradictions may require some form of _____ questions. These should be used _____ and _____ because they can easily _____ the other person.

10. _____ effective communication techniques can be used to help ancillary caregivers become better communicators.

Chapter 6 NUTRITION AND FLUID BALANCE/ MEETING NUTRITIONAL AND FLUID NEEDS

1. The energy available in food is measured in units called _____.

2. The amount of calories needed for each individual is based on:
   a.
   b.
   c.
   d.
   e.
   f.
   g.

3. Changes in the percentage of body fat and muscle lead to changes in the basal _____ rate.

4. Older adults should consume foods that are high in _____ but low in _____.

5. Foods rich in _____ are needed for tissue repair and healing.

6. Vitamins are a possible source of _____, which are suspected to be of value in blocking free radicals.

7. Vitamin B_{12} deficiency can affect the nervous system, causing changes in _____, _____, and _____.

8. Vitamin E appears to play a role in maintaining function of the _____ system.

9. Anemia in older adults is commonly a result of inadequate intake of the mineral _____, which can be found in foods such as _____, _____, _____, and _____.

10. Ingestion of vitamin _____ enhances the absorption of iron.

11. Older persons are likely to consume excessive amounts of _____, which contains the mineral _____, to compensate for a diminished sense of taste.

12. Potassium deficiency, or _____, is commonly a problem for older persons who are taking _____ or _____ medications.

13. Good sources of potassium are _____, _____, _____, and _____.

14. The most common symptom of potassium deficiency is _____.

15. Older adults have (more/less) body fluid than do younger adults. Most older adults require between _____ and _____ ml of fluid per day.

16. The nutritional status of older adults is affected by _____, _____, _____, and _____ factors.

17. When determining nutritional intake, the nurse needs to consider not only the amount but also the _____ of food and the _____ value of the food consumed.

18. Inadequate nutrition and fluid intake can result in serious problems such as _____ and _____. They can also contribute to the development of _____ and _____.

19. Factors that contribute to inadequate nutrition intake include:
    a.
    b.
    c.
    d.
    e.
    f.
    g.
    h.

20. Food _____ are often based on cultural experiences. Older adults may show improved appetite when the foods offered to them are _____.

21. Weight changes usually result from changes in the balance between _____ intake and _____ expenditure.

22. Inadequate intake of iron is likely to affect laboratory values for _____. Common forms of anemia observed in older adults include _____, _____, and _____.

23. Electrolyte imbalances in older adults commonly involve:
    a.
    b.
    c.

24. Inadequate nutritional intake is likely to contribute to tissue _____ and slow tissue _____.

25. Aging results in decreased production of _____, which can interfere with normal swallowing and lead to changes in _____ sensation.

26. When an individual is on a _____-restricted diet, beverages such as cola should be restricted.

27. Individuals with diverticulitis should avoid corn with _____.

28. Symptoms of deficient fluid volume include:
    a.
    b.
    c.
    d.
    e.
    f.
    g.
    h.
    i.
    j.

29. Symptoms of excess fluid volume include:
    a.
    b.
    c.
    d.
    e.
    f.
    g.
    h.
    i.

30. Difficulty swallowing is properly termed _____.

31. A person who has diminished gag or swallow reflexes is at increased risk for _____.

32. _____ position is used for individuals receiving tube feedings, because in this position _____ helps keep the solution in the stomach.

Chapter 7   MEDICATIONS AND OLDER ADULTS

1. Older adults must be cautious when taking medication because medications can alter their ability to perform normal _____, can result in _____ changes, and in the worst cases, can be life _____.

2. The study of how older adults respond to medications is called _____.

3. Drug absorption is affected by decreased gastric _____, _____, and _____.

4. Water-soluble drugs are likely to be present in (lower/higher) concentrations in the bloodstream of older adults, increasing the risk for _____.

5. Fat-soluble drugs are likely to become _____ in fatty tissues, resulting in (low/high) blood levels. These drugs are released slowly, resulting in _____ drug effects.

6. The likelihood of drug _____ is increased in malnourished older adults.

7. Drug metabolism is affected by altered _____ function.

8. Research has shown that _____ plays a role in the use and effectiveness of various drugs.

9. Response to medication is (more/less) predictable in older adults.

10. _____ is the term used to describe the use of multiple medications by older adults.

11. Factors that contribute to excessive use of medications by older adults include:
    a.
    b.
    c.
    d.

12. Cognitive problems that contribute to drug errors among older adults include the lack of:
    a.
    b.
    c.

13. Older adults must be aware that drugs purchased without a prescription, or over-the-counter medications, can _____ with other medications.

14. Before administering any medication, nurses must know why the person is receiving the medication. Nurses must also know the _____ of administration, the therapeutic _____, the therapeutic _____, the _____ effects, and signs of _____.

15. The rights of medication administration include the right:
    a.
    b.
    c.

d.

e.

f.

g.

16. _____ is a major nursing responsibility when an older person will be self-medicating.

17. Some precautions that older adults who live independently need to know include:

a.

b.

c.

d.

e.

18. For safety, medications used to promote sleep should not be kept _____.

Chapter 8   HEALTH ASSESSMENT OF OLDER ADULTS

1. Screenings are conducted to _____ older persons with significant findings and to _____ them to appropriate resources.

2. During a physical examination, the nurse should be careful to maintain the _____ set by each culture. In some cultures, a _____ may wish to be present during the examination or may request that only a nurse of the _____ perform the examination.

3. All of the information collected about an individual is called _____. This information can be _____ or _____.

4. _____ information is gathered using the senses. Examples of this type of information include _____, _____, _____ and _____. _____ information must be provided by the person being assessed. Examples of this include _____, _____, _____, and _____.

5. List some factors to consider when preparing the environment for an interview with an older person.

a.

b.

c.

d.

e.

6. Identify ways to establish rapport with older adults.

a.

b.

c.

d.

e.

f.

7. Commonly used assessment techniques include:

a.

b.

c.

d.

8. Temperature can be assessed by which routes? Identify the advantages/disadvantages of each.

a.

b.

c.

d.

9. When taking peripheral pulses, nurses should be careful to start with the most _____ pulse and compare pulses on each _____.

10. A decreased _____ rate may be an early indication of infection.

11. A blood pressure cuff that is too wide can result in falsely (low/high) readings. A cuff that is too narrow can result in falsely (low/high) readings.

12. Postural changes in blood pressure can result in a condition called _____. Symptoms of this problem include _____ or _____. When checking for this condition, blood pressure is first assessed with the patient _____, then _____, and then _____.

13. A federally developed assessment tool for extended-care facilities is called the _____, which is abbreviated MDS. This tool has special focus assessments called _____, or RAPs.

Chapter 9   MEETING SAFETY NEEDS OF OLDER ADULTS

1. Older persons make up 11% of the population but account for _____% of accidental deaths.

2. The four most common causes of accidental death among older adults are:

a.

b.

c.

d.

3. Changes in the senses of _____ and _____ increase the risk for accident and injury in older adults.

4. Risk for falls is increased because of physiologic factors, including:

a.

b.

c.

d.

e.

f.

g.

5. Cardiovascular changes, particularly those that result in postural hypotension, increase the risk for _____ and _____, both of which can lead to falls.

6. Classifications of medications that can contribute to falls include:
   a.
   b.
   c.
   d.
   e.
   f.

7. Physical _____ should be used only when other less restrictive methods have been used to prevent falls and found to be _____. They should never be used as a form of _____. _____ are necessary, and informed _____ should be obtained from the patient or legal guardian before restraints are used. The _____ device that provides protection should be used.

8. Emotional factors that increase the risk for injury include _____, _____, and _____.

9. Increasing the base of physical support can improve stability and help prevent falls. Devices that increase the base of support for older adults include _____ and _____.

10. Motor vehicle accidents are the _____ most common cause of accidental death among older adults.

11. Because of changes in thermoregulation, older adults are at increased risk for both _____ and _____.

12. Medications such as _____ and anti _____ drugs increase the risk for hyperthermia.

13. It is wise for older adults to take precautions, particularly when dealing with _____ or going to new _____. This is unfortunate because fear of _____ can make older persons prisoners in their own _____.

Chapter 10   COGNITION AND PERCEPTION

1. The term *perception* includes:
   a.
   b.
   c.

2. The term *cognition* includes:
   a.
   b.
   c.
   d.

3. Both perception and cognition rely on effective functioning of the _____ system, particularly sensory input from the senses of _____, _____, _____, _____, and _____.

4. Any disorder that affects the _____ is likely to affect perception and cognition.

5. Older individuals are likely to use _____ intelligence to make judgments. This form of intelligence is based on _____ and _____ gained over a lifetime.

6. The correct medical term for loss of the ability to understand or express oneself using language is _____ or _____. This should not be confused with _____, which is difficulty swallowing.

7. Intelligence does not normally decrease with aging, although responses tend to be _____ and more _____.

8. The _____-term memory of older persons tends to be affected more by aging than does _____-term memory.

9. _____ misperception should be ruled out before _____ disorders are suspected.

10. Confusion is defined as a mental state characterized by disorientation regarding _____, _____, or _____.

11. Confusion is categorized as:
    a.
    b.
    c.

12. Delirium can be caused by:
    a.
    b.
    c.
    d.
    e.
    f.
    g.
    h.
    i.
    j.
    k.
    l.

13. Acute delirium has a sudden onset measured in terms of _____ or _____.

14. Symptoms of acute delirium include:
    a.
    b.
    c.
    d.
    e.
    f.
    g.
    h.

15. Older adults suffering from acute delirium typically do not respond to _____ approaches because the problem has _____ causes.

16. Dementia has a _____, _____ onset.

17. Disease conditions that result in dementia include:
    a.
    b.
    c.
    d.
    e.
    f.
    g.
    h.
    i.
    j.

18. Common behaviors observed with dementia include:
    a.
    b.
    c.
    d.
    e.
    f.

19. Behaviors associated with dementia often _____ late in the day. This is referred to as _____ syndrome.

20. _____ therapy may decrease some of the _____ behaviors commonly associated with sundown syndrome.

21. Dementia affects up to _____% of the community-dwelling aging population. Estimates place the incidence of dementia in individuals older than age 85 at _____%.

22. _____ of care is important when caring for individuals with dementia. Physical and chemical _____ should be avoided because they can make behavior _____.

23. Positive effects of music therapy for patients experiencing dementia include:
    a.
    b.
    c.
    d.
    e.

24. Psychotropic medication should be kept at the _____ dose for the _____ period of time.

25. Older adults are at risk for _____ pain connected with disease processes. _____ or _____ pain can result in behavior changes.

26. Behavior changes observed with pain include:
    a.
    b.
    c.

Chapter 11   SELF-PERCEPTION AND SELF-CONCEPT

1. Self-identity is formed from the _____ and _____ a person holds of himself or herself. It originates in personal _____, life _____, and _____ with others. Much of a person's self-identity is affected by his or her _____ heritage.

2. People with good self-identity usually have strong _____ and a sense of _____ over their lives.

3. _____ feedback from others helps older persons maintain high self-esteem.

4. Nurses can assess a person's self-esteem level by observing:
    a.
    b.
    c.
    d.
    e.

5. Both _____ and _____ have a negative impact on self-image and self-esteem.

6. Placement in an _____ setting can contribute to loss of self-esteem by stripping older adults of their personal _____ and diminishing the amount of _____ older adults have over their lives.

7. Institutionalized older persons typically experience feelings of _____ or _____, which further diminish self-worth.

8. Nursing diagnoses that address loss of self-image and self-worth include:
    a.
    b.
    c.

9. Loss of physical health and/or deforming injuries are likely to affect an older person's body _____.

10. Nurses should encourage _____, or life review, to help the older person find _____ and _____ in his or her life. This process can also help older adults identify their _____ and _____ effective strategies they have used in the past.

11. Common fears experienced by older adults include those of:
    a.
    b.
    c.
    d.
    e.
    f.
    g.
    h.
    i.

12. A person experiencing fear or anxiety can manifest physical symptoms such as:
    a.
    b.
    c.
    d.
    e.
    f.
    g.
    h.

13. Physiologic stimulation caused by fear or increased anxiety is particularly dangerous to older people who have a history of diseases of the _____, _____, _____, or _____ system.

14. Hopelessness can lead an older person to engage in self-_____ behaviors, the most serious of which is _____.

15. Competent older persons often demonstrate a desire to retain control when they exercise the right to _____ treatments or procedures.

16. Methods of dealing with refusals include:
    a.
    b.
    c.
    d.

17. If older persons continue to object to or refuse care, nurses should:
    a.
    b.
    c.

Chapter 12   ROLES AND RELATIONSHIPS

1. People tend to establish their identities and describe themselves based on the _____ they play in life.

2. Roles are _____ and are given value by the _____ or _____ in which a person lives. Roles confer and carry various _____ that are communicated through _____, _____, and _____.

3. A _____ society has clear role expectations for all members. In a complex or _____ society, roles are not as clear; therefore role _____ and societal _____ are more likely to occur.

4. Aging often results in the _____ of familiar roles. These losses are likely to result in feelings of _____.

5. Typical life events that affect role identity include:
    a.
    b.
    c.

d.
e.

6. Stages of grieving include:
    a.
    b.
    c.
    d.

7. Dysfunctional grief can result in _____, _____, _____, and _____ changes.

8. A series of losses can lead to social _____ and impaired social _____.

9. An older person with adult children may have difficulty accepting change in the _____-_____ roles and relationships. This may lead to a nursing diagnosis of interrupted _____. This problem is particularly common when the older parent is _____ on the child for physical or financial support.

Chapter 13   COPING AND STRESS

1. Persons experience stress whenever they are faced with a _____ or _____ threat or a _____ or life-threatening change.

2. Stressors include external physical threats such as _____, _____, or _____; external emotional threats such as changes in _____ or social _____; and internal threats such as disturbing _____ or feelings.

3. Stress level is determined by the person's _____ of an event. Because stress is _____, several minor events can have the same impact as a single _____ event.

4. A very high stress rating for older adults is given to the _____ of a spouse.

5. The general _____ syndrome, proposed by _____, describes the physical response to stress. According to this theory, both the sympathetic and parasympathetic portions of the _____ nervous system are involved.

6. Physiologic signs of stress include:
    a.
    b.
    c.
    d.
    e.
    f.
    g.

7. Cognitive changes that are evident with severe stress include:
    a.
    b.
    c.

8. Emotional changes that are evident with severe stress include:

a.

b.

c.

d.

e.

f.

9. Behavioral changes that are evident with severe stress include:

a.

b.

c.

d.

e.

f.

10. Stress is closely related to the development of both _____ and _____ illness.

11. _____ strategies help people deal with stress. These strategies include _____, _____, _____, and _____.

12. A nontraditional intervention that may help decrease the physical side effects of stress is gentle _____.

13. Approaches that help decrease stress include:

a.

b.

c.

d.

14. Many of the stressors seen with aging are connected to _____ or _____. One specific problem related to loss or change of residence is called _____ stress.

Chapter 14   VALUES AND BELIEFS

1. A person's values and beliefs have their origins in _____, _____, _____, and _____.

2. Most values and belief patterns are established _____ in life.

3. _____ and _____ are likely to occur when people with differing values and experience interact.

4. To work effectively with a variety of people, nurses must be willing to try to _____ and _____ with the other person.

5. The _____ culture closely connects faith in the caregivers with the ability to recover and heal effectively. Inability to speak _____ is often perceived as a barrier to quality nursing and medical care.

6. Nonjudgmental interaction requires a high level of _____ and excellent _____ skills.

7. Common values and beliefs of today's older adult population include:

a.

b.

c.

d.

8. Religious _____ and _____ are very important to many older persons. Many wish to have _____ of religious significance available for comfort and _____.

9. _____ and _____ are inseparable for many American Indians. Elders are to be respected for their _____ and _____. They may verbalize a need to be alone to practice cultural rituals designed to maintain harmony of _____, _____, and _____.

10. Nurses must be careful to demonstrate _____ for the religious beliefs of older adults and to offer to contact a _____ counselor.

Chapter 15   END-OF-LIFE CARE

1. Medical _____ and _____ have extended life expectancy.

2. People older than age 65 account for _____% of deaths.

3. Death among older adults is most commonly a result of progression of _____.

4. The best time to have a discussion regarding end-of-life care is _____.

5. Opportunities to discuss end-of-life wishes include:

a.

b.

c.

6. Types of advance directives include _____ and _____.

7. Before making decisions about end-of-life care, the patient should gather information from the physician regarding:

a.

b.

c.

d.

e.

f.

g.

8. Four characteristics of a "good" death include _____, _____, _____, and _____.

9. Palliative care focuses on _____ or _____ the symptoms of disease without attempting to _____; it neither _____ nor _____ death.

10. At the end of life, it is important that family members and nurses spend _____ with the dying patient.

11. Some ways to demonstrate empathetic caring include:
    a.
    b.
    c.
    d.

12. Cultural sensitivity regarding death includes paying attention to:
    a.
    b.
    c.
    d.

13. Guidelines for meeting a dying patient's spiritual needs include:
    a.
    b.
    c.
    d.
    e.
    f.
    g.
    h.

14. A priority need for the dying patient is control of _____.

15. _____ can interfere with a dying person's ability to communicate and carry out end-of-life tasks.

16. As death nears, blood pressure _____, _____ are difficult to palpate, and the extremities _____.

17. Breathing changes that occur as death nears include _____ and _____.

18. Many patients experience episodes of _____ and other cognitive changes as death nears.

Chapter 16   SEXUALITY AND AGING

1. Sexual _____, _____, and _____ remain part of the lives of active older persons.

2. The major reason for lack of sexual activity is the _____ or _____ of a spouse.

3. Older women experience decreased vaginal _____ resulting from hormone changes. The tissues of the vagina become _____ and less _____.

4. Older men experience a _____ reaction to sexual stimuli and may take _____ to achieve an erection.

5. Medications likely to cause difficulty with sexual function include:
    a.
    b.
    c.
    d.
    e.

6. Many older persons refrain from sexual activity because of _____ of causing their partner _____ or worsening an existing _____.

7. Older individuals who reside in institutional settings should be provided with _____ so that they can conduct sexual activity without disturbance.

8. Vulnerable older adults should be protected from _____ sexual contact.

Chapter 17   CARE OF AGING SKIN AND MUCOUS MEMBRANES

1. Traumatic injuries to aging skin are common because the epidermal layer is _____ and there is less _____ padding.

2. Decreased _____ secretions contribute to dryness, which affects between _____% and _____% of those older than 65 years of age.

3. Dry skin is likely to result in itching, or _____, which further increases the risk for tissue damage and _____.

4. Common causes of rashes and skin irritation include:
    a.
    b.
    c.

5. The risk for pressure ulcers is increased in older adults who suffer from:
    a.
    b.
    c.
    d.
    e.

6. Common pressure points for individuals who spend extended periods of time sitting include:
    a.
    b.
    c.
    d.
    e.

7. Common foot problems in older adults include:
    a.
    b.
    c.
    d.
    e.
    f.

g.

h.

i.

8. To prevent excessive skin dryness in older adults, nurses can:

a.

b.

c.

9. To reduce shearing forces, the head of the bed should be elevated no more than _____ degrees. Care should be used to reduce _____ when moving or transferring older adults.

10. Special mattresses are used to decrease pressure over bony prominences. These devices work because they _____ over a larger area.

11. The nutrients _____ and _____ are particularly important for tissue repair.

12. High levels of bacteria in the mouth contribute to _____, _____, and _____ disease.

13. Dryness of the mouth, or _____, can be caused by age-related changes, _____, _____, or _____.

14. Oral mucous membranes can be affected by deficiencies of:

a.

b.

c.

15. Special attention should be paid to the gingiva of individuals receiving medication for _____ or other _____ disorders.

Chapter 18   ELIMINATION

1. The two major body systems involved in elimination of waste products are the _____ and _____ systems. The _____ plays a minor role in waste removal.

2. Elimination is affected by:

a.

b.

c.

d.

e.

f.

3. Most adults defecate every _____ to _____ days.

4. Most adults experience the urge to urinate when the bladder contains _____ ml of urine. Older individuals may experience this urge when only _____ ml is present.

5. Common elimination problems of older adults include:

a.

b.

c.

6. Factors that contribute to constipation include:

a.

b.

c.

d.

e.

f.

g.

h.

i.

j.

7. Medications that contribute to constipation include:

a.

b.

c.

d.

e.

f.

g.

h.

i.

8. A _____ is a hardened mass of feces that usually results from unrelieved _____. This problem should be suspected in individuals who do not have bowel movements for _____ days or when only _____ stool is passed without any formed material.

9. Common symptoms associated with severe constipation include:

a.

b.

c.

d.

e.

10. Digital examination should be used with caution on any older person who has a history of a _____ condition because such manipulation can result in a decreased _____, _____, or even loss of _____.

11. Caution must be used to administer adequate _____ to patients receiving a psyllium-based bulk former, or complications including _____ or _____ may occur.

12. High-fiber foods include:

a.

b.

c.

d.

13. Fluid intake of _____ ml/day helps reduce the risk for constipation.

14. Older persons with diarrhea are at risk for fluid volume _____. Fluids high in _____ are recommended to replace those lost through diarrhea.

15. Signs and symptoms of deficient fluid volume include:
    a.
    b.
    c.
    d.

16. Incontinence of bladder and/or bowel is likely to result in:
    a.
    b.
    c.

17. Urinary retention in older adults is commonly a result of:
    a.
    b.
    c.
    d.
    e.
    f.
    g.

18. Signs and symptoms of urinary retention include:
    a.
    b.
    c.
    d.
    e.
    f.

19. Types of urinary incontinence include:
    a.
    b.
    c.
    d.
    e.

20. Indwelling catheters should be used only when the _____ to the person outweigh the _____. Because urinary retention or _____ incontinence may occur after an indwelling catheter is removed, urinary _____ should be monitored closely.

Chapter 19   ACTIVITY AND EXERCISE

1. Activity requires interaction of the _____, _____, _____, and _____ systems.

2. Activity and _____ patterns established at a young age usually continue into older age, although there is typically a decrease in the _____, _____, and _____ of older persons.

3. Physical activity helps a person maintain _____ mobility and _____ tone.

4. _____ motor skills tend to remain intact longer than do _____ motor skills.

5. _____ exercises help maintain joint mobility.

6. Consultation with a _____ or _____ therapist can help identify

appropriate activities for an older person. These therapists can also recommend _____ devices designed to help older adults maintain optimal activity.

7. Exercise periods of _____ to _____ minutes at least _____ times per week are recommended for older adults.

8. Assessment of _____ provides a good indication of the ability of older persons to tolerate activity.

9. _____ often results in inadequate reserves of glucose, _____, and _____. Inadequate supplies of these nutrients can contribute to a reduced ability to perform _____ because of muscle _____ and decreased oxygen transport related to _____.

10. Emotional disorders, including _____, _____, and _____, can lead to decreased participation in normal activity.

11. Use of restraints should be _____, because by definition these devices limit _____ and cause joints and muscles to lose function. These changes ultimately increase the risk for _____.

12. _____ range-of-motion exercises help keep joints flexible but do little to maintain muscle strength. _____ range-of-motion or other types of exercise are needed to tone and strengthen muscles.

13. When an individual has one-sided weakness, assistive devices should be positioned on the _____ side.

14. Excessive respiratory secretions can reduce _____ intake and _____ the individual's ability to participate in activity. The most appropriate nursing diagnosis for an individual who is unable to clear secretions is ineffective _____.

15. Approaches designed to deal with excessive secretions include:
    a.
    b.
    c.
    d.
    e.

16. Medications that may aid individuals with excessive secretions include:
    a.
    b.
    c.

17. Analgesics and sedatives may make activity easier but should be used with caution because they can affect the _____ and _____ of respiration and can increase _____ risks.

18. Self-care deficits are often devastating to older adults because they lead to _____ and loss of _____, thereby affecting self-_____.

19. Older persons with self-care deficits should be _____ to perform as much self-care as possible. _____ helps maintain motivation.

20. Older adults should be encouraged to select diversional activities that they find _____.

21. A rehabilitative perspective credits older persons with _____ and _____ potential.

22. The long-term goal of rehabilitation is to help older adults achieve and maintain maximal _____, _____, and _____ health.

Chapter 20 SLEEP AND REST

1. Common behaviors connected to sleep deprivation include:
   a.
   b.
   c.
   d.
   e.
   f.
   g.
   h.

2. As many as _____ of independent-living older adults and _____ of institutionalized older adults are estimated to have sleep disturbances.

3. Sleep is under the influence of chemicals produced within the _____ system.

4. Deepest sleep occurs in stage _____ of non–rapid eye movement sleep.

5. Dreaming occurs during the _____ stage of sleep.

6. The average older person sleeps (more/less) than does the average younger adult.

7. Insomnia affects three phases of sleep and is categorized as:
   a.
   b.
   c.

8. Common factors that affect sleep include:
   a.
   b.
   c.
   d.
   e.

9. Nurses need to be aware that excessive noise from _____ or _____ should be minimized because this can further disturb the sleep of institutionalized older adults.

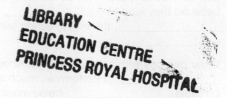